Augmentation Mastopexy

M. Bradley Calobrace
Bill G. Kortesis • Gaurav Bharti
Chet Mays
Editors

Augmentation Mastopexy

Mastering the Art in the Management of the Ptotic Breast

Springer

Editor-in-Chief
M. Bradley Calobrace, MD, FACS
Private Practice
CaloAesthetics Plastic Surgery Center
Louisville, KY
USA

Clinical Faculty
University of Louisville
Division of Plastic Surgery
Louisville, KY
USA

Clinical Faculty
University of Kentucky
Division of Plastic Surgery
Lexington, KY
USA

Co-editors
Bill G. Kortesis, MD, FACS
Hunstad/Kortesis/Bharti Plastic Surgery Center
Charlotte, NC
USA

Gaurav Bharti, MD, FACS
Hunstad/Kortesis/Bharti Plastic Surgery Center
Charlotte, NC
USA

Chet Mays, MD
Private Practice
CaloAesthetics Plastic Surgery Center
Louisville, KY
USA

University of Louisville
Division of Plastic Surgery
Louisville, KY
USA

ISBN 978-3-030-48225-1 ISBN 978-3-030-48226-8 (eBook)
https://doi.org/10.1007/978-3-030-48226-8

This Springer imprint is published by the registered company Springer Nature Switzerland AG
The registered company address is: Gewerbestrasse 11, 6330 Cham, Switzerland

Foreword

The concept of a plastic surgery textbook focused on augmentation mastopexy would have previously been viewed as overreaching. It would be perceived by most as too narrow and finite a topic to justify a full manuscript. As plastic surgery has evolved, concepts of augmentation mastopexy have grown considerably with additional methodologies, increased procedural detail, and overall expansion of the entire topic. A textbook of this combined topic is therefore not only justified but very welcome indeed.

The primary authors are all well known to me. They have all delved deeply into the concepts of augmentation mastopexy and expanded this field of interest through their contributions. All have significant experience with the topics discussed in this text and have been responsible for significant advancements in this area of breast surgery. Their thoughtful teachings as educators internationally and nationally have opened the minds of many plastic surgeons to the challenges and rewards of augmentation mastopexy.

At the risk of sounding mundane, it is an honor and privilege to write the foreword for this very comprehensive and timely compilation. The topic of augmentation mastopexy is one that is deserving of its own independent publication. This composition will serve as a reference for plastic surgeons to increase their understanding of and results with all categories of augmentation mastopexy.

Combining augmentation and mastopexy has been controversial and this text addresses these concerns from decision-making, methods and techniques, single stage procedures, staged procedures, and secondary procedures. Breast augmentation has been thoroughly presented herein including the anatomy, principles, technical specifics, implant selection, addressing anatomic variants, applications for the massive weight loss patient, as well as pitfalls and explantation.

Explantation is addressed throughout the book and is extremely germane in this era of concern with Anaplastic Large Cell Lymphoma and Breast Implant Illness. A careful review of this procedure in combination with mastopexy is extremely important for plastic surgeons because of the heightened interest and frequent demand for explantation with mastopexy in plastic surgery practices.

Prominent notable colleagues have provided their expertise in various chapters of this text, adding depth and complexity to this very important subject. The utilization of renowned experts beyond the primary authors further expands the breath of this manuscript.

This book has brought together many of the best-known authors in the field of breast surgery. Those that read and utilize this textbook will realize the significant effort that was placed into making this a truly comprehensive reference for augmentation mastopexy. I strongly believe that those who examine this work will benefit their individual practices improving overall understanding of the topic and most importantly overall patient results.

Joe Hunstad
Hunstad/Kortesis/Bharti Plastic Surgery
Charlotte, NC, USA

Contents

Contributors

William P. Adams Jr., MD University of Texas Southwestern, Department of Plastic Surgery, Dallas, TX, USA

Amy K. Alderman, MD, MPH Private Practice, Atlanta, GA, USA

R. Laurence Berkowitz, MD Aesthetx, Campbell, CA, USA

Gaurav Bharti, MD, FACS Private Practice Hunstad/Kortesis/Bharti Cosmetic Surgery, Charlotte, NC, USA

Louis P. Bucky, MD Private Practice, Bucky Plastic Surgery, Clinical Faculty, University of Pennsylvania School of Medicine, Division of Plastic Surgery, Philadelphia, PA, USA

M. Bradley Calobrace, MD, FACS Private Practice, CaloAesthetics Plastic Surgery Center, Louisville, KY, USA

Clinical Faculty, University of Louisville, Division of Plastic Surgery, Louisville, KY, USA

Clinical Faculty, University of Kentucky, Division of Plastic Surgery, Lexington, KY, USA

Ashley R. Chandler, MD Florida State University College of Medicine, Pensacola, FL, USA

Jeffrey R. Claiborne, MD Private Practice, Northshore Plastic Surgery, Mandeville, LA, USA

Robert Cohen, MD, FACS Beverly Hills Center, Beverly Hills, CA, USA

Scottsdale Center for Plastic Surgery, Paradise Valley, AZ, USA

Allen Gabriel, MD, FACS Department of Plastic Surgery, Loma Linda University Medical Center, Loma Linda, CA, USA

Private Practice, Vancouver, WA, USA

W. Grant Stevens, MD Private Practice Marina Plastic Surgery, Keck School of Medicine of USC, Division of Plastic Surgery, Marina del Rey, CA, USA

Elizabeth J. Hall-Findlay, MD, FRCSC Private Practice, Banff Plastic Surgery, Banff, AB, Canada

Dennis C. Hammond, MD Plastic Surgery, Spectrum Health Medical Education Partners, Grand Rapids, MI, USA

Partners in Plastic Surgery, Grand Rapids, MI, USA

Ziyad S. Hammoudeh, MD Private Practice Marina Plastic Surgery, Marina Plastic Surgery, Marina del Rey, CA, USA

Bill G. Kortesis, MD, FACS Private Practice, Hunstad/Kortesis/Bharti Cosmetic Surgery, Charlotte, NC, USA

G. Patrick Maxwell, MD, FACS Department of Plastic Surgery, Loma Linda University Medical Center, Loma Linda, CA, USA

Private Practice, Nashville, TN, USA

Chet Mays, MD Private Practice, CaloAesthetics Plastic Surgery Center, Louisville, KY, USA

Clinical Faculty, University of Louisville, Division of Plastic Surgery, Louisville, KY, USA

Evan Moore, MD Calobrace Aesthetic Surgery Fellowship, Louisville, KY, USA

James D. Namnoum, MD Private Practice, Atlanta Plastic Surgery, Emory University, Atlanta, GA, USA

Charalambos "Babis" Rammos, MD, FACS PSG Plastic Surgery, Peoria, IL, USA

Department of Surgery, Division of Plastic Surgery, University of Illinois, College of Medicine, Peoria, IL, USA

Kyle Sanniec, MD, MHA University of Texas Southwestern, Department of Plastic Surgery, Dallas, TX, USA

Michael R. Schwartz, MD Private Practice, Westlake Village, CA, USA

James M. Smartt Jr., MD Bucky Plastic Surgery, Philadelphia, PA, USA

Neil Tanna, MD, MBA, FACS Faculty, Northwell Health, Zucker School of Medicine, Division of Plastic Surgery, Great Neck, NY, USA

Bruce Van Natta, MD Private Practice, Meridian Plastic Surgery Owner/Partner, Indianapolis, IN, USA

Holly Wall Private Practice, The Wall Center for Plastic Surgery, Shreveport, LA, USA

Simeon Wall Jr., MD, FACS Private Practice, The Wall Center for Plastic Surgery, Shreveport, LA, USA

UT Southwestern Medical Center, Dallas, TX, USA

Kamakshi R. Zeidler, MD, FACS Aesthetx, Campbell, CA, USA

Anatomy of the Breast

1

Allen Gabriel and G. Patrick Maxwell

Introduction

Breast aesthetic surgery is one of the most common procedures performed by plastic surgeons [1]. The goal of surgery (augmentation mammoplasty, reduction mammoplasty, and mastopexy) is to improve breast shape, volume, and/or positioning, so as to improve the overall aesthetic appearance of the breast, without compromising functionality. For the safe and reliable performance of breast aesthetic procedures, a thorough and comprehensive understanding of breast anatomy, including surface anatomy, position and composition of nipple-areolar complex, soft tissue composition and distribution, connective and fascial supportive structures, vascular supply, innervation, and chest wall muscular anatomy is critical.

A. Gabriel (✉)
Department of Plastic Surgery, Loma Linda University Medical Center, Loma Linda, CA, USA

Private Practice, Vancouver, WA, USA

G. P. Maxwell
Department of Plastic Surgery, Loma Linda University Medical Center, Loma Linda, CA, USA

Private Practice, Nashville, TN, USA

M. B. Calobrace et al. (eds.), *Augmentation Mastopexy*,
https://doi.org/10.1007/978-3-030-48226-8_1

Surface Anatomy

Mature female breasts are conical or tear-drop shaped glands located toward the lateral aspect on either side of the chest wall between the subdermal layer of adipose tissue and the superficial fascia of the pectoralis major muscle. Anteriorly, the breast extends from just below the clavicle to the sixth rib and laterally from the sternum to the anterior border of the latissimus dorsi muscle (Fig. 1.1) [2]. Laterally, breast tissue also extends through the axillary fascia into the axillary fat pad as the "tail of Spence". The plane that extends from just below the clavicle to the nipple is the upper pole of the breast. At the center of the breast, at its greatest projection, lies the nipple-areolar complex. In the non-ptotic breast, the nipple-areolar complex is located above the inframammary fold and the breast mound, containing most of the breast volume, is located between the second and sixth ribs anteriorly and from the edge of the sternum to the anterior axillary line laterally.

Breast contour is defined by the upper pole superiorly, the inframammary fold inferiorly, the medial fold, and the lateral fold (Fig. 1.1). These breast borders, together with the position of the nipple-areolar complex, are important landmarks of the breast that define breast aesthetics. Further, breast aesthetics are defined by a set of ideal breast dimensions derived using statistical standards, which include a sternal notch to nipple distance of

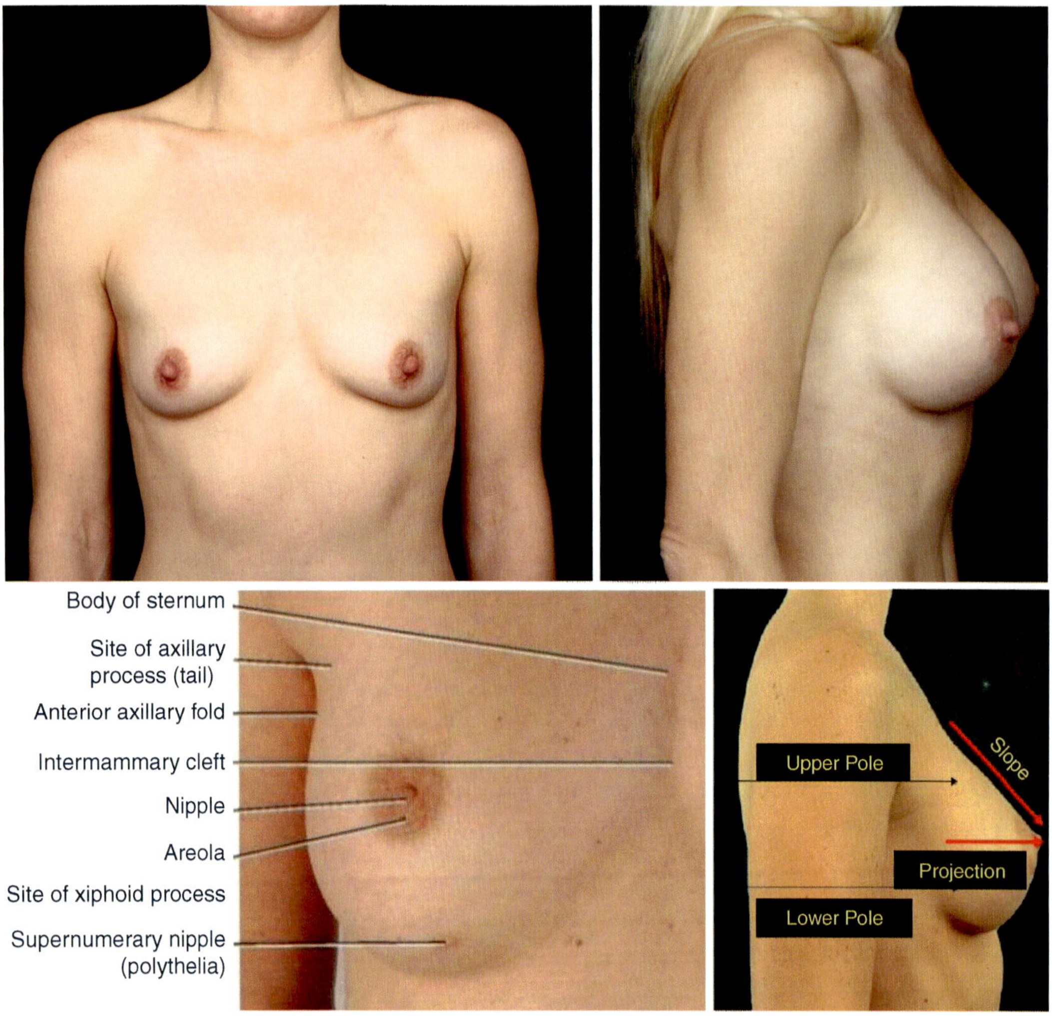

Fig. 1.1 Breast surface anatomy

19–21 cm, a midclavicular line to nipple distance of 19–21 cm, a nipple to inframammary fold distance of 5–6 cm, and a nipple to midline distance of 9–11 cm (Fig. 1.2) [3–5]. Based on these dimensions, an equilateral triangle formed between the nipples and sternal notch, averaging a distance of 21 cm per side, is representative of ideal symmetry, proportionality, and projection of the breasts (Fig. 1.2) [2]. It should be emphasized that these ideal breast dimensions are meant as a guide and may NOT be applicable to or achievable in all patients. Breast modifications in augmentation, reduction, or mastopexy procedures should be individualized taking into consideration individual patient's chest dimension; breast size, symmetry, and proportionality; posture, and preference.

Breast Tissue

The breast is composed primarily of glandular, connective, and adipose tissues [6]. Glandular tissue (or breast parenchyma) is the functional tissue of the breast that produces milk in the postpartum period. It consists of milk-producing lobules and a network of ducts that transport the milk to the nipple (Fig. 1.3). The lobules are clustered together into larger units, the lobes. Each breast contains about 20–25 lobes that are arranged in a spoke-wheel pattern, radiating outward and downward from the nipple-areolar complex. The lobes are non-uniformly distributed over the breast; the majority being located in the periphery

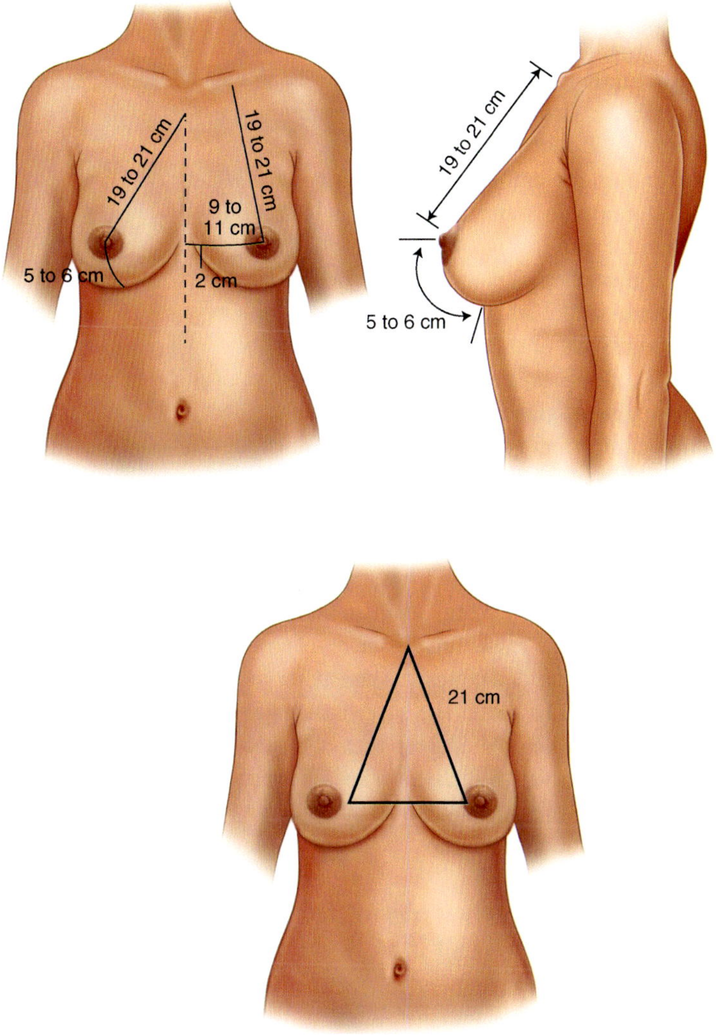

Fig. 1.2 Ideal breast dimension demonstrating symmetry, projection, and proportionality

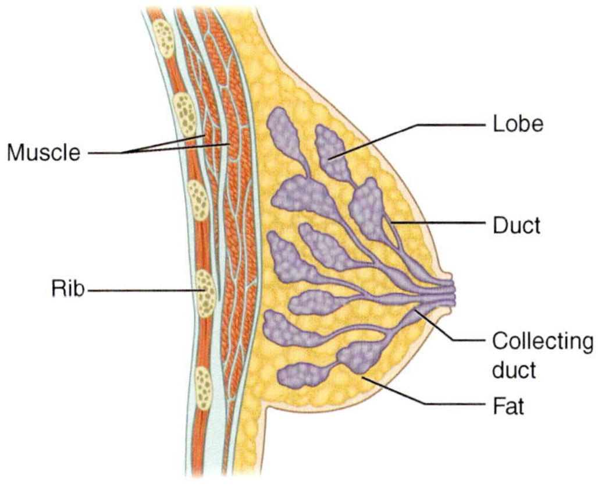

Fig. 1.3 Superficial fascial system of the breast and Cooper's ligaments

of the breast. The lobes empty into ducts which connect to form larger ducts that eventually converge into primary lactiferous ducts, which number approximately 20 per breast. The lactiferous ducts enter the nipple-areolar complex where they converge into 5–9 ducts and exit the nipple through 5–9 mammary ductal orifices [7]. Just before entering the nipple, under the areola, the lactiferous ducts dilate to form lactiferous sinuses. Each lactiferous sinus stores a milk droplet which is released when an infant suckles.

The duct entering each lobe branches into smaller ducts within the lobe and each terminal small duct enters a lobule (Fig. 1.3). Within the lobule, the terminal duct branches further into smaller ducts and ductules with each ductule ending in an acinus, which is the milk-producing gland. The acini, ductules, and its branches are embedded in specialized loose connective tissue (intralobular stroma) that contains capillaries, lymphocytes, and other plasma cells. The lobules, in turn, are embedded in denser connective tissue (interlobular stroma), which is less cellular than the intralobular stroma.

The glandular tissue is distributed within a substantial amount of adipose tissue. Adipose tissue is the predominant breast tissue and constitutes about 50–70% of total breast volume. The proportion of adipose tissue to glandular tissue, however, is highly variable among individuals. Adipose tissue gradually replaces glandular tissue as the latter involutes with age and menopausal hormonal changes.

The glandular and adipose tissues of the breast are supported and held in place by connective tissue. Breast connective tissue consists of an intricate fascial system and the suspensory ligaments of Cooper. The fascial system of the breast is derived from the superficial fascial system. The superficial fascia of the abdomen (fascia of Scarpa) extends cephalad and separates into a superficial layer and a deep layer at the sixth rib where the lower pole (inframammary fold) of the breast is (Fig. 1.3). The superficial layer and the deep layer of the superficial fascia engulf the breast tissues (glandular and adipose) and hold the breast to the chest wall. The superficial layer lies below the dermis and is separated from the dermis by the subcutaneous adipose tissue layer. The deep fascial layer lies on the deep surface of the breast above the pectoralis fascia. The deep fascial layer and the pectoralis fascia are separated by the retromammary space, containing loose tissue, small vessels, and lymphatics. The loose tissue allows the breast to move freely over the chest wall.

Cooper's ligaments are fibrous, elastic strands that run throughout the breast tissue, connecting the deep fascial layer to the superficial fascial layer. The ligaments insert perpendicularly into the superficial fascial layer and anchor the breast to the overlying skin and to the underlying deep fascia (Fig. 1.3). They provide structural support to the breast, maintain upward breast projection, and allow for the natural motion of the breast due to their elasticity. With age, however, the ligament suspension progressively attenuates, resulting in varying degrees of breast ptosis (Table 1.1) [8].

Table 1.1 Ptosis classification

Ptosis grade	Description	Schematic representation
Normal	Nipple lies above the IMF	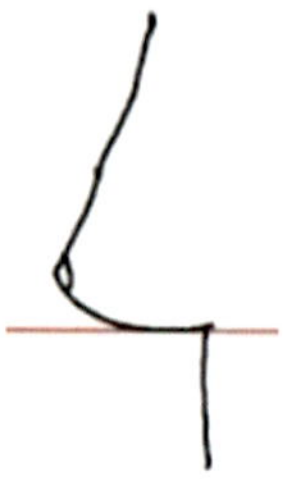
Mild (grade 1)	Nipple lies at the level of the IMF	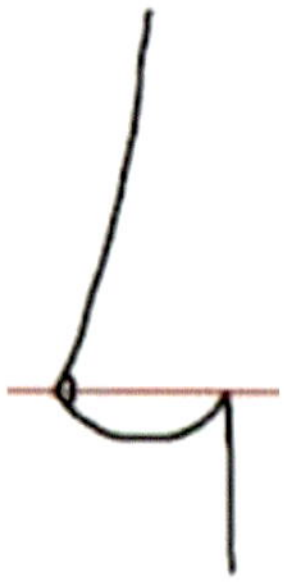
Moderate (grade 2)	Nipple lies below the IMF but above the lower contour of the breast	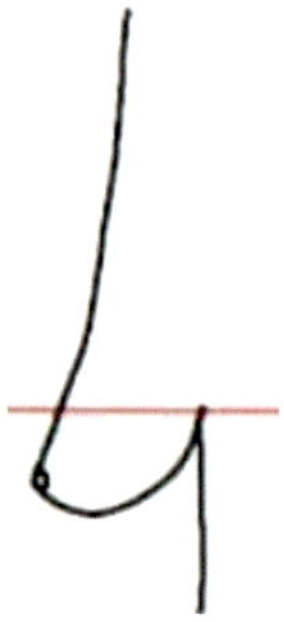
Severe (grade 3)	Nipple lies below the IMF and below the lower contour of the breast	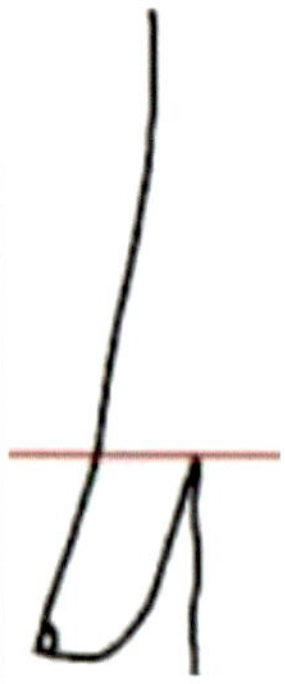
Pseudoptosis	Nipple lies above IMF but lower pole of the breast descends	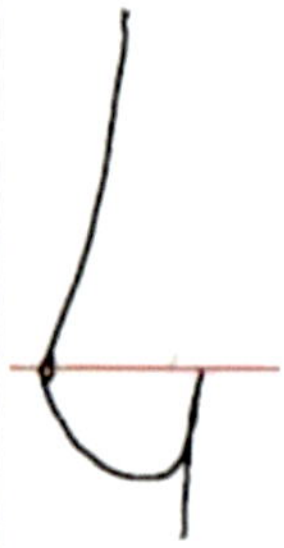

IMF inframammary fold

Nipple-Areolar Complex

The nipple-areolar complex is the central feature of the breast and an important landmark in breast surgery. The location of the nipple on the breast and its relationship to the inframammary fold contribute to mammary aesthetics.

The areola is a pigmented circular region of approximately 4–5 cm in diameter, situated over the fourth rib. The keratinizing, stratified, squamous epithelium of the areola is a continuation of the breast skin that contains sebaceous, sweat, and Montgomery's glands. The sebaceous glands are visible as raised bumps, the tubercle of morgani. The Montgomery's glands enlarge during pregnancy and become visible as the tubercles of Montgomery. They secrete a lipoid fluid that lubricates and protects the areola and the nipple during nursing. The areola contains two sets of smooth muscle fibers that are distributed circularly and radially (Fig. 1.4). The circular fibers are from the muscle of Sappey while the radial fibers are from the muscle of Meyerholz.

The nipple, or papilla, is a pigmented cylindrical projection that is located centrally on the areola with an average projection of about 4–12 mm and a diameter of 4–7 mm. The skin of the nipple is a continuation of the areolar skin consisting of sweat and sebaceous glands. As mentioned earlier, the nipple contains ductal orifices through which milk is released in lactating females. The 5–9 ductal orifices are distributed into two groups—one centrally and the other peripherally [7]. The centrally located ducts extend horizontally back toward the chest wall while the peripherally located ducts are arranged radially around the central ducts.

The nipple-areolar complex is devoid of a subcutaneous layer and rests on the areolar smooth muscle layer. The muscle fibers project into the nipple and are distributed as longitudinal and circular fibers which surround the mammary ducts and are supported by connective tissue. The contraction of these muscle fibers releases milk from the lactiferous sinuses. The muscle fibers are also responsible for nipple erection.

Vasculature

The breast has a rich, but redundant, arterial supply that is sourced by the subclavian, axillary, and intercostal arteries (Fig. 1.5). The internal mammary artery, also known as the internal thoracic artery, is the primary source of blood supply to the breast, providing approximately 60% of the blood supply. It is a paired artery arising from the subclavian artery that runs along either side of the sternum. Branches from this artery perforate the second to the sixth intercostal spaces before entering and perfusing the superomedial portion of the breast (upper inner quadrant), including the nipple-areolar complex. As they take a superficial course, the internal mammary artery perforators also send branches to the overlying skin.

The second main source of arterial supply to the breast is provided by the lateral mammary branches of the lateral thoracic artery, the pectoral branch of the thoracoacromial artery, and the subscapular artery. These arteries originate from the axillary artery and provide approximately 30% of the arterial blood supply to the breast. A prominent branch of the lateral thoracic artery (also referred to as the external mammary artery) primarily sources the superolateral portion of the breast (upper outer

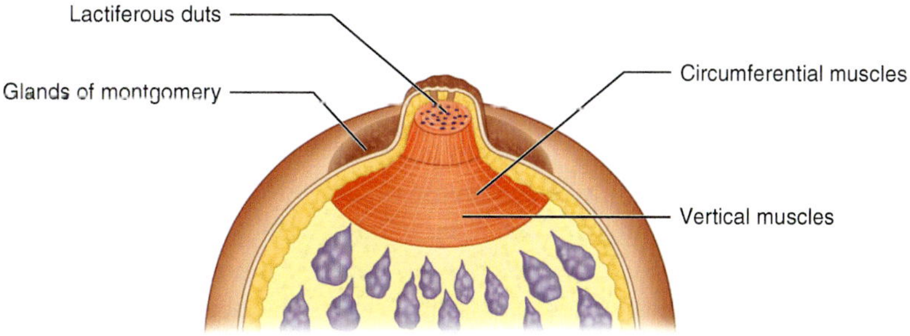

Fig. 1.4 Distribution of areolar muscular layer

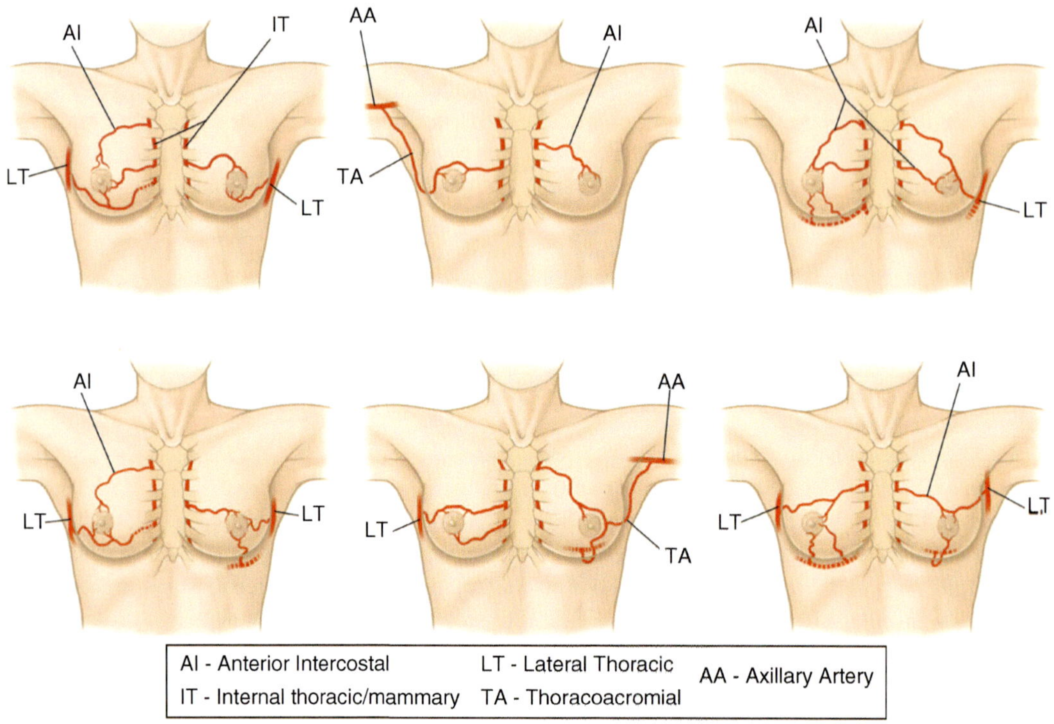

Fig. 1.5 Blood supply to the nipple areolar complex (NAC): The main blood supply is the internal thoracic/mammary artery and the lateral thoracic artery. The anterior intercostal perforators off the internal mammary provide specific branches of blood supply that can be designed as pedicles when performing mastopexies, reductions or other various flaps. With permission of Wolters Kluwer. Abbreviations: *AI* Anterior Intercostal, *IT* Internal thoracic/mammary, *LT* Lateral thoracic, *TA* Thoracoacromial, *AA* Axillary Artery

quadrant). This artery courses the lower border of the pectoralis minor muscle and around the lateral border of the pectoralis major muscle before entering the breast. The pectoral branch of the thoracoacromial artery, which runs between the pectoralis major and minor muscles, provides blood supply to the superior aspect of the breast.

A third source of blood supply to the breast is provided by the branches of the intercostal arteries. Branches of the anterolateral intercostal arteries perfuse the lateral aspect of the breast and the overlying skin. Blood supply to the inferior central portion of the breast, below the nipple-areolar complex, as well as the nipple-areolar complex, is provided by the anteromedial intercostal branches.

The redundancy in blood supply to the breast ensures adequate perfusion of the breast tissues as well as the overlying skin. The skin, in addition, is sourced by the subdermal plexus which arises from the vascular system within the breast. From a surgical standpoint, the redundancy allows the safe partition of breast tissue in breast reduction. Any one of the arterial pathways can be preserved which will also assure the viability of the nipple-areolar complex. Surgeons have a choice of selecting from any of the techniques for the preservation of the superior, medial, lateral, or inferior pedicle blood supplies. It is critical to be aware of the blood supply and which pedicle will be utilized. The superior and medial pedicles are generally speaking preferred since the lower pole and lateral tissue are removed to improve the shape of the breast. In revision surgery where prior mastopexy or reduction was performed, the superior and medial pedicles are still utilized regardless of the prior pedicle use. If circumareolar surgery is at least 6–12 months postoperative, then it is safe to proceed with another pedicle if it is needed. It is important to select patients carefully and avoid operations on patients with comorbidities that lead to decreased blood supply to the existing nipple-areolar complex (i.e. smoking and uncontrolled diabetes mellitus).

Venous drainage from the breast is mediated via two systems—a superficial system and a deep system. The superficial system involves the subdermal venous plexus, situated above the superficial fascia. Veins from the subdermal venous plexus anastomose extensively with the deep system and drain into the internal mammary vein and the anterior superficial jugular vein The deep system consists of the corresponding paired veins of the arterial system that drain into the tributaries of the internal mammary vein, tributaries of the intercostal veins, and the vertebral system. The internal mammary vein drains into the brachiocephalic vein and the lateral thoracic veins drain into the axillary vein and then into the superior vena cava. Venous drainage from the areola occurs via the internal thoracic, axillary, and intercostal veins.

Lymphatic System

The breast has an extensive network of lymphatic channels that course through the breast parenchyma, the skin, and the nipple-areolar complex. Lymph drainage from the breast occurs via two main pathways that feed into the axillary nodes and the internal mammary (or parasternal) nodes. The majority of the lymphatic drainage passes into the axillary nodes. There are about 20–30 axillary lymph nodes that are arranged into 6 groups: axillary vein or lateral group, external mammary or pectoral or anterior axillary group, subscapular group, central group, subclavicular or apical group, and the Rotter's group or interpectoral group. The external mammary group of nodes receives the bulk of the lymphatic drainage from the breast. In addition to the axillary and parasternal nodes, the breast also has other accessory lymphatic networks such as the transmammary and paramammary vessels. The former connects to the contralateral breast while the latter connects to the hepatic lymph nodes and subdiaphragmatic nodes.

Knowledge of the breast lymphatic system is extremely important for understanding breast cancer dissemination. Further, knowledge of lymph nodes is critical for successful performance of sentinel lymph node biopsy.

Innervation

The breast is innervated by the lateral and anterior cutaneous branches of the thoracic intercostal nerves and the supraclavicular branch of the superficial cervical plexus. The former is responsible for the majority of breast sensation. Branches of the third to sixth lateral intercostal nerves innervate the lateral breast while branches of the second to sixth anterior intercostal nerves innervate the medial breast. Both sets of nerve branches innervate the breast glandular tissue, the overlying skin, and the nipple-areolar complex. The cervical plexus runs superficially along the subcutaneous tissue, innervating the superior medial breast.

Preservation of breast innervation is critical while performing breast augmentation or reduction so as not to compromise breast sensation. Branches of the cervical plexus are usually unperturbed when the upper breast flap is elevated. Care is taken when a dissection is performed laterally when an implant is placed to minimize the trauma to the nerve supply of the nipple-areolar complex.

Musculature

Chest and abdominal wall muscles that are of relevance to breast anatomy include the pectoralis major, serratus anterior, rectus abdominis, and the external oblique muscles. Breast tissue is attached to these muscles.

The pectoralis major muscle is a broad, triangular-shaped muscle that extends from its origins in the medial clavicle, lateral sternum, and second to sixth ribs to its insertion in the intertubercular groove of the humerus. Most of the breast surface lies on this muscle. The pectoralis major is responsible for the flexion, adduction, and medial rotation of the arm. The muscle is innervated by the medial and lateral portions of the pectoral nerves. Blood supply to the muscle is provided primarily by the thoracoacromial artery and secondarily by the lateral thoracic artery, intercostal perforators, and internal mammary perforators.

Pectoralis major is an important muscle in breast reconstructive and aesthetic surgery for it provides implant coverage and support when a subpectoral approach is undertaken. In reconstructive surgery, the muscle is elevated and typically covers the upper two-third of the implant. In this setting, the muscle provides a layer of tissue to cushion the implant from the overlying skin and subcutaneous tissue which are usually attenuated after a mastectomy. Subpectoral placement attenuates the risk of implant exposure, palpability, and wrinkling and capsular contracture but may cause animation deformity as the muscle contracts. Releasing the inferior and medial attachments of the muscle ameliorates animation deformity and also serves to lower the implant positioning which is aesthetically more appealing.

In breast augmentation, when a dual plane approach is planned, the origins of the pectoralis major are released and care is taken not to cross to the sternal border. The different levels of release of the pectoralis major from the glandular tissues determine the level of the dual plane that is created based on patient's presenting anatomy. It is also important not to violate the pectoralis minor or serratus anterior muscles during this dissection.

The serratus anterior muscle spans the anterolateral chest wall, lying below the lateral aspect of the breast. It originates as muscle strips on the surface of the first eight ribs which converge and insert into the medial margin of the scapula. The muscle pulls the scapula forward and around the rib cage and permits the forward rotation of the arm. It is innervated by the long thoracic nerve. The superior aspect of the muscle is supplied by the lateral thoracic artery and the inferior aspect by the thoracodorsal artery perforators.

The serratus anterior may be recruited in the subpectoral approach of breast reconstructive surgery. Elevation of the pectoralis major muscle laterally for implant insertion can lead to the partial elevation of the serratus anterior as well. Additionally, in the instance where complete muscle coverage of the implant is needed, the serratus anterior is elevated to provide lateral implant coverage. With the introduction of acellular dermal matrices for breast reconstruction, the need for serratus anterior recruitment has diminished. In breast augmentation, the serratus anterior is generally not elevated for subpectoral implant placement.

The rectus abdominis muscle is an elongated muscle that spans over the anterior abdominal wall, extending from the pubis to the inferior margin of the fifth to seventh costal cartilages. Attachment of breast tissue to the superior limit of the rectus abdominis demarcates the inferior border of the breast. The linea alba, a thick band of connective tissue, interconnects the rectus abdominis muscle on either side of the abdomen. The muscle is responsible for compression of the abdominal wall and flexion of the spine. It is innervated by the seventh through twelfth intercostal nerves. Arterial blood flow to the muscle is predominantly via the superior and inferior epigastric arteries, which source the superior and inferior portion of the muscle, respectively, forming a rich network of anastomoses between them.

The rectus abdominis muscle is an important muscle in autologous breast reconstructive surgery where it is used in the transverse rectus abdominis myocutaneous (TRAM) flap approach. In prosthetic breast reconstruction, the fascia of the rectus abdominis muscle may be recruited to establish lower pole coverage of the implant. Elevating the fascia also allows the more caudal placement of the implant. In breast augmentation, caudal placement of the implant below the rectus abdominis fascia attachment is usually not advocated.

The external oblique muscle is a broad thin muscle that spans the anterolateral abdomen, bordering the inferolateral aspect of the breast. Its muscular portion covers the lateral abdomen while its aponeurosis covers the anterior abdominal wall. It originates from the lower eight ribs (fifth to twelfth ribs) and inserts along the anterior half of the iliac crest, the pubic tubercle, and the aponeurosis of the linea alba from the xiphoid to the pubis. The function of the muscle is to compress the abdominal cavity which depresses the ribs downwards, permit lateral (same-side) bending, and lateral rotation of the spine. The muscle is innervated by branches of the lower six intercostal nerves and the subcostal nerve. The lower eight posterior intercostal arteries provide blood supply to the muscle.

In breast augmentation, inferior placement of the implant usually does not surpass the fascia of the external oblique muscle or the fascia of the rectus abdominis muscle. Placing the implant behind the fascia produces a "high-riding" implant which may lead to "waterfall" deformity.

Thoracic Wall

As breasts lie on the anterior thoracic wall, structural deformities of the thoracic wall affect breast shape, projection, and symmetry. Pectus excavatum and pectus carinatum are the two most common chest wall deformities, although they are rare conditions. In pectus excavatum, the abnormal development of the sternum and rib cage result in a sunken appearance of the chest Pectus carinatum is characterized by a protrusion of the sternum and ribs due to abnormal or uneven growth of intercostal cartilage. Poland syndrome, another chest wall deformity, is characterized by missing or underdevelopment of the pectoralis major muscle on one side of the chest wall (Fig. 1.6). Breast and nipple abnormalities as well as thoracic cage abnormalities (shortened ribs) may also occur. As a result of the underdeveloped or missing pectoralis major muscle, the chest wall has a concave appearance. Abnormal spinal curvature such as scoliosis may be another source of beast asymmetry.

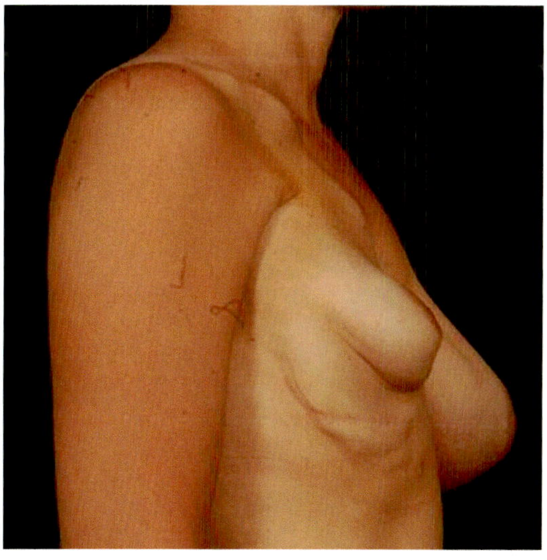

Fig. 1.6 Poland syndrome: absence or underdevelopment of the underlying pectoralis major muscle

Although structural deformities of the chest wall and the spine are beyond the scope of breast surgeons, it is nonetheless important that surgeons evaluate for such deformities at the preoperative planning stage. As spinal curvature and chest wall deformities can affect breast symmetry and projection postoperatively, the patient should be informed of the deformity and its impact on postoperative breast aesthetics so as to set realistic expectations for the planned breast surgery.

Conclusion

Breast aesthetics are determined by volume, soft tissue composition and distribution, shape/contour, tissue elasticity, location and appearance of the nipple-areolar complex, and proportionality of the breast with respect to the thoracic wall and the body. As there is substantial inter-patient and intra-patient variability in breast shape and size, breast modifications to improve aesthetic appearance should be individualized. A comprehensive knowledge of breast anatomy and chest wall structure facilitates surgical planning and execution, minimizes complications, and ensures successful outcomes.

References

1. American Society of Plastic Surgeons. 2019 Plastic surgery statistics report. https://www.plasticsurgery.org/documents/News/Statistics/2019/plastic-surgery-statistics-full-report-2019.pdf
2. Maxwell GP, Gabriel A. Breast reconstruction. In: Aston SJ, Steinbrech DS, Walden JL, editors. Aesthetic plastic surgery. Philadelphia: Elsevier; 2009, chap 57.
3. Liu YJ, Thomson JG. Ideal anthropomorphic values of the female breast: correlation of pluralistic aesthetic evaluations with objective measurements. Ann Plast Surg. 2011;67:7–11.

4. Tepper OM, Unger JG, Small KH, Feldman D, Kumar N, Choi M, et al. Mammometrics: the standardization of aesthetic and reconstructive breast surgery. Plast Reconstr Surg. 2010;125:393–400.
5. Vandeput JJ, Nelissen M. Considerations on anthropometric measurements of the female breast. Aesthet Plast Surg. 2002;26:348–55.
6. Hunt KK, Mittendorf EA. Diseases of the breast (chapter 34). In: Townsend CM, Beauchamp RD, Evers BM, Mattox KL, editors. Sabiston textbook of surgery, The biological basis of modern surgical practice. Philadelphia: Elsevier; 2016. p. 820–64.
7. Love SM, Barsky SH. Anatomy of the nipple and breast ducts revisited. Cancer. 2004;101:1947–57.
8. Regnault P. Breast ptosis: definition and treatment. Clin Plast Surg. 1976;3:193–203.

Principles of Breast Augmentation: The Process of Augmentation Mastopexy and Criteria for Staging

2

Kyle Sanniec and William P. Adams Jr.

Introduction

Augmentation mastopexy has evolved over the years since first being described by Gonzalez-Ulloa [1] and Regault [2]. The number of patients requesting augmentation mastopexy has also increased with this evolution. The conflict between increasing breast volume and expanding this skin envelope with an augmentation while simultaneously reducing the skin envelope and breast parenchyma during a mastopexy presents a challenge with a slim margin for error. The conflicting goals/forces of tightening and reducing the breast and skin envelope while increasing the breast volume with an implant have led to a high reported operation rate in the literature ranging from 8.7% to 23.2% [3–7].

Moreover, even if they do not require a reoperation, patients may be less satisfied with their post-operative result and desire additional procedures on their breast [8]. This decrease in satisfaction and high operation rate has even led some to encourage staging of <u>all</u> augmentation mastopexy procedures and in any case cautionary accounts have been told [9]. While staging the operation does lead to less wound breakdown and tissue distortion, it requires a second operation with the added cost to the patient, both financially and emotionally. This two-stage operation runs counter to what most patients seeking a rejuvenated breast want, as the push in aesthetic surgery is toward combining operations to get more done under one anesthetic.

Given the complexities of the surgery, the high litigation rate [9, 10] and the above average revision rates, many authors have provided various techniques to produce a reliable, reproducible and predictable result in single stage augmentation mastopexy [11–13].

The Process of Augmentation Mastopexy

Similar to The Process of Breast Augmentation [14] that re-defined the approach to the breast augmentation patient and optimized outcomes, augmentation mastopexy benefits from a process approach; this process primarily manages the preoperative planning and intraoperative approach, and is invaluable to deliver the optimal result in this complicated patient population. In treating the deflated, volume deficient breast, our process involves utilizing quantifiable numbers from the patient's native anatomy/tissues, defined patient goals, and methodical criteria to get a predictable result. The senior author (WPA Jr.) has developed a process-oriented approach to augmentation mastopexy [12, 15] with a low revision rate around 3% [16]. The

K. Sanniec · W. P. Adams Jr. (✉)
University of Texas Southwestern, Department of Plastic Surgery, Dallas, TX, USA
e-mail: wpajrmd@dr-adams.com

M. B. Calobrace et al. (eds.), *Augmentation Mastopexy*,
https://doi.org/10.1007/978-3-030-48226-8_2

preoperative planning and the intraoperative steps that are critical in achieving a reliable result with a low revision rate will be discussed further. All our patients undergo the same validated process that consists of an extensive organized patient education, an assessment based on their own tissues, and a refined surgical technique followed by a clearly defined postoperative regimen.

The Tissue Based Triad

As with all techniques, this should serve as an infrastructure for the surgeon to help organize their evaluation of an augmentation mastopexy patient. Surgeons have typically used the Regnault classification [17] to determine which patients require an augmentation mastopexy versus solely an augmentation. The problem is the Regnault classification is very non-specific. Classically, a patient with grade 2 ptosis has been deemed a candidate requiring an augmentation mastopexy; however, the classification requires surgeon interpretation that is far from objective. For example, in this case demonstrating a patient with Grade 2 ptosis (Fig. 2.1), using the Regnault classification would be relegated to an augmentation mastopexy procedure; however, using the tissue-based triad concepts we prefer to

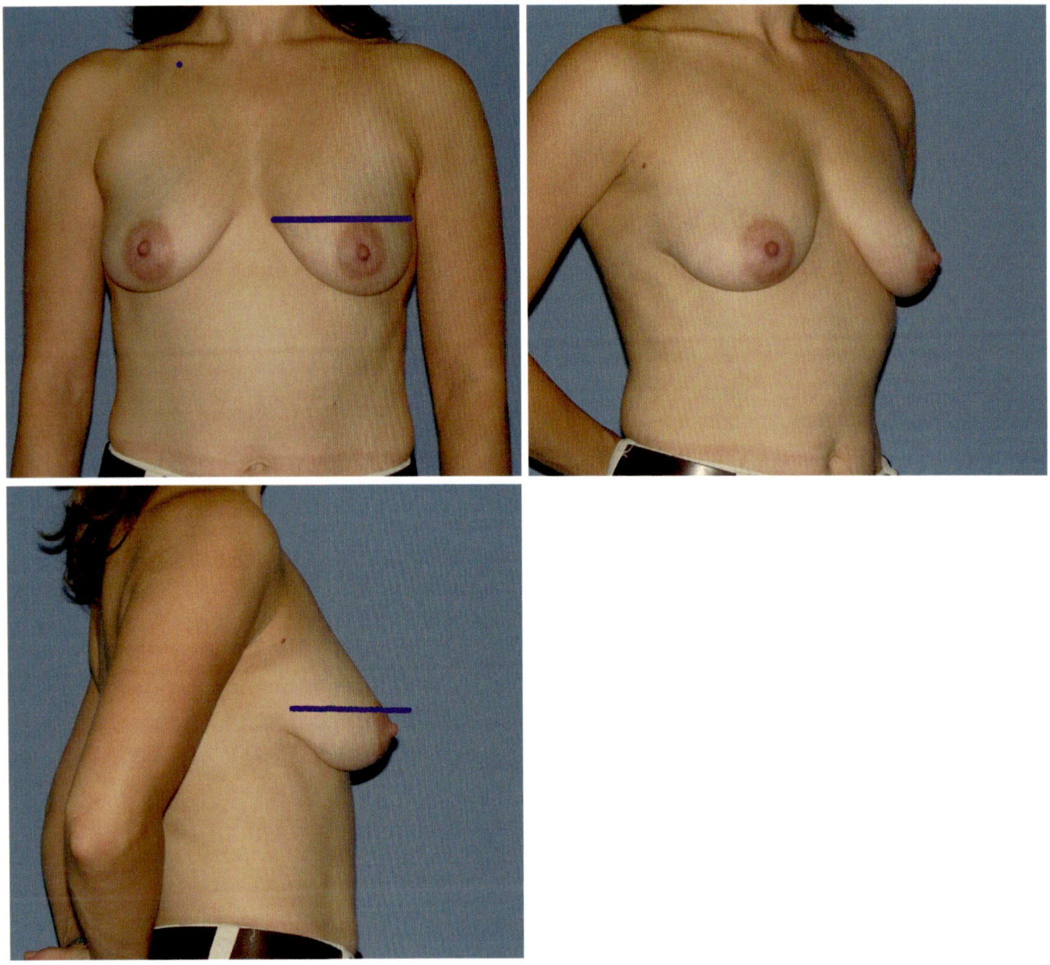

Fig. 2.1 Preop evaluation comparing tissue based triad and traditional Regnault classification. The blue line represents her native IMF, and the nipple is clearly below the fold demonstrating grade 2 ptosis. Using the Regnault classification, this patient would require an augmentation mastopexy, as she presents with grade 2 ptosis. However, using the tissue-based triad, her skin stretch is 3.5 cm and her nipple to fold distance is 9.5 cm, indicating moderate laxity that can be treated with an augmentation alone

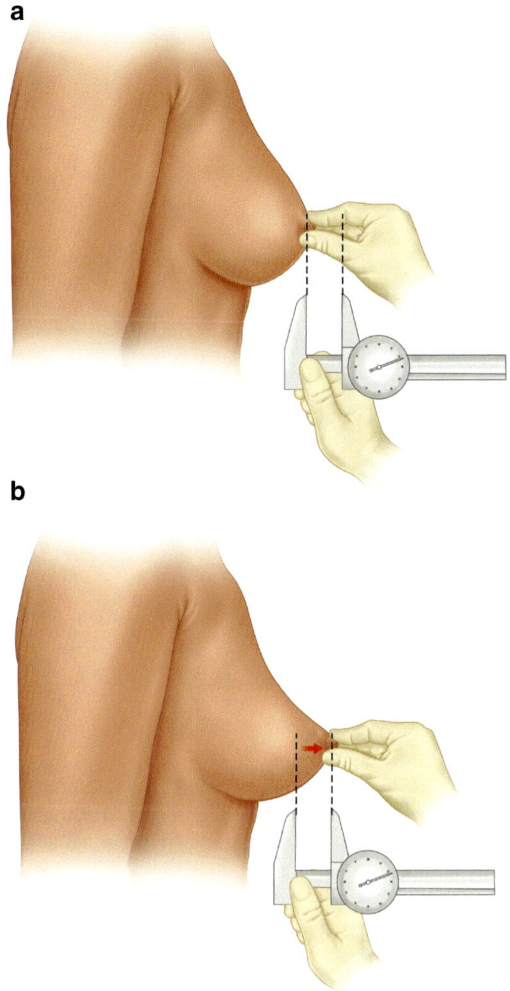

Fig. 2.2 Skin stretch measurement. The anterior displacement of the nipple is measured from resting position to determine the amount of skin stretch

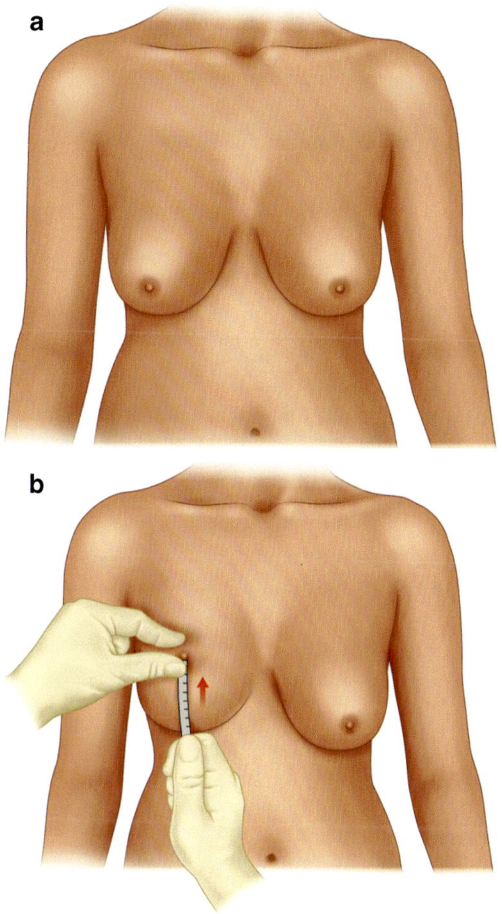

Fig. 2.3 Nipple to fold measurement on stretch. The current nipple to fold is measured on maximum stretch by placing superior traction on the breast and measuring from the nipple position to the current IMF

measure the global laxity in the breast starting with a skin stretch (SS) (Fig. 2.2) and Nipple to Fold under max stretch (NIMF) (Fig. 2.3). These 2 measurements better define what patient can be treated with breast augmentation and what patient needs an augmentation mastopexy.

In this example the SS = 3.5 cm and NIMF = 9.5 (Fig. 2.4) and the patient underwent an augmentation alone without the need for a mastopexy. If the SS < 4 **and** the NIMF<10 this indicates moderate laxity and the patient can be treated with breast augmentation alone. If the patient's nipples are down pointing a peri-areolar nipple repositioning can be performed as well. In this example the patient was treated with a standard dual plane breast augmentation with a 2-year result shown.

In the next case example, the skin stretch is >4 and/ or the NIMF >10, The next measurement in the tissue-based triad planning process is Vertical Excess (VE) (Fig. 2.5). The VE measurement is utilized to objectively determine who will need a two-stage operation versus who can achieve good results with a single stage operation. The VE is a measurement of global laxity in the breast as well as incorporating information on the surgical plan. It is measured by picking the new nipple position and then measuring the desired/planned nipple to fold length. The remaining skin from the inferior aspect of the nipple to fold planned length to the

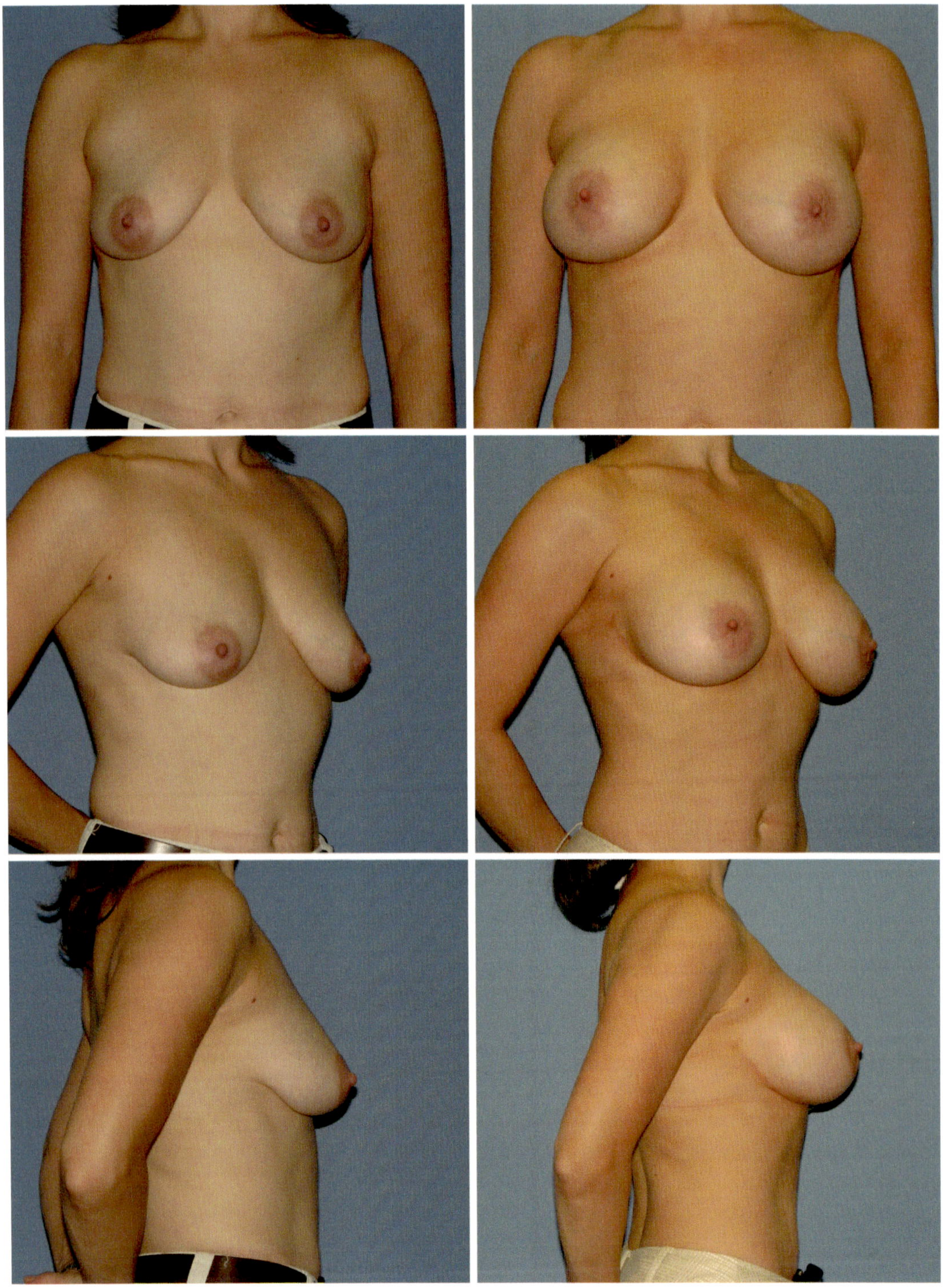

Fig. 2.4 Patient from Fig. 2.1 with before and after photos following single stage augmentation alone. Preoperative and postoperative images at 2 years out from single stage augmentation with (Allergan 410MM 320 cc implants). Note the improved aesthetic result without the need for a mastopexy

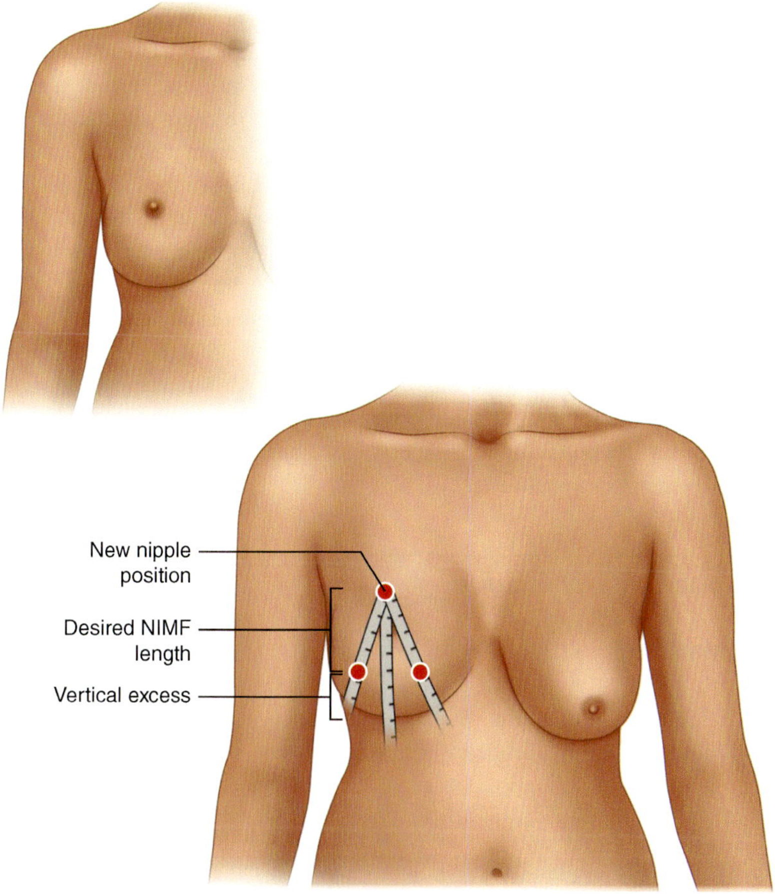

Fig. 2.5 Vertical Excess Measurement. Illustration showing how to determine the vertical excess. The new nipple position is marked from Pitanguy's point and the desired nipple to fold length (from red dot to red dot) is marked to create the new nipple to fold position both medially and laterally from the breast meridian, with each point along the fold equally measuring the ideal NIMF distance. The remaining breast skin inferior to this new fold position is the vertical excess

existing IMF is the vertical excess. Single stage augmentation mastopexy procedures are reserved for VE < 6 and 2 stage procedures for VE > 6 performing a mastopexy first followed by a breast augmentation at 4–6 months post-op.

The benefit of the tissue-based triad is its straightforwardness. The measurements can be performed in 15 seconds.

Once the patient is deemed an appropriate candidate for a single staged augmentation mastopexy based on the above tissue-based criteria, the implant is selected based on the patient's breast parenchyma and overall volume. If the patient has minimal breast tissue, the goal for this patient is to provide volume that is missing from the absent breast tissue, and a more projecting higher fill implant is needed. If the patient has breast tissue but it is simply ptotic, the goal is simply to provide upper pole fullness, as the native breast parenchyma will provide the volume and a lower profile implant that will fill the upper pole is used.

The implant size is typically determined by the patient's preoperative breast width less 1 cm to account for the mastopexy. A low profile implant equal to this dimension will give the patient optimal fill [18]. In general, a slightly wider implant is preferable, as the key dimension in providing upper pole fill is the height of the implant which corresponds to the implant width in a round implant. Additionally, the use of 3D imaging assists the patient and surgeon in selecting the implant that meets the patients desired aesthetic result while still staying with an implant that will fit their tissues.

In our practice, the key to implant selection is related to the height of the implant. We utilize lower profile enhanced cohesive gel Generation 6 implants, as the patients typically have breast tissue, and therefore do not need projection, but fill and control of the distribution of fill especially in the upper pole. The primary deficiency with high profile implants is the lack of fill into the upper pole. These implants, typically, are narrower and shorter. They are more projected, but they don't provide the desired control of the distribution of fill in the upper pole as lower profile implants will.

The goal of this chapter is to provide a thorough description of our technique to guide both the novice and experienced plastic surgeon. Long term data has shown our revision rates at the lower end of the published literature, with no statistical difference in wound complication rates between our mastopexy and single stage augmentation mastopexy patients.

Pre-operative Evaluation

The Markings

We utilize a modification of the mastopexy markings reported by Tebbetts [19, 20]. In the preoperative suite, all patients are marked in an upright position (Fig. 2.6a, b). The patient's midline, breast meridian and inframammary fold are all marked. Pitanguy's point is utilized to get a rough estimate of the appropriate nipple position, the nipple is then raised superiorly to a level that is the most aesthetically pleasing on the breast then release the breast and mark where the nipple was on the patient's breast. Sternal notch to nipple measurement confirms symmetry of the nipple positions. The two main differences with our modification, is that we doubly confirm the nipple position by a nipple drop technique and utilizing Pitanguy's point and the top of our marking is planned as the nipple proper not the superior border of the areola as Tebbetts described [19].

The breast is then placed on maximal stretch and the ideal nipple to fold length is measured from the previously marked new nipple location. The desired nipple to fold length is measured and marked, with an added 0.5 cm increase to account for the discrepancy in true

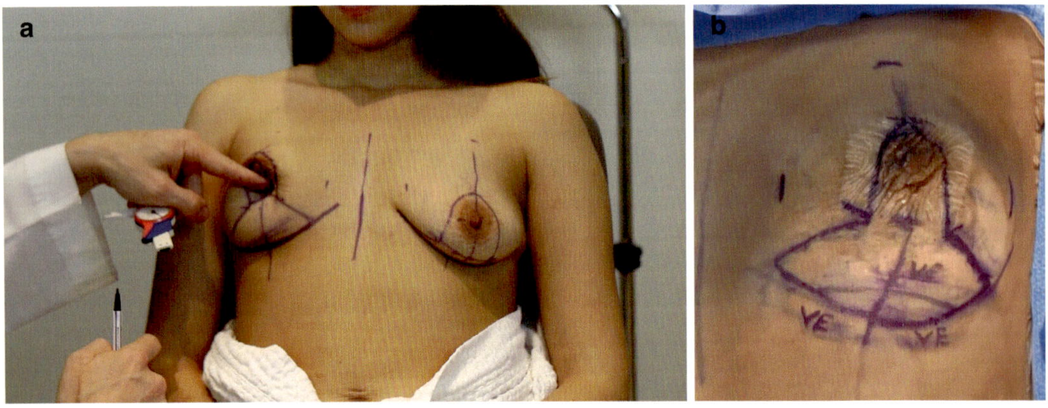

Fig. 2.6 (**a**) Preoperative markings. A photo of a patient with markings immediately prior to the operating room. The hash marks on the periphery of the breast demonstrate the width and height of the selected implant. These correspond to the base width in round implants. The implant pocket dissection should not veer outside these marking to maintain a tight pocket. An arc is draw from the new nipple position, the apex of the vertical incision, to the new desired inframammary fold. All points along the arc are equidistant to the new nipple position. (**b**) Intraoperative markings. The distance from the new inframammary fold to the current inframammary fold is the vertical excess. The vertical excess is measured and a horizontal mark twice the vertical excess is created for the inferior incision. The Adams Dermal Flap is also marked

maximal stretch versus the maximal stretch that can be achieved in the preoperative area. From the new nipple location, an arc is drawn, which will be the new inferior border of the breast. All points along the arc are equal to the nipple to fold distance.

The distance between the desired nipple to fold and the current inframammary fold is the vertical excess. This excess determines the width of the marking. The incision width is the superimposed vertical excess distance medially and laterally to the breast meridian. The new fold arc and the existing fold are marked at the point the vertical excess length connects the two horizontal markings [20].

The vertical limbs are marked just outside of the areola from the ideal nipple position to where the medial and lateral width of the horizontal excision goes. The width and height of the implant pocket is also marked on the breast. The width is equal to the ideal breast width and the height is the base width distance from the inframammary fold.

Surgical Approach

Intraoperative Steps

Section 1 – Augmentation The procedure is split into two sections to completely separate exposure of the implant to breast parenchymal contaminants. The augmentation is performed first, through an inframammary incision that is performed within the mastopexy marks and slightly above the current inframammary fold. A classic four-part dual plane dissection (Fig. 2.7) is performed [21, 22].

A modified inframammary incision is made with the electrocautery preserving an inferiorly based dermal flap (used later in closure), the dissection is carried down similar to an IMF augmentation with electrocautery to the pectoralis major muscle. The inferior origins of the muscle are divided **(part 1)** with prospective hemostasis. The retractor is utilized to tent up the pectoralis major fascia to afford confidence that you are

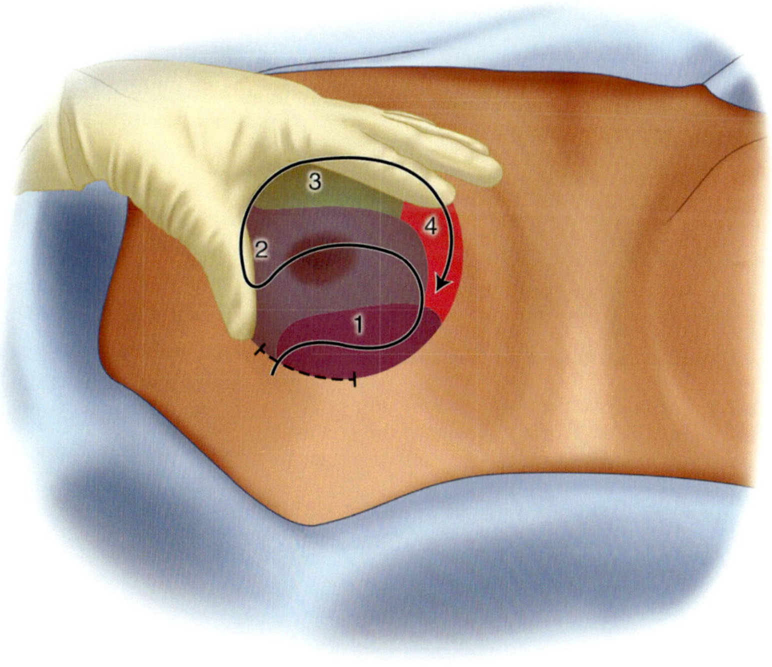

Fig. 2.7 Pocket Dissection Part. The pocket is dissected initially inferiorly (1), then laterally to the lateral border of the sub-pectoral pocket (2), followed by superior dissection equal to the height of the implant (3), and lastly medially (4) to the level of the accessory pectoralis major insertions

truly incising through pectoralis muscle rather than serratus or intercostal muscle, as this will not tent up (Fig. 2.8). The dissection is carried around to the edge of the muscle laterally and the sub-pectoral plane is entered prior to dividing the inferior margins. The division is stopped at the medial mark for the base width. It is critical to incise the inferior pectoral origins full thickness without stopping at the parasternal region but must use caution not to over-divide the medial sternal attachments.

The dissection is then swept laterally to define the lateral border of the sub-pectoral pocket **(part 2)**. Pectoralis minor is identified and protected. The dissection continues until reaching the lateral breast width mark from our preoperative markings. This is the extent of the lateral pocket dissection.

The dissection then continues superiorly to make the height of the dissection equal to the height of the selected implant **(part 3)** which is guided by the preoperative superior guide mark in the cranial caudal direction. Lastly the medial pocket dissection is performed **(part 4)** dividing any tendinous or accessory origins of the pectoralis major that are identified. Care is taken to not divide any of the main body of the medial origins of the muscle. Once the pocket dissection is completed, a dual plane 2 [22] adjustment is performed.

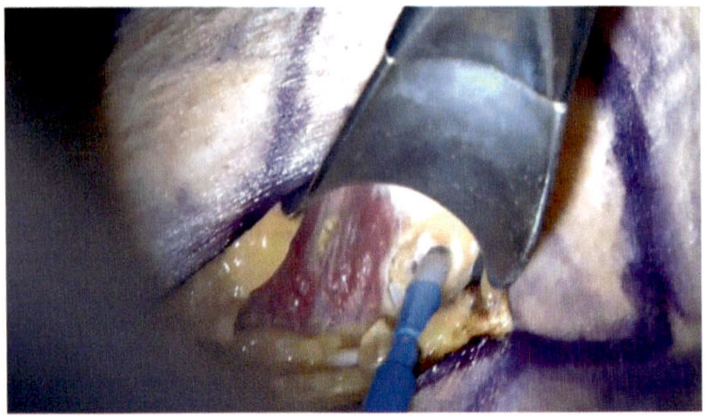

Fig. 2.8 Pocket Dissection. Intraoperative close up demonstrating use of the retractor to tent up the pectoralis major fascia to ensure incision only through pectoralis major muscle

The pocket is then prepared for implant insertion including irrigation with 150 cc saline and then betadine triple ((50 cc Betadine, 1gm cefazolin, 80 mg gentamycin, 500 cc NS), the external skin around the incision is re-prepped with chlorhexidine, and betadine triple solution is used to dip and clean the instruments in accordance with previously published guidelines and the 14-point plan to decrease bacterial load on the implant [23]. Gloves are changed immediately prior to implant handling and insertion.

The implant is sealed off from the rest of the wound by closing the superficial fascia with a running 3-0 PDS suture, with the 2nd layer going slightly outside the incision to plicate the fascia and ensure a water tight closure. A dermal flap will be designed during the mastopexy, that will further reinforce this closure and provide an additional layer between the implant and the skin.

Section 2 – Mastopexy Once the implant pocket has been closed, the mastopexy markings are again confirmed with a central mound configuration. A simple skin pinch is used to confirm that the skin resection has not been over planned (surgeons with less experience can do simple tailor tacking if desired).

A 38 mm cookie cutter is utilized to incise around the nipple. The rest of the incisions are then incised. The area around the nipple are de-epithelialized as well as a central inferior dermal flap with a scalpel. This inferiorly based dermal flap will be inset later to protect the incision site at the T point should delayed wound healing occur (Fig. 2.9). The dermal flap typically has a 2.5 cm height and a 4 cm base. It needs to have enough height to be able to be pulled cranially to unify the lateral and medial limbs of the breast Slight undermining between the dermis and the parenchyma is performed to prevent tethering of the flap.

The inferior skin is then excised directly with electrocautery. The amount of undermining is minimal. The level of undermining is slightly deep to the superficial fascia which is important for the IMF fixation suture closure at the IMF, and if the undermining is continued it is taken more superficial just above the superfi-

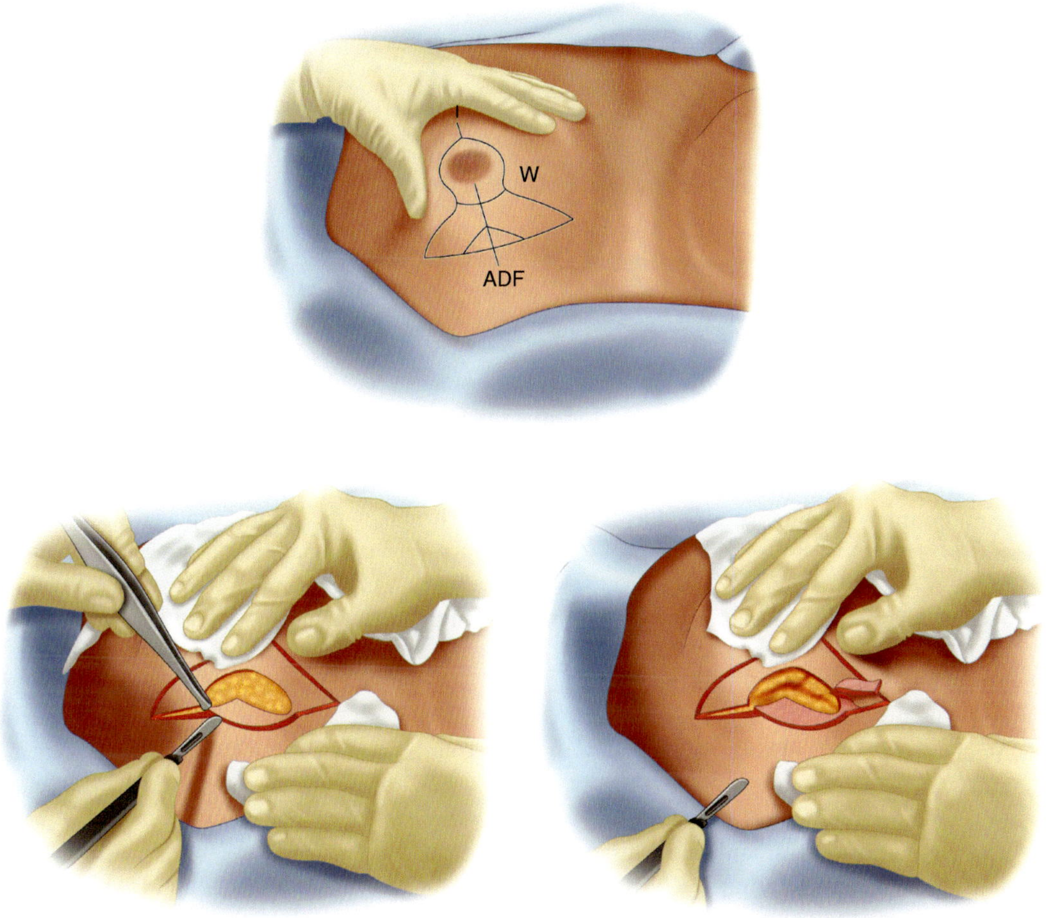

Fig. 2.9 Adams Dermal Flap Part 1 (CH02-Adams dermal flap-A). The Adams Dermal Flap is an inferiorly based dermal flap with a 2.5 cm height and 4 cm width. The flap is de-epithelialized and will be pulled cranially during closure to unify the lateral and medial skin flaps of the breast

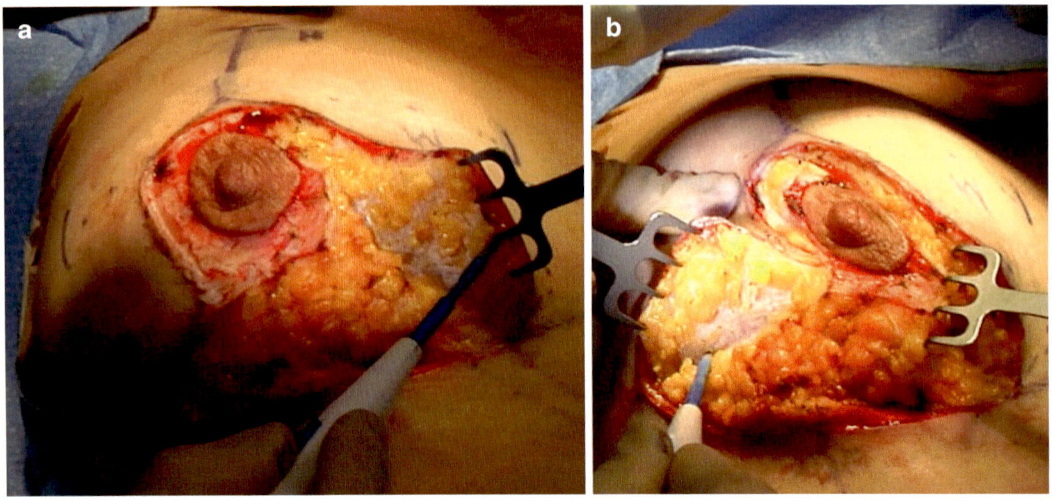

Fig. 2.10 (**a**, **b**) Elevation of medial and lateral limbs. The medial (**a**) and lateral (**b**) limbs are undermined with electrocautery just deep to the superficial fascia initially and then transitioned superficial to this fascia. This is raised just enough to provide a tension free closure at the T point

cial fascia (Fig. 2.10a, b) A diamond wedge of parenchyma in generally removed in the lower pole and this can be customized depending on the clinical situation to prevent crowding at the T point. Four key sutures are placed as follows (Fig. 2.14a–e):

1. 3-point dermal 3-0 Monocryl at T point (Fig. 2.11)
2. 2 IMF fixation 3-0 PDS - 1 medial and 1 lateral (Fig. 2.12)
3. 3-point fixation 3-0 PDS inferiorly based dermal flap (Fig. 2.13)

The nipple position is confirmed utilizing a bottom up technique. The nipple to fold relationship in an augmentation mastopexy for most breasts is shown in the table (Table 2.1). While not an exact science, however the planning is based on known relationships between the breast width and nipple to fold length. In general, the nipple needs to be relatively higher on the breast to be in an aesthetic location since the upper pole is being filled as well (which makes the nipple appear lower on the breast). For most patients this is 8–10 cm from the IMF. A higher nipple position is critical in an augmentation mastopexy where you are filling the upper pole and changing the ratio of the inferior pole to the superior pole in relation to the nipple.

Using skin hooks on the superior and inferior portion of the vertical limbs, the vertical dimension is placed on maximal stretch (Fig. 2.15a, b). The ideal nipple to fold distance is measured, though this usually corresponds between 8.5 to 9.5 cm. This technical step including placing the skin between the nipple and fold on max stretch and measuring from the fixed IMF to bottom of the areola are

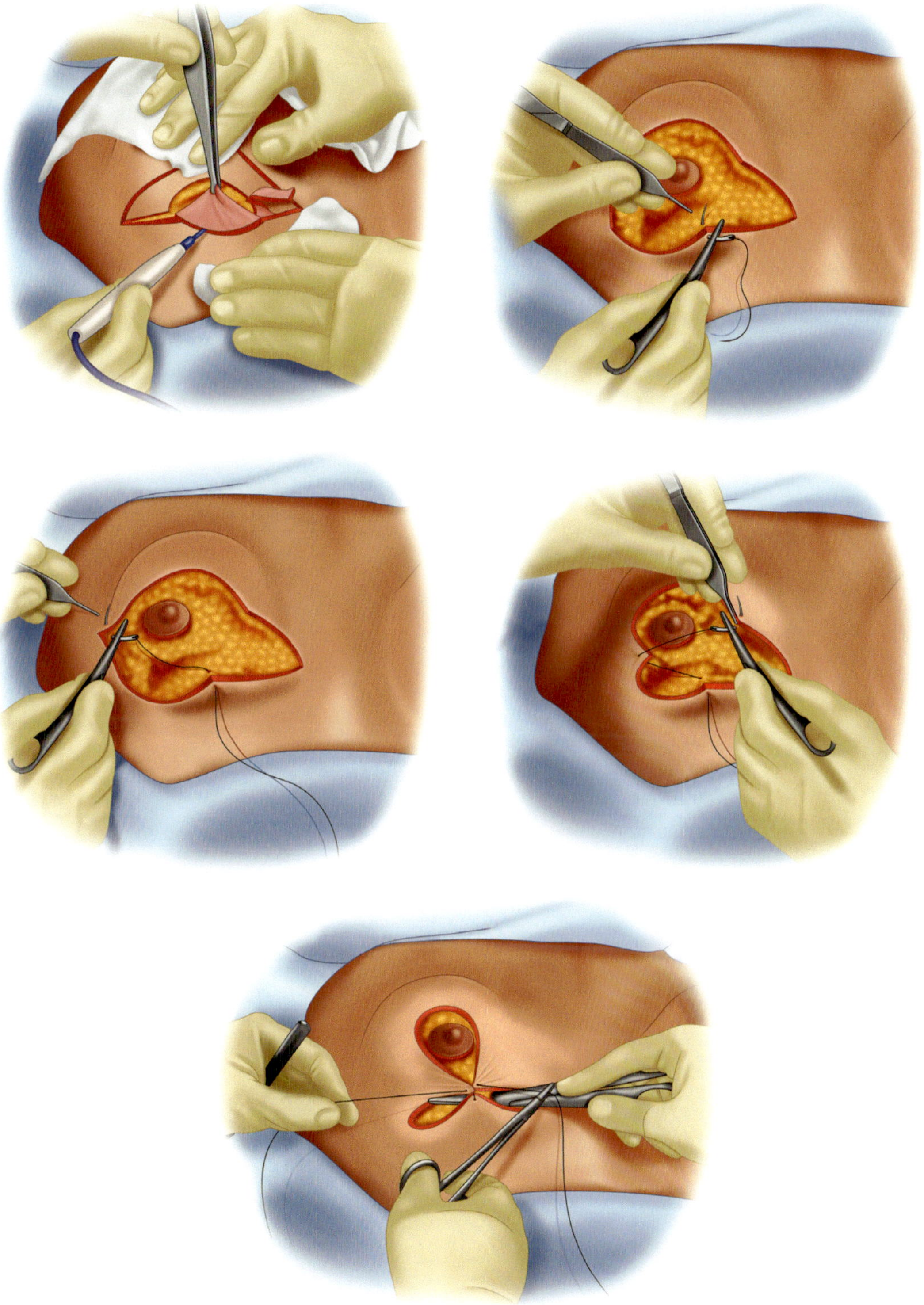

Fig. 2.11 Adams Dermal Flap Part 2 (Ch02_Adams Dermal Flap-B). After completion of the skin and breast parenchyma resection, a suture from the inferior incision at the interface of the chest wall skin and the dermal flap is place connecting the inferior incision with the lateral and medial breast incisions. The dermal flap is pulled cranially underneath this suture

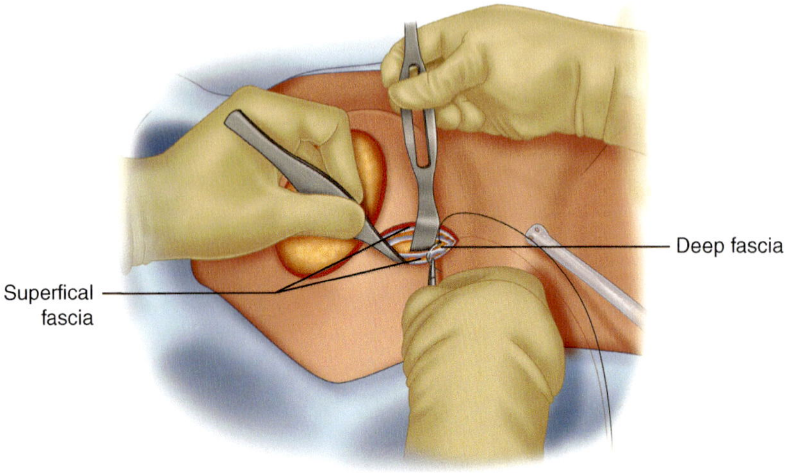

Fig. 2.12 IMF fixation suture (Ch 02_IMF Fixation Suture –**a**/**b**/**c**). A 3-point fixation suture is placed medially and laterally to secure the IMF. The suture is placed by grabbing the deep fascia (**a**) then from the deep fascia to the inferior superficial fascial system (**b**) and then to the superior superficial fascia system (**c**). This is sutured down to secure and set the IMF and prevent bottoming out

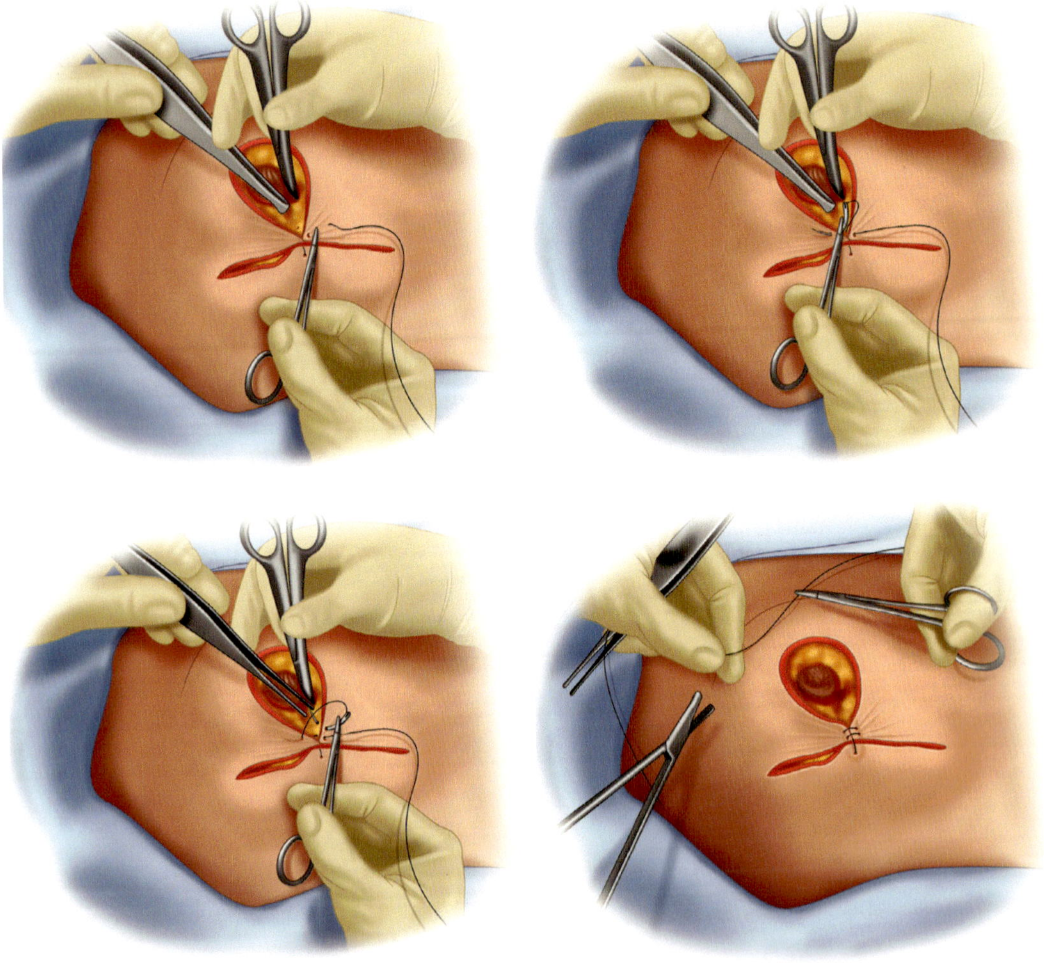

Fig. 2.13 Adams Dermal Flap Part 3 (Ch02_Adams dermal flap-C). The dermal flap is then sutured to the lateral and medial aspect of the vertical incision to support the inferior portion of the breast and to provide well vascularized tissue over the implant pocket as well as the T-point in the event of wound breakdown, so the implant is not exposed

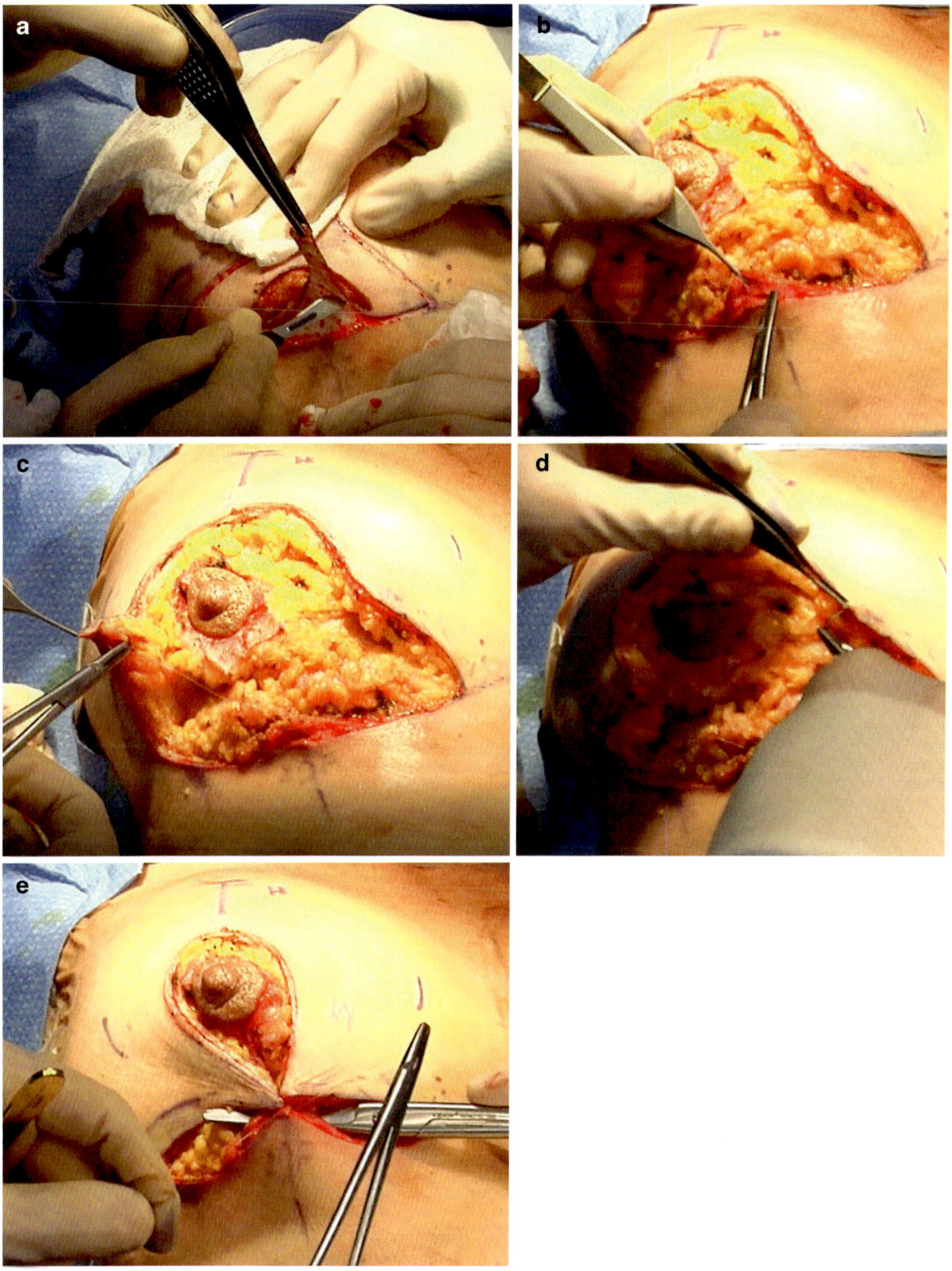

Fig. 2.14 (**a**–**e**) Intraoperative photos of Adams Dermal Flap. The flap is de-epithelialized (**a**) at the start of the mastopexy portion of the procedure to be used later for the closure and to cover the implant incision. A suture is then used to anchor the inferior flap (**b**) to the lateral (**c**) and medial limb (**d**) and finally is tied down to bring the flap entirely underneath the T point (**e**) to take tension off and provide dermal tissue underneath this area in the event of wound breakdown

Table 2.1 Nipple-fold index in augmentation mastopexy in relation to breast base width

BW pre	Planned breast width post	Aug-Masto NIMF index
10.5	9	7.3
11	9.5	7.65
11.5	10	8
12	10.5	8.35
12.5	11	8.7
13	11.5	9.05
13.5	12	9.4
14	12.5	9.75

BW breast width, *NIMF* nipple to inframammary fold

key to achieving predictability. The 38 mm cookie cutter is then placed on this mark and it should correlate to the most projecting portion of the breast (Fig. 2.16). By marking the nipple at the end using a bottom up technique this allows for better control of the nipple position to optimize its placement on the breast mound.

The vertical and horizontal limbs have a deep dermal closure and then a running subcuticular closure. The nipple is closed in a running fashion.

Dressings Steri-strips are placed square around the areola and then at 45-degree square around the areola on top of the previous steri-strips to allow for equal compression around the areola incision. Steri-strips are placed longways over the vertical and horizontal components of the incision. The bandages are removed 7 days after surgery and scar therapy is started with Mepiform (Molynlycke Health Care, Oakville, Ontario) and Biocorneum (Sientra, Santa Barbara, CA).

Adjunctive Procedures

Fat grafting has further improved treatment in patients seeking larger breast sizes than the patient's base width would normally allow. Fat

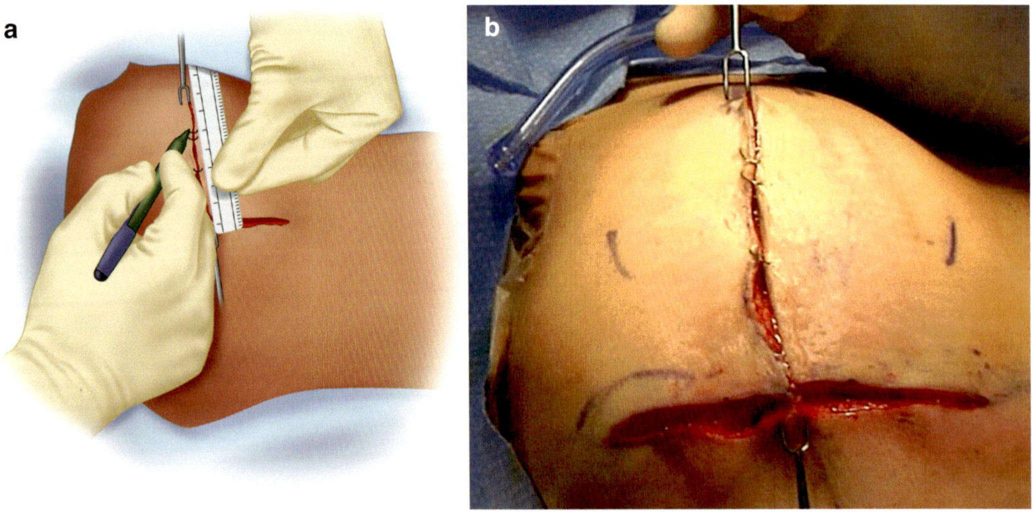

Fig. 2.15 (**a**) Bottom up technique for Nipple position Part 1. The vertical incision is placed on stretch from the fixed IMF position to the bottom of the areola. The ideal nipple position in relation to the fold is marked. In general, this should be between 8.5 and 9.5 cm. (**b**) Intraoperative photo demonstrating the bottom up technique, notice the vertical incision is placed on maximum stretch with the use of skin hooks to ensure precise nipple location

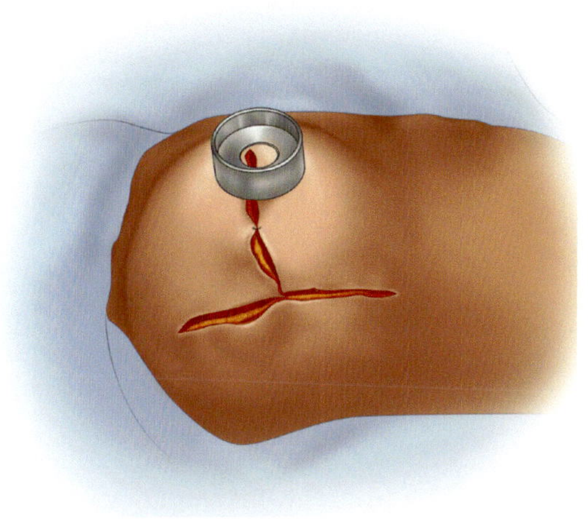

Fig. 2.16 Bottom up technique for Nipple position Part 2. Placement of a cookie cutter on the breast at the level of the marked nipple position, to ensure the nipple will be at the most projecting portion of the breast. The cookie cutter should be flush with the skin if truly on the most projecting portion

grafting allows the patient to have increased size and shape in multiple dimensions without taxing the breast tissue with the weight of a larger implant.

Depending on the patient's skin quality, the use of biologic adjunctive support is often needed. The senior author (W.P.A.), now routinely offers Galaform (Galatea Surgical, Lexington, MA) to all patients seeking augmentation mastopexy in the setting of massive weight loss, thin tissue, multiple stretch marks, patients prone to soft tissue stretch or those seeking larger implants that would increase the likelihood of stretch on the breast.

Conclusion

The use of a sound tissue-based planning strategy can allow for safe and reliable one stage augmentation mastopexy. By utilizing the technical refinements obtained over the senior authors career, patient results are improved (Figs. 2.17, 2.18, and 2.19), and complications rates are significantly decreased. This has led to increased consistency in delivering high quality results to patients in a procedure fraught with challenges.

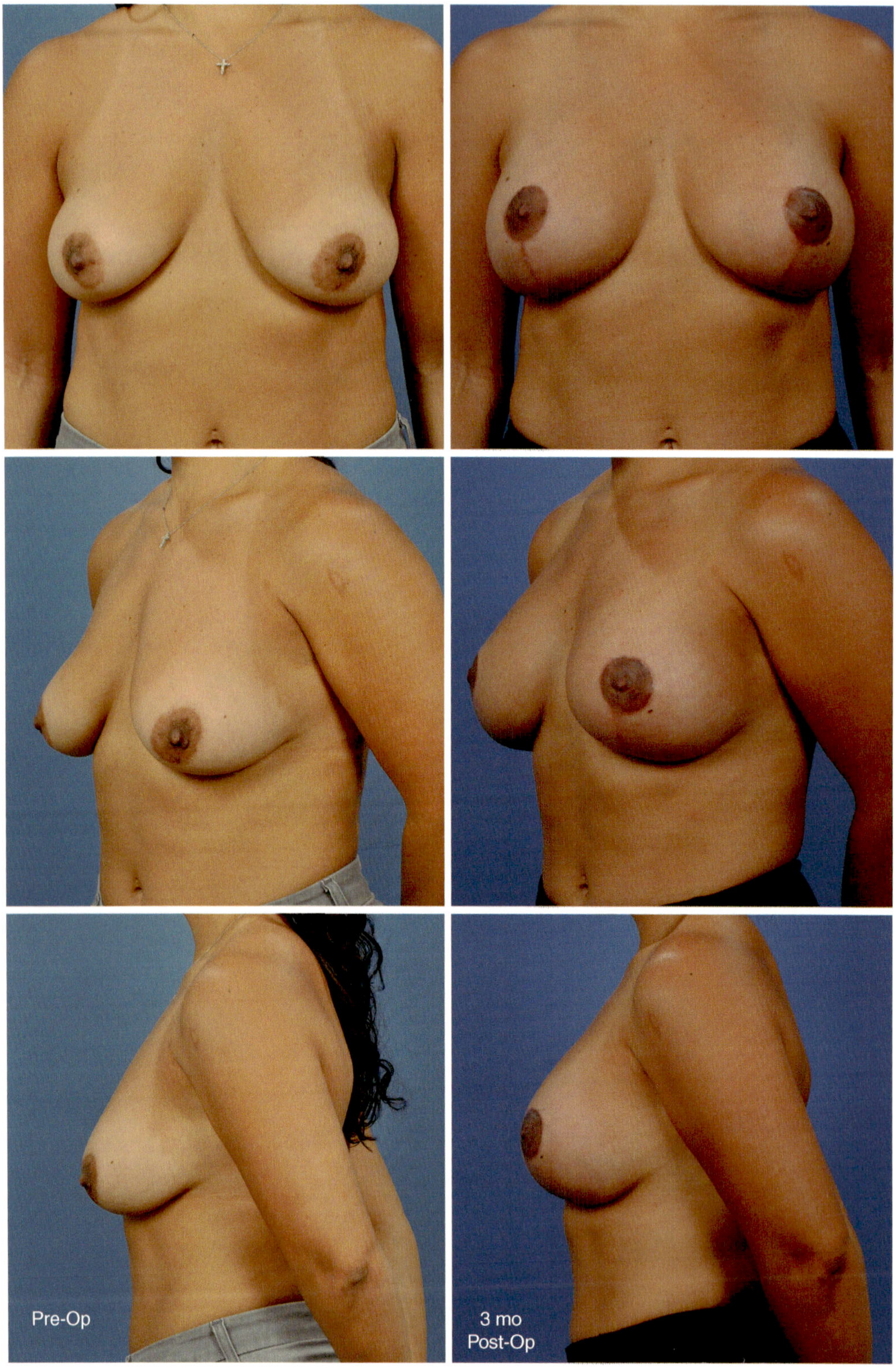

Fig. 2.17 Preoperative and Postoperative images at 3 months out. Single stage augmentation mastopexy patient with asymmetry and placement of SRL 230 on the left and 260 cc on the right

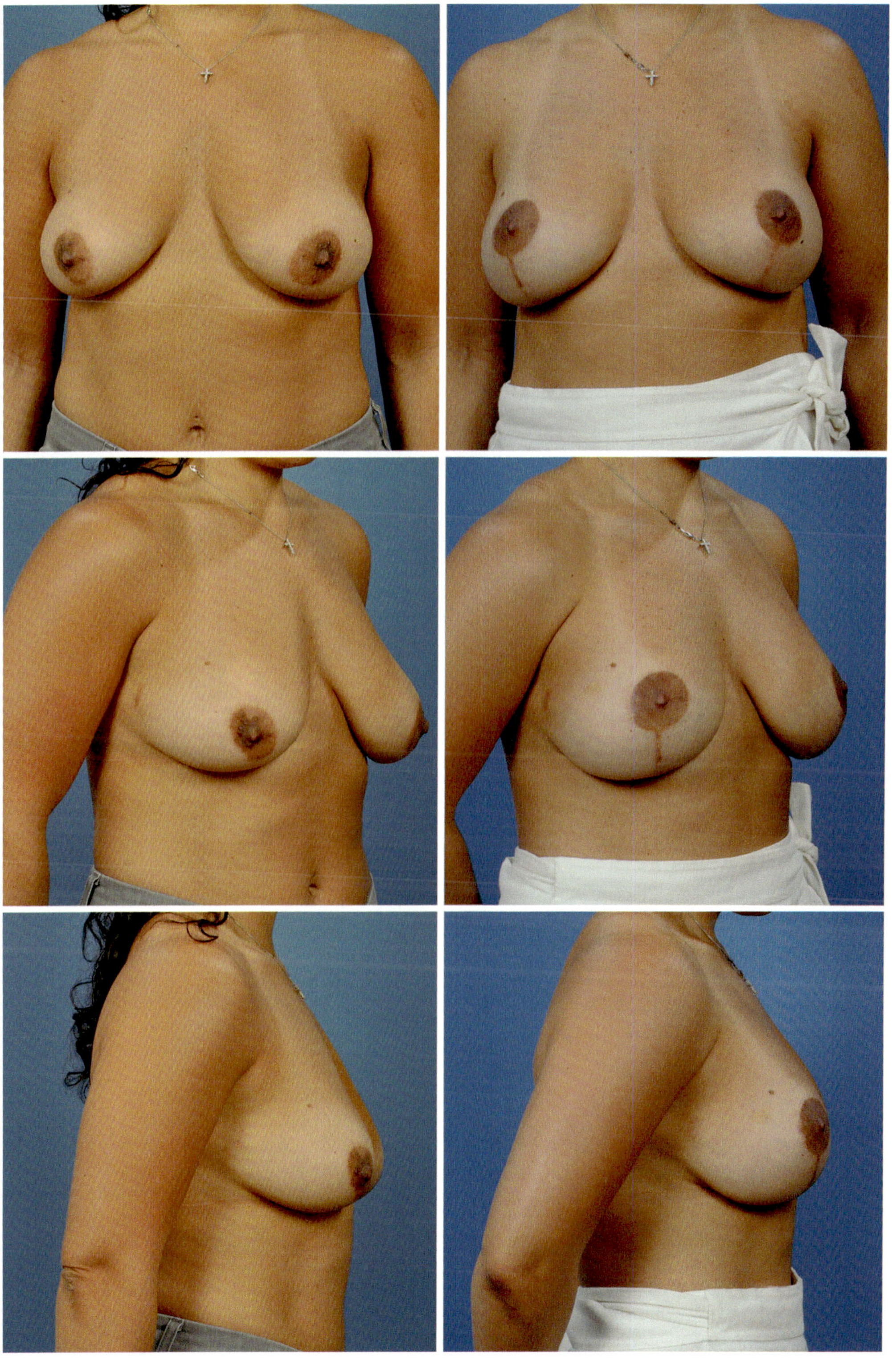

Fig. 2.18 Preoperative and Postoperative images at 1 year out from same patient in Fig. 2.14. Single stage augmentation mastopexy patient with asymmetry and placement of SRL 230 on the left and 260 cc on the right

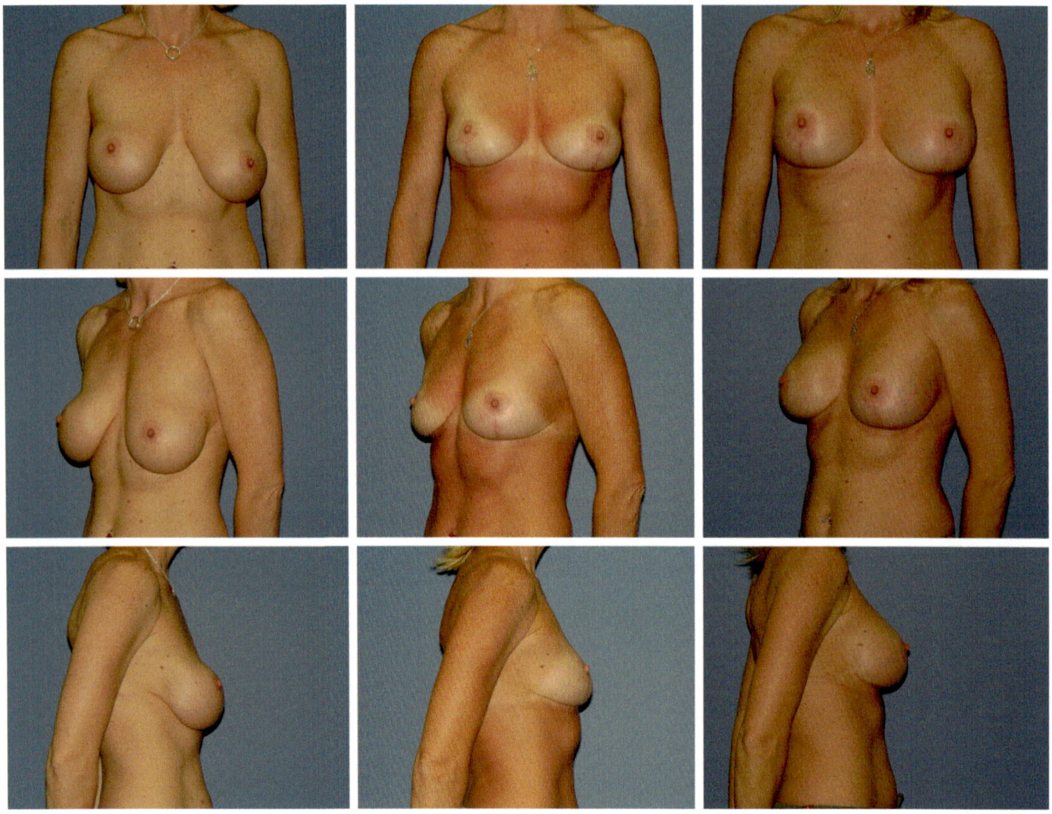

Fig. 2.19 Preoperative and postoperative images at 1 year out from two stage augmentation mastopexy. Two stage augmentation mastopexy with mastopexy performed first followed by augmentation (Allergan 410 FM 310 cc implant) 3 months after the mastopexy

References

1. Gonzalez-Ulloa M. Correction of hypotrophy of the breast by means of exogenous material. Plast Reconstr Surg Transplant Bull. 1960;25:15–26.
2. Regnault P. The hypoplastic and ptotic breast: a combined operation with prosthetic augmentation. Plast Reconstr Surg. 1966;37(1):31–7.
3. Calobrace MB, Herdt DR, Cothron KJ. Simultaneous augmentation/mastopexy: a retrospective 5-year review of 332 consecutive cases. Plast Reconstr Surg. 2013;131(1):145–56. https://doi.org/10.1097/PRS.0b013e318272bf86.
4. Castello MF, Silvestri A, Nicoli F, Dashti T, Han S, Grassetti L, et al. Augmentation mammoplasty/mastopexy: lessons learned from 107 aesthetic cases. Aesthet Plast Surg. 2014;38(5):896–907. https://doi.org/10.1007/s00266-014-0388-1.
5. Khavanin N, Jordan SW, Rambachan A, Kim JY. A systematic review of single-stage augmentation-mastopexy. Plast Reconstr Surg. 2014;134(5):922–31. https://doi.org/10.1097/prs.0000000000000582.
6. Spear SL, Boehmler JH 4th, Clemens MW. Augmentation/mastopexy: a 3-year review of a single surgeon's practice. Plast Reconstr Surg. 2006;118(7 Suppl):136S–47S; discussion 148S–149S, 150S–151S.
7. Stevens WG, Macias LH, Spring M, Stoker DA, Chacon CO, Eberlin SA. One-stage augmentation mastopexy: a review of 1192 simultaneous breast augmentation and Mastopexy procedures in 615 consecutive patients. Aesthet Surg J. 2014;34(5):723–32. https://doi.org/10.1177/1090820x14531434.
8. Spear SL, Pelletiere CV, Menon N. One-stage augmentation combined with mastopexy: aesthetic results and patient satisfaction. Aesthet Plast Surg. 2004;28(5):259–67.
9. Spear S. Augmentation/Mastopexy: "surgeon, beware". Plast Reconstr Surg. 2003;112(3):905–6. https://doi.org/10.1097/01.prs.0000072257.66189.3e.
10. Hoffman S. Some thoughts on augmentation/mastopexy and medical malpractice. Plast Reconstr Surg. 2004;113(6):1892–3.
11. Beale EW, Ramanadham S, Harrison B, Rasko Y, Armijo B, Rohrich RJ. Achieving predictability

in augmentation mastopexy. Plast Reconstr Surg. 2014;133(3):284e–92e. https://doi.org/10.1097/prs.0000000000000079.
12. Lee MR, Unger JG, Adams WP Jr. The tissue-based triad: a process approach to augmentation mastopexy. Plast Reconstr Surg. 2014;134(2):215–25. https://doi.org/10.1097/PRS.0000000000000387.
13. Spring MA, Hartmann EC, Stevens WG. Strategies and challenges in simultaneous augmentation mastopexy. Clin Plast Surg. 2015;42(4):505–18. https://doi.org/10.1016/j.cps.2015.06.008.
14. Adams WP Jr. The process of breast augmentation: four sequential steps for optimizing outcomes for patients. Plast Reconstr Surg. 2008;122(6):1892–900. https://doi.org/10.1097/PRS.0b013e31818d20ec.
15. Adams WP Jr, Small KH. The process of breast augmentation with special focus on patient education, patient selection and implant selection. Clin Plast Surg. 2015;42(4):413–26. https://doi.org/10.1016/j.cps.2015.06.001.
16. Sanniec K, Adams WP Jr. The tissue-based triad in augmentation mastopexy: single-stage technical refinements. Aesthet Surg J. 2019;39:1331–41. https://doi.org/10.1093/asj/sjz006.
17. Regnault P. Breast ptosis. Definition and treatment. Clin Plast Surg. 1976;3(2):193–203.
18. Tebbetts JB, Adams WP. Five critical decisions in breast augmentation using five measurements in 5 minutes: the high five decision support process. Plast Reconstr Surg. 2005;116(7):2005–16.
19. Tebbetts JB. A process for quantifying aesthetic and functional breast surgery: I. quantifying optimal nipple position and vertical and horizontal skin excess for mastopexy and breast reduction. Plast Reconstr Surg. 2013;132(1):65–73. https://doi.org/10.1097/PRS.0b013e318291 0b0a.
20. Tebbetts JB. A process for quantifying aesthetic and functional breast surgery: II. Applying quantified dimensions of the skin envelope to design and preoperative planning for mastopexy and breast reduction. Plast Reconstr Surg. 2014;133(3):527–42. https://doi.org/10.1097/01.prs.0000438470.23249.27.
21. Tebbetts JB. Dual plane breast augmentation: optimizing implant-soft-tissue relationships in a wide range of breast types. Plast Reconstr Surg. 2001;107(5):1255–72.
22. Tebbetts JB. Dual plane breast augmentation: optimizing implant-soft-tissue relationships in a wide range of breast types. Plast Reconstr Surg. 2006;118(7 Suppl):81S–98S; discussion 99S–102S.
23. Adams WP Jr, Culbertson EJ, Deva AK, Magnusson RM, Layt C, Jewell ML, Mallucci P, Heden P. Macrotextured breast implants with defined steps to minimize bacterial contamination around the device: experience in 42,000 implants. Plast Reconstr Surg. 2017;140(3):427–31. https://doi.org/10.1097/prs.0000000000003575.

Principles of Mastopexy

3

Amy K. Alderman and Elizabeth J. Hall-Findlay

General Principles of Mastopexy

Mastopexy is a key component to both aesthetic and reconstructive breast surgery. Without mastering this technique, the surgeon is limited in his or her ability to adequately address anatomical issues associated with aging, childbirth and weight loss and create a youthful appearing breast. It is important to understand what a mastopexy can and cannot do to the existing breast footprint. Adding volume is not always the answer. The aesthetic breast surgeon must master the techniques associated with skin envelope modification, selective parenchymal resection and nipple areolar repositioning if true rejuvenation of the breasts is to be performed.

Mastopexy has two primary purposes: correction of glandular and nipple ptosis. It is important to understand that all of "lift" in a mastopexy occurs in how the ptosis is corrected. A mastopexy cannot move the base of the breast (the footprint) up the chest wall. The goal of a mastopexy is to correct unwanted descent of the nipple and parenchyma.

A. K. Alderman (✉)
Private Practice, Atlanta, GA, USA

E. J. Hall-Findlay
Private Practice, Banff Plastic Surgery, Banff, AB, Canada
e-mail: ehallfindlay@banffplasticsurgery.ca

Key Principles

1. Breast parenchyma must be addressed to prevent recurrent glandular ptosis. The skin envelope alone cannot be used to provide long-term correction of glandular ptosis. Nipple ptosis is more easily corrected and must be evaluated separately from glandular ptosis.
2. Internal sutures do not provide long-term results. The sutures, even permanent ones, help with initial wound healing but do not contribute to long-term breast shape. The breast parenchyma must be rearranged.
3. Wait 1 year to assess your result. Mastopexy results will change over the first postoperative year as the skin envelope relaxes. Glandular ptosis often reoccurs if not addressed with the surgical procedure.

Breast Anatomy

It is important to understand breast anatomy, in particular the breast footprint, and the changes that can and cannot be accomplished with aesthetic breast surgery [1]. Each woman has a particular breast footprint that is unique to her. The footprint is defined by the upper breast border superiorly, the inframammary fold inferiorly, cleavage medially and lateral breast border. Achieving good, consistent results in mastopexy is dependent on the surgeon's understanding of

M. B. Calobrace et al. (eds.), *Augmentation Mastopexy*,
https://doi.org/10.1007/978-3-030-48226-8_3

what can and cannot be changed with the footprint and setting appropriate patient expectations (Figs. 3.1 and 3.2).

In Fig. 3.1, the above patient has a normal footprint. The arrow shows the upper breast border – which does not change postoperatively. Mastopexy is all about control of the glandular (and nipple) ptosis. This patient did not have any parenchyma removed; an inferior Ribeiro-type of flap [2] was used to rearrange the ptotic gland.

In Fig. 3.2, the patient had a low footprint with poor upper pole fullness. Both the nipple and the glandular ptosis was corrected, but the breast footprint was not moved up on the chest wall.

The *upper breast border* is easily identified by the lateral crease near the axilla and extending that point medially towards the sternum. It can also be noted by gently folding the breast upward and noting the transition of tissue from breast to chest wall (Fig. 3.3). The upper breast border can

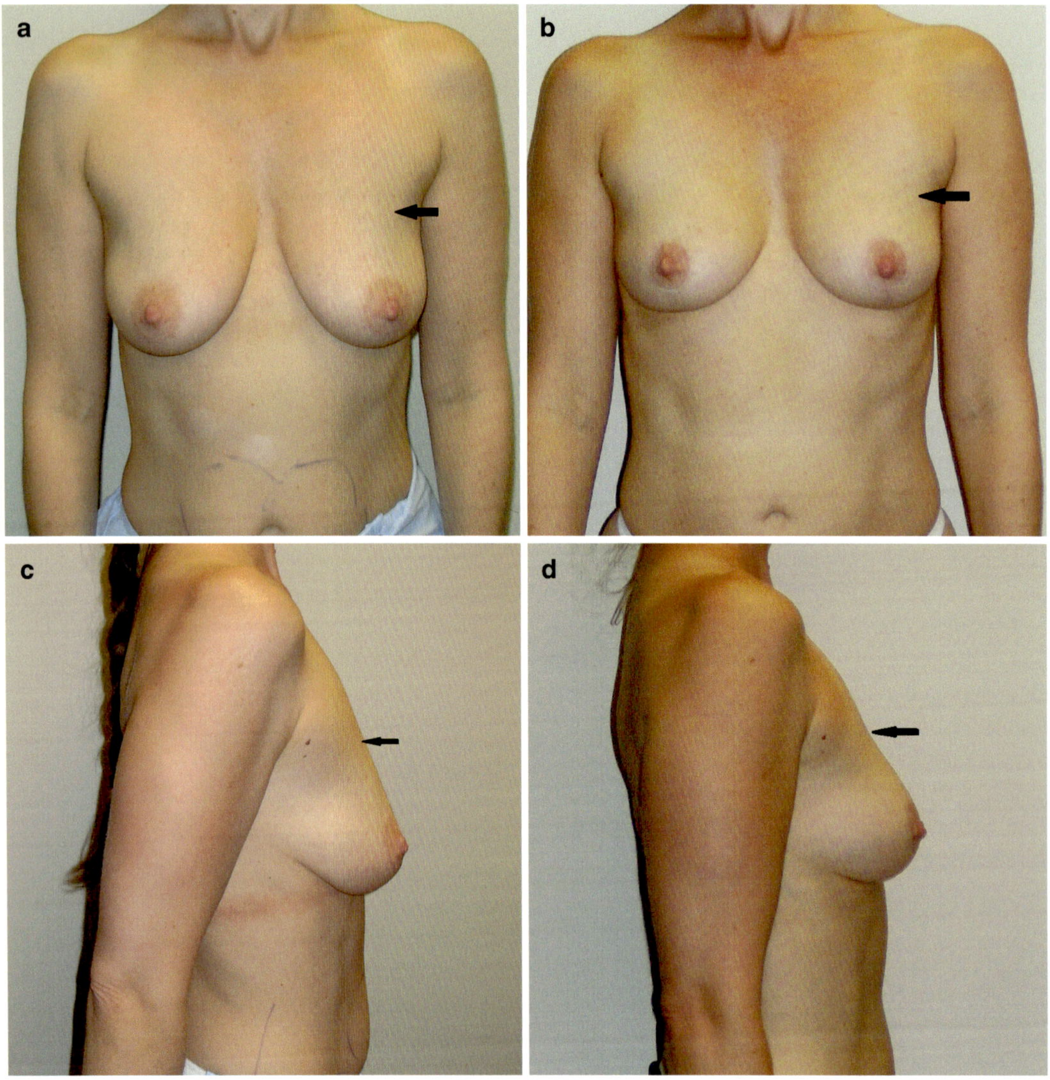

Fig. 3.1 (**a**–**d**) This patient has a normal footprint. The arrow shows the upper breast border – which does not change postoperatively. Mastopexy is all about control of the glandular (and nipple) ptosis. This patient did not have any parenchyma removed; an inferior Ribeiro-type of flap was used to rearrange the ptotic gland. (Figure courtesy of Elizabeth Hall-Findlay, copyright reserved)

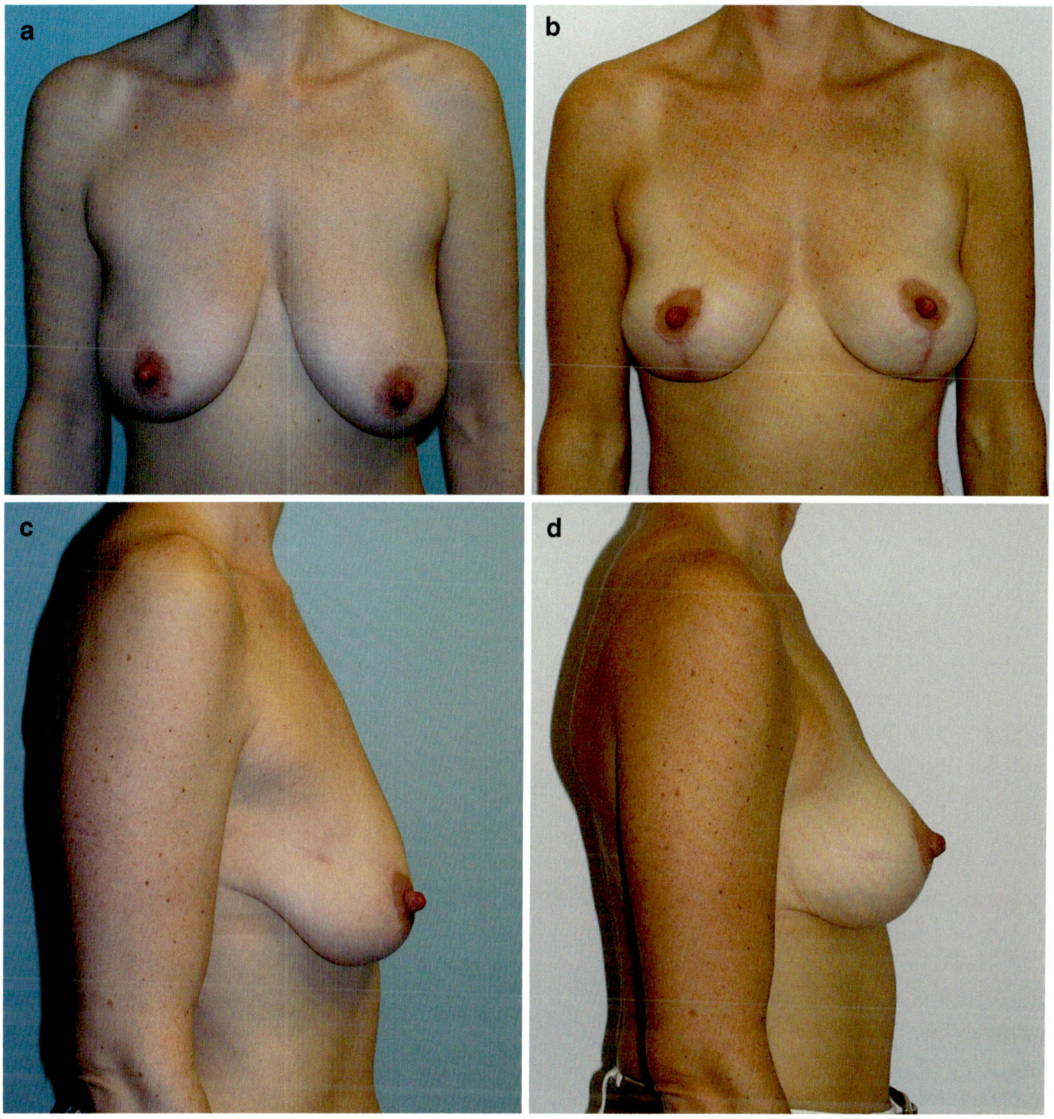

Fig. 3.2 (**a–d**) This patient had a low footprint with poor upper pole fullness. Both the nipple and the glandular ptosis was corrected, but the breast footprint was not moved up on the chest wall. (Figure courtesy of Elizabeth Hall-Findlay, copyright reserved)

only be elevated by adding volume with an implant, and in general, can be raised about 2–3 cm. Mastopexy and a breast reduction do not change the upper breast border. Mastopexy with auto-augmentation can slightly raise the upper breast border, but not nearly as much as with an implant.

In Fig. 3.3, the upper breast border is at the junction of the preaxillary fold and the breast. It can be easily seen if the breast is folded up on the chest wall. Just pushing the breast up will not work.

The *lower breast border*, or inframammary fold, is lowered with procedures that add weight to the breasts and raised with procedures that remove tissue in the lower pole of the breasts. Breast augmentation and breast augmentation with mastopexy both have added weight due to

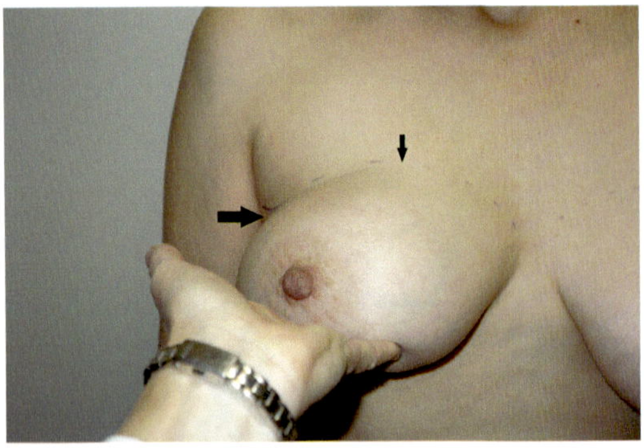

Fig. 3.3 The upper breast border is at the junction of the preaxillary fold and the breast. It can be easily seen if the breast is folded up on the chest wall. Just pushing the breast up will not work. (Figure courtesy of Elizabeth Hall-Findlay, copyright reserved)

the implant, and in both cases, the inframammary fold will be lowered. A breast reduction or mastopexy that involves removal of lower pole tissue will unweight the lower pole of the breasts and cause the inframammary fold to rise. A breast reduction that keeps lower pole tissue, such as with an inferior pedicle technique, will often result in lowering of the inframammary fold in the long-term due to the weight of the lower breast. This can be seen in wise pattern breast reductions where the inframammary scar tends to rise up on the breast and the lower breast parenchyma descends below the scar (pseudoptosis). Understanding this concept is important when planning your surgical incisions. The vertical scar of a mastopexy or breast reduction that removes lower pole tissue should stop 2–3 cm above the fold in order to avoid ending up with a scar below the (newly raised) inframammary fold.

When the inferior vertical wedge of skin and breast tissue is either "removed" as in a breast reduction or "moved" as in a mastopexy, good control of the horizontal base diameter of the breast can be achieved (Fig. 3.4).

The *base width* of the breast can be expanded with an implant or narrowed with a vertical breast reduction or mastopexy (Fig. 3.4). Removing or moving tissue in the central lower aspect of the breast allows the medial and lateral breast pillars to rotate centrally and narrow the base diameter

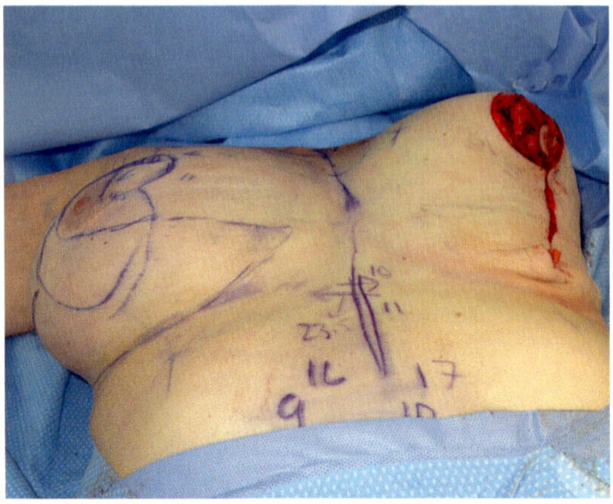

Fig. 3.4 When the inferior vertical wedge of skin and breast tissue is either "removed" as in a breast reduction or "moved" as in a mastopexy, good control of the horizontal base diameter of the breast can be achieved. (Figure courtesy of Elizabeth Hall-Findlay, copyright reserved)

of the breast. An inferior pedicle breast reduction or mastopexy will not change the base diameter as much as a vertical reduction since the majority of the parenchymal resection is from the superior pole of the breasts in an inferior pedicle approach.

How to Decide if a Mastopexy Is the Best Surgical Approach

Regnault's classification of ptosis has been the long-term standard for whether mastopexy is clinically indicated. This concept is founded on the relationship between the nipple and the inframammary fold, but this can occasionally be misleading.

- Grade 1 (minor): Nipple is at the inframammary fold
- Grade 2 (moderate): Nipple is below the level of the inframammary fold but above the lower contour of the breast
- Grade 3 (major): Nipple is below the inframammary fold and at the lower breast contour

Mastopexy is indicated if the nipple is below the inframammary fold when using Regnault's classification. Unfortunately, always using the inframammary fold for clinical decision-making can be problematic. The inframammary fold can vary dramatically across individuals, such as constriction in tuberous breast patients, and when present there can be significant asymmetry within the same patient. The upper breast border tends to be a more predictable breast measurement with the decision for mastopexy. When using the upper breast border, the nipple position and glandular ptosis are assessed separately.

- Nipple ptosis: nipple position lower than two-thirds the distance down the ideal breast mound, measured from the upper breast border
- Glandular ptosis: excess gland in the lower pole of the breast
- Pseudoptosis: unacceptable bottoming out of the inframammary fold

Nipple Ptosis

The ideal breast shape includes having the nipple areolar complex (NAC) centered on the breast meridian and located near the midpoint of breast mound height. Some variation exists in where it is believed to be the ideal position, with Europeans preferring a position a bit higher on the breast mound at 50–55% of height and Americans generally preferring a slightly lower position at 45–50% height. It is important to realize that it is much easier to correct a slightly lower than desired NAC position than a high NAC position, and that lowering the NAC is nearly impossible without unwanted upper breast scars. It is also important to realize that an overly high NAC can negatively impact a woman's quality of life and cause embarrassment if the NAC is seen above a bra, bathing suit or other low-cut clothing options. In addition, an overly high NAC can create an odd appearance to the breast especially if the nipple is pointing upwards and on the upper slope of the breast.

It's important to realize that the only way to elevate the nipple areolar complex is with a mastopexy or reduction technique. The dual plane technique has been mistaken as an option for elevating the NAC with breast augmentation. However, if you measure NAC position before and after dual plane augmentation, the NAC actually drops on average 2 cm from sternal notch due to the weight of the implant. The dual plane procedure helps facilitate fill of the lower pole tissue and stretching of the lower skin of the breast. This creates the visual effect of NAC elevation as more breast skin is seen below the NAC. But it is important to understand that the NAC is actually not elevated.

Surgeons have used different landmarks to mark the new NAC position with mastopexy or breast reduction. One of the outdated concepts is to use a standard distance from the sternal notch, usually around 18 cm. However, using a set distance is a flawed concept as it does not take into consideration variations in the location of the breast footprint on the patient's chest wall. Some patients have an inherently high footprint, with the inframammary fold and upper breast border closer to the sternal notch and some patient have a lower footprint with the breast sitting closer to the location of the elbow crease. Using a set distance from the sternal notch to mark with NAC will result in an overly high NAC position in a low footprint patient that cannot be easily corrected.

The inframammary fold (IMF) is another landmark used by surgeons to mark the new NAC position. This landmark will work 80% of the time and will account for variations in breast footprints. A mastopexy with an implant will raise the upper breast border, and therefore, the NAC can be set slightly higher than a mastopexy-only procedure where the upper breast border is not changed. A good rule of thumb is to set the NAC 4 cm above the IMF for an augmentation mastopexy and 3 cm for a mastopexy or breast reduction. The reason why this technique does not work in every case is that sometimes the inframammary fold can be constricted and overly high or have significant asymmetry between the two breasts.

The newest concept in setting the new NAC position is to use the upper breast border. This landmark can be found by folding the breast upward (Fig. 3.3) and seeing the transition between the breast and the upper chest along with looking for lateral axillary crease and extending that point across the upper breast. The benefits of using the upper breast border is that it is usually symmetric between the breasts and not distorted in constricted breasts. A good rule of thumb is to set the nipple 8–10 cm inferiorly from the upper breast border at the breast meridian for most C-D cup breasts. Using both the IMF and the upper breast border to set the new NAC position is a good check and balance system. Occasionally, the IMF position will lead to an overly high NAC position if the fold is constricted, and the upper breast border is a more reliable landmark.

The key to good, predictable mastopexy result is to control (move or remove) the glandular ptosis (Fig. 3.5). The upper breast border (arrow) cannot be elevated without the addition of an implant and it serves as a better landmark than the inframammary fold. The new nipple position is determined by how much of the glandular ptosis will be corrected.

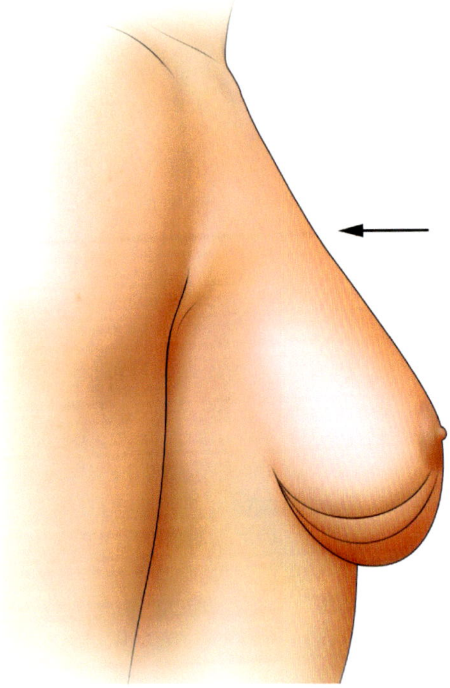

Fig. 3.5 The key to good, predictable mastopexy result is to control (move or remove) the glandular ptosis. The upper breast border (arrow) cannot be elevated without the addition of an implant and it serves as a better landmark than the inframammary fold. The new nipple position is determined by how much of the glandular ptosis will be corrected. (From Hall-Findlay [1]. Image used with permission)

Glandular Ptosis

Glandular ptosis occurs when there is too much parenchyma in the lower pole of the breast; this is independent of the location of the inframammary fold. The solution is to either remove the tissue or relocate the tissue higher on the chest wall (Fig. 3.5). Using the skin brassiere to elevate the gland will fail, as the skin will stretch over time due to the weight of the tissue. The decision to remove or relocate the tissue is often made by the patient's desired breast volume. For patients who desire slightly smaller breasts, the lower central tissue is removed, which will unweight the breasts and provide a longer lasting lift. For patients who are happy with their current breast volume, the lower tissue can be relocated behind the NAC to help add upper pole volume and projection.

Pseudoptosis

Pseudoptosis is bottoming out of the inframammary fold. The nipple position will appear too high, whether or not it actually is anatomically too high. The problem is that there is too much glandular volume below the nipple. Correction is achieved by removal of some of the lower pole tissue, creating a better ratio of breast gland to nipple position. The inframammary fold will rise (Fig. 3.6) along with reduction of the lower pole and both of these changes mean that the nipple will appear lower, even though it has not actually been moved.

The inframammary fold can be elevated by removing the weight in the lower pole of the breast (Fig. 3.6).

Types of Mastopexy

Just as with a breast reduction, mastopexy procedures can be categorized by how the skin and parenchyma are addressed, and the two can be independent of each other. Key components to a good outcome are correction of NAC malposition, correction of glandular descent, and correc-

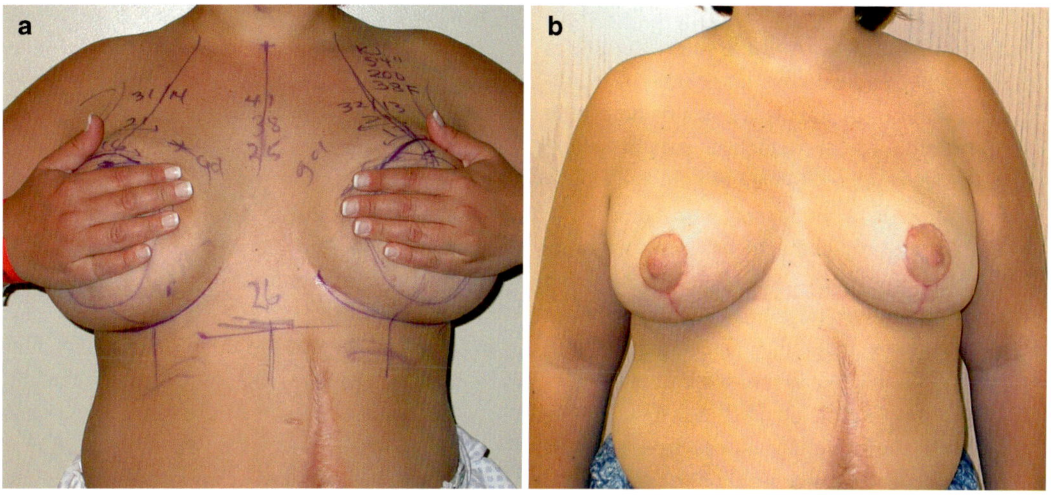

Fig. 3.6 (**a**, **b**) The inframammary fold can be elevated by removing the weight in the lower pole of the breast. (Figure courtesy of Elizabeth Hall-Findlay, copyright reserved)

tion of skin excess while optimizing scar outcomes. It is important to remember that modifying the skin envelope alone is not enough to create a long-lasting correction of glandular ptosis.

1. Periareolar mastopexy:

   The mastopexy technique with the least scarring is a peri-areolar approach. This technique is appealing to both surgeon and patient due to the limited scarring, however, this approach does not correct parenchymal ptosis and is limited in the amount of nipple ptosis that can be corrected. The nipple can be elevated a maximum of 2–3 cm. If too much tension is placed on the scar, the result will be in a wide scar and an oddly stretched out NAC. Unfortunately the "donut" mastopexy also tends to flatten the breast resulting in decreased projection. Benelli modified this approach by releasing the skin from the lower pole of the breast, allowing modification of the lower pole tissue through either resection or imbrication [3]. This technique is not recommended in cases of moderate nipple or glandular ptosis. The surgeon should be aware that unacceptable scarring and blunting of breast projection will occur if these approaches are used too aggressively to correct nipple or glandular ptosis.

2. Inverted T, inferior pedicle mastopexy:

   The Wise pattern [4] or anchor approach to mastopexy has the most scarring of all procedures and does not address gland malposition. The concept is that the longer scars help address the excess skin, and results will be improved if the skin envelope is maximally tightened. This approach is flawed in that the parenchyma of the lower pole remains, which will contribute to recurrent glandular ptosis. The skin envelope alone cannot be used to create long-term correction of ptosis. However, if there is too much redundancy of the skin envelope then it will need to be excised in an inverted T manner – but it is important to understand that the skin is not being used to shape the gland. In addition, the horizontal base diameter of the breast footprint is not modified with this approach, and this can often result in a 'boxy' post-operative appearance.

3. Liposuction-only mastopexy:

   Liposuction has a very limited role in correcting breast ptosis. The advantages are limited scarring and preservation of neurovascular structures. But for the majority of patients, the disadvantages of the procedure far outweigh the advantages. Only fat, not gland, can be removed. The nipple is not repositioned but a slight elevation can be achieved (Fig. 3.7).

The final result can look empty with a lack of upper pole fullness. And the final outcome is dependent on skin quality and extent of retraction. However, this approach can be helpful in the revision breast reduction patient where breast size is related to weight gain and vascularity to the NAC will be preserved. Liposuction-only can also be used to correct pseudoptosis where the inframammary fold has bottomed-out. Removing the weight from the inframammary fold can elevate the fold. It is actually a mistake to remove inframammary skin because it pulls the IMF down.

Removal of weight by liposuction-only can elevate both the lower pole of the breast and the nipple position, but it can leave an empty appearance in the breast (Fig. 3.7).

4. Vertical mastopexy:

   There are numerous pedicles that can be used to achieve a mastopexy while limiting the scar to the vertical approach. The vertical mastopexy with a superior or superior-medial pedicle is our preferred technique. It has the benefit of less scarring than the Wise pattern, allows for correction of parenchymal malposition, and helps to narrow the breast footprint and provide added breast projection. Minimal tension is placed on the NAC scar, which helps prevent spreading of the nipple postoperatively. The technique allows for the flexibility of reducing breast volume if desired or repositioning the lower pole tissue if added volume behind the NAC is advantageous to overall breast shape. The excess skin correction can usually be performed without extending the scar along the IMF.

   (a) Superior pedicle extension flaps:

   The superior pedicle has an excellent blood supply and the pedicle can be extended to include the inferior vertical wedge of breast tissue that is excised in a breast reduction. That superior pedicle extension flap is then turned up under the pedicle in an effort to not only reposition the ptotic gland but also to give more upper pole fullness (Fig. 3.8). Unfortunately, this cannot be effectively achieved and the flap will tend to flip back into a more inferior position.

   As shown in Fig. 3.8, a superior pedicle extension flap did work as a mastopexy but a few months after her surgery she felt "something give" on both sides and she lost some of her correction.

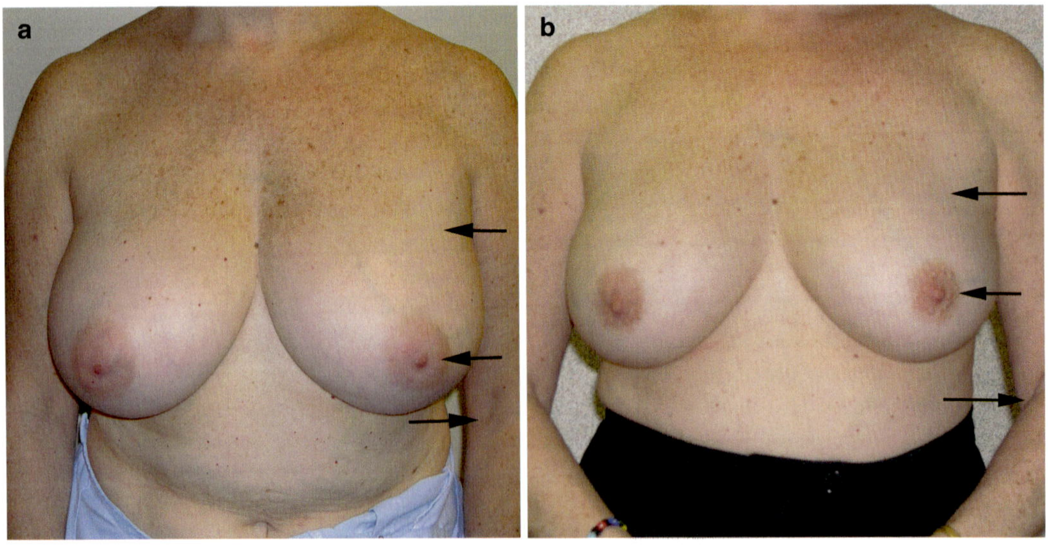

Fig. 3.7 (**a**, **b**) Removal of weight by liposuction-only can elevate both the lower pole of the breast and the nipple position, but it can leave an empty look to the breast. (Figure courtesy of Elizabeth Hall-Findlay, copyright reserved)

(b) Medial Pedicle Extension flaps:

A medial pedicle [5] can also be used to recruit that inferior wedge of breast tissue and it can be rotated up to try to fill the upper pole. Although this does help rearrange the breast parenchyma, it is usually not long enough to achieve the desired results (Fig. 3.9).

In Fig. 3.9, Medial pedicle extension flaps were used in the patient. The correction was not as good as desired and the upper pole was not adequately filled.

(c) Combination of medial and lateral flaps:

The inferior gland that needs to be rearranged can be moved with a combination of medial and lateral flaps. Much like the medial pedicle extension flap, the main advantage of these flaps is the rearrangement of breast parenchyma so that

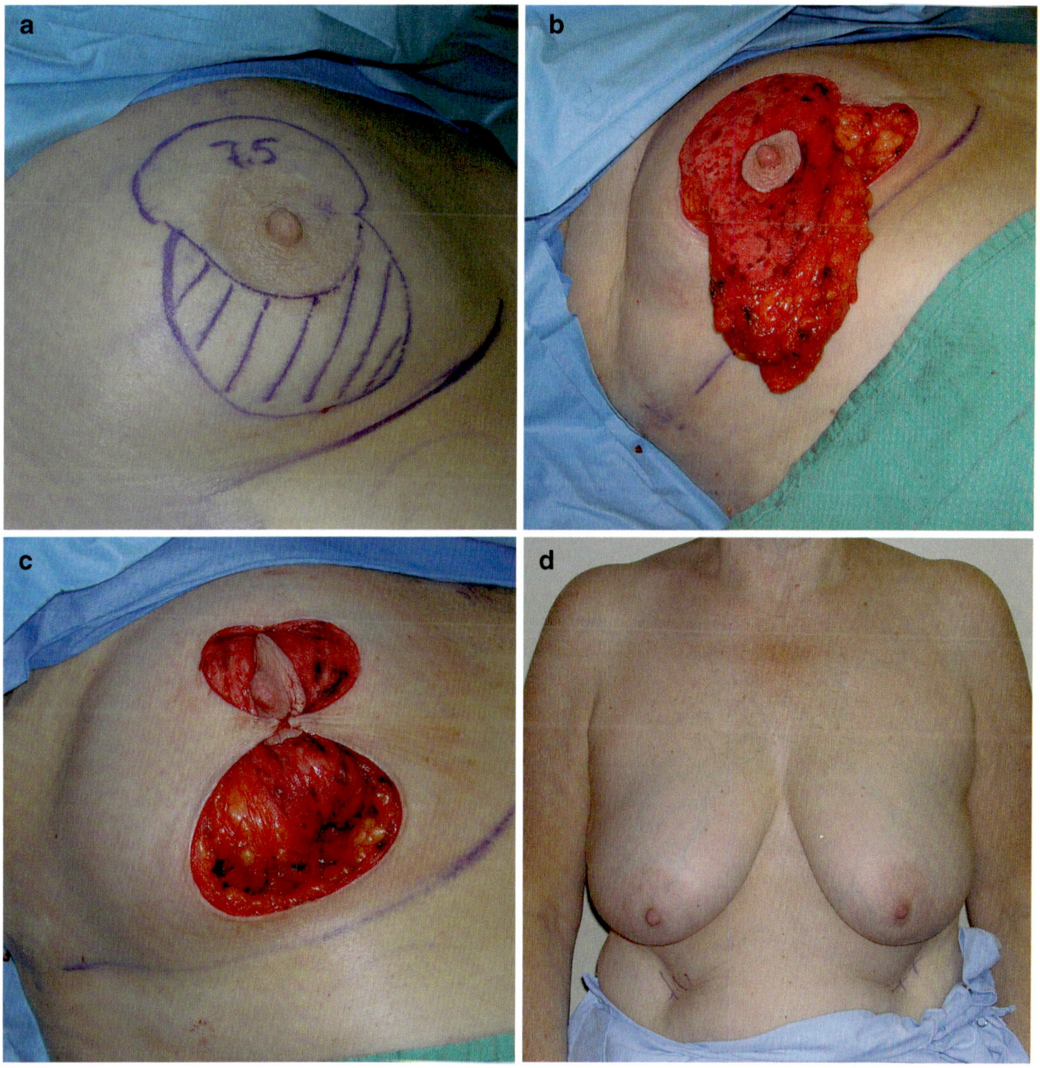

Fig. 3.8 (**a**–**c**) A superior pedicle extension flap is often described as a good way to perform a mastopexy. It can be difficult to turn the flap under the pedicle without pulling the nipple downward. (Figure courtesy of Elizabeth Hall-Findlay, copyright reserved). (**d**–**g**) A superior pedicle extension flap did work as a mastopexy but a few months after her surgery she felt "something give" on both sides and she lost some of her correction. (**d**, **e**) Preoperative photos. (**f**, **g**) Postoperative photos. (Figure courtesy of Elizabeth Hall-Findlay, copyright reserved)

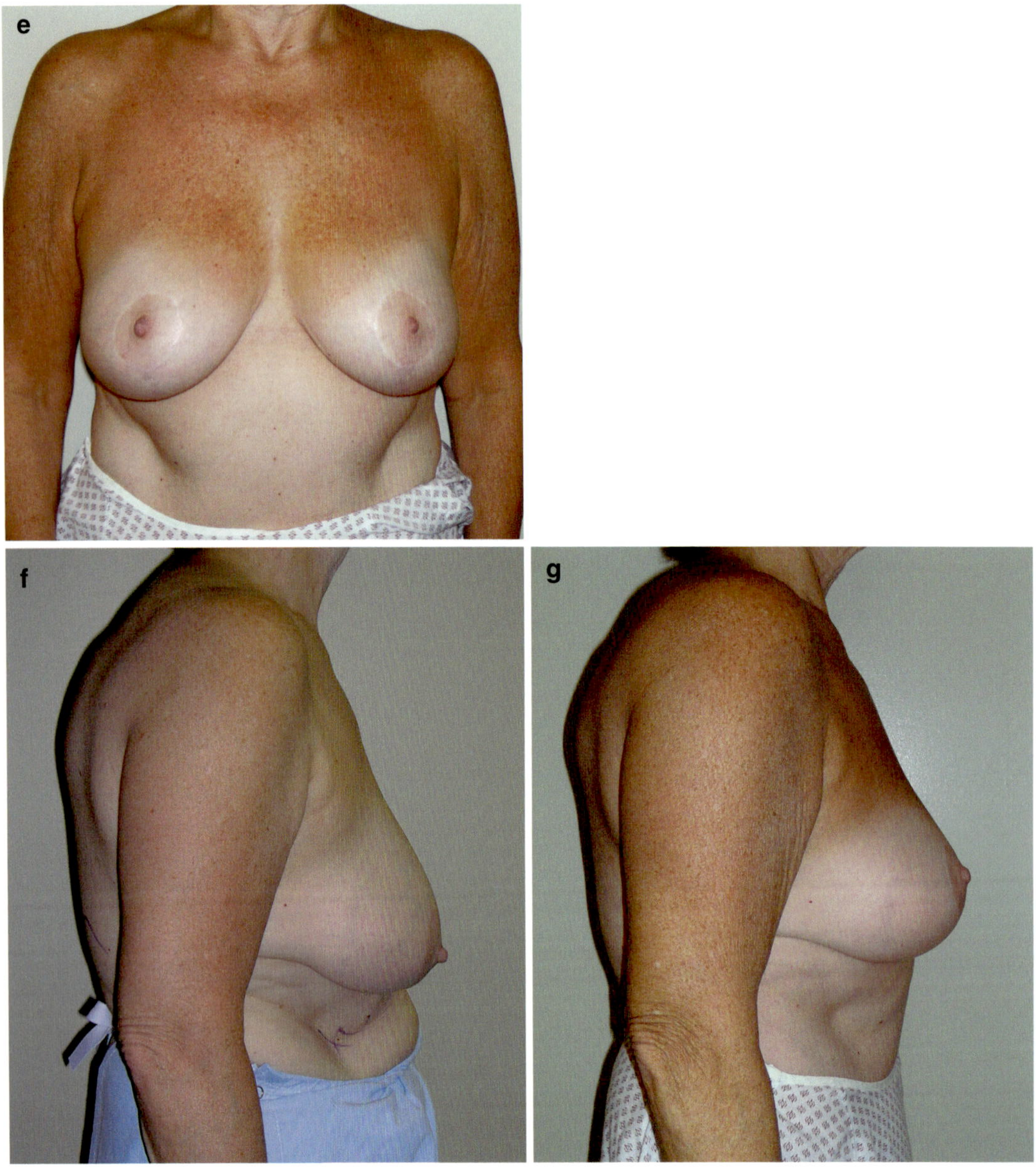

Fig. 3.8 (continued)

the skin envelope is not being relied upon to hold up the breast (Fig. 3.10).

As shown in Fig. 3.10, rearranging the inferior breast tissue with medial and lateral flaps could achieve some improvement but the Ribeiro flap (below) gives better, more consistent results.

(d) Inferior flap (Ribeiro):

Repositioning the lower parenchyma behind the NAC with the vertical mastopexy is often referred as an 'auto-augmentation' and was first described by Liacyr Ribeiro [2]. In his technique, the lower flap of parenchyma is mobilized and sutured to the upper chest wall behind a superior or superomedial pedicle. The medial and lateral breast pillars are brought together inferiorly caudal to the flap . Sutures to hold the inferior flap up do not end up healing to the pectoralis fascia but the flap is held in place long enough so that the anterior surface of the flap heals to the posterior surface of the pedicle. Daniel [6] and Graf [7] modified the technique by using a strip of pectoralis as an added measure to hold the flap in place. The vascularity of the flap is supplied by a deep chest wall-based artery and vein that perforate the pectoralis muscle just above the 5th rib and just medial to the breast meridian (Fig. 3.11).

Figure 3.11 The inferior flap is a chest wall based flap. The blood supply comes from the fourth interspace and this is the only artery and vein that goes through the breast parenchyma to the nipple. There are lateral branches but the main blood supply to the nipple is superficial with the veins just under the dermis and the arteries about 2 cm deep to the skin surface

The various other pedicle extensions that have been described above are not as successful or

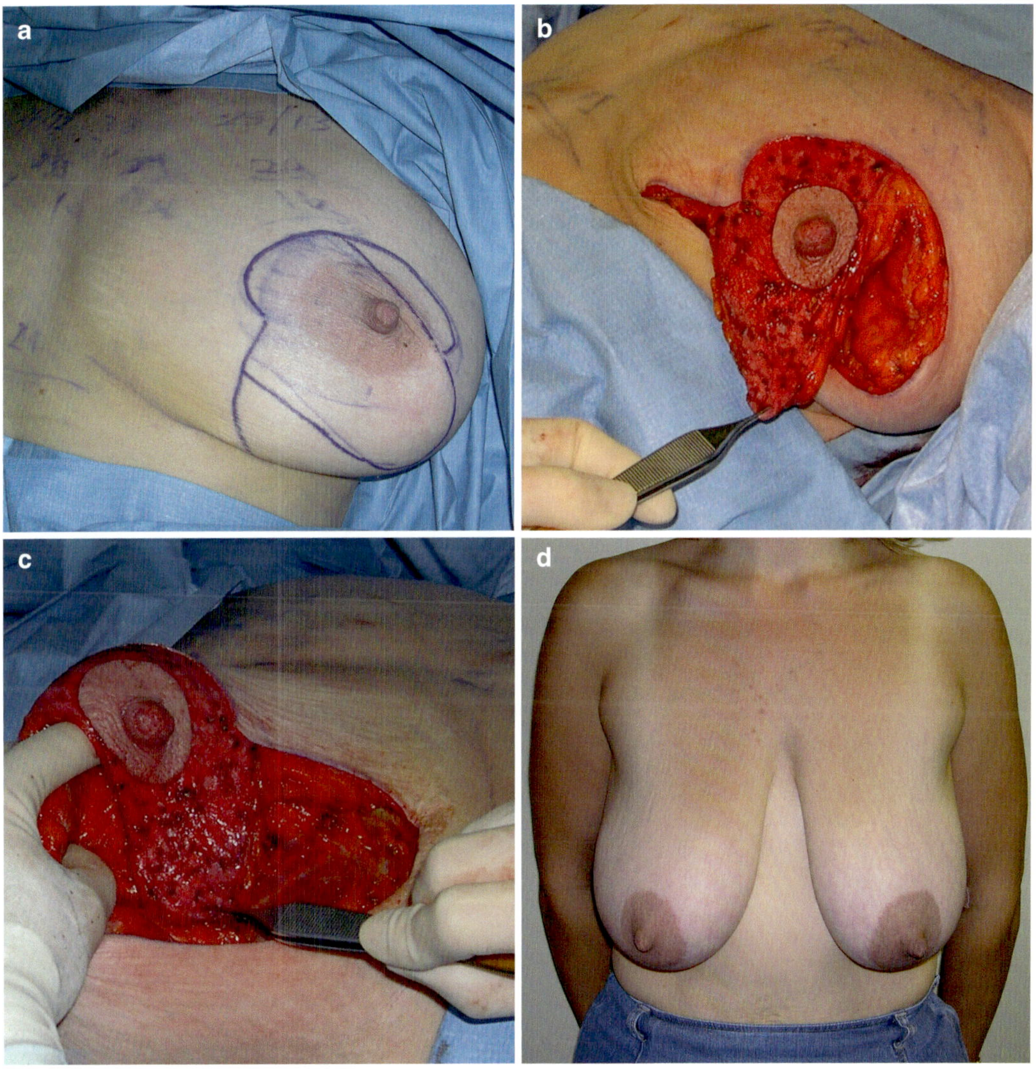

Fig. 3.9 (**a–c**) Medial pedicle extension flaps are an alternate method of performing a mastopexy. (**d–g**) Medial pedicle extension flaps were used in this patient. The correction was not as good as desired and the upper pole was not adequately filled. (**d**, **e**) Preoperative photos. (**f**, **g**) Postoperative photos. (Figure courtesy of Elizabeth Hall-Findlay, copyright reserved)

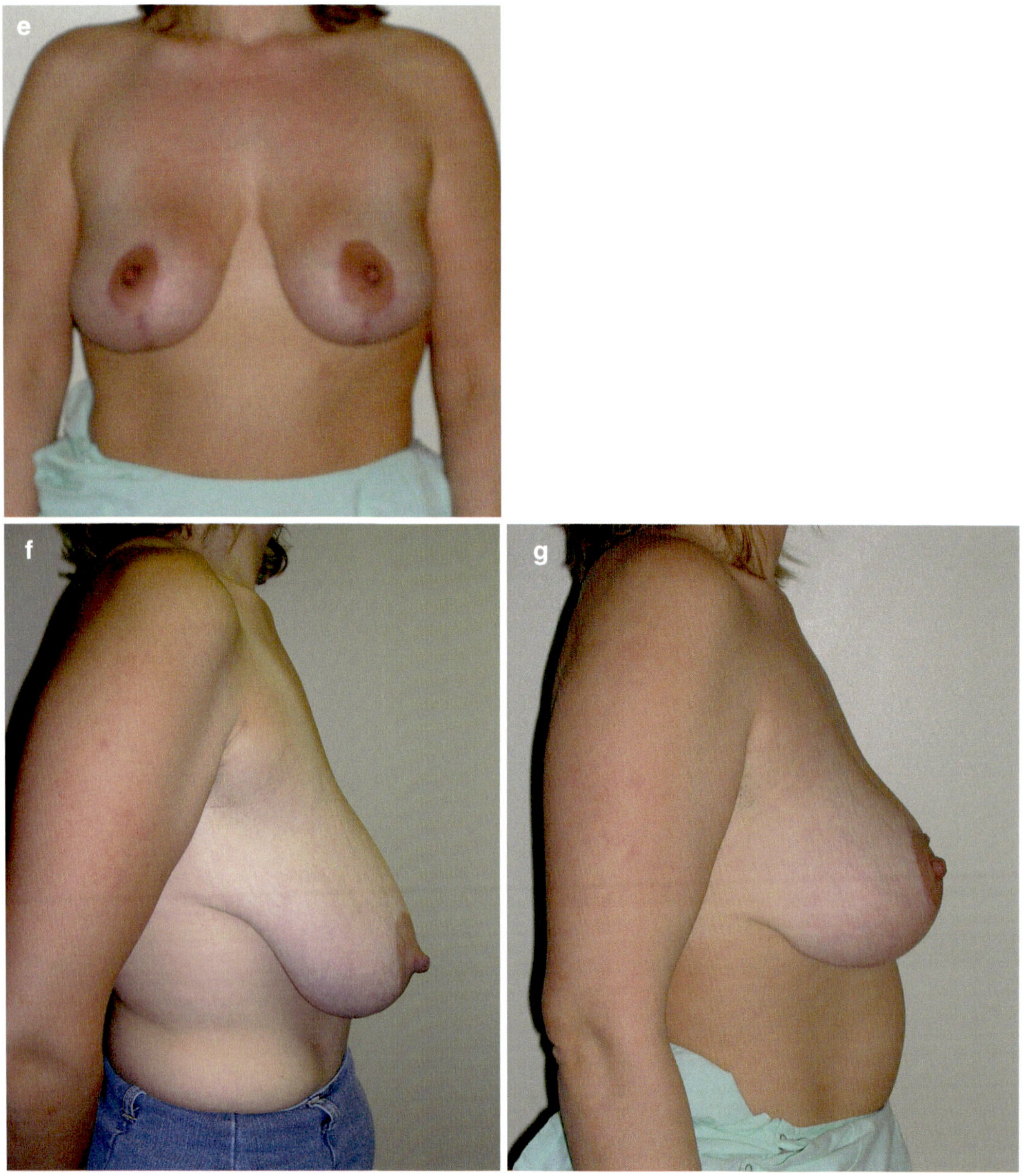

Fig. 3.9 (continued)

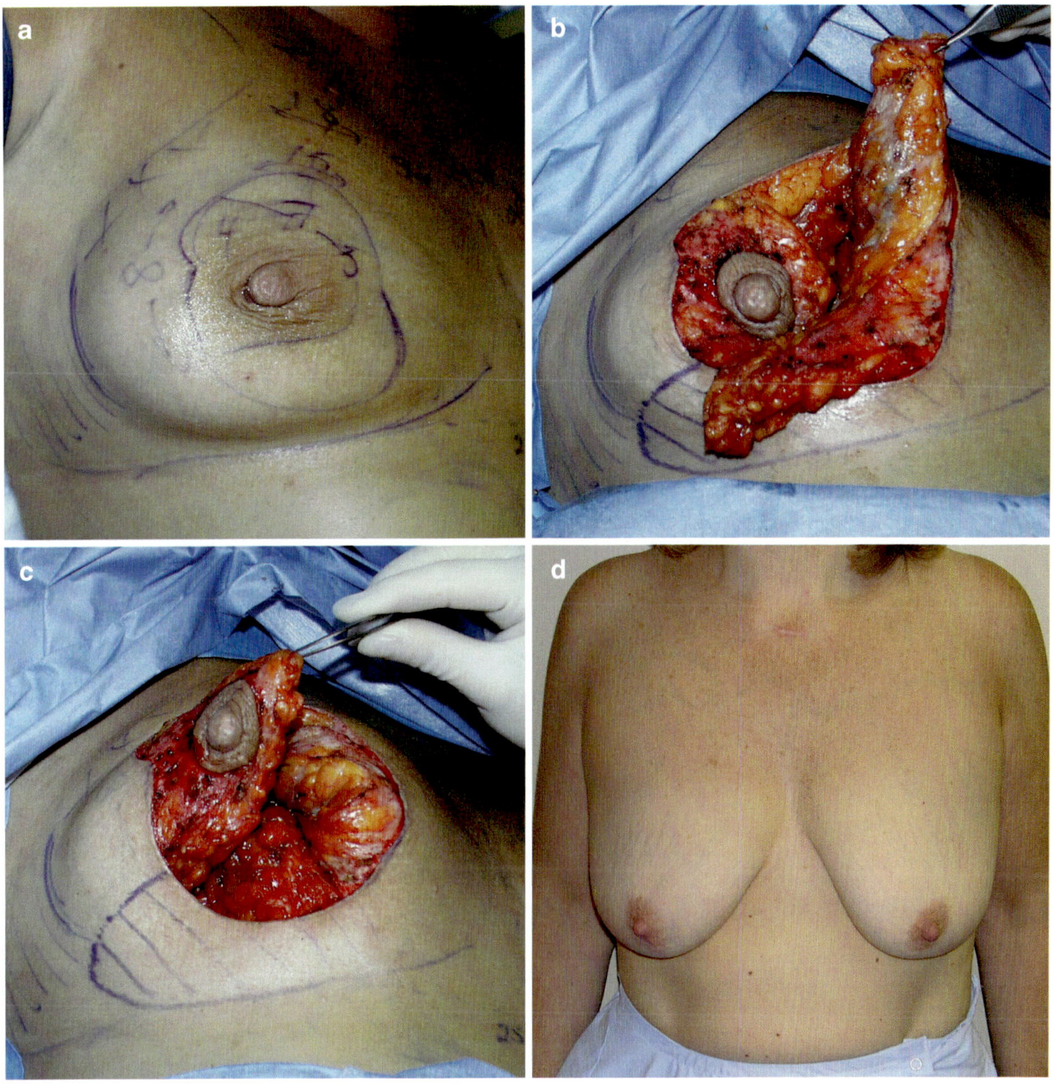

Fig. 3.10 (**a**–**c**) Rearranging the inferior breast tissue with medial and lateral flaps is an effective method of performing a mastopexy but the flaps cannot be mobilized to a significant degree. (**d**–**g**) The results are acceptable but the major improvement is the correction of nipple ptosis. The Ribeiro flap (below) gives better, more consistent results. (**d**, **e**) preoperative photos. (**f**, **g**) postoperative photos. (Figure courtesy of Elizabeth Hall-Findlay, copyright reserved)

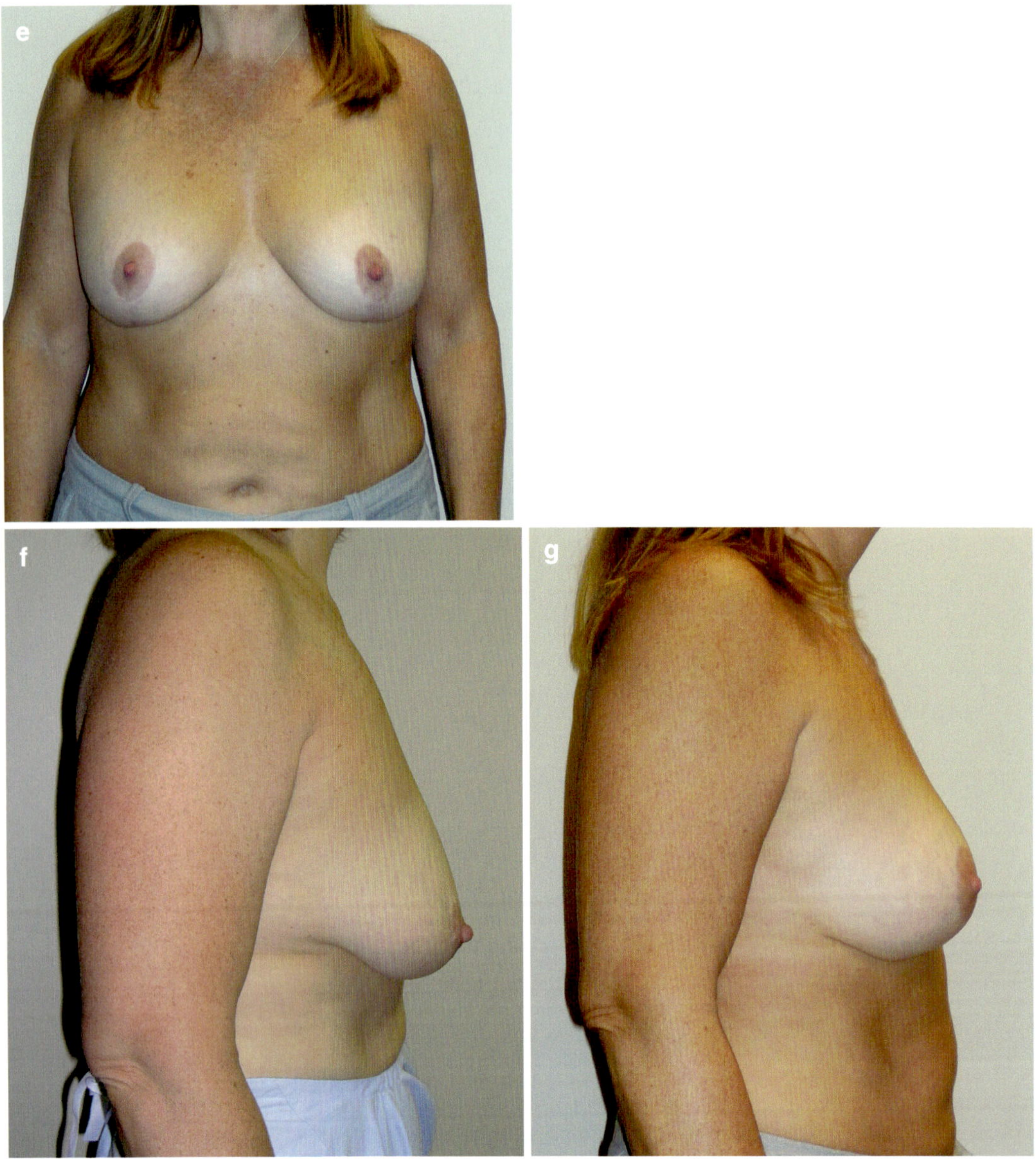

Fig. 3.10 (continued)

predictable as this inferior flap. The Ribeiro flap with or without the pectoralis strip is the most predictable (Fig. 3.12).

As shown in Fig. 3.12a, b Liacyr Ribeiro used a superior pedicle and he then mobilized the inferior flap and moved it up (while still attached as a chest-wall-based flap) under the superior pedicle. It can be held up with a pectoralis sling but the advantage of this is the extent of mobilization that is achieved compared to the other methods.

The inferior flap (which is usually removed in a breast reduction) is de-epithelialized. The flap is then mobilized on all four sides and left as a chest wall-based flap. Note how much mobilization can be achieved. The anterior surface of the flap then heals to the posterior surface of the pedicle which gives a good long-lasting result.

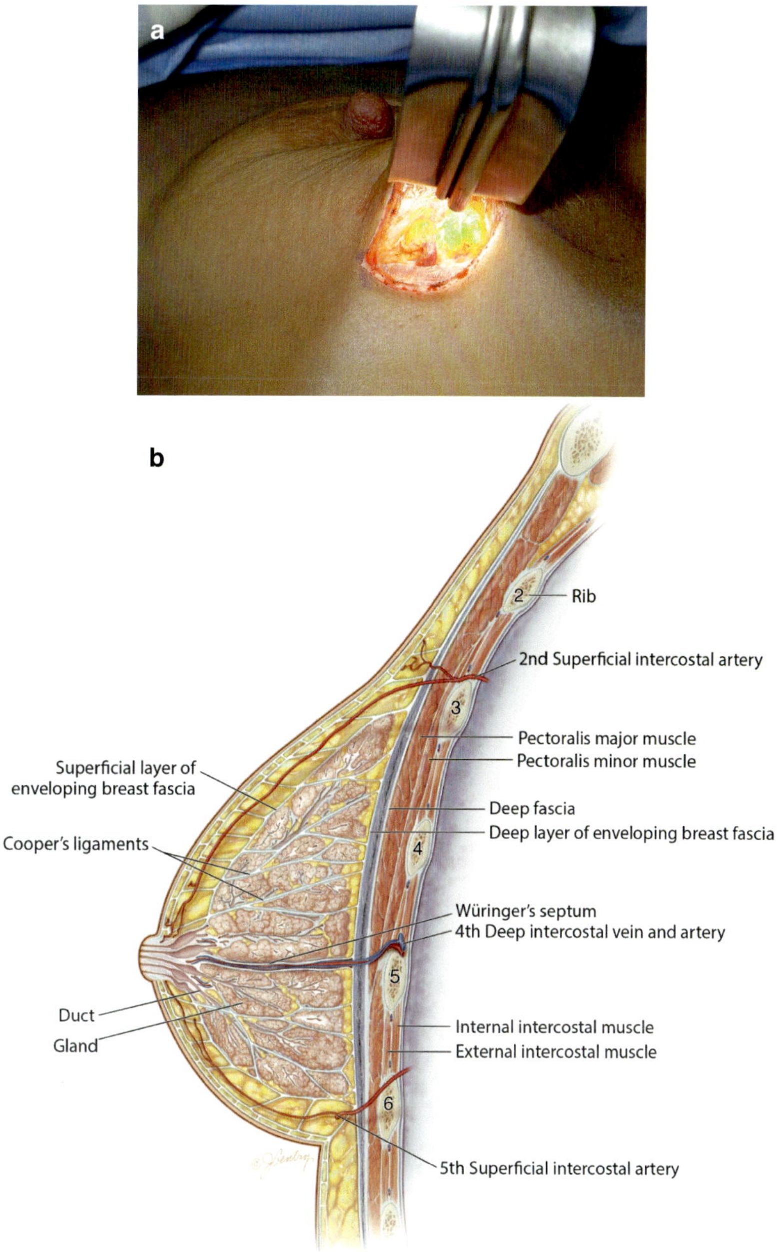

Fig. 3.11 (**a**, **b**) The inferior flap is a chest wall-based flap. The blood supply comes from the fourth interspace and this is the only artery and vein that goes through the breast parenchyma to the nipple. There are lateral branches but the main blood supply to the nipple is superficial with the veins just under the dermis and the arteries about 2 cm deep to the skin surface. (**a** Figure courtesy of Elizabeth Hall-Findlay, copyright reserved. **b**, From Hall-Findlay [1]. Image used with permission)

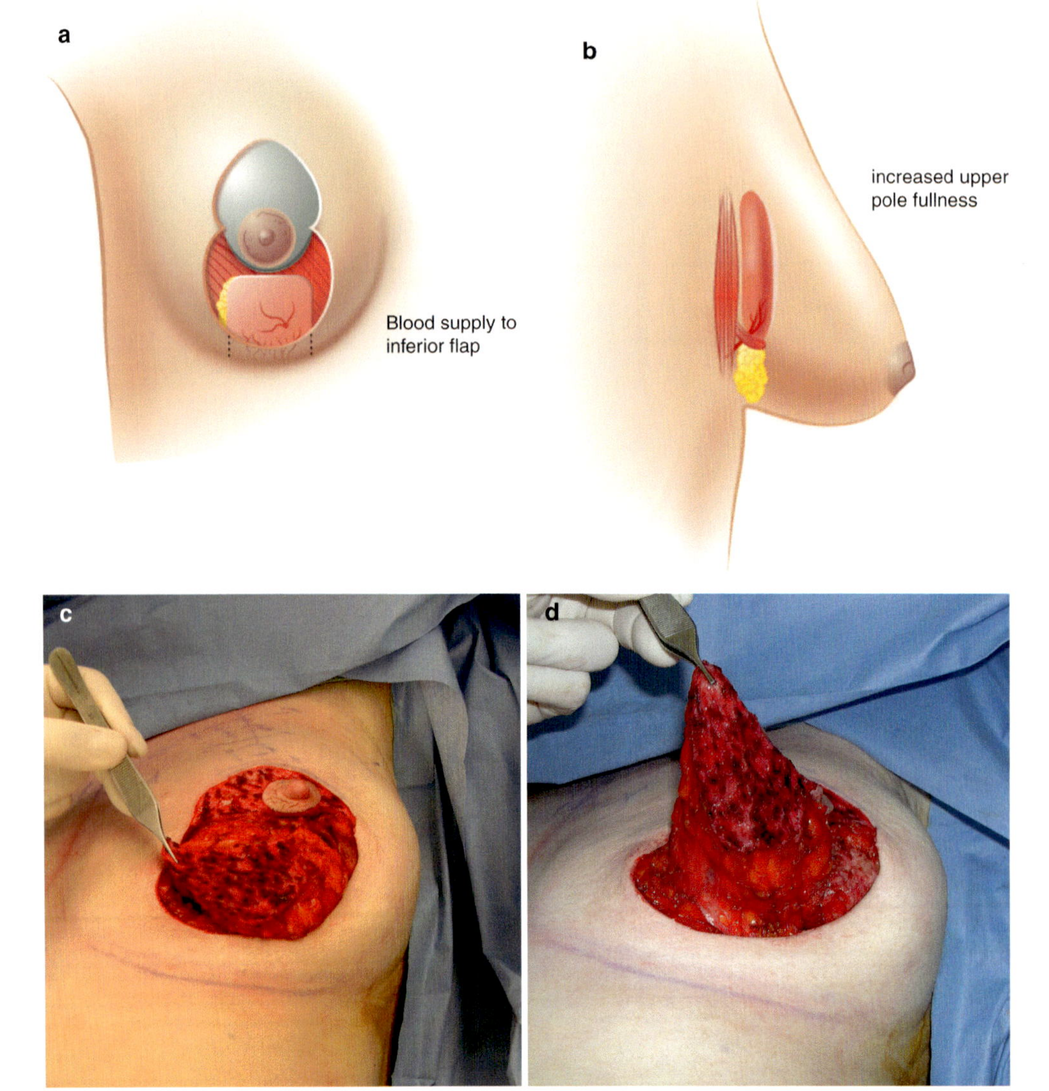

Fig. 3.12 (**a**, **b**) Liacyr Ribeiro used a superior pedicle and he then mobilized the inferior flap and moved it up (while still attached as a chest-wall-based flap) under the superior pedicle. It can be held up with a pectoralis sling but the advantage of this is the extent of mobilization that is achieved compared to the other methods. (From Hall-Findlay [1]. Image used with permission). (**c**–**e**) The inferior flap (which is usually removed in a breast reduction) is de-epithelialized. The flap is then mobilized on all four sides and left as a chest wall-based flap. Note how much mobilization can be achieved. The anterior surface of the flap then heals to the posterior surface of the pedicle which gives a good long-lasting result. (Figure courtesy of Elizabeth Hall-Findlay, copyright reserved)

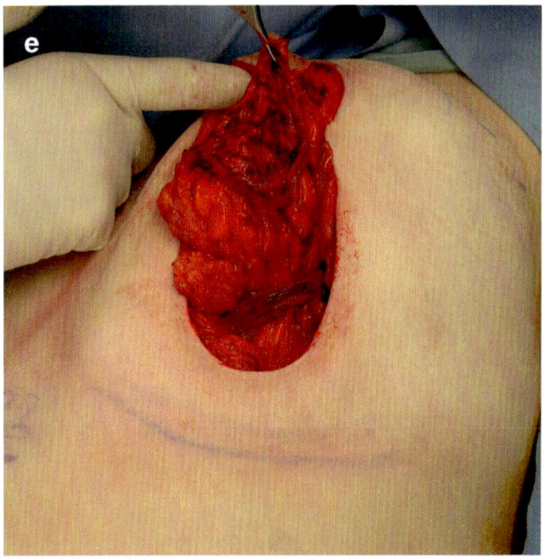

Fig. 3.12 (continued)

Key Elements to the Pre-operative Workup

Although a mastopexy is a fairly low risk operation, a few key elements should be followed to ensure patient safety and optimize outcomes. It is recommended to follow the American Cancer Society guidelines for mammogram screening and ensure patient compliance before any elective breast surgery. In addition, a thorough breast exam should be performed by the surgeon prior to surgery.

Smoking status should always be confirmed with the patient, especially with breast procedures that involve repositioning of the NAC or incisions that may be under tension. The risk of nipple loss and wound breakdown is significantly increased with current use of nicotine. Patients should be advised to stop using nicotine for a minimum of 2–4 weeks before and after surgery. A urine cotinine test is an easy way to ensure patient compliance. Of note, second hand smoke can be detected on a urine cotinine test, and patients should be warned of that exposure.

Patients should be screened for any medical issues that are associated with impaired wound healing. Some risk factors for poor healing include long-term steroid use, collagen vascular disorders and previous breast radiation for cancer treatment. Elective breast surgery should often be avoided in these settings. In addition, the surgeon should be aware that patients with gastric bypass surgery are often at risk for being deficient in iron, thiamin, B12, vitamin D3, calcium and protein [8].

Pre-operative Breast Markings for Vertical Mastopexy (Figs. 3.13 and 3.14)

The key elements when marking a vertical breast reduction include:

- Midline of the chest starting from the sternal notch
- Midpoint of clavicle, usually 7 cm from sternal notch. From that point, mark the breast meridian through the desired nipple position. It is important to ignore the existing nipple position because it can be too lateral or too medial for an ideal result. An ideal nipple is about 10 cm from the breast meridian (on a straight line, not curved around the breast).
- Inframammary fold
- Mark 3 cm above the inframammary fold and translocate that mark on the breast meridian as potentially the new NAC location. Be aware that the IMF can be misleading in patients with long or short vertical footprints.
- Mark the upper breast border. You can find this from a slight notch just inferior to the axillary fullness and translocate that point medially or by folding the breasts up superiorly and finding the transition between the chest wall and the breast.
- Next mark the NAC position from the upper breast border. For a C-D cup breast, the nipple is generally 8–10 cm from the upper breast border, making the top of the NAC 6–8 cm from the upper breast border. Evaluate how this mark corresponds to your mark 3 cm superior to the IMF. If these marks to not correspond, it is generally more accurate to use

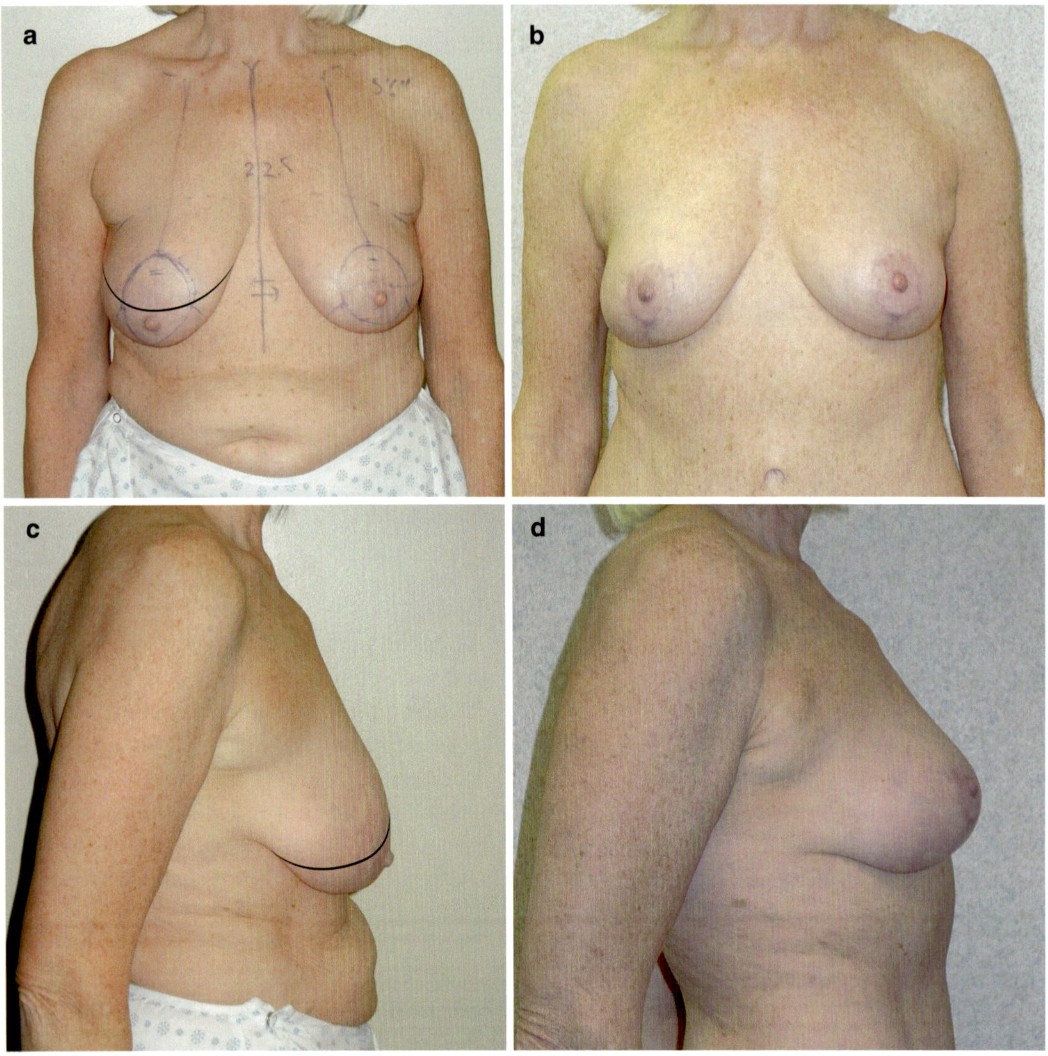

Fig. 3.13 (**a**–**d**) The surgeon can visualize the result that can be achieved by rearranging the breast tissue when performing a mastopexy. The upper breast border is marked with a dotted line. In this patient, the breast meridian did line up with the existing nipple position, but it should always be placed in the desired position and not necessarily existing position. Mastopexies are all about controlling the glandular (and nipple) ptosis. (Figure courtesy of Elizabeth Hall-Findlay, copyright reserved)

the upper breast border as a guide because the upper breast border will not change after a mastopexy.

- The shape for the areola can be drawn freehand so that it closes as a circle. An ideal areolar circumference is 14–16 cm to leave a 4–5 cm diameter areola.
- The tissue resection is determined by displacing the breast medially and laterally against the breast meridian line. The vertical lines tend to follow the same position as an inverted T, Wise pattern but it is important not to make the resection too wide or the closure will be tight resulting in a shape with a concave inferior pole.
- Always stop the vertical incision 2–4 cm above the inframammary fold. This is important to ensure that the incision does not extend below the new inframammary fold. With a vertical technique, the lower pole of the breast is unweighted as tissue is removed. The new IMF will be higher in location than the original fold.

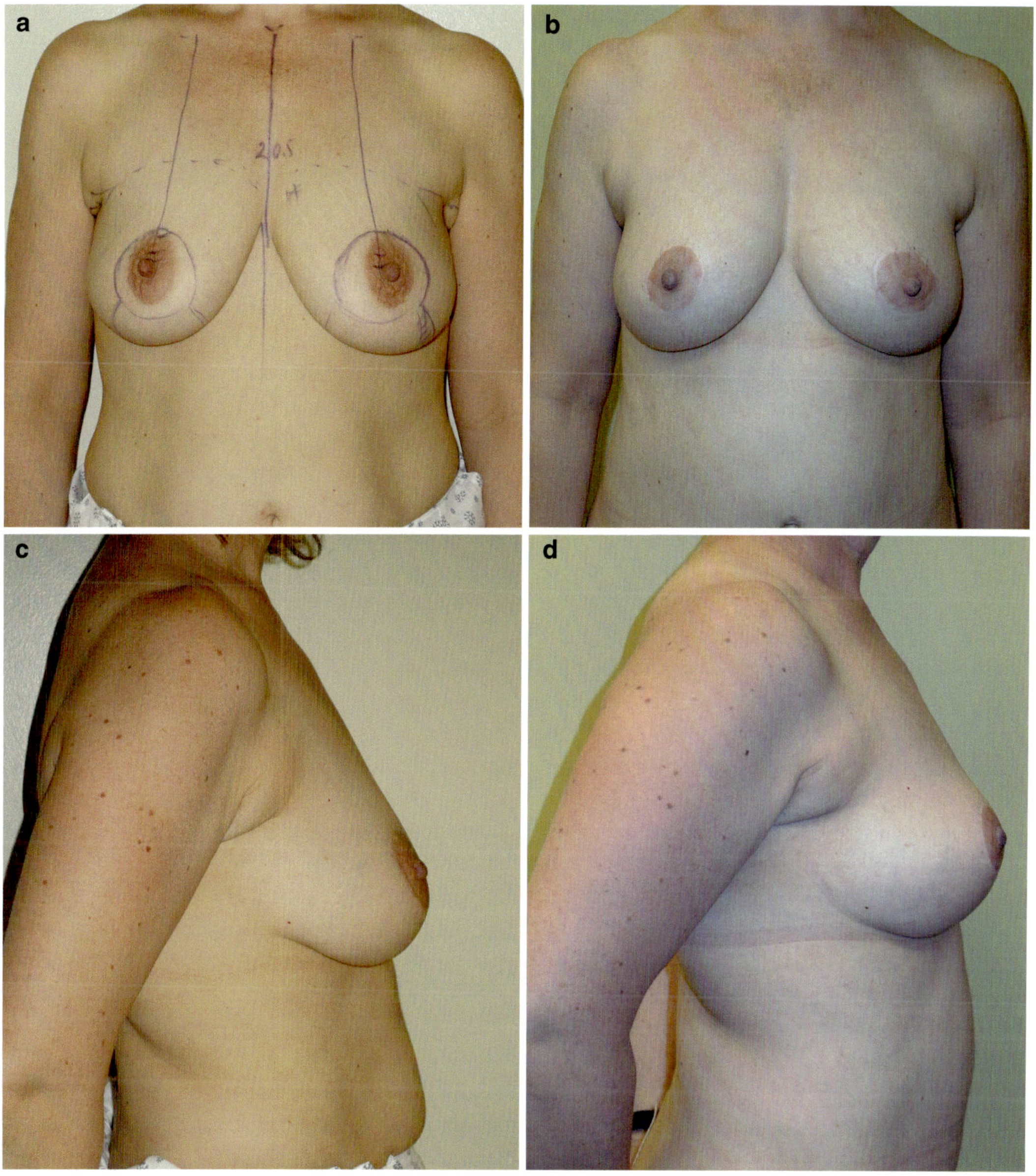

Fig. 3.14 (**a–d**) This patient did not have nipple ptosis but did have glandular ptosis. This was corrected with an inferior (Ribeiro) flap mobilized under a superior pedicle. (Figure courtesy of Elizabeth Hall-Findlay, copyright reserved)

Intra-operative Details and Clinical Pearls

The surgery is performed under general anesthesia. A preoperative dose of antibiotics delivered within an hour of incision is standard of care to reduce surgical site infections. Prior to incision, a field block of bupivacaine will decrease the need for intra-operative narcotics and assist with post-operative pain control.

A 42 mm nipple marker is used to outline around the NAC. It is important to recognize that the areolar skin is very elastic and it will stretch to fit the areolar skin opening. The type of pedicle is determined. If the nipple is within the upper NAC marks of the areolar opening, a superior pedicle is easiest for NAC elevation. A true superomedial pedicle may be required if the nipple is significantly inferior to the new NAC location. The skin of the pedicle is de-epithelialized, making sure to not damage the underlying veins and avoid venous congestion to the nipple.

The parenchyma outlined in the lower pole skin resection will either be removed if the patient desires a smaller breast or translocated superiorly if an auto-augmentation is planned. If a smaller breast is desired, the surgeon has the flexibility of just removing an inferior vertical wedge of parenchyma. If the surgeon wants to use the inferior flap but still reduce the breast volume, the excess is best removed from under the lateral flap. The blood supply enters the inferior flap just medial to breast meridian at the fourth interspace. If resection is performed beyond the skin resection, it is advised to leave some thickness to the flaps of about 3 cm so that the initial layers of sutures are in the breast parenchyma and not only the dermis. Closing in layers with the least tension on the superficial skin layer will help minimize spreading of the scar.

If an auto-augmentation is planned, it is important to dissect all the way down to the chest wall on all 4 sides of the flap in order for the flap to translocate superiorly. It is also helpful in the dissection to have the base of the flap a bit wider than the top, which will provide added safety with incorporating the intercostal perforator. If there is any residual tethering of the inferior flap to the inframammary fold, it will cause a postoperative deformity. It must be completely released (Fig. 3.12).

The breast parenchyma superior to the flap is then elevated off the chest wall just above the pectoralis fascia, allowing the flap to be inset within the breast meridian and slightly above the new NAC position. The flap is secured to the chest wall with 2 or 3 PDS sutures. It is important that these inferior flaps are secured at the same height on both breasts. This can be determined by sitting the patient upright before skin closure and evaluating the height of each inset flap.

Occasionally the inferior flap can be placed in a more medial direction to help fill the inferior medial defect of a tuberous breast type of deformity.

The potential complication of the auto-augmentation is flap necrosis. It is important to have a wide footprint of the flap in order to incorporate the intercostal perforator and it is important to create a large enough space for insetting, so the flap is not compressed. The use of a pectoralis sling can further compromise vascular flow to the pedicle, and therefore, it is advised to use the sling with caution.

Final shape and contour can be assessed prior to skin closure by sitting the patient in an upright position and using a temporary staple closure. Minor adjustments to skin resection can be made at this point. Closure should be performed in multiple layers, starting with the underlying breast pillars which are closed with PDS or Monocryl.

We have found that using the antibacterial coated sutures has resulted in less suture spitting around the NAC post-operatively. Drains are rarely used unless aggressive liposuction has been performed in the bra roll or lateral breast and the liposuction communicates with the area of parenchymal resection. Often a separate small incision can be made laterally away from the parenchymal resection, keeping the spaces separate and eliminating the need for a drain to collect fluid from the liposuction.

Figure 3.13 The surgeon can visualize the result that can be achieved by rearranging the breast tissue when performing a mastopexy (Fig. 3.13). The upper breast border is marked with a dotted line. In this patient, the breast meridian did line up with the existing nipple position, but it should always be placed in the desired position and not necessarily in the existing position. Mastopexies are all about controlling the glandular (and nipple) ptosis.

In Fig. 3.14, the patient did not have nipple ptosis but did have glandular ptosis. This was corrected with an inferior (Ribeiro) flap mobilized under a superior pedicle.

Postoperative Care

At the time of surgery, patients can be fitted with a surgical bra or the surgeon can create a foam tape bra. The benefit of the foam tape bra is controlled support laterally and inferiorly and allows the patient a few days to swell before the surgical bra is fitted. The surgical bra is worn for 6 weeks, and after that, the patient can wear any type of brassiere she desires.

Patients can be advised to ice on the lateral sides and tops of the breasts for the first 2 to 4 days, but no ice on or near the nipples. Ibuprofen can be started either the night of surgery or the next morning, and patients are advised to take 600 mg 3 times a day around the clock for the first week. Another approach is to give the patient acetaminophen and celecoxib preoperatively and to continue both on a regular basis for about 5 days postoperatively. We have found that aggressive use of non-steroidal anti-inflammatory medication and regular use of acetaminophen significantly reduces the use of opioid narcotics.

Patients are generally advised to refrain from lifting more than 5 lbs for 6 weeks but can begin cardiovascular exercise 3 weeks postoperatively. They can begin driving 4–5 days postoperatively if off narcotics.

Scar care involves a regimen of tape for 6 weeks followed by silicone strips or gel for another 3–4 months. Steri-strips can be applied horizontally across the vertical scar in order to take tension off of the scar, which may help prevent spreading of the scar. An alternative to steristrips is to place paper tape on the incisions which lasts in place for 3–4 weeks. Patients are advised to refrain from sun exposure for the first year after surgery. Patients who appear to be scarring abnormally are aggressively treated with IPL, fractional CO2 laser or steroids as appropriate.

Complications

Preoperative Planning

The majority of complications can be avoided with proper pre-operative planning. It is important to manage patient expectations by evaluating the individual footprint and emphasizing to the patient that the mastopexy will not elevate the breast up the chest wall. All of the "lift" effect is in rearranging the breast parenchyma and taking care of the glandular ptosis.

Preoperative Markings

Complications related to aesthetic outcome can be avoided with thoughtful, precise pre-operative markings. Setting appropriate nipple position on the breast mound is crucial. Lowering a nipple which has been placed too high cannot be corrected without scars above the NAC location and can lead to significant patient dissatisfaction and embarrassment and will limit patients' clothing options.

Intraoperative Execution

Other complications can be the result of poor planning. The surgeon must decide what to do with the lower pole breast tissue. If the tissue is left, the lower pole is not unweighted, and recurrent ptosis is likely. The lower tissue can either be removed if the patient desires a smaller breast volume or relocated under the NAC to increase upper pole projection. However, leaving the tissue is not ideal. If an auto-augmentation is performed, it is recommended to bevel the dissection, leaving a wider base to the lower pole flap. By beveling out, the surgeon increases with chances of capturing perforating vessels needed for flap vascularity.

It is important to remember that it is the breast parenchyma, not the skin envelope, that should be used to create the breast shape. It is an easy tendency to think that tightening the skin is the key to a long-lasting lift. However, that is incorrect. Too much tension on the skin results in stretching of the skin (skin expansion) and hypertrophic scarring. Tension should be placed in the support sutures approximating the medial and lateral pillars of breast parenchyma, not the final skin closure.

The vertical scar should not be cinched in order to shorten the scar. The vertical scar will be longer with a vertical mastopexy or reduction compared to a Wise pattern skin resection due to the added projection of the breast mound. It is perfectly acceptable to have vertical limbs as long as 11–12 cm. Attempting to cinch and shorten the vertical limb results in tissue ischemia, potential skin necrosis and poor scarring.

The incision around the NAC can also be prone to having sutures spit 6–12 weeks after surgery, resulting in a small abscess or raised scar. This most likely results from the incision being very superficial around the NAC and, as a result, the sutures closer to the surface. In our experience, using an antibacterial coated suture such as Monocryl-Plus will decrease the incidence of sutures abscesses.

Nipple necrosis is one of the most devastating complications with breast surgery. Fortunately, this is a rare complication with a vertical mastopexy. It is important, however, not to undermine the NAC when dissecting around the lower pole tissue. The arterial supply to the NAC in the superior pedicle is from the superficial branch of the second branch of the internal mammary artery and is located about 2 cm deep to the skin. The NAC can be raised off of the pectoralis fascia without compromising the superficial blood supply, but thinning the parenchyma too close to the NAC may compromise the vascular supply. It is also important to resect the skin around the new NAC position superficially, preserving the dermis and underlying veins. Loss of nipple sensation is rare since the nipple has multiple sources of innervation, both superficially and deep from both the medial and lateral intercostal nerves.

Infection with mastopexy is extremely rare. Preoperative antibiotic is standard of care for all patients. In our experience, we have also found that irrigating the surgical site with an antibiotic provides additional protection. Be cautious if the patient has significant acne on her chest. This should be medically treated prior to surgery as this does increase the risk of infection from propionobacterium acnes infection. Hematoma and seroma are also rare events, and drains are not recommended for a standard mastopexy.

References

1. Hall-Findlay EJ. Aesthetic breast surgery: concepts and techniques. St. Louis: Quality Medical Publishing; 2011. p. 429–514.
2. Ribeiro L. A new technique for reduction mammoplasty. Plast Reconstr Surg. 1975;55:330–4.
3. Benelli L. A new periareolar mammoplasty: the 'round block' technique. Aesthet Plast Surg. 1990;14:99.
4. Wise RJ. A preliminary report on a method of planning the mammoplasty. Plast Reconstr Surg. 1956;17:367–75.
5. Losken A, Holtz DJ. Versatility of the superomedial pedicle in managing the massive weight loss breast: the rotation-advancement technique. Plast Reconstr Surg. 2007;120:1060–8.
6. Daniel MJB. Mammaplasty with pectoral muscle flap. Presented at the sixty-fourth scientific meeting of the American Society of Plastic and Reconstructive Surgeons, Montreal, Oct 1995.
7. Graf RM, Mansur AE, Tenius FP, et al. Mastopexy after massive weight loss: extended chest wall-based flap associated with a loop of pectoralis muscle. Aesthet Plast Surg. 2008;32:371–4.
8. Seeniann J, Hoegerl C. Nutrional deficiencies after gastric bypass surgery. J Am Osteopath Assoc. 2009;109:601–4.

4 Breast Augmentation for Early Ptosis

Chet Mays and M. Bradley Calobrace

Introduction

Breast augmentation is the most commonly performed plastic surgery procedure worldwide [1]. In breast surgery, the surgeon is often faced with patients whom not only have micromastia but also some degree of ptosis. The challenge is often in determining the optimal procedure for the patient's problem that is going to yield the best cosmetic result. When moderate to severe ptosis is present, the best procedure to correct this is often a mastopexy. These patients have an option for a mastopexy alone or in combination with an augmentation to improve long-term upper pole fullness. An augmentation alone for these patients is inadequate and would simply correct the upper pole without adequately addressing the lower pole. Potentially, the even more challenging decisions are in patients requiring an augmentation but whom also have some degree of ptosis. The question to be answered is whether an augmentation alone will provide adequate rejuvenation and meet the patient's aesthetic goals or is an augmentation mastopexy required for a successful outcome. This decision is always accompanied by the knowledge that most patients would prefer not to have a breast lift, often because of dislike of mastopexy scars and financial considerations. Mastopexy with a simultaneous augmentation is more technically challenging with significantly higher complication rates compared to a breast augmentation alone. Perioperative decision making is critical to a successful outcome. In this chapter, we will review our approach to decision making with a focus on pocket and implant selection to optimize breast aesthetics in patients with varying degrees of ptosis. The goal is to provide a foundation for decision making that will provide optimal results in the patients who forego a mastopexy thus utilizing the pocket selection, implant choice, and dual plane techniques to provide a lift to the breast without the extra incisions of a mastopexy effectively performing the "no lift, lift".

C. Mays (✉)
Private Practice, CaloAesthetics Plastic Surgery Center, Louisville, KY, USA

Clinical Faculty, University of Louisville, Division of Plastic Surgery, Louisville, KY, USA
e-mail: drchet@calobrace.com

M. B. Calobrace
Private Practice, CaloAesthetics Plastic Surgery Center, Louisville, KY, USA

Clinical Faculty, University of Louisville, Division of Plastic Surgery, Louisville, KY, USA

Clinical Faculty, University of Kentucky, Division of Plastic Surgery, Lexington, KY, USA

Pre-operative Evaluation

Determining the appropriate procedure for the patient with ptotic breast begins with a thorough evaluation to determine the optimal surgical approach. The evaluation should begin with a

M. B. Calobrace et al. (eds.), *Augmentation Mastopexy*,
https://doi.org/10.1007/978-3-030-48226-8_4

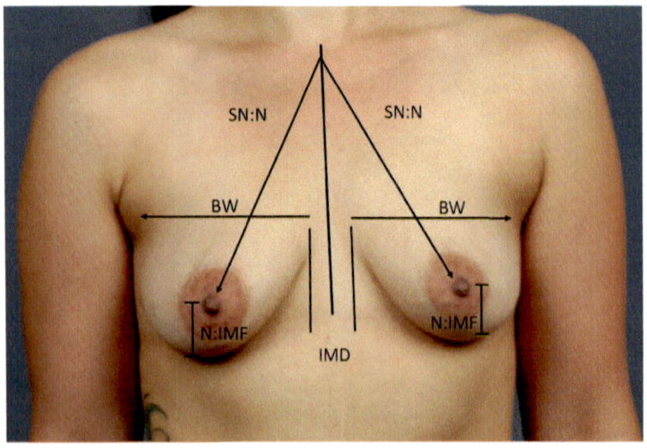

Fig. 4.1 Breast measurements: The Sternal notch to Nipple (SN: N), Breast width (BW), nipple to Inframammary fold (N:IMF), Intermammary distance (IMD)

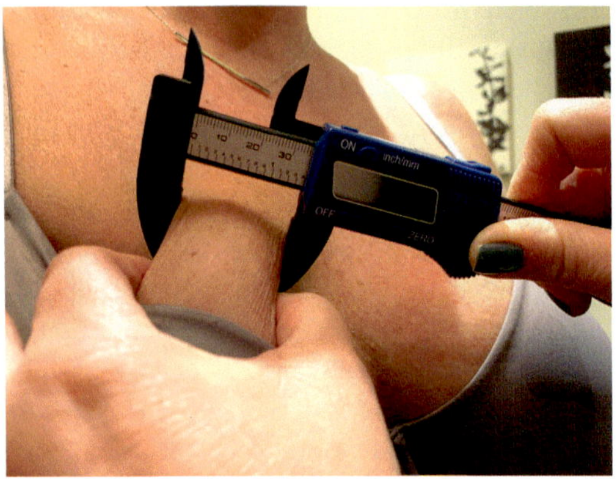

Fig. 4.2 The skin pinch test to assess the thickness of the overlying soft tissue)

Table 4.1 Assessment of breast ptosis

Relationship of the NAC to the IMF (Regnault's degree of ptosis)
Grade 1: nipple at the level of the inframammary fold, above the lower contour of the gland
Grade 2: nipple below the level of the inframammary fold, above the lower contour of the gland
Grade 3: nipple below the level of the inframammary fold, at the lower contour of the gland
Pseudoptosis: nipple at or above inframammary fold, but breast hangs below the fold
Amount of breast tissue overhanging the fold
Location of the NAC on the breast mound
Amount of vertical excess and horizontal excess
Footprint of the breast on the chest wall – low, medium, high
Quality and quantity of breast parenchyma and skin

breast exam with breast measurements including the base width, sternal notch to nipple distance, nipple to inframammary fold distance (at rest and under maximal stretch) and the intermammary distance (Fig. 4.1).

The amount of breast ptosis present should also be assessed. The varying degrees of ptosis have classically been described as per Regnault based on the relationship of the NAC to the inframammary fold [2]. Further assessment should also include evaluation of the skin thickness and elasticity, the quantity and distribution of subcutaneous fat, and the composition and firmness of the breast parenchyma. Soft tissue coverage is assessed by measuring and documenting the skin pinch in the upper pole, medial breast and lateral breast (Fig. 4.2). This will provide guidance in determining the optimal pocket for implant placement. Additionally, special attention should be given to the laxity of the breast. This can be determined by performing a skin stretch test. It also can be assessed by determining the difference between the N-IMF distance at rest and under maximal stretch. One can also evaluate generically, as in the Bodylogic system, defining it as tight, moderate, loose and/or with ptosis [3]. This can provide some understanding as to the quality of the skin envelope and its response to an augmentation only.

A more complete assessment of ptosis is summarized in Table 4.1. All of these aspects of the assessment must be considered when deciding the appropriate surgical procedure to perform because each will influence the shape of the breast, the ability to "lift" the breast with an augmentation only and ultimate the success of the operation (Figs. 4.3 and 4.4).

When evaluating patients, the vertical excess is assessed to help determine the amount of excess tissue present and whether a patient is a better candidate for an augmentation, an augmentation mastopexy or a staged augmentation mastopexy. It measures the excess skin present based on the planned breast augmentation and/or mastopexy. In other words, if performing a mastopexy, the amount of skin necessary for coverage of the implant is determined with the new nipple position, the vertical excess would be the amount of vertical extra skin left in the lower pole. If performing an augmentation only where the NAC is

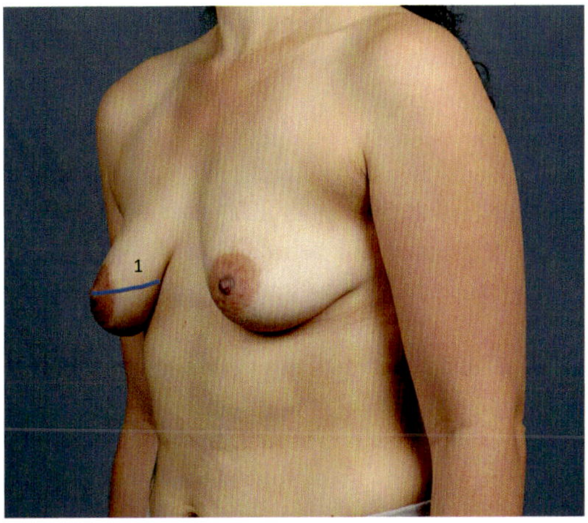

Fig. 4.3 Grade 1 ptosis. The nipple is at the level of the inframammary fold, above the lower contour of the gland

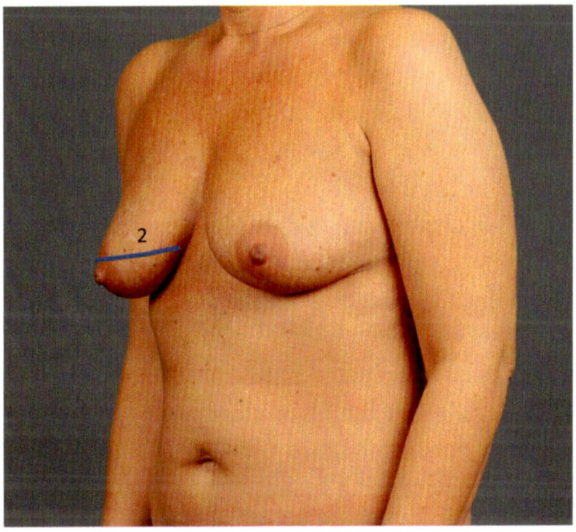

Fig. 4.4 Grade 2 ptosis. The nipple is below the level of the inframammary fold, above the lower contour of the gland

not being elevated, the vertical excess would represent the Nipple to fold distance under stretch minus the amount of skin optimally needed for any given implant.

Perioperative Decision Making

There are many options available for the correction of breast ptosis and the appropriate surgical approach is based on a myriad of variables. (Table 4.2)

Table 4.2 Surgical options for breast ptosis

Options for breast posis
Mastopexy only
Breast augmentation only
Mastopexy with a staged augmentation
Augmentation with a staged mastopexy
Simultaneous augmentation mastopexy

In determining the most appropriate approach, the goal is to select the procedure with the least morbidity that will achieve the aesthetic goals of the patient. Thus, if possible, achieving a successful outcome in a ptotic breast with only augmenting the breast would be optimal, eliminating scarring, morbidity and the additional expense. However, performing an augmentation in a patient with ptosis whom is not a good candidate and would have been better served with a mastopexy should be avoided. Thus, analyzing the breast based on the assessment of multiple characteristics as discussed will provide guidance in selecting the appropriate patient for a breast augmentation only. In general, a breast augmentation would be reserved for patients with minimal ptosis, including pseudoptosis and grade 1 ptosis. These patients are where we rely on pocket selection, implant optimization, fold adjustments and a varying level of dual plane to yield the best results. The challenge lies in determining which grade 1 or pseudoptosis patients can have optimal aesthetic results without performing a mastopexy. Most grade 2 and 3 ptotic patients are not considered for an augmentation only and are best served with a mastopexy to provide elevation of the breast and NAC. There is an occasional patient with up to grade 2 ptosis that may be a candidate, but generally this would be in a patient with some type of constricted breast deformity.

In the gray area or "in-between" patients with pseudoptosis or grade 1 ptosis, there are many characteristics or considerations that provide guidance on whether to perform an augmentation alone or an augmentation mastopexy. Patients with different grades of ptosis per the Regnault's classification may have completely different breast compositions including the quality of breast tissue and skin, the quantity of breast tissue present and the vertical excess present. All these aspects of the breast composition influence the shape of the breast and ultimately the outcome after the augmentation. The amount of expansion of the breast that can occur with the placement of an implant is a key component in breast augmentation. Tightness to the breast or a constricted breast will behave differently than a mobile, expansive breast. Conversely, tissue that is lax with breasts that are deflated with minimal breast tissue will be more likely to expand under the influence of the implant. Heavy, dense breasts are, however, less likely to expand adequately increasing the risk of postoperative waterfall deformity.

Additionally, vertical excess that is too significant may require a mastopexy for correction. A good rule of thumb is if the nipple-to-fold distance does not exceed 9.5–10 cms, a breast augmentation alone without a mastopexy may provide satisfactory correction and meet the patient's goal [4].

The pocket decision will also impact the success of ptosis correction with augmentation only. Placing the implant in either a submuscular, subfascial or subglandular pocket can have different degrees of impact on the overlying breast and correction of the ptosis. The subglandular pocket will expand the lower pole maximally whereas the subfascial pocket will be similar but with a slightly reduced ability to expand the breast, especially if the fascial layer is well-developed. The use of these pockets requires an upper pole pinch test of at least 2 centimeters to avoid the possibility of implant visibility or traction wrinkling. These pockets are commonly used around the world, especially with the use of more cohesive and/or textured devices. In the United States, smooth implants are most commonly used and placed in the submuscular breast pocket [5]. The majority of surgeons prefer subpectoral implant placement to achieve greater tissue coverage, a more natural appearance, less wrinkling, and possibly less risk of capsular contracture [6, 7]. This can liberalize the use of many different pockets in selected patients. However, the submuscular pocket is restrictive in the lower pole and does not allow significant expansion. The dual plane technique, providing a submuscular pocket in the upper breast and subglandular pocket in the lower breast has allowed the submuscular breast augmentation to be used successfully in patients with grade 1 ptosis and pseudoptosis. In the dual plane technique, the breast tissue is released from the caudal edge of the underlying pectoralis major muscle (PMM) and the muscle will retract upward (cephalad) freeing the breast tissue, allowing the NAC to rise and the lower pole to expand. Whereas the appearance is one of NAC elevation with centralization of the implant on the breast, the correction is simply the expansion of the lower pole that improves the NAC position, not a true elevation of the NAC position [8]. When utilizing the dual plane, different levels of release allow increased levels of expansion of the lower pole with correction of the pseudoptosis.

Implant characteristics including implant fill, shell texturization, silicone gel cohesiveness, gel-to-shell fill ratios, projections and shape can all impact the success of the operation and will have different levels of impact based on the breast pocket utilized [9, 10].

When considering a candidate for an augmentation vs an augmentation mastopexy, other issues may be under consideration, especially if either procedure would be appropriate based on the clinical setting and patient expectations. One consideration is the issue of smoking. Smokers are also poor candidates for a mastopexy, especially those refusing to quit prior to surgery, The effects of smoking on the soft tissue and vascularity can be detrimental leading to delayed wound healing and increased complications [11]. The augmentation mastopexy patient is at a significant risk of healing problems due to the incisions interfering with blood supply. The incisions and breast flaps that are needed in a breast lift compared to an augmentation creates a higher oxygen demand for the tissue during wound healing which can be delayed with the vasoconstrictive property of nicotine. Additionally, the expansion pressure of the underlying implant compresses the vessels, increasing the risk of ischemia and necrosis. Longer operative times needed to perform the mastopexy compared to an augmentation also put smokers at higher risk for other medical complications [12].

Patient Expectations

In planning the operative approach, it cannot be overstated the importance of patient education and the need to spend some time understanding the patient's desired outcome and expectations with the operation. Patients with ptosis are more likely to have undergone changes to the breast from weight loss or postpartum and suffer the sequalae of increased laxity of the tissue, stria, nipple and breast ptosis, and loss of parenchymal volume and/or firmness. They need to understand the challenges faced and what a breast augmentation alone can and cannot do. Does the patient want the NAC in the center of the breast mound? Is there a desire for the areola to be smaller? Is the patient unwilling to make her breasts large enough to fill out the extra skin present? If so, these will not be adequately corrected with a breast augmentation and the patient may be best suited for a mastopexy.

The breast augmentation's ability to correct the NAC positioning is key to determining the success of the operation. There are many opinions on the most aesthetically pleasing breast in relation to position of the NAC with varying amounts of breast tissue above or below. When it comes to the general population, when polled, men prefer a NAC position with 45% of breast tissue above and 55% below the NAC. Women prefer a lower NAC position with 55% of breast tissue above and 45% of breast below [13]. Counseling the patient that the nipple areolar complex may be low on the breast mound is key to managing expectations. Additionally, patients that are low breasted need to understand their breast will still be positioned low on the chest wall. It is important to understand the mastopexy will not improve the position of the breast on the chest wall, it will only improve the NAC position and excess skin. Thus, if the breast is low but upper pole volume is lacking, a breast augmentation may be adequate and provide maximal benefit.

Patients need to understand the limitations in achieving a desired look to the breast when performing breast augmentation alone. The results of an augmentation are not the same as an augmentation mastopexy in most patients [14]. However, if they can achieve a satisfactory outcome, avoidance of the scars can be worthwhile. In a study where they compared breast augmentation patients to augmentation mastopexy patients, breast augmentation patients were significantly more satisfied with the aesthetic outcome and the quality of life on many psychosocial aspects. The augmentation mastopexy patients reported dissatisfaction with shape, scarring, symmetry and the nipple-areolar complex [14].

Based on the patient's desired outcome, the operative approach can be adjusted to create different aesthetics. A patient desiring a more natural look may benefit more from a subpectoral implant, a less cohesive implant or a shaped device, whereas a patient desiring more volume and roundness in the upper pole may require a more cohesive higher profile implant and potentially the implant placed above the muscle. There are limitations in what can be achieved in breast augmentation in patients with minimal grade 1 ptosis and pseudoptosis. Good perioperative decision making with an operative approach specifically designed to meet the patient's goals is more likely to provide optimal results for each patient.

Operative Approach: Breast Augmentation for Early Ptosis

Patient positioning Patients are placed on the operating room table in the supine position. The arms are secured to the arm board with soft gauze wraps at 45 degrees to stabilize the patient in the upright position (Fig. 4.5). This relaxes the pectoralis muscle providing a more accurate assessment of the implant position and the redraping of the overlying breast tissue. Alternatively, some surgeons prefer placing the arms alongside the patient on the operative table, but an arm board at 90 degrees should be avoided as it does not allow accurate assessment of the breast when the patient is placed in the upright position.

Infiltration of Local Prior to surgical preparation, 50 ml of a local field block is injected of 1/4% lidocaine, 1/8% bupivicaine, 1:400,000 epi-

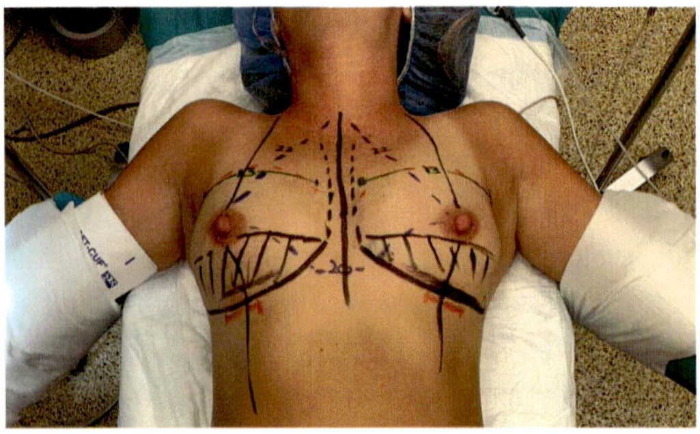

Fig. 4.5 patient positioning on the table with arms abducted at 45 degrees

Table 4.3 Breast local anesthetic formula

1/2% Lidocaine plain	25 ml
1/2% Lidocaine/1:200,000 epinephrine	25 ml
1/2% bupivacaine/1:200,000 epinephrine	25 ml
Injectable saline	25 ml
1/4% lidocaine, 1/8% bupivacaine, 1:400,000 epinephrine	100 ml

nephrine (Table 4.3). The injection is placed in the dermis along the planned incision line, and as a field block with injections along the inframammary fold, the medial pectoral border, the anterior axillary line and finally deep to the breast parenchyma in a fanning fashion throughout the area of planned pocket creation. These injections provide not only assistance in operative hemostasis, but also in the management of postoperative pain.

Surgical Prep and Sterile Draping After local infiltration, nipple shields (created by placing a small piece of Tegaderm over each nipple-areolar complex) provide a barrier against potential bacterial contamination [15] (Fig. 4.6).

The patient is prepped with chlorhexidine and draped to provide a sterile field with the entire chest and bilateral breasts visible for assessment during the procedure. The sterile dressings must be secured to prevent disruption in the sterile field while placing the patient in the upright position.

Inframammary Incision The inframammary fold has become the preferred incision location for most surgeons today. The size of the incision increases with increases in implant size, gel cohesiveness, optimal fills and texturization of

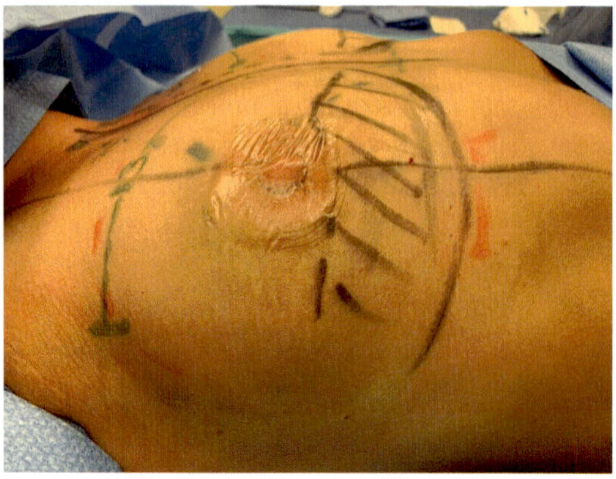

Fig. 4.6 Placement of Tegaderm nipple shields over the NAC

the implant and should be large enough not to injure the implant. Incision length ranges include: 3–4.5 centimeters for saline implants, 4–6 centimeters for silicone round implants and 4.5–7 centimeters for shaped cohesive silicone implants.

Inframammary Fold Positioning When correcting some forms of low NAC position and ptosis but with constricted lower poles, the correction with a breast augmentation is accomplished in part by lowering the IMF to place NAC more centralized over the implant. Predicting the final position of the inframammary fold is critical to determining the placement of all breast incisions, but especially the inframammary incision. This can be a challenging task as so many variables contribute to the final position of the fold. The inframammary fold is formed by the fusion of the anterior and posterior leaves of the superficial fascia which is intimately associated with the dermis at the lowest aspect of the inferior pole of the breast [16].

During preoperative markings, the native inframammary fold is identified and marked in the sitting position. The true IMF position is determined by performing an IMF expansion test. The breast is grasped and auto-rotated inferiorly to identify the inferior extent of the attachments of the inframammary fold (Fig. 4.7). This is the best predictor of where the fold will naturally sit after breast augmentation. The amount of lower pole skin required and the ultimate position

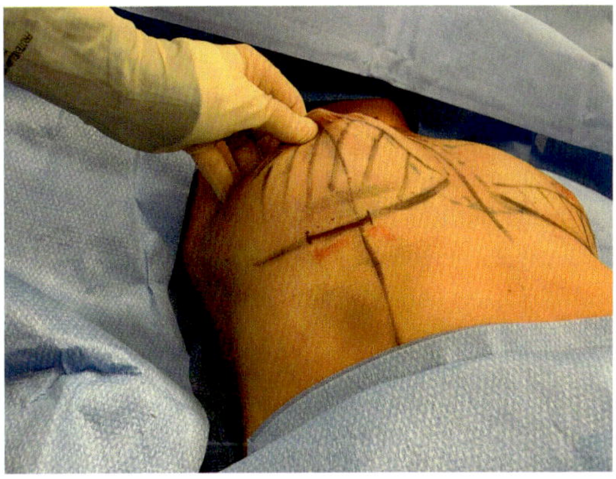

Fig. 4.7 Downward pressure on the breast with the expansion test helps identify the native or true IMF of the breast

Table 4.4 Formula to determine optimal nipple to inframammary fold (IMF) distance

Optimal N-IMF distance = ½ implant projection + ½ implant height

Table 4.5 Quick reference for determining the optimal nipple to inframammary fold (IMF) distance using the implant base diameter or fill volume

Optimal N-IMF distance (cms)	Base Diameter (cms)	Volume (cc)
7	11	200
8	12	300
9	13	400

cms centimeters

of the fold is a function of many factors, including the type of implant (saline vs silicone, round vs shaped), size of implant, pocket location and the strength and stability of the soft tissue of the lower pole. The distance measured from the nipple to true fold under maximal stretch assesses the amount of lower pole skin available to accommodate the selected implant.

In determining fold position, our team has found three alternative methods extremely useful. One method is using a formula to determine optimal N-IMF distance with a formula using implant projection and height (Table 4.4).

The other methods involve using either the base diameter or fill volume of the implant to determine the optimal N-IMF distance (Table 4.5). If the current N-IMF is shorter than the optimal distance, the fold will need to be lowered.

Table 4.6 Characteristics associated with less stretching of the lower pole

Textured implants
Cohesive implants
Shaped implants
Silicone compared to saline implants
Lower profile implants
Smaller implants
Tight, firm breast skin

If the desired N-IMF distance is equal or less than the measured N-IMF distance, then the fold does not require lowering. It is important to recognize that inframammary fold lowering is less often required when placing a larger smooth silicone or saline implant, especially if higher profile, secondary to the lower pole stretch that is seen over time [17, 18].

However, when implant choice or soft tissue characteristics predict less lower pole stretching, inframammary fold lowering may be required [19, 20]. This is very important when treating a ptotic patient with a breast augmentation because it is the lower pole stretching and IMF repositioning that create the desired results. Likewise, shaped implants are not only textured but also have a greater volume of a more cohesive gel present in the lower pole of the implant, thus requiring more lower pole skin to accommodate the implant [21–26]

There are certain implant and soft tissue characteristics that may be associated with greater need to lower the inframammary fold due to less postoperative stretching of the lower pole (Table 4.6) [17–27].

Incision After determining the inframammary fold position (either the native true fold position or the planned lowered position), a paramedian line is drawn through the center of the breast and bisects the newly drawn inframammary fold. The incision's medial extent begins one centimeter medial to the paramedian line and extends laterally for the appropriate distance as previously described (Fig. 4.8).

The initial incision is made with a 15-blade scalpel and then dissection is then carried out with electrocautery through the skin and subcutaneous

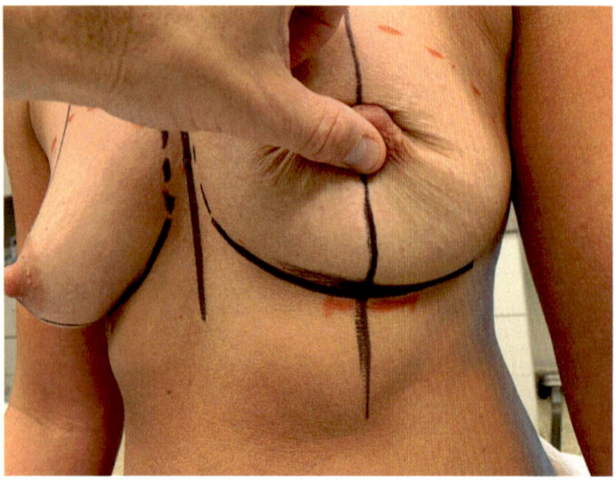

Fig. 4.8 Surgical incision shown as solid red line just below the black inframammary fold line (IMF). Medial extent begins one centimeter medial to paramedian line and extends laterally

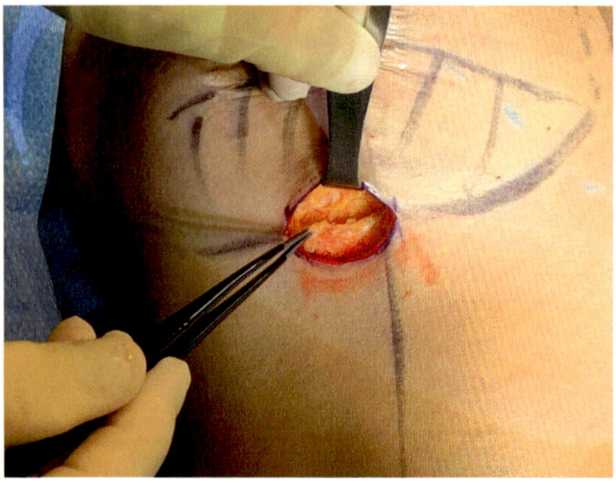

Fig. 4.9 Small cuff of superficial fascia preserved during the initial dissection of the pocket. Superficial fascia being held with forceps

tissue beveling upward while rotating the breast off of the chest wall. The dissection proceeds subcutaneous for approximately one centimeter and then deep through the superficial fascia and towards the lateral pectoral border deep on the chest wall. This technique preserves a small cuff of superficial fascia at the incision which helps to protect the IMF and will prove useful during closure (Fig. 4.9).

Implant Pocket At this point, the dissection is continued to create the desired pocket that will optimally correct the breast, including enhancing the volume and correcting the early ptosis that is present. There continues to be divergent thought as to the optimal pocket for breast implants. In the borderline patients with pseudoptosis, grade 1 and early grade 2 ptosis, a subglandular or subfascial pocket can provide horizontal and vertical expansion of the breast and lifting of the NAC. The subglandular/subfascial pocket is also the most natural for the implant with avoidance of animation deformities seen with submuscular implants, enhanced correction of constricted breast or ptotic breasts, ease of dissection and less postoperative discomfort for the patient [28–31].

The submuscular pocket advantages have included lower capsular contracture rates, enhanced coverage of the implant minimizes issues of wrinkling, provides a more natural upper pole and provides enhanced support for the breast implant [19, 32–34].

No matter which pocket is selected, it is helpful during the marking process to identify as accurately as possible the pocket size necessary to accommodate the selected implant. This will provide a pocket that maintains the implant in a controlled position and minimizes the risk of postoperative implant malposition. In breast augmentation with round implants, the accurate placement of the inframammary fold and control of the medial and lateral extent of the pockets provide ideal implant positioning to achieve the desired cleavage and minimizes lateral migration of the implant [20]. When using a shaped implant, a controlled pocket including the superior extent is even more essential to minimize the risk of implant rotation postoperatively [24–26].

Dual-plane Submuscular Pocket The importance of optimizing soft tissue coverage in breast augmentation cannot be overstated. Inadequate coverage, often combined with oversized implants, can lead to parenchymal atrophy and skin stretching resulting in wrinkling and palpability of the implants and other associated breast deformities [17, 18].

The dual-plane, initially described by Tebbetts, can be an effective technique for treating patients with ptotic breast who require muscle coverage due to inadequate soft tissue coverage (upper pole pinch less than 2 centimeters). The muscle

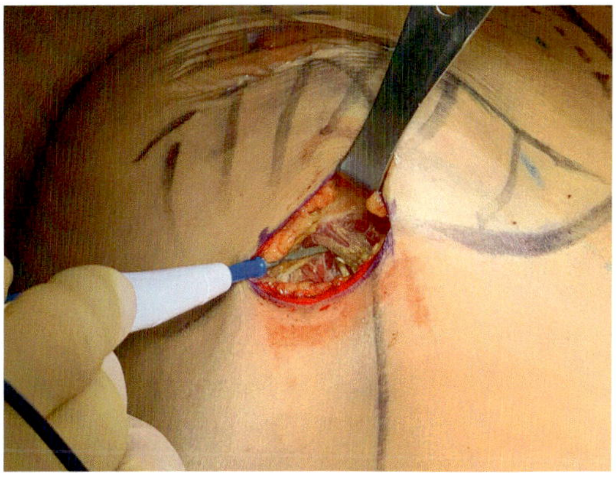

Fig. 4.10 Elevation of the lateral border of the pectoralis major muscle

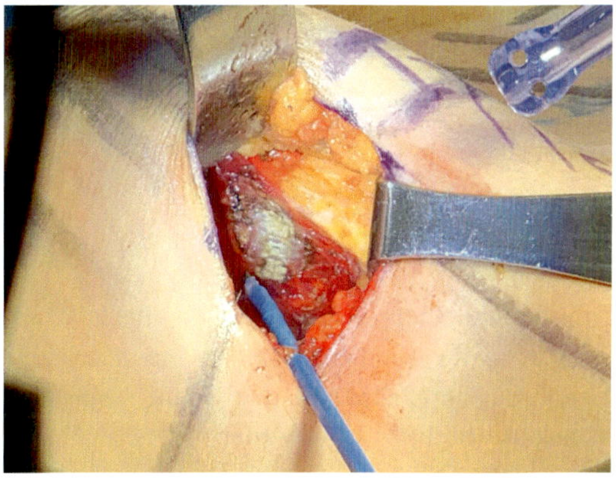

Fig. 4.11 Release of the pectoralis major muscle staying 1 cm superior to the inframammary fold

provides the coverage while allowing expansion of the subglandular lower pole [34].

When performing a dual-plane pocket, the lateral pectoral border is identified, and fascia incised to expose the underlying muscle. Upward retraction of the breast tissue will usually elevate the lateral border allowing further dissection and placement of the retractor beneath the overlying pectoralis muscle (Fig. 4.10). A very helpful "rule" is to never cut through the muscle that cannot be elevated. The inability to tent the muscle up off the chest wall may indicate that the muscle fascia is extremely adherent, but more likely that the identified muscle is actually not the pectoralis, but rather the serratus, rectus or an intercostal muscle. Continuing the dissection through an intercostal could inadvertently penetrate the pleural space resulting in a pneumothorax.

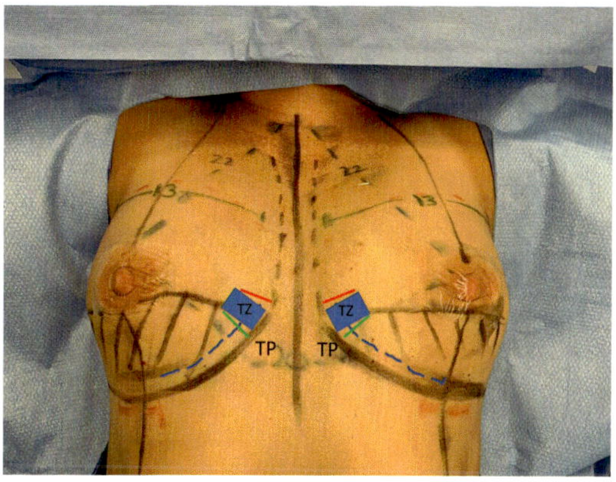

Fig. 4.12 Transition Zone (TZ-blue square region), Transition Point (TP-solid green line lateral to the TZ). Blue dashed line represents pectoralis major muscle release medially up to the TP

Once the edge of the pectoralis is safely elevated and the subpectoral space is identified, dissection is carried upward centrally to the superior extent of the pocket. Dissection is then carried laterally to identify the pectoralis minor and then carried directly over the its fascia until the lateral border of the pocket is reached. Dissection is then continued along the lateral border of the pocket, identifying and staying superficial to the serratus muscle until the inferior extent of the pocket at the inframammary fold is reached. The muscle is then released along the planned inframammary fold, staying one-centimeter superior to the fold to account for post-operative caudal muscle descent (Fig. 4.11). Dissection directly at the fold will often lead to a fold that is lower than planned as the muscle retracts inferiorly.

As you carry your dissection medially along the IMF it is critically important to stop the dissection at the most medial extent along the sternum. Preservation of the most caudal attachment of the pectoralis muscle at the Transition Point (TP) along the sternum is critical to minimize the chance of window shading of the pectoralis with subsequent medial implant exposure and animation deformities. A Transition Zone (TZ) of tapered muscle release connects the transition point to the main body of medial pectoral muscle along the sternum (Fig. 4.12).

The extent of the pocket is completed by defining the medial pectoral border, dividing the accessory slips of pectoralis muscle that insert

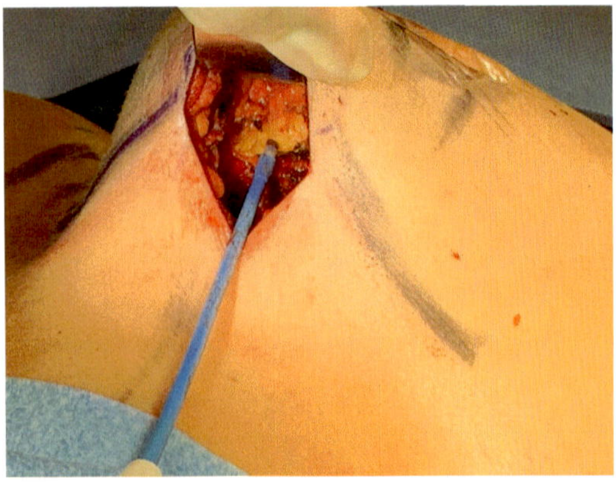

Fig. 4.13 Creation of the dual plane as the breast tissue is being released off the underlying pectoralis major muscle

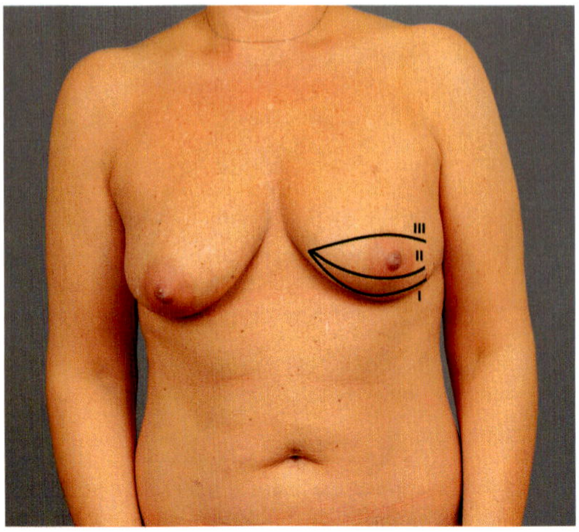

Fig. 4.14 Dual plane levels. Dual plane I is complete division the pectoralis major muscle (PMM) along the IMF. Dual plane II is release of the breast tissue off the PMM up to the lower areola. Dual plane III is release of the breast tissue off the PMM up to the upper border of the areola

along the ribs and preserving the main body of the muscle as it inserts along the sternum. Dividing these muscles with electrocautery rather than blunt dissection improves postoperative cleavage and maintains prospective hemostasis.

The dual plane approach ultimately creates a subglandular pocket in the inferior breast pocket. The levels of dual plane represent the amount of muscle released from the inferior breast tissue and resultant inferior subglandular pocket. Division of the inferior pectoralis muscle just above the inframammary fold during initial pocket dissection creates a dual plane level 1. The level of dual plane required varies and each surgery can be tailored to provide the optimal level based on soft tissue requirements and implant selection. In general, creating a subglandular pocket inferiorly is required to either re-drape the skin or breast tissue more accurately over the implant of the ptotic breast. The release of the caudal edge of the muscle is performed incrementally, creating the least amount of release that will adequately address the ptosis (Fig. 4.13).

As the breast tissue is released from the underlying pectoralis major muscle, the muscle will slide superiorly allowing the breast tissue to distribute around the implant. As the tissue re-drapes, the goal is to have the NAC lying over the most prominent portion of the implant. This will create horizontal and vertical expansion of the breast tissue subsequently elevating the NAC.

Placement of a retractor into the breast pocket and elevating superiorly while rocking the breast tissue over the retractor will assist in assessing the effects of the implant on the overlying skin and breast tissue once placed in the pocket. The different dual levels are based on the level of release of the breast tissue off the pectoralis major muscle (PMM). A dual plane level 1 is release of the PPM off its inferior costal attachments as you approach the sternum during a submuscular augmentation. A dual plane level 2 is release of the breast tissue off the PMM up to just below the NAC. A dual plane 3 is release of the breast tissue off the PMM to above the NAC. The more you release the breast tissue the more that the overlying tissue will be able to expand over the implant and provide support to the lax tissue and elevate the NAC slightly. When performing augmentation alone the dual plane release can be aggressive to provide necessary expansion of the breast tissue (Fig. 4.14).

Subglandular/Subfascial Pocket A subfascial pocket can be utilized if the upper pole pinch is 2 centimeters or greater. The subglandular pocket should be reserved for those with upper pole pinch of 3 centimeters or greater and is more appropriate for round implants. These are only guidelines and many other factors contribute to pocket decisions, including not only the thickness of the soft tissue coverage, but also the quality of the tissue. Importantly, the implant choice in subglandular/subfascial pockets can impact results as larger devices may increase the development of a stretch deformity when placed without muscular support. Also, implants with greater cohesiveness, optimal fills and possibly texture, provide a more optimal implant for limiting lower pole stretch over time and maintaining upper pole volume.

The subglandular or subfascial pocket can be easily developed through the inframammary incision and the dissection is performed without the need for muscle division or dual plane creation. Once the incision is made and the lateral pectoral border has been identified, the dissection is carried out either above (subglandular) or deep to (subfascial) the pectoralis fascia. As the dissection is carried medially in the subglandular plane, the midline can quickly be violated due to the lack of sternal muscle attachments that usually limits your dissection in the submuscular plane. When dissecting the subfascial pocket, the fascial attachments assist in limiting the medial dissection. This is important as inadvertent over dissection can lead to implant medialization, visibility and potentially symmastia. The pocket dissection then proceeds to the extent of the desired pocket. The subfascial plane can be a more challenging dissection as there is no natural plane present for this dissection. The subfascial pocket is often preferred over a subglandular pocket when shaped implants are used as it potentially provides a more precise and stable pocket in the upper pole to avoid implant rotation.

Implant Selection The implant selection can significantly impact the outcome in breast augmentation which is why we have so many options when it comes to size, style, texture and composition. The implant choice has an important role in augmentation with lax soft tissue envelopes. When a mastopexy is not going to be performed, stretched, thinned out tissue with stria will be less tolerant to the effects of the underlying implant.

Implant Profile and Size Tissue-based planning proves very beneficial in breast augmentation [27]. The base width of the breast provides

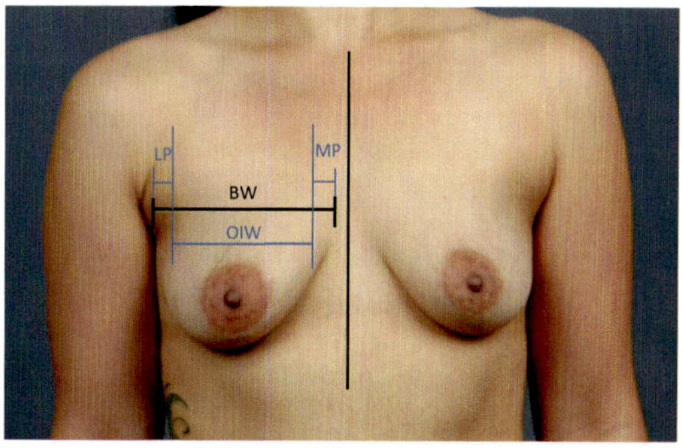

Fig. 4.15 Defining the optimal implant width (OIW) based on the breast width (BW) minus the medial pinch (MP) and Lateral pinch (LP)

Table 4.7 Optimal implant width

Optimal implant width (OIW) = Desired Breast width (BW) – (1/2 medial pinch (MP) + 1/2 Lateral pinch(LP)

a general guide as to the appropriate sizing of the implant for the breast. In considering implant width, critical to that calculation is determining how much the native breast itself will contribute to the final width of the breast. Optimal implant width (OIW) is calculated by determining the desired final breast width (BW) (usually anterior axillary line to 1 cm from the midline of the chest) minus the soft tissue contribution from medial (MP) and lateral pinch (LP) of the breast tissue (Fig. 4.15, Table 4.7).

In a patient with ptosis but with a thin skin brassiere, the implant determination should remain on the smaller side to prevent even more thinning of tissue. In patients who want larger breast, sometimes when trying to achieve a desired volume with limited base width, a higher profile implant may be necessary. The effect of higher profile implants on the skin envelope immediately and over time with potential for stretch deformity must be balanced against the patients desire for more volume [18]. In the heavier breasted patient requiring an augmentation, an implant is often selected with a lower profile and more width/height to add volume to the upper pole but to minimize the impact on the overlying breast. Because of stretch and weight of the implant on the overlying breast tissue, the authors prefer silicone implants over saline implants as saline leads to greater lower pole stretch, palpability, visibility and higher revision rates [5].

Smooth vs Textured Implants Not only the size and profile, but also the implant shell can affect the final outcome. Silicone implants are available as smooth or textured devices. In the United States, smooth implants are utilized in most cases, whereas textured implants predominate in the rest of the world. More recently, textured implants have been associated with BIA-ALCL leading to a growing trend towards use of smooth or nanotextured devices. Smooth implants have several advantages, including a natural mobility and an extremely low risk of wrinkling or palpability. The implants tend to settle at the bottom of the breast pocket and continue to descend with the overlying breast tissue naturally. Due to the laxity of the skin envelopes, surgeons often cite the mobility of the implants as an advantage when there is instability in the overlying breast envelope. This can be very helpful when treating the borderline case as the smooth implant will fill out the skin allowing for expansion and "lift" of the breast.

Textured implants have more stability in the breast pocket. Whereas it has been proposed that adherence of the implant is necessary for stability, it appears that frictional coefficient alone created by the texture provides significant stability [35]. There are many different textures and currently only the less aggressively textured implants that depend on this frictional stability are available. The stability imparted seems to create less lower pole stretch deformity over time. Nanotexture, however, acts as a smooth implant and reduces capsule formation, and is more likely to result in greater lower pole expansion compared to other textured implants and possibly even more than smooth implants.

Thus, when selecting between a smooth, nanotexture or textured device, the challenge is in trying to determine the optimal implant for each patient while minimizing unwanted sequalae. Patients with firm parenchyma and good soft tissue coverage are ideal for a textured implant. When the laxity is too great, as in a weight loss patient, it can be challenging to stabilize the skin envelope adequately over the textured implants. In patients you are trying to lift the breast without performing a lift, the correction of the breast requires expansion of loose breast tissue and this may be better accomplished with a smooth or nanotextured device. However, shaped implants provide a point of maximal projection lower than a round implant which may allow improved expansion of the lower pole and nipple positioning with an augmentation alone, especially when placed above the muscle. The stability and lack of lower pole expansion associated with a more stable textured implants can result in a waterfall (snoopy) deformity with descent of the breast tissue over the implant (Fig. 4.16). Textured devices have additional concerns, including traction wrinkling, double capsule formation, late seromas, and BIA-ALCL (breast implant associated-anaplastic large cell lymphoma) and the future of these devices is uncertain [36–38].

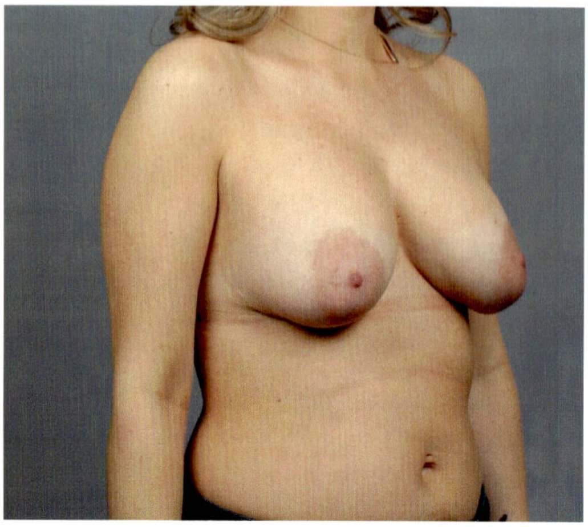

Fig. 4.16 Oblique view of a waterfall deformity

Additional Implant Characteristics Silicone implants have continued to evolve over the last few years, providing enhanced choices for the surgeon. The performance of an implant is multifactorial and dependent on many features. The design of the implant, the shell, the fill ratio, the gel cohesiveness and the gel-to-shell interaction all affect the ultimate performance of the implant in-vivo [9, 10]. Silicone implants are now available as 4th generation and 5th generation devices, based on the cohesiveness of the gel within the implant. Round implants can either be 4th generation, such as the Allergan Natrelle or Mentor MemoryGel implants, or 5th generation, such as the Sientra HSC and HSC+ or Allergan Soft touch and Cohesive implants. The greater the cohesiveness, the more stable the gel is within the device [10]. This greater stability improves the implants performance, expanding lower pole tissue through its increased cohesiveness and yet improved maintenance of upper pole volume. An additional feature has been a trend to increase the gel-to-shell volume ratio, optimizing the fill of the implants. This, likewise, can create a more stable volume in the upper pole as well, in addition to potentially reducing the amount of wrinkling seen with any given implant. All manufacturers have developed and offer implants with optimal fill ratios. In the "no-lift, lift" patients, the optimally filled implants may provide a much more predictable result, allowing lower pole expansion and lift to the breast with less upper pole failure and wrinkling of the implant.

Implant Placement

- Once the pocket has been created, it is irrigated with triple antibiotic betadine solution (50 ml of povidone-iodine, one gram of Cefazolin sodium, 50,000 units of bacitracin mixed in 500 ml of normal saline) or 50% povidine-iodine saline solution and hemostasis is assessed [39]. It is the goal during the operation to achieve prospective hemostasis with minimal blood staining, however a final assessment is mandatory prior to implant placement. The implants are soaked in the irrigation solution prior to insertion. Gloves are changed and rinsed with the irrigation solution to remove any lint or powder.

The implant is then placed either manually or with the assistance of an insertion sleeve such as the Keller funnel [40] (Fig. 4.17).

The opening of the funnel should be cut large enough to allow the implant to pass easily through the funnel. The funnel provides a "minimal to no touch" technique which has been associated with lower capsular contracture rates [41]. The funnel allows for easier implant placement with potentially smaller incision requirements compared to manual placement. Once the implant is in the pocket, a finger-assisted assessment and manipulation of the implant within the pocket is necessary to confirm its proper placement and assure appropriate redraping of the breast parenchyma over the implant. This maneuver is especially important with textured device as these implants are less mobile and less likely to stretch the pocket and thus a distortion or wrinkling of the implant in a tight pocket may be permanent if not resolved prior to closure. Repeated removal and insertions of the implant should be avoided to minimize implant or incision damage, potential contamination and pocket over-dissection.

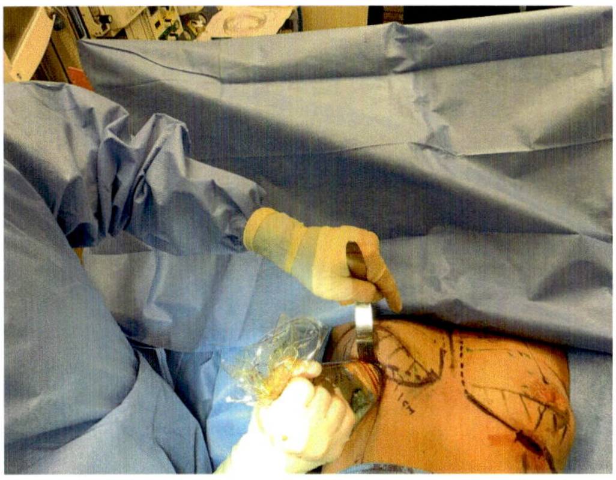

Fig. 4.17 Insertion of the implant with a Keller funnel using the no-touch technique

Closure

- Prior to incision closure, the patient should be placed in the upright position to assess implant position, fold position, symmetry and the adequacy of the dual plane. Any additional adjustments of the dual plane can be accomplished after placed back in the recumbent position by simply retracting the breast tissue superiorly off the implant, identifying the caudal edge of the muscle, and releasing it incrementally off the overlying breast tissue to the desired level.

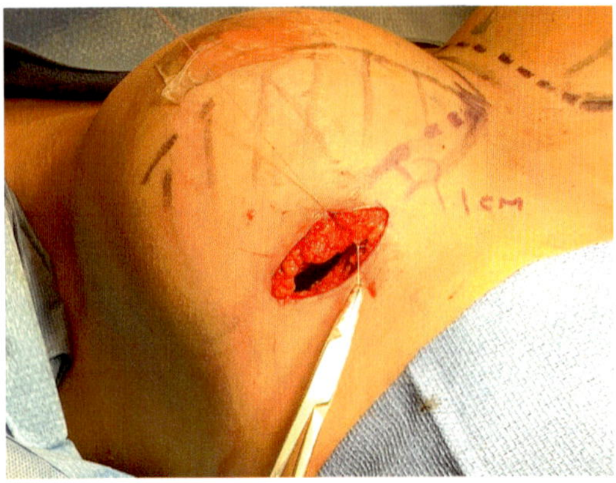

Fig. 4.18 Locking the IMF, requires securing the superficial (Scarpa's) fascia to the underlying deep fascia with a 2–0 Vicryl suture

A significant advantage of the inframammary approach is the ability to accurately and effectively control the fold position during closure of the incision. The cuff of superficial fascia that was preserved during the initial incision is utilized to secure the fold during closure. Although in our practice all inframammary folds are "locked-down" during incisional closure, it could be argued that a well-developed stable IMF that has not been violated or lowered during the procedure is potentially stable and may only require a more superficial closure. However, when the fold is unstable due to either inherent weakness in the fold structure or from disrupting it with fold lowering, closure should include stabilization of the fold structure. This is accomplished by securing caudal edge of the superficial (Scarpa's) fascia present on the lower incisional edge to the underlying deep fascial structures with an absorbable suture such as a 2-0 Vicryl (Fig. 4.18).

This is usually done by simply incorporating the superficial and deep fascia together during a running closure. It may also be performed by first placing 3 to 4 interrupted sutures on the lower flap securing the superficial (Scarpa's) fascia to the underlying deep fascia followed by closure of the skin incision. The skin incision is closed with interrupted deep dermal absorbable suture (4-0 PDS) and a running subcuticular absorbable (4-0 PDS) suture to complete the 3-layer closure of the breast augmentation.

Post-operative Management

Patients are wrapped in an ace wrap for the first 24 hours followed by a sports bra to be worn 23 hours a day for the next 4 weeks. Early range of motion beginning in the recovery room is initiated for all patients which includes shoulder rolls in both directions as well as elevation of the arms outward to the sides and over the head. With smooth devices, implant massage begins postoperative day 4 and includes displacing the implant upward and downward in the pocket, crossing the arms and pulling the implants inward to create cleavage and downward pressure on the implants to stretch the lower pole. Implant massage is contraindicated with textured surface devices as it can irritate the pocket and potentially create serous fluid around the implant or a double capsule formation. The textured implants are placed in a controlled pocket with the implant positioned appropriately at the base of the pocket and displacement with massage or activity could lead to implant malposition or in the case of shaped devices, rotation of the implant. Limited arm movement other than range of motion is recommended for the first week. It is also advisable to limit strenuous exercise for 6–12 weeks with textured implants to avoid early seroma formation Patients can resume regular bras after 4 weeks but should continue with sports bra during bedtime for an additional 2–4 weeks to limit lateral implant migration while recumbent. Normal activity resumes within a few days after surgery, but exercise and high impact activity should be delayed for 3–4 weeks. Whereas smooth implants often seem high initially and often require downward massage and/or the use of breast bands or bandeaus, textured devices that are appropriately seated in the base of the breast pocket and should only occasionally require such maneuvers.

Conclusion

The treatment for breast ptosis and loss of volume involves appropriate evaluation by the plastic surgeon and consideration of the patient's goals regarding her breasts. The techniques of breast augmentation and mastopexy are helpful in treating breast ptosis and loss of volume. A concomitant augmentation mastopexy is a powerful procedure to improve the size and shape of the breast. Some patients defer the mastopexy to avoid the scaring and some patient factors make the mastopexy contraindicated. The ""in-between" patients with pseudoptosis up to an early grade 2 ptosis can be a challenge when trying to expand and lift the breast without performing the mastopexy. Performing the "no lift, lift" while optimizing the implant choice, pocket location and dual plane techniques during breast augmentation for the ptotic breast patient can achieve a satisfactory result and avoid the unnecessary scars of a mastopexy and minimize the morbidity of the operation.

Case Examples Are Given in Figs. 4.19, 4.20, 4.21, and 4.22

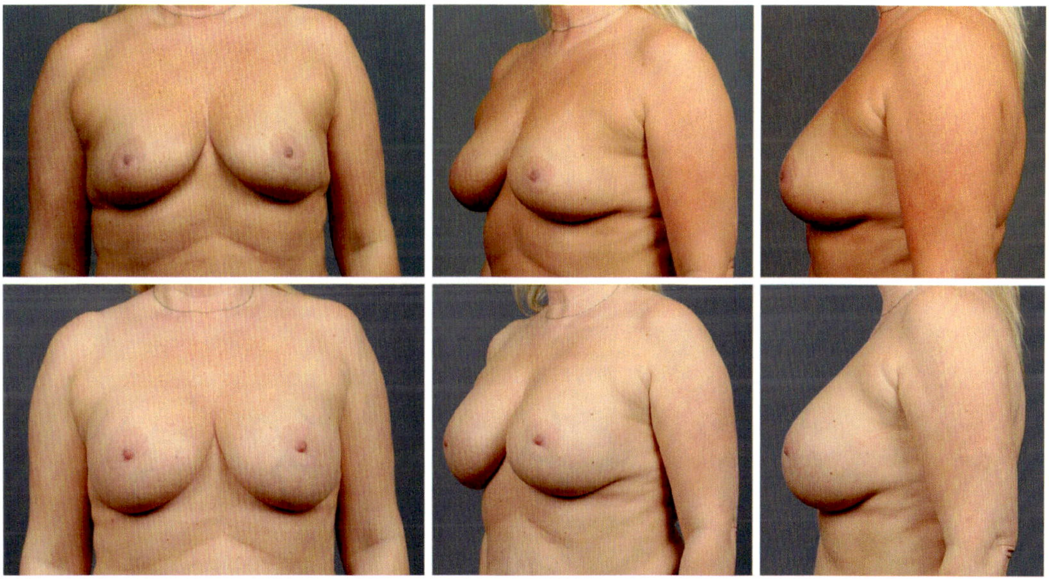

Fig. 4.19 Case 1. 40-year-old female with bilateral grade I ptosis underwent bilateral subglandular augmentation mammoplasty with 435 cc moderate plus textured round silicone implants

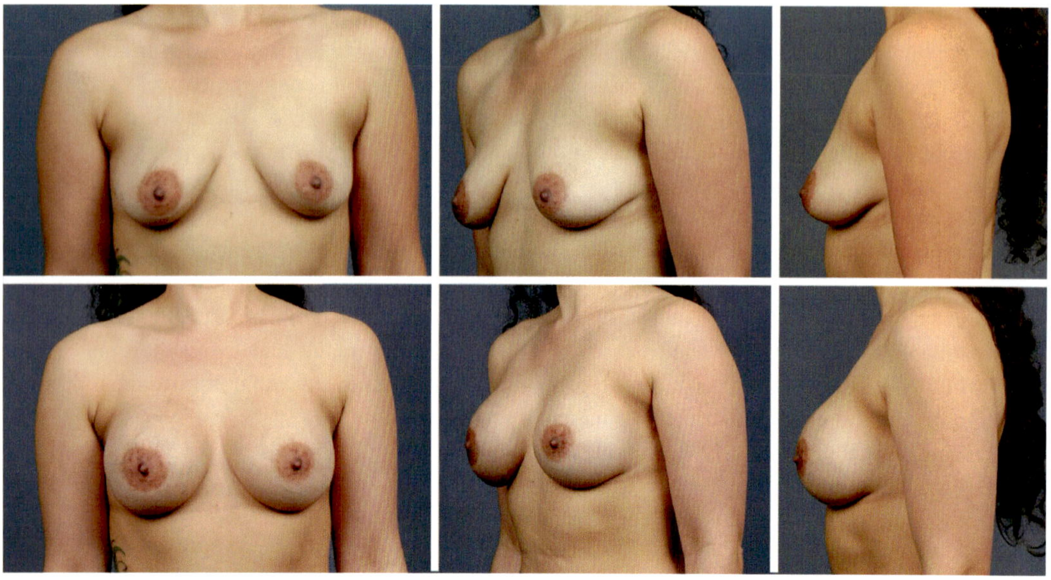

Fig. 4.20 Case 2. 31-year-old female with grade II ptosis on the right and grade I ptosis on the left underwent bilateral subglandular augmentation mammoplasty with 355 cc moderate plus textured round silicone implants

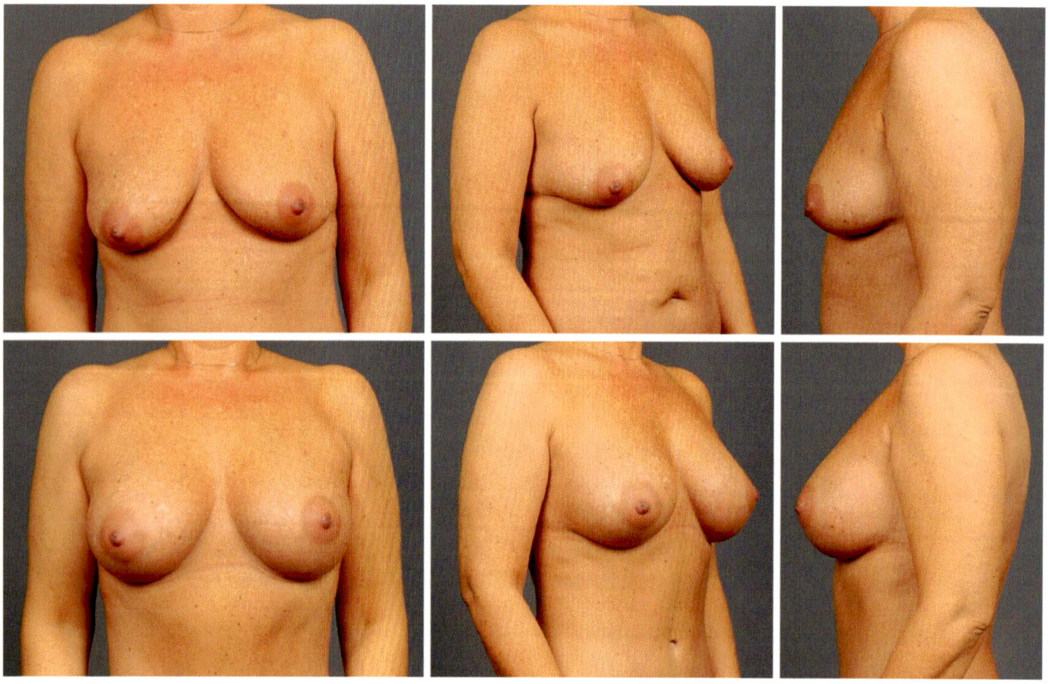

Fig. 4.21 Case 3. 41-year-old female with grade II ptosis on the right and grade I ptosis on the left underwent bilateral subfascial augmentation mammoplasty with 355 cc moderate plus textured round silicone implants

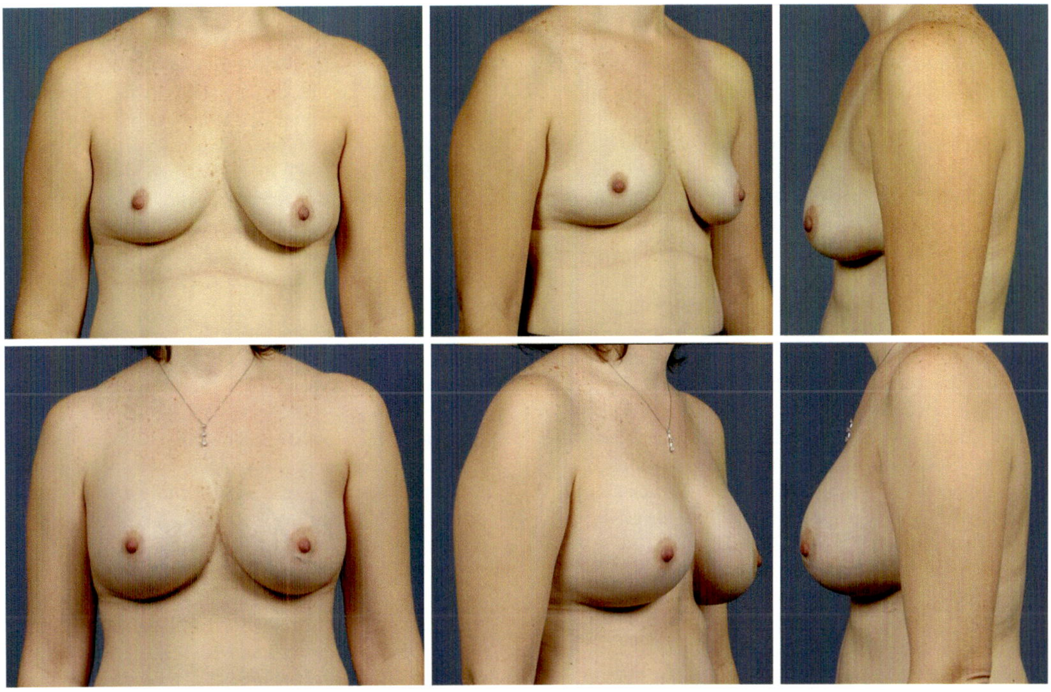

Fig. 4.22 Case 4. 35-year-old female with grade I ptosis on the right and grade II ptosis on the left underwent bilateral submuscular augmentation mammoplasty with a dual plane 3 on the left using a 375 cc moderate plus smooth round silicone implant. On the right she underwent a dual plane 2 with a 425 cc high profile smooth round silicone implant

References

1. 2019 American Society for Aesthetic Plastic Surgery 2019 statistic report. Aesthetic Plastic Surgery National Data Bank; 2019. https://www.surgery.org/sites/default/files/Aesthetic-Society_Stats2019Book_FINAL.pdf.
2. Regnault P. Breast ptosis. Definition and treatment. Clin Plast Surg. 1976;3:193–203.
3. Choudry U, Kim N, Cunningham B. BodyLogicTM System: Intelligent implant selection in primary breast augmentation. J Surg Res. 2014; 186(2):672.
4. Lee MR, Unger JG, Adams WP. The tissue-based triad: a process approach to augmentation mastopexy. Plast Reconstr Surg. 2014;134:215–225.19.
5. Calobrace MB, Schwartz M, Kamakshi Z, Pittman T, Cohen R, Stevens G. Long term safety of textured and smooth breast implants. August: Aesthetic Surgery Journal; 2017.
6. Namnoum JD, Largent J, Kaplan HM, et al. Primary breast augmentation clinical trial outcomes stratified by surgical incision, anatomical placement and implant device type. J Plast Reconstr Aesthet Surg. 2013;66(9):1165–72.
7. Calobrace MB, Stevens WG, Capizzi PJ, et al. Risk factor analysis for capsular contracture: a 10-year Sientra Study using round, smooth, and textured implants for breast augmentation. Plast Reconstr Surg. 2018;141(4S):20S–8S. 26, 27.
8. Gryskiewicz J. Dual-plane breast augmentation for minimal ptosis pseudoptosis (the "in-between" patient). Aesthet Surg J. 2013;33(1):43–65.
9. Tebbetts JB. Form stability of the style 410 implant: definitions, conjectures, and the rest of the story. Plast Reconstr Surg. 2011;128:825–6.
10. Calobrace MB, Capizzi PJ. The biology and evolution of cohesive gel and shaped silicone implants. Plast Reconstr Surg. 2014;134(1S):6S–11S.
11. Coon D, Tuffaha S, Christensen J, Bonawitz SC. Plastic surgery and smoking: a prospective analysis of incidence, compliance, and complications. Plast Reconstr Surg. 2013 Feb;131(2):385–91. https://doi.org/10.1097/PRS.0b013e318277886a.
12. Goltsman D, Munabi NC, Ascherman JA. The association between smoking and plastic surgery outcomes in 40,465 patients: an analysis of the American College of Surgeons National Surgical Quality Improvement Program Data Sets. Plast Reconstr Surg. 2017 Feb;139(2):503–11.
13. Lewin R, Amoroso M, Selvaggi G. The aesthetically ideal position of the nipple-areola complex on the breast. Aesthet Plast Surg. 2016;40(5):724–32.
14. Kalaaji A, Dreyer S, Brinkmann J, et al. Quality of life after breast enlargement with implants versus

augmentation mastopexy: a comparative study. Aesth Surg J. 2018;38(12):1304–15.
15. Wixtrom RN, Stutman RL, Burke RM, et al. Risk of breast implant bacterial contamination from endogenous breast flora, prevention with nipple shields, and implications for biofilm formation. Aesthet Surg J. 2012;32:956–63.
16. Muntan CD, Sundine MJ, Rink RD, Acland RD. Inframammary fold: a histological reappraisal. Plast Reconstr Surg. 2000;105:549–56.
17. Adams WP. The process of breast augmentation: four sequential steps for optimizing outcomes for patients. Plast Reconstr Surg. 2008;122:1892–900.
18. Tebbetts JB, Teitelbaum S. High- and extra-high-projection breast implants: potential consequences for patients. Plast Reconstr Surg. 2010;126:2150–9.
19. Namnoum JD, Largent J, Kaplan HM, Oefelein MG, Brown MH. Primary breast augmentation clinical trial outcomes stratified by surgical incision, anatomical placement and implant device type. J Plast Reconstr Aesthet Surg. 2013;66(9):1165–72.
20. Calobrace MB, Kaufman DL, Gordon AE, et al. Evolving practices in augmentation operative techniques with Sientra HSC round implants. Plast Reconstr Surg. 2014;134(Suppl 1):57S–67S.
21. Hammond DC, Migliori MM, Caplin DA, et al. Mentor contour profile gel implants: clinical outcomes at 6 years. 2012;129:1381–91.
22. Maxwell GP, Van Natta BW, Murphy DK, et al. Natrelle style 410 form-stable silicone breast implants: Core study results at 6 years. Aesthet Surg J. 2012;32:709–17.
23. Jewell ML, Jewell JL. A comparison of outcomes involving highly cohesive, form-stable breast implants from two manufacturers in patients undergoing primary breast augmentation. Aesthetic Surg J. 2010;30:51–65.
24. Hammond DC. Technique and results using MemoryShape implants in aesthetic and reconstructive breast surgery. Plast Reconstr Surg. 2014;134(Suppl 3):16S–26S.
25. Schwartz MR. Algorithm and techniques for using Sientra's silicone gel shaped implants in primary and revision breast augmentation. Plast Reconstr Surg. 2014;134(Suppl 1):18S–27S.
26. Caplin DA. Indications for the use of MemoryShape breast implants in aesthetic and reconstructive breast surgery: long-term clinical outcomes of shaped versus round silicone breast implants. Plast Reconstr Surg. 2014;134(3S):27S–37S.
27. Tebbetts JB, Adams WP. Five critical decisions in breast augmentation using five measurements in 5 minutes: the high five decision support process. Plast Reconstr Surg. 2005;116:2005–16.
28. Strasser EJ. Results of subglandular versus subpectoral augmentation over time: one surgeon's observations. Aesthet Surg J. 2006;26:45–50.
29. Goes JCS, Landecker A. Optimizing outcomes in breast augmentation: seven years of experience with the subfascial plane. Aesth Plast Surg. 2003;27:178–84.
30. Serra-Renom J, Garrido MF, Yoon T. Augmentation mammoplasty with anatomic soft, cohesive silicone implant using the transaxillary approach at a subfascial level with endoscopic assistance. Plast Reconstr Surg. 2005;116:640–5.
31. Graf R, Pace DT, Damasio RC, et al. Subfascial breast augmentation. Chapter 50. In: Innovations in plastic and aesthetic surgery. New York: Springer; 2008. p. 406–13.
32. Stevens WG, Nahabedian MY, Calobrace MB, Harrington JL, et al. Risk factor analysis for capsular contracture: a 5-year Sientra study analysis using round, smooth and textured implants for breast augmentation. Plast Reconstr Surg. 2013;132(5):1115–23.
33. Schaub TA, Ahmad J, Rohrich RJ. Capsular contracture with breast implants in the cosmetic patient: saline versus silicone. A systematic review of the literature. Plast Reconstr Surg. 2010;126:2140–9.
34. Tebbetts JB. Dual plane breast augmentation: optimizing implant-soft-tissue relationships in a wide range of breast types. Plast Reconstr Surg. 2001;107:1255–72.
35. Derby BM, Codner MA. Textured silicone implant use in primary augmentation: core data update and review. Plast Reconstr Surg. 2015;135:113–25.
36. Hall-Findlay EJ. Breast implant complication review: double capsules and late seromas. Plast Reconstr Surg. 2011;127:56–66.
37. Spear SL, Rottman SJ, Glicksman C, et al. Late seromas after breast implants: theory and practice. Plast Reconstr Surg. 2012;130(2):423–35.
38. Loch-Wilkinson AL, Beath KJ, Knight RJW, et al. Breast implant-associated anaplastic large cell lymphoma in Australia and New Zealand: high surface-area textured implants are associated with increased risk. Plast Reconstr Surg. 2017;140(4):645-654.28-30–54.
39. Adams WP, Rios JL, Smith S. Enhancing patient outcomes in aesthetic and reconstructive breast surgery using triple antibiotic breast irrigation: six-year prospective clinical study. Plast Reconstr Surg. 2006;118(Suppl 7):46S–52S.
40. Moyer HR, Ghazi B, Saunders N, Losken A. Contamination in smooth gel breast implant placement: testing a funnel versus digital insertion technique in a cadaver model. Aesthet Surg J. 2012;32(2):194–9.
41. Mladick RA. "No-touch" submuscular saline breast augmentation technique. Aesth Plast Surg. 1993;17:183–92.

Preoperative Assessment in Augmentation Mastopexy

5

M. Bradley Calobrace and Chet Mays

Introduction

Breast ptosis is one of the most common issues seen for evaluation in a plastic surgeon's office. It can be developmental or more commonly acquired, secondary to weight loss, hormonal changes, pregnancy and aging. When evaluating a patient with ptosis, it is important to determine the volume status of the breasts. A mastopexy alone is reserved for a patient in whom the major concern is breast ptosis and not an issue of breast volume or upper pole fullness, as the procedure repositions the breast with only limited removal or transposition of breast tissue. Patients with volume deficiencies or desiring significant upper pole volume often require placement of an implant with the mastopexy.

In certain clinical scenarios, staging an augmentation and mastopexy may provide the safest option with potentially a more optimal outcome [1–3]. However, a simultaneous mastopexy is an excellent option in many patients and can be performed safely with high patient satisfaction [4–8]. The surgical approach to the patient with ptotic breast desiring or requiring a breast implant for correction is determined following a thorough evaluation. Appropriate breast measurements, breast tissue density, quality of skin, NAC (nipple areolar complex) and breast ptosis, chest wall characteristics, breast footprint and the patient's expectations all must be considered in planning for the procedure. For the patient with limited ptosis, a breast augmentation alone may provide adequate rejuvenation. If a mastopexy is deemed necessary with the augmentation, many types of mastopexy techniques described to address the ptotic breast can be utilized, including circumareolar, circumvertical, circumvertical with IMF wedge, inframammary technique or the inverted-T scar technique [9–13].

In preoperative planning, one must plan the implant pocket including dual-plane submuscular, subfascial or subglandular. The pocket selection can impact the surgical approach, the vascularity of the skin flaps and NAC and long-term outcome. Likewise, a wide variety of breast implants options are available to optimize final results. Implant characteristics including implant fill, shell texturization, silicone gel cohesiveness, gel-to-shell fill ratios, projections and shape can impact the final results [14, 15].

M. B. Calobrace (✉)
Private Practice, CaloAesthetics Plastic Surgery Center, Louisville, KY, USA

Clinical Faculty, University of Louisville, Division of Plastic Surgery, Louisville, KY, USA

Clinical Faculty, University of Kentucky, Division of Plastic Surgery, Lexington, KY, USA
e-mail: drbrad@calobrace.com

C. Mays
Private Practice, CaloAesthetics Plastic Surgery Center, Louisville, KY, USA

Clinical Faculty, University of Louisville, Division of Plastic Surgery, Louisville, KY, USA

M. B. Calobrace et al. (eds.), *Augmentation Mastopexy*,
https://doi.org/10.1007/978-3-030-48226-8_5

Perioperative decision making is critical to a successful outcome in augmentation mastopexy surgery. In this chapter, we will review our approach to decision making with a focus on patient selection, determination of mastopexy approach, pocket and implant selection in hopes of providing a foundation for decision making that will provide optimal results in the augmentation mastopexy patient.

Pre-operative Evaluation

The evaluation should begin with a breast exam with breast measurements including the base width, sternal notch to nipple distance, nipple to fold distance (at rest and under maximal stretch) (Fig. 5.1).

The amount of ptosis present should also be assessed. Ptosis has classically been described as per Regnault based on the relationship of the NAC to the inframammary fold [16]. Although this provides some information about the degree of breast ptosis, it in of itself is insufficient to describe the true extent of breast ptosis. A more complete assessment of ptosis is summarized in Table 5.1 and Fig. 5.2.

Patients with different grades of ptosis per the Regnault's classification may have completely

Table 5.1 Assessment of breast ptosis

Relationship of the NAC to the IMF (Regnault's degree of ptosis)
(a) **Grade 1**: Nipple at the level of the inframammary fold, above the lower contour of the gland
(b) **Grade 2:** Nipple below the level of the inframammary fold, above the lower contour of the gland
(c) **Grade 3:** Nipple below the level of the inframammary fold, at the lower contour of the gland
Amount of breast tissue overhanging the fold
Location of the NAC on the breast mound
Amount of vertical excess and horizontal excess
Footprint of the breast on the chest wall – Low, medium, high
Quality and quantity of breast parenchyma and skin

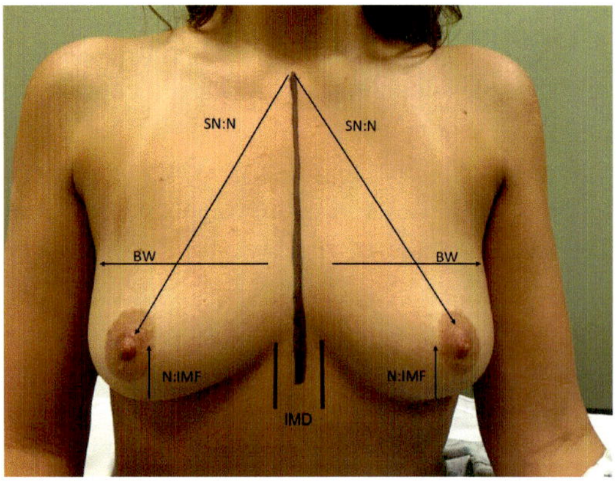

Fig. 5.2 Breast measurements

Fig. 5.1 Regnault Classifications of Ptosis

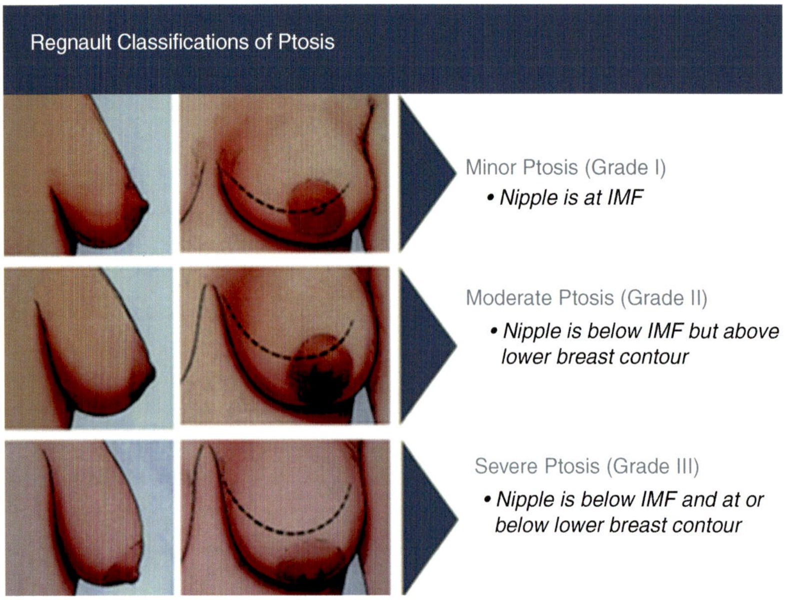

different breast compositions including the quality of breast tissue and skin, the quantity of breast tissue present and the vertical excess present as shown in Figs. 5.3 and 5.4 (see also Table 5.2).

Assessment should also include evaluation of the skin thickness and elasticity, the quantity and distribution of subcutaneous fat, the composition and firmness of the breast parenchyma, the integrity of the Cooper's ligaments, the nature and position of the underlying musculature and the shape and slope of the underlying chest wall. All these aspects of the breast composition influence the shape of the breast and ultimately the outcome after the augmentation mastopexy.

Blood Supply as Impacts Decisions in Mastopexy and Pocket Selection

When performing an augmentation mastopexy, an understanding and assessment of the vascular anatomy is critical to performing the procedure safely [17]. The breast has a rich blood supply from multiple sources, including the internal mammary artery perforators, the lateral thoracic arteries, the thoracoacromial and the anterolateral and anteromedial intercostal perforators. Implant selection, pocket selection, mastopexy performed and the extent of skin undermining all impact the blood supply to the NAC and breast skin flaps.

The inferior pedicle and central pedicle are supplied by the fourth branch of the IMA that courses deeply across the medial breast to enter through Wuringer's septum just above the 5th rib and medial to the breast meridian approximately 1–2 cm above the IMF. The Inferior pedicle also has additional blood supply through contribution from intercostal perforators along the IMF. In the augmentation mastopexy procedure, the implant pocket development always includes division of the 4th branch of the IMA and thus the central pedicle and a significant portion of the inferior pedicle blood supply has been sacrificed.

To insure the most reliable blood supply to the NAC and skin flaps, the superior pedicle and occasionally the superomedial pedicles are utilized. The superior pedicle is supplied by the second branch of the internal mammary artery (IMA) that emerges deep from the second interspace and courses superficial across the medial upper breast to enter the NAC slightly medial to the midline and approximately one centimeter deep. The medial pedicle is supplied by the third branch of the IMA that emerges from the third interspace and similarly courses superficially across the breast parenchyma to the medial aspect of the NAC. The superficial position of these vessels in the upper pole allow the implant placement and mastopexy without interfering with the blood supply. However, these vessels take origin along the sternal border in the medial aspect of the implant pocket and can be inadvertently sacrificed when aggressive medial pectoral muscle division is performed.

Additionally, implant and pocket selection affect the blood supply to the overlying breast. The subpectoral pocket maintains the musculocutaneous perforators (unless an extensive dual plane is performed) and is less likely to interfere with the blood supply compared to a subglandular/subfascial pocket. Likewise, larger implants placed in any pocket, but especially the subglandular/subfascial pocket, that results in undue tension on the mastopexy closure can also create vascular compromise to the NAC or overlying skin flaps, resulting in skin or NAC necrosis.

Patient Expectations

In planning the operative approach, it cannot be overstated the importance of patient education is and the need to spend some time understanding the patient's desired outcome and expectations with the operation. Patients requiring an augmentation mastopexy are more likely to have undergone changes to the breast from weight loss or postpartum and suffer the sequalae of increased laxity of the tissue, stria, nipple and breast ptosis,

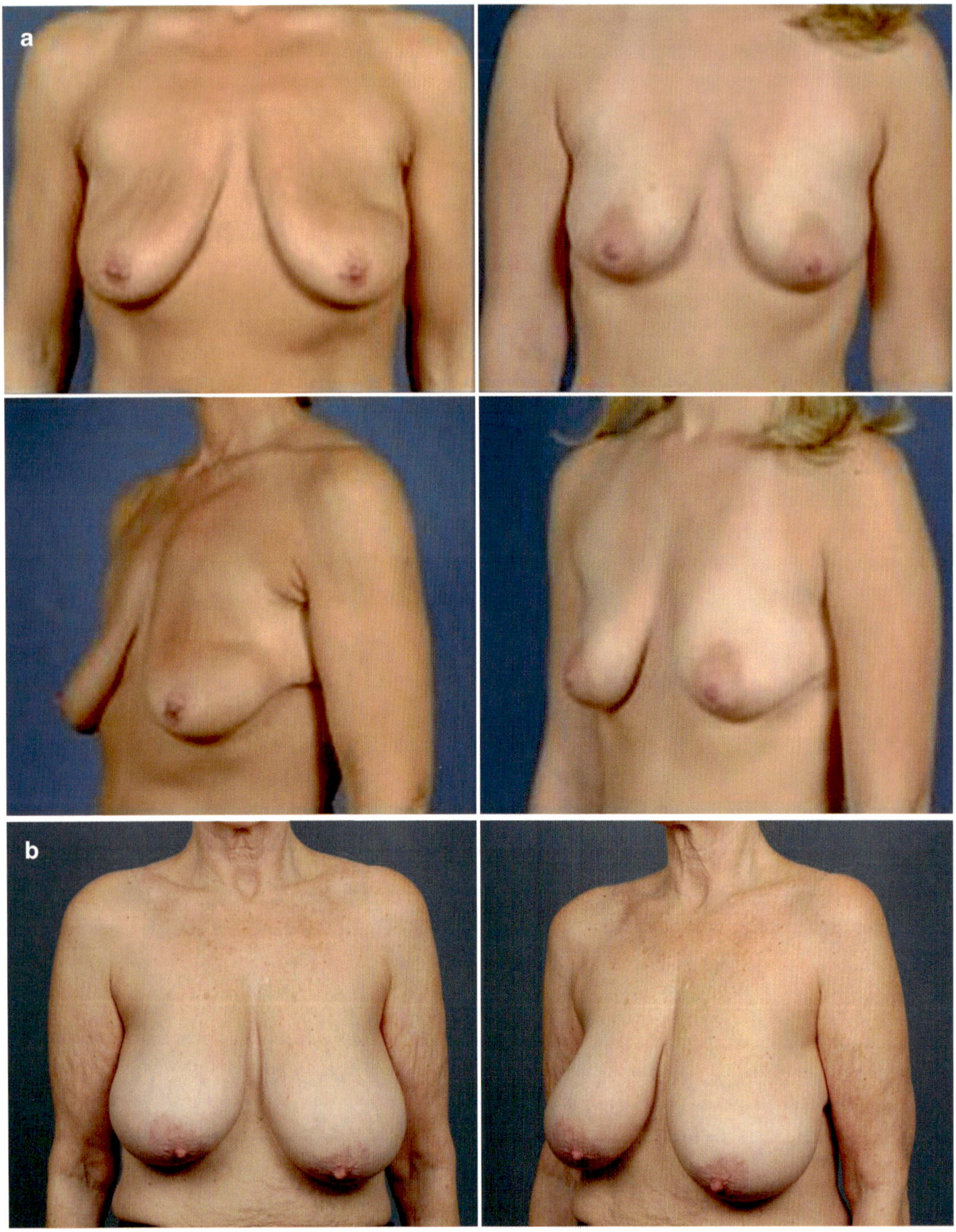

Fig. 5.3 (**a**) Two patients shown with Grade 2 ptosis. The nipple is below the IMF but above the lower breast contour. Note although both patients have the same level of ptosis, the patient on the left has much greater vertical excess. (**b**) One patient shown with Grade 3 ptosis. The nipple is below the IMF and below the lower breast contour. Vertical excess on the left breast is >10 cm which makes her a good candidate for a staged augmentation mastopexy

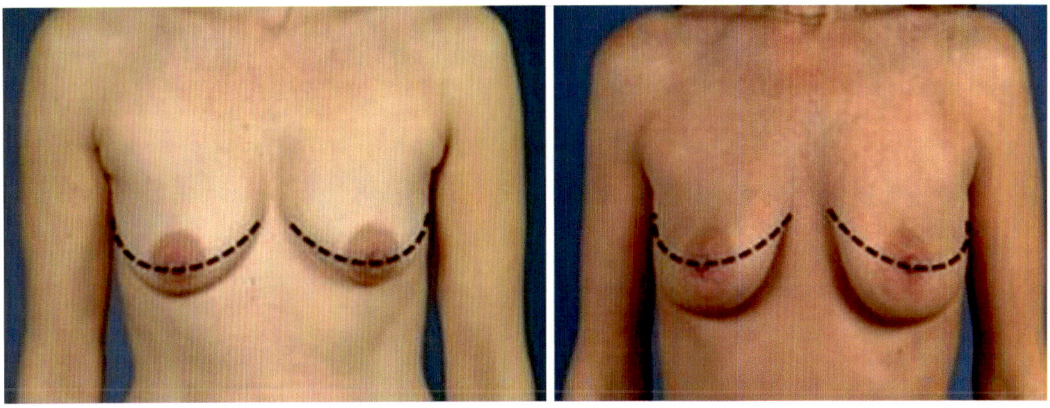

Fig. 5.4 Grade 1 Ptosis - The dotted line represents the reflection of the inframammary fold with the nipple position at the fold (Grade 1 ptosis), and yet the vertical excess in much greater on the patient to the right

Table 5.2 Formula for determination of vertical excess

Vertical excess (VE)
VE = new nipple to actual IMF – New N to new IMF
VE > 8-10 cm consider staging augmentation mastopexy

and loss of parenchymal volume and/or firmness. Thus, managing expectation and these challenging cases in paramount.

Patients often are unaware of asymmetries, the significant atrophy of the breasts, and differences in the chest wall that affect the final outcome. During the evaluation, it is important to determine what "look" the patient would desire, especially in terms of nipple position and volume in the upper pole. Patients need to understand the limitations in achieving a desired look to the breast compared to a breast augmentation alone. In a recent quality of life study comparing breast augmentation patients to augmentation mastopexy patients, breast augmentation patients were significantly more satisfied with the aesthetic outcome and the quality of life on many psychosocial aspects. The augmentation mastopexy patients reported dissatisfaction with shape, scarring, symmetry and the nipple-areolar complex [18]. Based on the patient's desires, the operative design considers the patient's desires in an effort to achieve a satisfactory result for the patient. A patient desiring a more natural look may benefit more from a subpectoral implant, a less cohesive implant or a shaped device, whereas a patient desiring more volume and roundness in the upper pole may require a more cohesive higher profile implant and potentially the implant placed above the muscle. Undoubtedly, there are limitations in what can be achieved in augmentation mastopexy but good perioperative decision making with an operative approach specifically designed to meet the patient's goals is more likely to provide optimal results for each patient.

Patients should be educated on their specific clinical findings, with a frank discussion not only about the anticipated results, but also the limitations of the procedure. The results of an augmentation mastopexy are not the same as a breast augmentation in most patients [18]. The unique challenges need to be understood by the patient, with an understanding that a revision may be necessary to achieve the final outcome. The procedure can be formidable because it requires enlarging the breast with the augmentation and simultaneously reducing the breast and skin envelope with the mastopexy. All issues related both to the mastopexy and the augmentation must be discussed including the associated complications. These patients will have scars on the breast, which at times can heal unpredictably, and a clear understanding of the location of the scars and anticipated outcome should be discussed.

Selection of Procedure

Breast Augmentation Patients with deflated breasts often describe their breasts as "droopy" and often come to the consultation with the impression they need a breast lift. If the patient has pseudoptosis or grade 1 ptosis and the stretched nipple-to-fold distance does not exceed 9.5–10 cm, a breast augmentation alone without a mastopexy may provide satisfactory correction and meet the patient's goals [7]. Based on the clinical setting, the NAC may be positioned slightly lower and the upper pole less full depending on implant and pocket selection. The subglandular/subfascial pocket may facilitate expansion and lift of the breast in borderline cases. In these patients, there must ultimately be congruity in the volume of the breast and the overlying skin envelope. If the patient's desired breast size is less than what can satisfactorily fill out the skin envelope or if the NAC position desired is greater than what can be accomplished with the breast augmentation alone, some type of mastopexy may be required. Thus, the desired look of the patient can determine the surgical approach, which might be quite different for patients with similar preoperative breast appearance.

Mastopexy The ideal candidate for a mastopexy alone is a patient that is relatively satisfied with her volume and is mainly looking for correction in her breast ptosis and improvement in breast shape. The ideal candidate has adequate breast volume and enough ptosis to warrant a mastopexy and the scars associated with these procedures. The patient is looking for a more natural upper pole; a more rounded upper pole with significant cleavage is not a goal of these patients.

Augmentation Mastopexy A patient desiring considerably more volume or significant upper pole volume and cleavage would be better served with an augmentation mastopexy technique. The exception would be the patient desiring those attributes, but the simultaneous procedure is deemed inappropriate or unsafe. (Table 5.3) In these cases, a mastopexy can be performed at the initial procedure, followed at least 6 months to 1 year later with a staged breast augmentation (see Fig. 5.3b).

Table 5.3 Indications for Staged Augmentation Mastopexy

Indications for staged augmentation Mastopexy
Obesity: BMI >30
Large, pendulous breasts - needs volume reduction
Significant breast ptosis - NAC elevation >5-6 cm
Vertical excess >8–10 cm
Unrealistic expectations understand reoperation rate > 20%
Smokers who refuse to quit

Mastopexy Selection

When determined that a simultaneous augmentation mastopexy is deemed appropriate, the approach to the mastopexy is based on the preoperative evaluation. The assessment of the level of ptosis (see Table 5.1) guides the surgeon in assessing the need for NAC elevation as well as skin envelope reduction and possibly parenchymal excision.

Circumareolar Patients with borderline ptosis, grade 1 ptosis or pseudoptosis (N-IMF under maximal stretch 10 cm), low NAC (such as constricted breast deformity) or tuberous breast deformity may benefit from a circumareolar mastopexy. This can elevate the NAC modestly (2 cm or less) and can reduce the areolar diameter. There should be minimal overhang of breast over the fold and limited horizontal laxity. The circumareolar mastopexy should be used very selectively, as it can create widening and flattening of the breast, which may prove beneficial in a tuberous breast deformity but undesirable in a deflated, flattened breast.

Circumvertical Patients with moderate ptosis, grade 1 or 2, requiring NAC elevation of usually less than 4 cm, with modest amounts of breast overhanging the fold can be addressed with a circumvertical mastopexy with or without removal of a small amount of skin along the fold (horizontal wedge). These patients tend to have more horizontal laxity requiring breast narrowing with only a modest amount of reduction in the vertical component.

Circumvertical with Inverted-T Skin Excision For patients with more severe ptosis, grade 2 or 3, with significant vertical excess and overhang over the fold, a circumvertical with inverted-T skin excision is more appropriate to achieve optimal results. The greater the vertical excess and laxity, the greater the horizontal wedge and the longer the incision becomes along the inframammary fold.

When planning the type of mastopexy, it is important to distinguish between the pedicle design and the skin excision design of the mastopexy [19]. In augmentation mastopexy, the design of the more ptotic breast is always a circumvertical approach with the superior or occasional the superomedial pedicle as the pedicle blood supply. The only difference in the approach is whether skin needs to be excised along the fold. Thus, even in the more ptotic breasts with significant laxity requiring an inverted-T skin pattern excision, the parenchymal and pedicle design is still a circumvertical approach with a superior pedicle. In these patients, if the breasts are heavy with excessive ptotic parenchyma, a lower pole parenchymal resection along with the skin excision is optimal to reduce the likelihood of recurrent ptosis post-operatively [20].

Lower pole Mastopexy There is an occasional patient, especially in secondary cases, in which the NAC is in satisfactory position but a significant amount of glandular ptosis or pseudoptosis is present. These patients may benefit from simply an inframammary fold resection (smile mastopexy) or vertical-horizontal resection (sailboat mastopexy) without transposing the NAC [21]. This can address both vertical and horizontal laxity without jeopardizing NAC circulation and placing an unnecessary scar around the areola.

Implant Selection

In augmentation mastopexy, implant selection can significantly impact the final outcome in an augmentation mastopexy case. The implant selection has greater impact as the augmentation is performed in the face of a mastopexy with soft tissue envelopes which are more lax, stretched, thinned with stria and less tolerant to the effects of the underlying implant.

Implant Profile and Size Tissue-based planning proves very beneficial in augmentation mastopexy just as it does in augmentation alone [7]. The base width of the breast provides a general guide as to the appropriate sizing of the implant for the breast. In considering implant width, critical to that calculation is determining how much the native breast itself will contribute to the final width of the breast. Optimal implant width is calculated by determining the desired final breast width (usually anterior axillary line to 1 cm from the midline of the chest) minus the soft tissue contribution from the native breast using the medial and lateral pinch (see Table 5.4).

In a patient with ptosis but with a thin skin brassiere, the implant determination will be identical to a straightforward breast augmentation. In breasts with more significant volume and heavier breasts, this calculation might lead to a smaller implant compared to a breast augmentation alone. When trying to achieve a desired volume with limited base width, a higher profile implant may be deemed as appropriate in these patients. However, the skin envelope laxity with the planned mastopexy must be taken into consideration. The effect of a high-profile implant on the skin envelope immediately on the skin flaps and over time with potential for stretch deformity must be balanced against the patients desire for more volume [22]. In the heavier breasted patient requiring an augmentation and mastopexy, an

Table 5.4 Determining optimal implant width

Optimal implant width = desired breast width – (1/2 medial pinch + 1/2 lateral pinch)

implant is often selected with a lower profile and more width/height to add volume to the upper pole but to minimize the impact on the overlying breast. Oversized implants not only create long term effects, the undue tension created when mastopexy flaps are closed around a larger implant can impact circulation to the NAC and overlying breast skin flaps, leading to ischemia and necrosis. The pocket selection with these implants can also impact circulation. Because of stretch and weight of the implant on the overlying breast tissue, the author prefers silicone implants over saline implants as saline leads to greater lower pole stretch, palpability, visibility and higher revision rates.

Smooth vs Textured Implants Not only the size and profile, but also the implant shell that makes up a silicone implant can affect the final outcome. Silicone implants are available as smooth or textured devices. In the United States and currently in our practice, smooth implants are utilized in the vast majority of cases, whereas textured implants predominate in the rest of the world. Smooth implants have several advantages, including a natural mobility and an extremely low risk of wrinkling or palpability. The implants tend to settle at the bottom of the breast pocket and continue to descend with the overlying breast tissue naturally. When performing a mastopexy with the augmentation, the smooth implants can be translocated superiorly taking the tension off the closure and will naturally descend over time back into the newly lifted skin envelope. Due to the laxity of the skin envelopes, surgeons often cite the mobility of the implants as an advantage when there is instability in the overlying breast envelope.

Textured implants have more stability in the breast pocket. Whereas it has been proposed that adherence of the implant is necessary for stability, it appears that frictional coefficient alone created by the texture provides significant stability [23]. It is mostly agreed that in cosmetic procedures, even the most aggressively textured device rarely actually achieves adherence and depends mostly on friction for its stability. It is important to understand each of the textures and what impact these implants might have on the final result. Implant texturization can be considered in gradients 1–4, with the most aggressively textured implants being a 4 such as polyurethane foam. Grade 3 texture is seen in salt-loss processing (such as the Biocell implant) or with the ammonium carbonate processing (Sientra), grade 2 with implant imprinting process (Siltex of Mentor), and grade 1 with Nano-texturing (such as the Motiva) and a smooth implant [24] (see Table 5.5).

Table 5.5 Implant texture levels

Grade	Method	Brand
4	Polyurethane foam coating	Bristol-Meyers Squibb (removed from US market 1991)
3	Salt-loss processing	Biocell of Allergan
3	Ammonium carbonate processing	Sientra
2	Imprinting process	Siltex of Mentor
1	Nanotexturing	Motiva

The more aggressive the texture, in general, the more stable the implant. In the author's opinion, textured implants can significantly improve the quality of results in many augmentation mastopexy patients. The stability imparted seems to create less lower pole stretch deformity over time. Textured implants allows not only for placement of round implants, but also the possibility of using an anatomic shaped implant. The textured devices, when placed subglandular or subfascial, has been correlated with a lower capsular contracture rate compared to smooth devices [25, 26]. This can liberalize the use of many different pockets in selected patients.

When selecting between a smooth and textured device, the challenge is in trying to determine the optimal implant for each patient while minimizing unwanted sequalae. In the author's experience, textured devices can provide excellent stability in an otherwise unstable breast envelope and is the implant of choice in many patients. Patients with sloping chest walls are also ideal for textured devices as the texture sta-

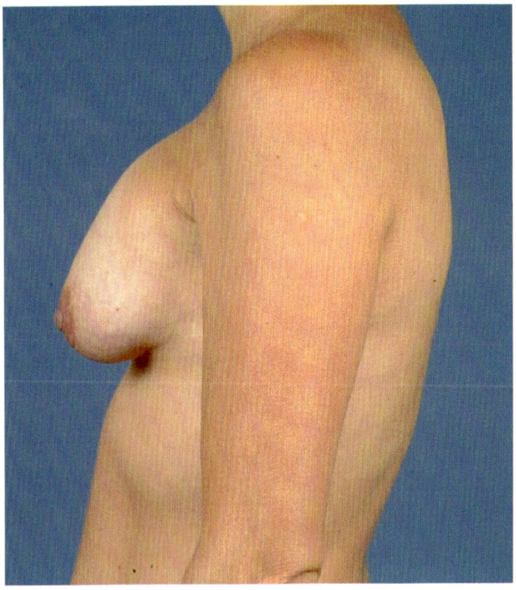

Fig. 5.5 Waterfall deformity

bilizes the implant and minimizes migration, especially lateral slip of the implant into the axilla. Patients with firm parenchyma and good soft tissue coverage are ideal for a textured implant. When the laxity is too great, as in a weight loss patient, it can be challenging to stabilize the skin envelope adequately over the textured implants. There is an increased risk of waterfall deformity when textured implants are placed under very lax skin envelopes, and the benefits of stability have to be weighed against this possibility (Fig. 5.5).

Textured implants are more likely to wrinkle compared to a smooth silicone implant. When the skin envelope is thin and wrinkling is a possibility postoperatively, a smooth device may prove advantageous. The newer, more cohesive implants with optimal fills have significantly decreased the amount of wrinkling seen, thus the difference between smooth and textured as it relates to wrinkling may be more theoretical than reality. Textured devices have additional concerns, including double capsule formation, late seromas, and the emerging relationship to BIA-ALCL (breast implant associated-anaplastic large cell lymphoma) [27–29]. The advantages of the textured device in any clinical situation must therefore be weighed against the possibilities of these unfortunate sequela and the possibilities discussed openly and frankly as part of the consent process. Currently, in light of all issues related to textured implants, smooth implants have increasingly been the implant of choice in augmentation mastpexy procedures. If additional stability is required and a textured device is not possible, a stabilizing mesh reinforcement is utilized with the smooth implant as an alternative.

Shaped Implants Shaped implants can provide advantages in certain types of patients and may be appropriate in an augmentation mastopexy. Of course, all shaped implants are textured so the advantages and disadvantages of textured devices apply when considering a shaped device.

There are many varieties of shaped devices and all the manufacturers have a matrix of choices available to accommodate different shaped breasts and chest walls. Shaped implants in general create a more natural sloping upper pole. Due to the increased cohesiveness of the gel, however, the upper pole volume is more stable compared to other implants. An implant that is taller than it is wide can provide a nice volume distribution for a long-chested patient with a low breast footprint without over augmenting the breast. A patient with a high foot print or a very wide base width can benefit from a shaped implant that is wider than it is tall, allowing improved cleavage without over-augmenting the breast and/or upper poles of the breast.

Shaped implants are uniquely beneficial when performing an augmentation mastopexy on patients with constricted breast or tuberous breast deformities. These augmentations are often performed in conjunction with a circumareolar mastopexy to optimize results. The shaped implant provides a point of maximal projection lower than a round implant allowing improved expansion and nipple positioning with the augmentation. The increased cohesiveness of the gel and the texturization of the implant provides stability that tends to improve the expansion of the lower pole.

Additional Implant Characteristics Silicone implants have continued to evolve over the last few years, providing enhanced choices for the surgeon. The performance of an implant is multifactorial and dependent on many features. The design of the implant, the shell, the gel cohesiveness, the gel-to-shell fill ratio, the gel cohesiveness and the gel-to-shell interaction all affect the ultimate performance of the implant in-vivo [14, 15]. Silicone implants are now available as 4th generation and 5th generation devices, based on the cohesiveness of the gel within the implant. All shaped devices are 5th generation devices. Round implants can either be 4th generation, such as the Allergan Natrelle or Mentor MemoryGel implants, or 5th generation, such as the Sientra HSC and HSC+ or Allergan Soft touch and Cohesive implants. The greater the cohesiveness, the more stable the gel is within the device [15]. This can impact the appearance of the upper pole, stabilizing the sloping look of a shaped device or the rounded look of a round device. The 4th generation gels will provide less stability in the implant shape, leading to a more natural upper pole or even failure to maintain the volume in the upper pole over time.

An additional feature has been to increase the gel-to-shell volume ratio, optimizing the fill of the implants. This can create a more stable volume in the upper pole as well, in addition to potentially reducing the amount of wrinkling seen with any given implant. All manufacturers have developed and offer implants with optimal fill ratios. In the augmentation mastopexy patients with more lax, thinner skin, the optimally-filled implants have provided a much more predictable result with less upper pole failure and wrinkling of the implant.

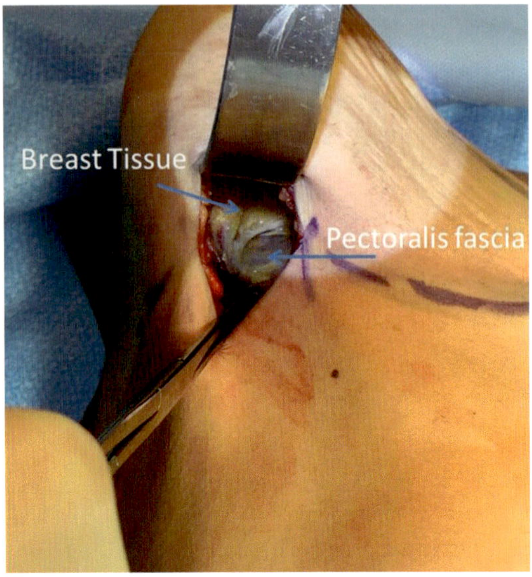

Fig. 5.6 Subglandular pocket creation noting the breast tissue being lifted off of the pectoralis major muscle

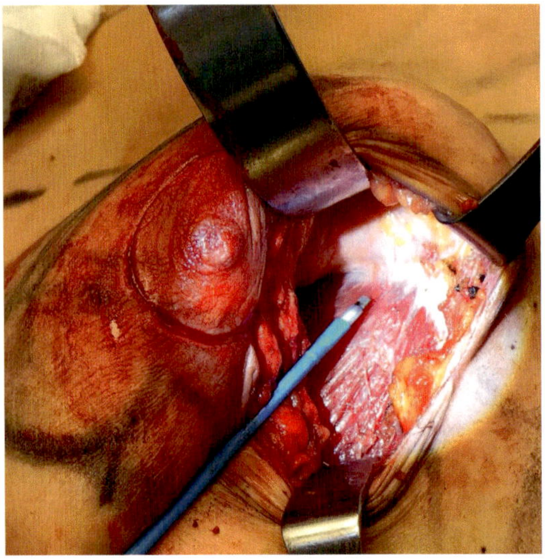

Fig.5.7 Subfascial pocket creation. Note the elevation of the fascia off of the underlying pectoralis major muscle

Pocket Selection

Pocket selection for the augmentation mastopexy is often one of the most overlooked aspects and may have the greatest impact on the final results. The pocket choices include the submuscular, subfascial and subglandular. The dual plane submuscular pocket is by far the most common implant pocket utilized (see Figs. 5.6, 5.7, 5.8, and 5.9).

The dual plane pocket allows for submuscular pocket with additional coverage and support in the upper portion of the breast while being subglandular and allowing for greater expansion in the lower poles of the breast [27].

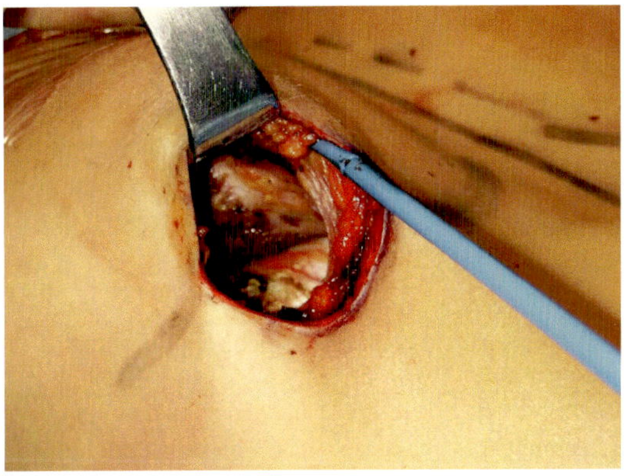

Fig. 5.8 Submuscular pocket creation. Note the elevated pectoralis major muscle with underlying ribcage. The dual plane submuscular pocket is mandatory if the upper pole pinch test is less than 2 cm in order to avoid upper pole implant visibility and wrinkling

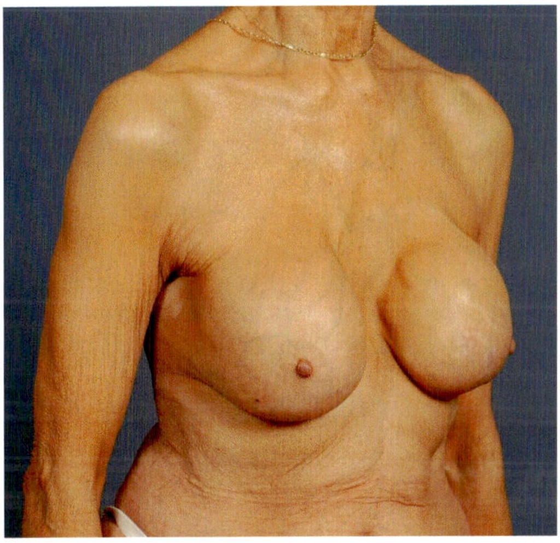

Fig. 5.9 Patient shown with upper pole visibility and wrinkling

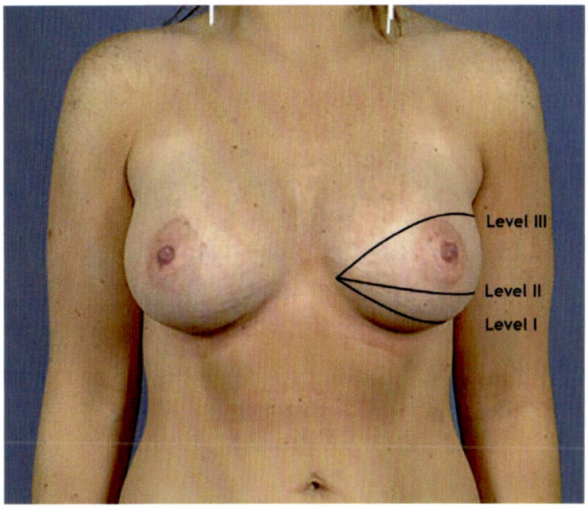

Fig. 5.10 Dual plane levels shown based on the level of the release of the breast tissue. Dual plane 1 is release of the pectoralis off of the inferior costal attachments seen with all submuscular augmentations. Dual plane 2 is release of the breast tissue off of the pectoralis muscle to just below the NAC. A dual plane 3 is release of the breast tissue to above the NAC

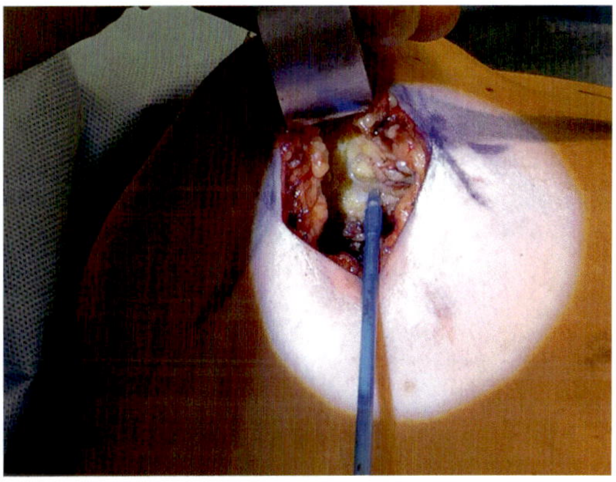

Fig. 5.11 Creation of a dual plane with release of the breast tissue off of the underlying cut edge of the pectoralis muscle

Interestingly, the tighter or looser the lower pole, the greater the level of dual plane needed. The constricted, lower pole breast requires greater dual plane, level 2 or 3, to allow for maximal expansion of the tight lower pole (see Figs. 5.10 and 5.11).

Muscle in the lower pole would limit the amount of expansion possible in this tight tissue envelope. The additional parenchymal exposure with the dual planes allows for parenchymal expansion techniques such as radial scoring. The very lax, loose breast also requires greater expansion for correction. Whereas, one might think this is not necessarily due to the overlying mastopexy that is capable of tightening the tissue over the implant, the very lax breast even after a mastopexy will often fall off of the under expanded lower pole and implant, leading to a waterfall deformity. The ability of the implant to have some influence over the overlying breast tissue is an important and yet often misunderstood concepts for achieving long-term success in augmentation mastopexy. The most lax and thin breast envelopes, such as the weight loss patients, require the lifting effect of the implant to avoid a waterfall deformity with time.

A subfascial pocket is possible if the upper pole pinch is 2 cm or greater. In the author's opinion, the subglandular pocket should be reserved for those with upper pole pinch of 3 cm or greater. These are guidelines and many other factors contribute to pocket decisions, including not only the thickness of the soft tissue coverage, but also the quality of the tissue. Additionally, the implant decision impacts the appropriateness of placing the implant above the muscle. There is good evidence that when a subglandular/subfascial pocket is utilized, a textured device has a lower capsular contracture rate compared to a smooth implant. Likewise, the size of the implant can impact the development of a stretch deformity when placed without muscular support. Finally, implants placed above the muscle have less coverage in the upper pole compared to submuscular implants. Thus, when above the muscle, implants with greater cohesiveness, optimal fills and possible texture, provide a more optimal implant for limiting lower pole stretch over time and maintaining upper pole volume.

Conclusion

The treatment for breast ptosis and loss of volume involves appropriate evaluation by the plastic surgeon taking into account the patient's goals regarding her breasts. The upper pole volume of the breast after a mastopexy alone can often still be deficient even though the shape and contour have been improved. The addition of an implant can adequately fill this upper pole deficit. The implant type, pocket location and mastopexy approached are dictated by a variety of patient factors that must be considered. Knowing which patients are candidates for a staged vs. simultaneous augmentation mastopexy is key to a great outcome with low revision rates in a procedure that is challenging and historically known for higher revision rates.

Summary Box – Pearls for Success

Analyze the ptotic breast
Determine patient goals for aesthetic appearance of the breast
Determine single vs. staged augmentation mastopexy
Determine mastopexy technique and pedicle choice, most commonly superior or superomedial.
Avoid large implants to prevent stress on the soft tissue envelope.
Consider texture or smooth implants with mesh reinforcement when a sloping chest wall is present

Case Examples

Case 1 (Fig. 5.12)

Twenty-five-year-old female with grade III ptosis. Bilateral augmentation vertical mastopexy with submuscular smooth round saline implants filled to 420 cc on the right and 450 cc on the left.

Case 2 (Fig. 5.13)

Thirty-five year old female with grade III ptosis. Bilateral Periareolar vertical mastopexy with subfascial augmentation with 325 cc moderate profile textured round silicone implants.

Case 3 (Fig. 5.14)

Twenty-four year old female with grade III ptosis. Bilateral Inverted-T mastopexy with submuscular round smooth moderate profile 325 cc silicone implants.

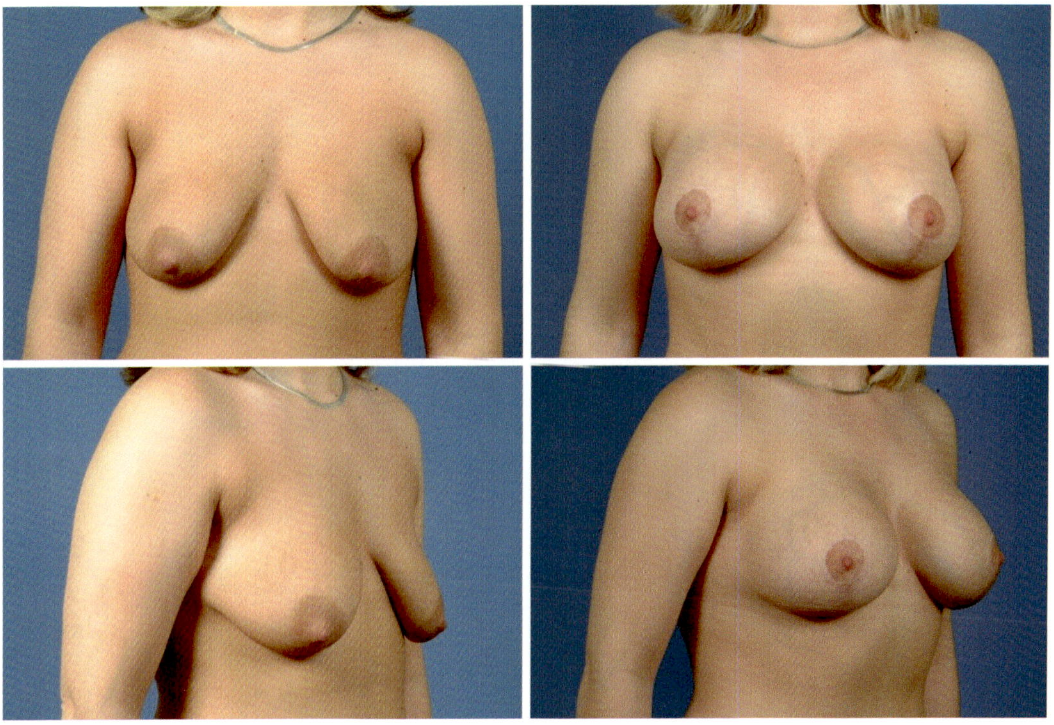

Fig. 5.12 Case 1: 25-year-old female with grade III ptosis. Bilateral augmentation vertical mastopexy with submuscular smooth round saline implants filled to 420 cc on the right and 450 cc on the left

Case 4 (Fig. 5.15)

Twenty-four year old female with grade III ptosis. Bilateral augmentation periareolar vertical mastopexy with 400 cc textured shaped moderate profile implants.

Case 5 (Fig. 5.16)

Forty-three year old female with grade III ptosis. Bilateral periareolar short horizontal submuscular augmentation mastopexy with 375 cc moderate profile smooth round silicone implants.

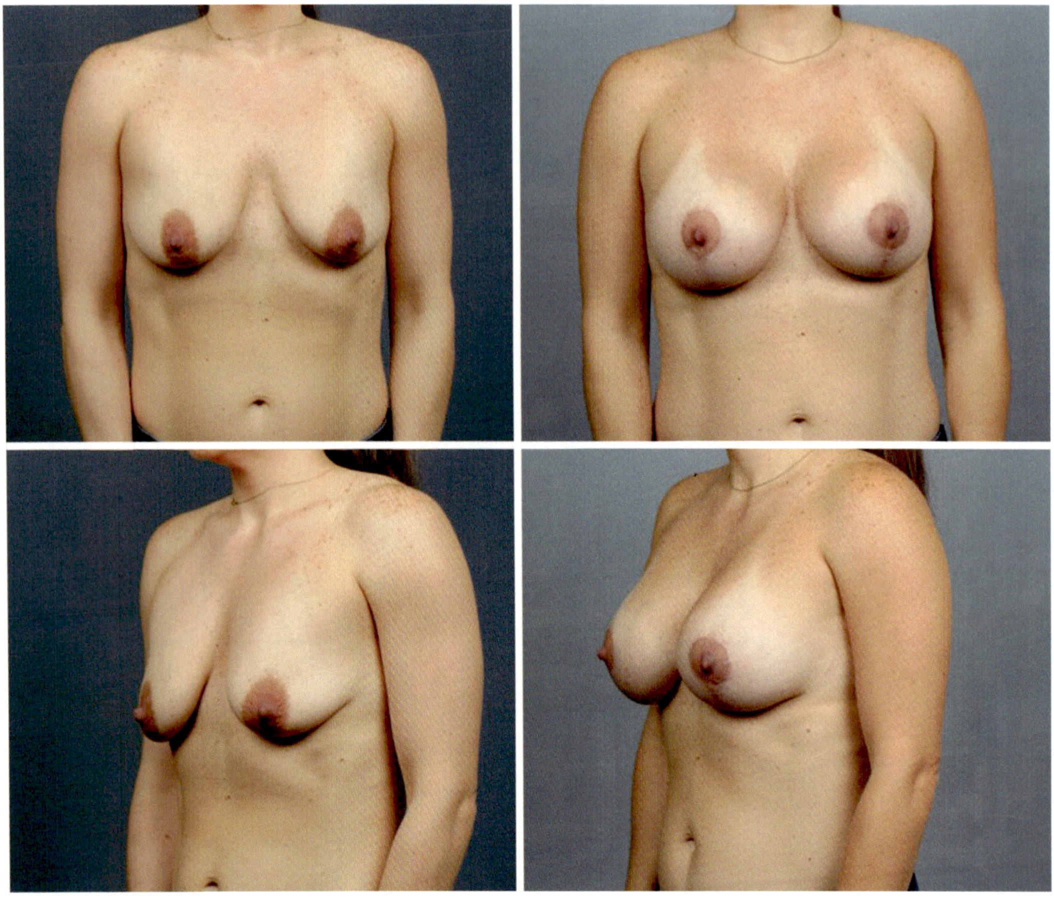

Fig. 5.13 Case 2: 35 year old female with grade III ptosis. Bilateral Periareolar vertical mastopexy with subfascial augmentation with 325 cc moderate profile textured round silicone implants

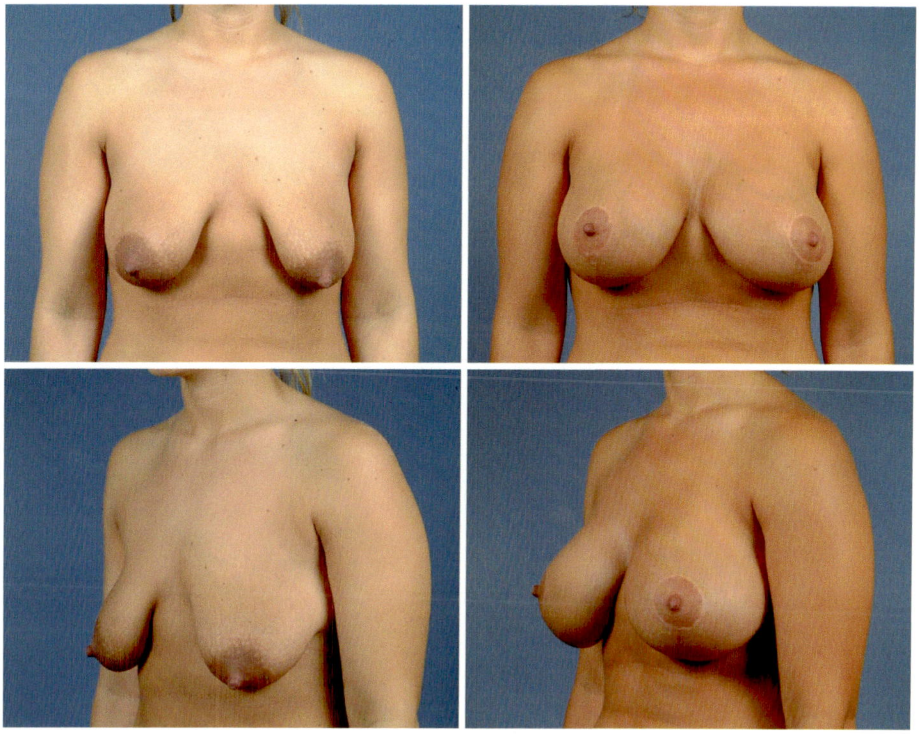

Fig. 5.14 Case 3: 24 year old female with grade III ptosis. Bilateral Inverted-T mastopexy with submuscular round smooth moderate profile 325 cc silicone implants

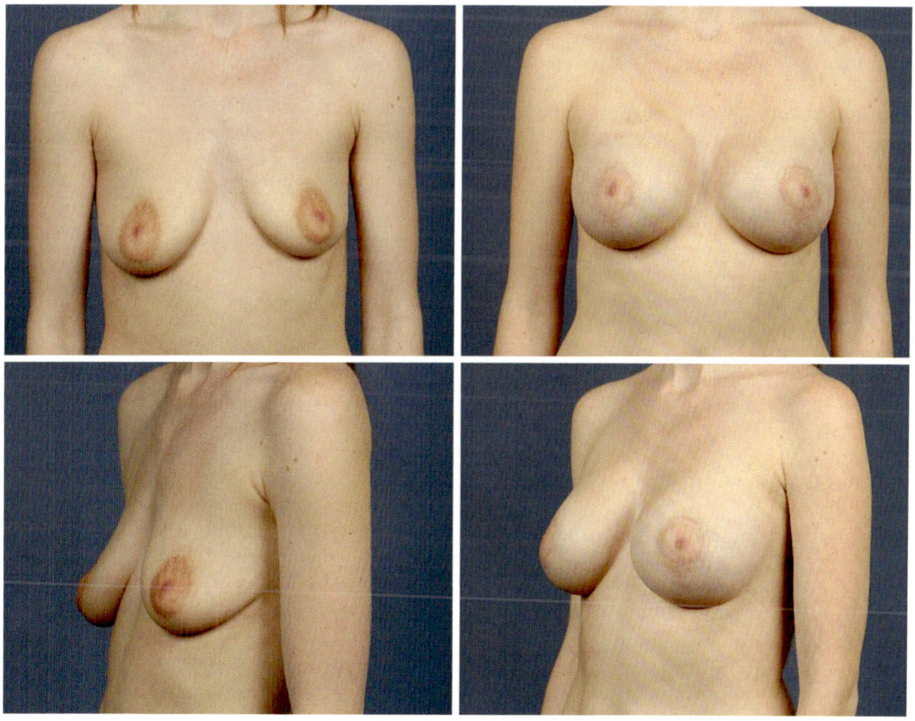

Fig. 5.15 Case 4: 24 year old female with grade III ptosis. Bilateral augmentation periareolar vertical mastopexy with 400 cc textured shaped moderate profile implants

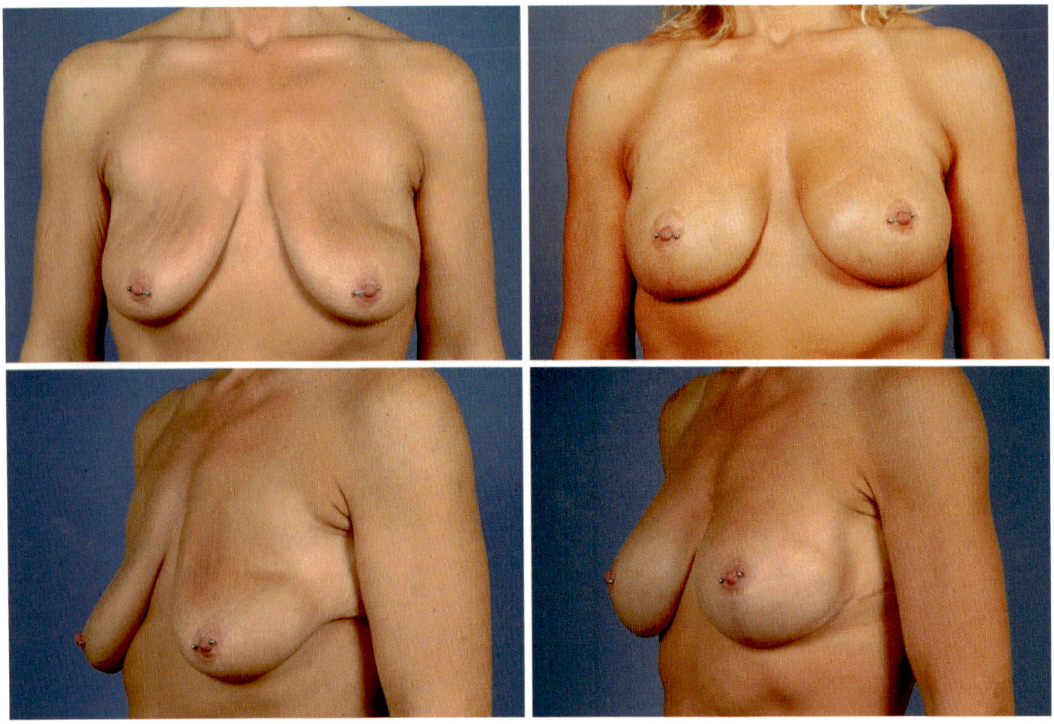

Fig. 5.16 Case 5: 43 year old female with grade III ptosis. Bilateral periareolar short horizontal submuscular augmentation mastopexy with 375 cc moderate profile smooth round silicone implants

References

1. Hoffman S. Some thoughts on augmentation/mastopexy and medical malpractice. Plast Reconstr Surg. 2004;113:1892–3.
2. Nahai F, Fisher J, Maxwell GP, Mills DC II. Augmentation Mastopexy: to stage or not. Aesthet Surg J. 2007;27:297–305.
3. Spears SL. Augmentation mastopexy: "Surgeon beware". Plast Reconstr Surg. 2003;112:905–6.
4. Stevens WG, Macias LH, Spring M, et al. One-stage augmentation mastopexy: a review of 1192 simultaneous augmentation and mastopexy procedures in 615 consecutive cases. Aesthet Surg J. 2014;34:723–32.
5. Calobrace MB, Herdt DR, Cothron KJ. Simultaneous augmentation/mastopexy: a retrospective 5-year review of 332 consecutive cases. Plast Reconstr Surg. 2013;131:145–56.
6. Tessone A, Millet E, Weissman O, et al. Evading a surgical pitfall: mastopexy-augmentation made simple. Aesthet Plast Surg. 2011;35:1073–8.
7. Lee MR, Unger JG, Adams WP. The tissue-based triad: a process approach to augmentation Mastopexy. Plast Reconstr Surg. 2014;134:215–25.
8. Persoff MM. Mastopexy with expansion-augmentation. Aesthet Surg J. 2003;23:34–9.
9. Binelli L. A new periareolar mammoplasty: the "round block" technique. Aesth Plast Surg. 1990;14:93–100.
10. Lejour M. Vertical mammoplasty for breast reduction and mastopexy. In: Spear SL, editor. Surgery of the breast: principles and art. Philadelphia: Lippincott-Raven; 1998. p. 73.
11. Hall-Findlay EJ. Pedicles in vertical breast reduction and mastopexy. Clin Plast Surg. 2002;29:379–91.
12. Wise RJ. Treatment of breast hypertrophy. Clin Plast Surg. 1976;3:289–300.
13. Marchac D, Olarte G. Reduction mammoplasty and correction of ptosis with a short inframammary scar. Plast Reconstr Surg. 1982;69:45–55.
14. Tebbetts JB. Form stability of the style 410 implant: definitions, conjectures, and the rest of the story. Plast Reconstr Surg. 2011;128:825–6.
15. Calobrace MB, Capizzi PJ. The biology and evolution of cohesive gel and shaped silicone implants. Plast Reconstr Surg. 2014;134(1S):6S–11S.
16. Regnault P. Breast ptosis. Definition and treatment. Clin Plast Surg. 1976;3:193–203.
17. Hall-Findlay EJ. Applied anatomy: key concepts for modern breast surgery. In: Hall-Findlay, editor. Aesthetic breast surgery: Thieme Publishers New York, concepts and techniques.
18. Kalaaji A, Dreyer S, Brinkmann J, et al. Quality of life after breast enlargement with implants versis augmen-

tation mastopexy: a comparative study. Aesth Surg J. 2018;38(12):1304–15.
19. Hall-Findlay EJ. Discussion: inferiorly based parenchymal flap mammaplasty a safe, reliable, and versatile technique for breast reduction and mastopexy. Plast Reconstr Surg. 2012;130:126e–7e.
20. Regnault P, Daniel RK, Tirkanits B. The minus-plus mastopexy. Clin Plast Surg. 1988;15:595–600.
21. Spring MA, Macias LH, Nadeau M, Stevens WG. Secondary augmentation-Mastopexy: indications, preferred practices, and the treatment of complications. Aesthet Surg J. 2014;34(7):1018–40.
22. Tebbetts JB, Teitelbaum S. High- and extra-high-projection breast implants: potential consequences for patients. Plast Reconstr Surg. 2010;126(6):2150–9.
23. Derby BM, Codner MA. Textured silicone implant use in primary augmentation: core data update and review. Plast Reconstr Surg. 2015;135:113–25.
24. Jones P, Mempin M, Hu H, Chowdhury D, Foley M, Cooter R, Adams WP, Vickery K, Deva AK. The functional influence of breast implant outer shell morphology on bacterial attachment and growth. Plast Reconstr Surg. 2018;142(4):837–49.
25. Namnoun JD, Largent J, Kaplan HM, Oefelein MG, Brown MH. Primary breast augmentation clinical trial outcomes stratified by surgical incision, anatomical placement and implant device type. J Plast Reconstr Aesthet Surg. 2013;66:1165–72.
26. Calobrace MB, Stevens WG, Capizzi PJ, et al. Risk factor analysis for capsular contracture: a 10-year Sientra study using round, smooth, and textured implants for breast augmentation. Plast Reconstr Surg. 2018;141(4S):20S–8S.
27. Hall-Findlay EJ. Breast implant complication review: double capsules and late seromas. Plast Reconstr Surg. 2011;127:56–66.
28. Spear SL, Rottman SJ, Glicksman C, et al. Late seromas after breast implants: theory and practice. Plast Reconstr Surg. 2012;130(2):423–35.
29. Loch-Wilkinson AL, Beath KJ, Knight RJW, et al. Breast implant-associated anaplastic large cell lymphoma in Australia and New Zealand: high surface-area textured implants are associated with increased risk. Plast Reconstr Surg. 2017;140(4): 645–54.

Technique in Simultaneous Augmentation Mastopexy

6

M. Bradley Calobrace and Chet Mays

Introduction

Evaluation of a patient with ptotic breasts can be challenging and the options available to the plastic surgeon are quite varied, as are the ultimate results. When a mastopexy is deemed necessary, this can be performed alone or in conjunction with placement of a breast implant. These patients often desire to be larger and almost universally desire improved volume in the upper poles of their breasts with improved cleavage. To achieve these objectives, the most predictable result includes a mastopexy and a breast augmentation, either as a simultaneous or staged procedure. Much controversy has existed over the years as to the safety of doing this procedure as one-stage [1–3]. Distractors believe a two-stage procedure produces superior aesthetic results and is a much safer approach compared to a one-stage procedure. Over the past many years, significant data and reports have emerged demonstrating the safety and efficacy of these procedures being performed simultaneously [4–8].

Of course, not only is patient education and perioperative decision making vitally important in achieving a successful outcome. The operative approach which is based on all the decisions leading up to the surgery is likewise of immense importance in achieving success. The operative approach should prioritize safety without compromising the final aesthetic result. In this chapter, the details of the surgical technique will be explored with a focus on the use of a variety of mastopexy designs, pockets, implants and the modifications required in the technique to optimize the outcome with each of the different options available to the surgeon. It is the marriage of decision making with expert execution that leads to the highest level of safety, optimal aesthetic outcomes and high patient satisfaction.

Preoperative Evaluation

The initial consultation always begins a discussion of patient's goals and desire results with the procedure. A good medical history should be obtained as including personal or family history of breast cancer, medical or psychiatric conditions. A history of previous breast procedures, such as aesthetic procedures, biopsies or irradiation should be elicited in planning as these have

M. B. Calobrace (✉)
Private Practice, CaloAesthetics Plastic Surgery Center, Louisville, KY, USA

Clinical Faculty, University of Louisville, Division of Plastic Surgery, Louisville, KY, USA

Clinical Faculty, University of Kentucky, Division of Plastic Surgery, Lexington, KY, USA
e-mail: drbrad@calobrace.com

C. Mays
Private Practice, CaloAesthetics Plastic Surgery Center, Louisville, KY, USA

Clinical Faculty, University of Louisville, Division of Plastic Surgery, Louisville, KY, USA

M. B. Calobrace et al. (eds.), *Augmentation Mastopexy*,
https://doi.org/10.1007/978-3-030-48226-8_6

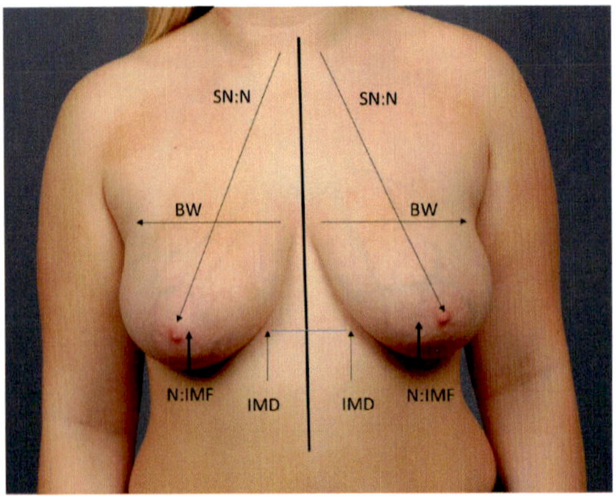

Fig. 6.1 Breast measurements

significant implications when designing the surgical approach. Previous surgery can impair breast vascularity and radiation therapy impacts healing and the long-term outcome. If possible, any medical records should be obtained to gain more knowledge and understanding of the exact procedures performed prior to finalizing the surgical approach.

The evaluation should begin with a breast exam with breast measurements, including (Fig. 6.1):

1. Breast base width (BW)
2. Sternal notch-to-nipple distance (SN-N)
3. Breast Height (BH)
4. Intermammary distance (IMD)
5. Nipple-t-fold distance (N-IMF) at rest and under maximal stretch
6. Intermammary Distance (IMD)

An assessment of the breast should include details on the ptotic nature of the breast and should include details that impact the decision on mastopexy technique, including those in Table 6.1.

Determining the amount of vertical excess that is present will assist in determining the type of mastopexy that should be accomplished. It also can assist in determining the appropriate patients for staging (Vertical excess >8–10 cm) [7] (See Table 6.2).

The assessment should also include evaluation of the skin thickness and elasticity, the quantity and distribution of subcutaneous fat, the composition and firmness of the breast parenchyma, the integrity of the Cooper's ligaments, the nature and position of the underlying musculature, and the shape and slope of the underlying chest wall. All these aspects of the breast composition influence the shape of the breast and ultimately the outcome after the mastopexy. Any asymmetries should be noted as they exist in most patients and will often become apparent post-operatively.

Lastly, the footprint of the breast should be noted [9]. Whereas this procedure can be performed on any footprint, a breast augmentation with the mastopexy is most beneficial the lower the footprint of the breast. In the low-breasted footprint patient, mastopexy alone does not elevate the upper breast border appreciably and an implant is advantageous in adding volume to a long, empty upper chest.

Table 6.1 Assessment of breast ptosis

Relationship of the NAC to the IMF (Regnault's degree of ptosis) (a) Grade 1: nipple at the level of the inframammary fold, above the lower contour of the gland (b) Grade 2: nipple below the level of the inframammary fold, above the lower contour of the gland (c) Grade 3: nipple below the level of the inframammary fold, at the lower contour of the gland
Amount of breast tissue overhanging the fold
Location of the NAC on the breast mound
Amount of vertical excess and horizontal excess
Footprint of the breast

Table 6.2 Formula for determining breast vertical excess

Vertical excess (VE)
VE = new nipple to actual IMF – New N to new IMF
VE > 8–10 cm consider staging augmentation mastopexy

Blood Supply

When performing a augmentation mastopexy, an understanding and assessment of the vascular anatomy is critical to performing the procedure safely. Figure 6.2 shows breast blood supply.

The breast has a rich blood supply from multiple sources, including the internal mammary artery perforators, the lateral thoracic arteries, the thoracoacromial and the anterolateral and anteromedial intercostal perforators [10]. In the augmentation mastopexy, the superior pedicle is used as the blood supply to the NAC. The superior pedicle is supplied by the second branch of the internal mammary artery (IMA) that emerges deep from the second interspace and courses superficial across the medial upper breast to enter the NAC slightly medial to the midline and approximately 1 cm deep.

The superficial position of these vessels in the upper pole allow the entire breast to be elevated off the muscle and chest wall for placement of the breast implant without compromising NAC vascularity, whether above or below the muscle. The superior pedicle's second branch emerges along the sternal border and great care should be taken not to inadvertently divide the vessel during development of the implant pocket. The inferior pedicle and central pedicle are supplied by the fourth branch of the IMA that courses deeply across the medial breast to enter through Wuringer's septum approximately 1–2 cm above the IMF and just medial to the breast meridian. Figure 6.3 shows vessel coursing through Wuringer's septum.

The Inferior pedicle also has additional blood supply through contribution from intercostal perforators along the IMF [11]. In an augmentation mastopexy procedure, the deep fourth branch that supplies the central pedicle and most of the infe-

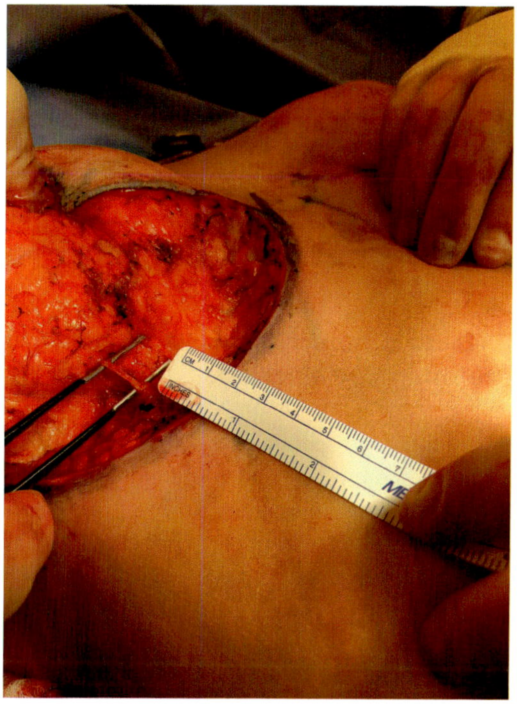

Fig. 6.3 Vessel coursing through Wuringer's septum

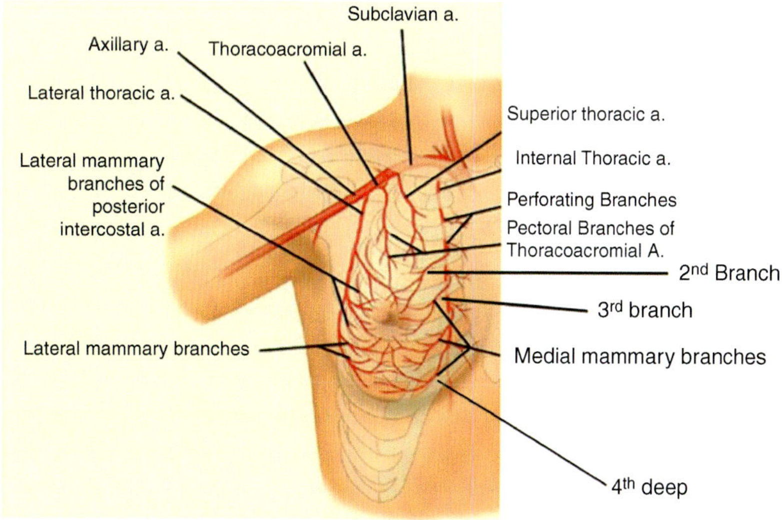

Fig. 6.2 Breast blood supply

rior pedicle is divided while developing the implant pocket. The incision in the IMF often divides the remaining blood supply to the inferior pedicle. It is important to understand that performing an augmentation mastopexy with an inferior pedicle is not truly supplied by pedicle blood supply in most cases, and the best one can hope for is random blood supply. If the remainder of the mastopexy is performed dividing deep into the flaps with an assumption that the inferior pedicle will provide circulation, the division of much needed superficial perforators both medially and laterally can lead to devastating consequences including loss of NAC or breast flap viability and resultant necrosis.

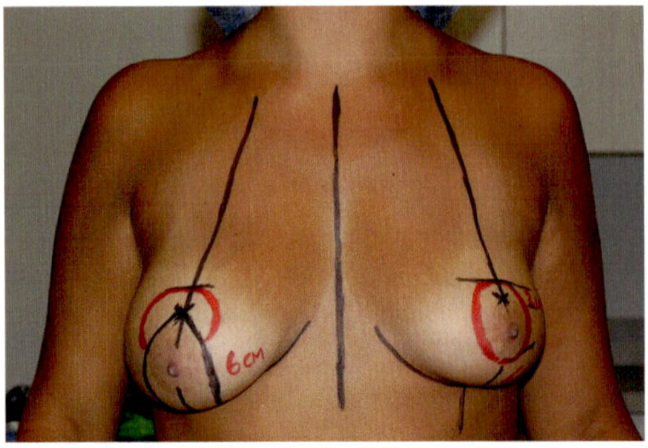

Fig. 6.5 Pre-op markings in an asymmetry case showing location of the new nipple position (black X) which is within 2 cm of the reflected inframammary fold. The Red circles represent the proposed new NAC location. The left breast will be a periareolar mastopexy and the right breast will be a periareolar vertical with possible short horizontal along the IMF. Be sure to keep the distance from the IMF to new NAC 6–8 cm

Pre-operative Markings

Appropriate preoperative markings provide a roadmap and are essential to planning and performing an augmentation mastopexy. The markings guide the surgeon in providing symmetrical NAC placement and mastopexy design. The patient is sitting upright during the markings. A line is initially drawn along the midline of the breasts and bilaterally down the meridians. The meridian lines bisect the breast equally and may not intersect though the nipple if there is NAC malposition. The inframammary folds are then drawn, noting any asymmetries to be addressed at surgery. Figure 6.4: pre-op marking of the midline and breast meridian.

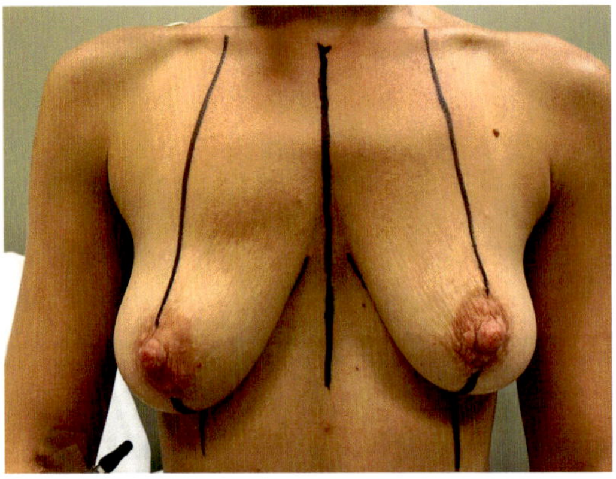

Fig. 6.4 Pre-op marking of the midline and breast meridian

The position of the IMF is then drawn on the anterior breast through the meridian incision. This augmentation mastopexy is based on a superior pedicle blood supply and is not dependent on the final skin excision pattern. Decision on nipple placement is performed is based on the location of the fold and expectation on the location of the new lifted breasts with an underlying implant. This can be approximated by simulating the mastopexy and identifying the probable location of the NAC. The nipple position is marked along the breast meridian at or within 2 cm of the reflected inframammary fold.

Figure 6.5 shows pre-op markings in an asymmetry case showing location of the new nipple position (black X) which is within 2 cm of the reflected inframammary fold. The Red circles represent the proposed new NAC location. The left breast will be a periareolar mastopexy and the right breast will be a periareolar vertical with possible short horizontal along the IMF. Be sure to keep the distance from the IMF to new NAC 6–8 cm.

In the circumareolar approach, the proposed location of the new areolar opening is marked, starting approximately 2 cm above the nipple position and 6–8 cm above the inframammary fold based on implant size. An oval line is then

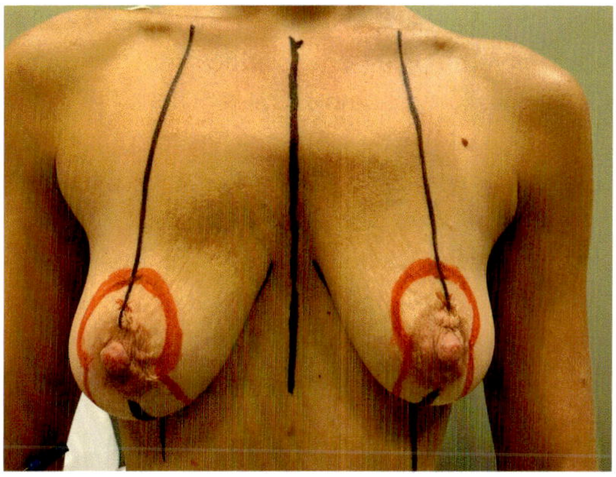

Fig. 6.7 Red "x" is the reflected IMF or new nipple position and the thick red oval is the new proposed areolar opening

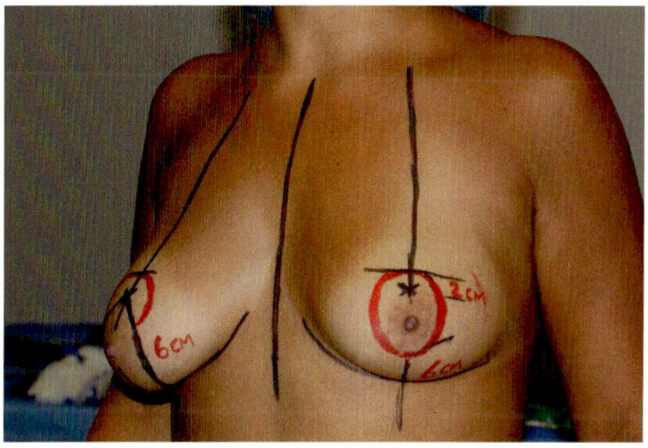

Fig. 6.6 Circumareolar (periareolar) markings shown with the new upper NAC position marked 2 cm above the new nipple position and the lower NAC position marked 6 cm above the IMF

drawn from the two points extending around the areola to create the desired shape and skin excision.

Figure 6.6 shows circumareolar (periareolar) markings shown with the new upper NAC position marked 2 cm above the new nipple position and the lower NAC position marked 6 cm above the IMF.

When a vertical or inverted-T mastopexy is planned, the areola is drawn from the planned superior areola opening extending around the areola to produce an areolar opening of approximately 42 millimeters.

In Fig. 6.7, ted "x" is the reflected IMF or new nipple position and the thick red oval is the new proposed areolar opening.

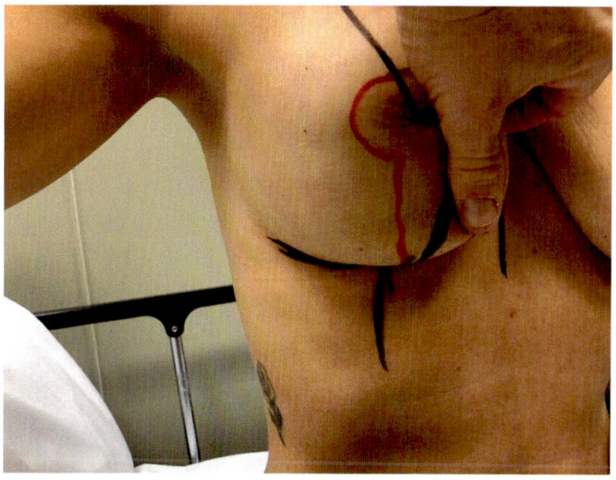

Fig. 6.8 Right breast rotated medially to marking location of lateral vertical incision shown in red

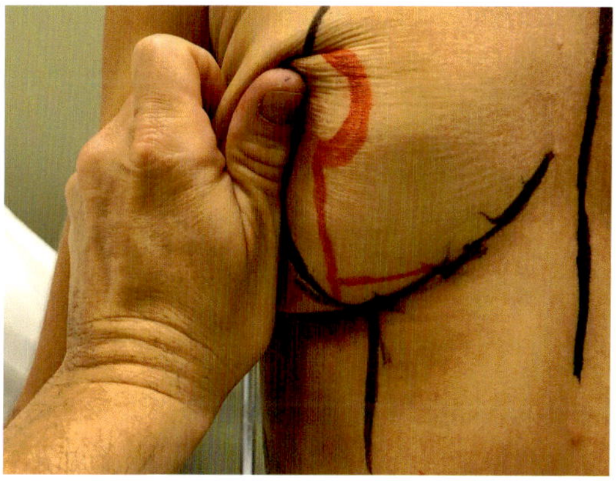

Fig. 6.9 Pre -op drawing of vertical medial incision and anticipated Horizontal wedge excision shown as horizontal red line above the IMF to shorten the vertical limb of the mastopexy

The breasts are then rotated medially and laterally to mark the location of the vertical incisions, recognizing that the placement of the implant will add volume, thus requiring less skin excision than would be required with mastopexy designed without an implant.

Figure 6.8 shows the right breast rotated medially to marking location of lateral vertical incision shown in red.

If the vertical limbs are deemed excessively long, the design can be modified to include additional skin excision around the areola (circumvertical mastopexy) or along the inframammary fold.

Figure 6.9 is a pre -op drawing of vertical medial incision and anticipated Horizontal wedge excision shown as horizontal red line above the IMF to shorten the vertical limb of the mastopexy.

Patients with greater ptosis will often require more significant excision of skin and elevation of the NAC. This can range from a long wise-pattern excision down to a very short horizontal wedge based on the amount of skin excess. These markings are made along the inframammary fold and intersect with a line drawn from the vertical limbs extending in a curved fashion down to the fold markings. When planning an augmentation mastopexy, these drawings should be conservative allowing for adjustments once the implant has been placed. All the markings made preoperatively are made as a guideline for the operation, but the final NAC placement and skin excision required will be determined in surgery after the breast implant has been placed.

Surgical Technique

The patient is placed on the operating room table with the arms secured to the sides at 45 to 60 degrees.

Figure 6.10 shows pre-op positioning on the OR table with arms secured at 45–60 degrees.

Once the patient is prepped with Chloraprep and draped appropriately, the markings and incision location are confirmed and reinforced with a surgical pen to avoid loss of markings during the prep. The operative field is then injected with 50cc per side of local anesthetic of 0.25% lidocaine, 0.125% Marcaine, 1:400,000 epinephrine. The concentrations of each local anesthetic is shown in Table 6.3.

Figure 6.11 shows pre-op injection of breast analgesic with a 20cc syringe and spinal needle.

Each breast is placed under maximal stretch and the areolas are marked with a 42 mm cookie-cutter (range 38–45 mm depending on desired aesthetics) and incised with a 15-blade scalpel.

Figure 6.12 shows an incision of NAC with 15-blade scalpel.

Pocket Development

Once the areolas are incised, access to the breast pocket is determined. For circumareolar mastopexies, the access is either through the

Table 6.3 Concentration of breast local anesthetic

Breast local anesthetic formula	
½% lidocaine plain	25 ml
½% lidocaine/ 1:200,000 epinephrine	25 ml
½% bupivicaine/1:200,000 epinephrine	25 ml
Injectable saline	25 ml
TOTAL concentration:	**Total volume:**
¼% lidocaine, 1/8% bupivicaine, 1:400,000 epinephrine	100 ml

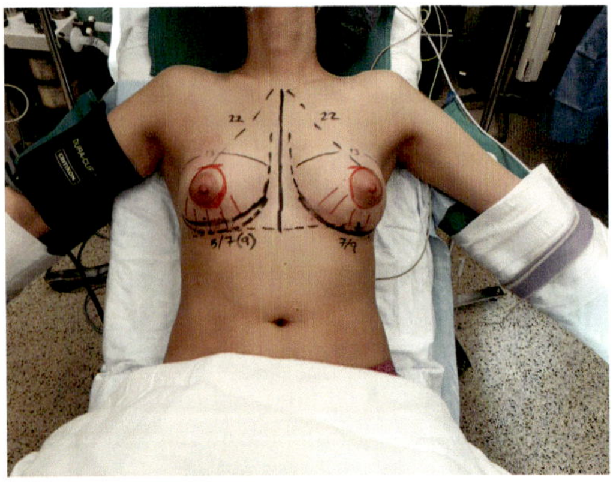

Fig. 6.10 Pre-op positioning on the OR table with arms secured at 45–60 degrees

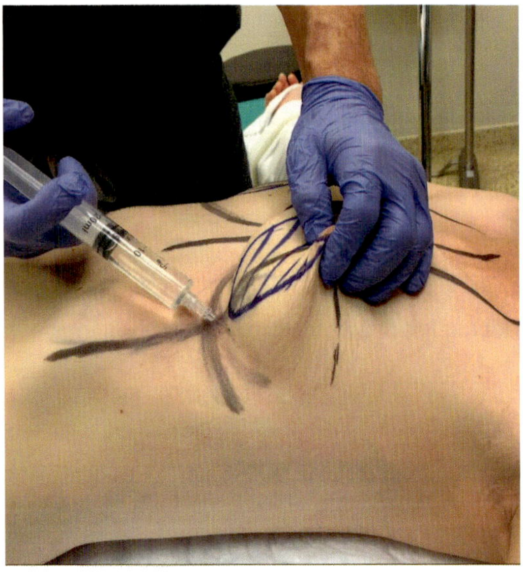

Fig. 6.11 Pre-op injection of breast analgesic with a 20cc syringe and spinal needle

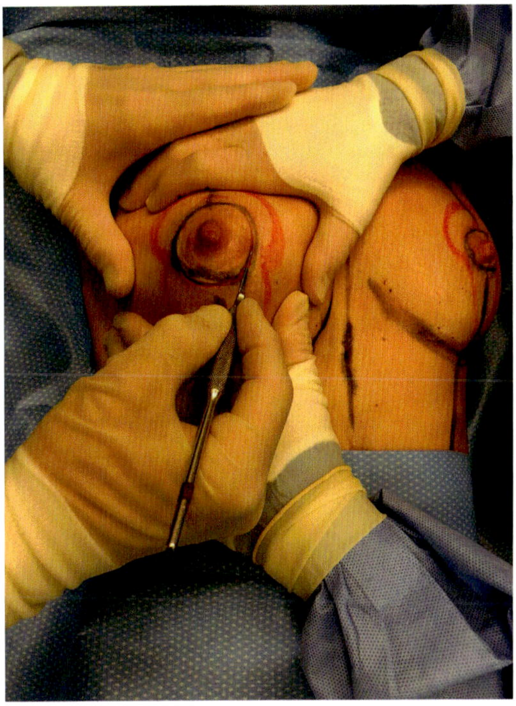

Fig. 6.12 Incision of NAC with 15-blade scalpel

inferior areola in the area of planned de-epithelization or through a counter-incision in the IMF. The advantages of going through the areola is eliminating the need for an additional scar in the IMF. It also has been proposed that when lowering the fold, the dissection from above can allow for fold lowering incrementally, obviating the need to determine its new position preoperatively. However, the preferred access currently is with an IMF incision. This provides improved exposure and visualization of the pocket, is associated with lower capsular contracture rates, and allows for IMF control sutures to be placed to stabilize the new fold position. In the circumareolar approach, the skin edges are retracted inferiorly and superiorly and dissection is carried down towards the pectoralis fascia either directly through the breast tissue (transparenchymal) or inferiorly under the skin (subcutaneous) until the fascia is reached at the fold.

Figure 6.13 is a periareolar incision showing dissection planes; transparenchymal, periareolar and subcutaneous (SubQ).

The author prefers the transparenchymal approach. If access is through an IMF counter incision, the dissection is carried through Scarpa's (superficial) fascia leaving a small cuff on the inferior incision, and then dissected under the breast directly onto the pectoralis fascia.

Figure 6.14 shows a small cuff of Scarpa's fascia at the IMF incision.

When a vertical or inverted-T skin incision is planned, access to the breast pocket can be made via the periareolar, vertical or the inframammary approach. However, a vertical access or inframammary approach is utilized in the vast majority of cases. In the vertical approach, the breast is divided down the midline extending from the inferior areola to at least 2 cm above the inframammary fold to gain access to the desired pocket. Figure 6.15 shows the vertical incision access approach to the breast. The incision is made inferior to the NAC

It is extremely important to not carry this incision all the way down to the fold as this lower area of the breast, the "No-Go Zone", will provide a protective cuff of tissue during closure.

Figure 6.16 shows vertical dissection to just above the IMF leaving a cuff of tissue (no-go-zone) to protect implant at the T-point.

Once through the breast tissue, the pocket is created based on preoperative decision making.

Submuscular Dual Plane Pocket Dissection is carried down toward the chest wall while maintaining a constant upward retraction of the breast tissue, ultimately exposing the lateral edge of the pectoralis muscle. The upward retraction of the breast tissue is key as the suspensory ligaments of the breast will concomitantly elevate the muscle. It is imperative to not cut the muscle unless you can elevate the muscle off the chest wall. Inability to elevate the muscle most likely indicates that the identified muscle is not the pectoralis, but rather the serratus, rectus, or an intercostal muscle. Once the lateral border of the pectoralis is identified, the fascia is incised to expose the underlying muscle. After the subpectoral space is entered, dissection is carried upward centrally to the superior extent of the pocket. Dissection is then carried laterally just superficial to the pectoralis

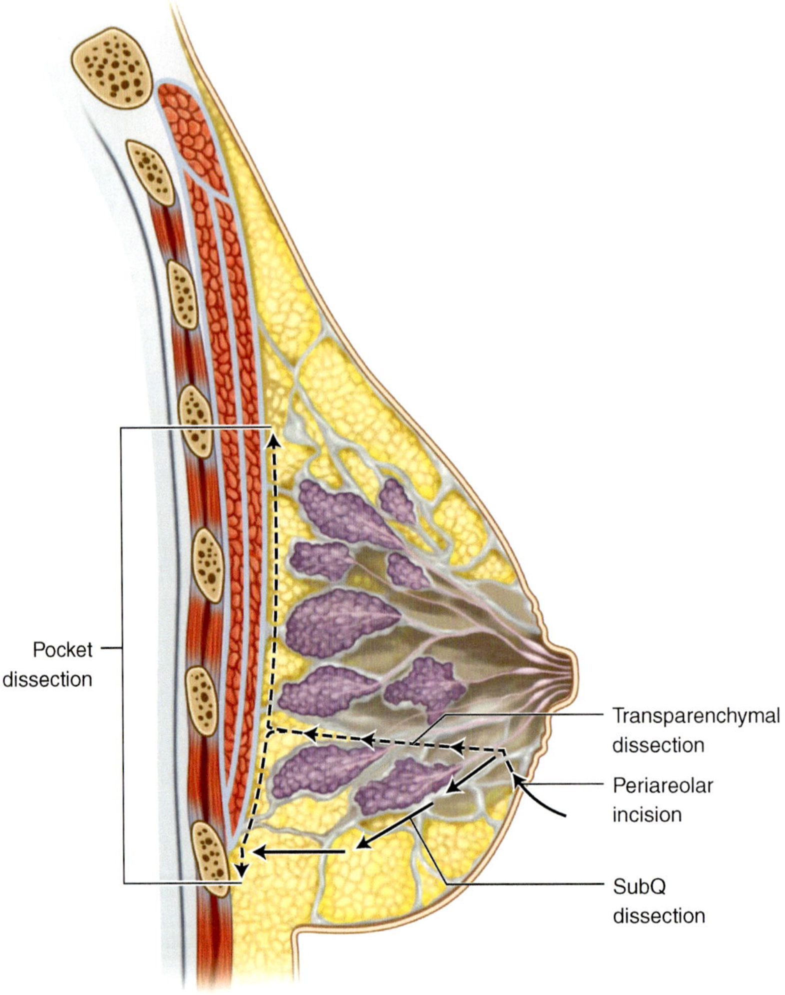

Fig. 6.13 Periareolar incision showing dissection planes; transparenchymal, periareolar and subcutaneous (SubQ)

minor and serratus anterior until the lateral border of the pocket is reached. Lateral pocket dissection should be performed bluntly with minimal cautery to avoid injury to the lateral cutaneous nerves resulting in sensory changes to the NAC. Especially important in augmentation mastopexy cases, dissection of the pocket laterally should be minimized to facilitate optimal medial projection of the implant.

The pectoralis is then released along the planned IMF, staying 1 cm superior to the fold to account for caudal muscle descent.

Figure 6.17 shows dissection of pectoralis major staying at least 1 cm above the IMF.

Dissection directly at the fold will often lead to a fold that is lower than planned as the muscle retracts inferiorly. As you carry your dissection medially along the IMF it is critically important to stop the dissection at the most medial extent along the sternum. Preservation of the most caudal attachment of the pectoralis muscle at the Transition Point (TP) along the sternum is critical to minimize the chance of window shading of the pectoralis with subsequent medial implant exposure and animation deformities. A Transition Zone (TZ) of tapered muscle release connects the transition point to the main body of medial pectoral muscle along the sternum.

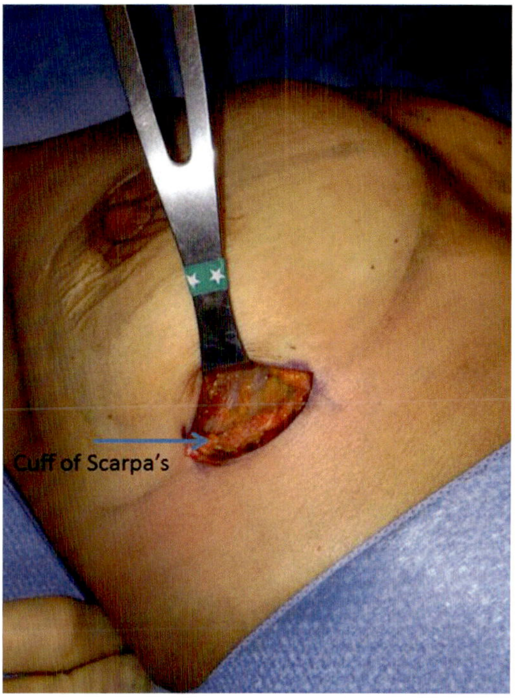

Fig. 6.14 Small cuff of Scarpa's fascia at the IMF incision

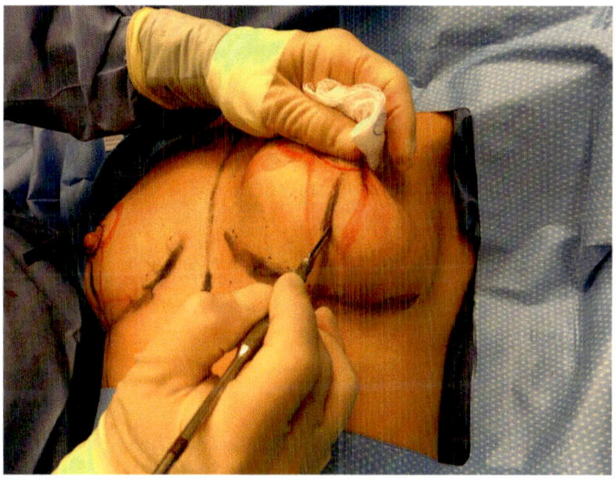

Fig. 6.15 The vertical incision access approach to the breast, incision is made inferior to the NAC

In Figure 6.18a, TP is the transition point where the pectoralis major is no longer completely released from costal attachments. The TZ, is the Transition Zone as the pectoralis major is thinned from the TP to the sternum.

Figure 6.18b is a schematic showing the TP, transition point and TZ, transition zone.

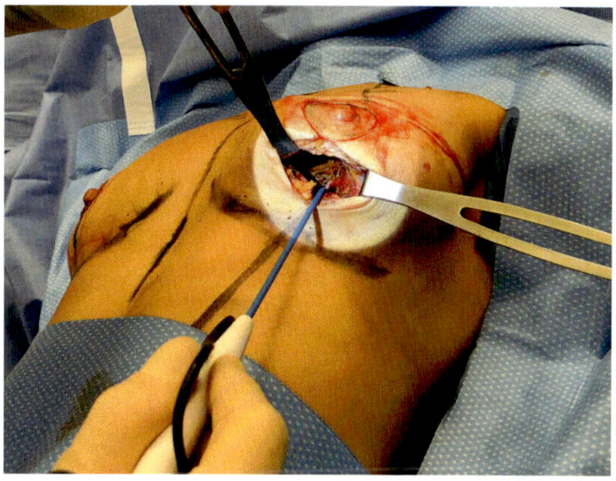

Fig. 6.16 Vertical dissection to just above the IMF leaving a cuff of tissue (no-go-zone) to protect implant at the T-point

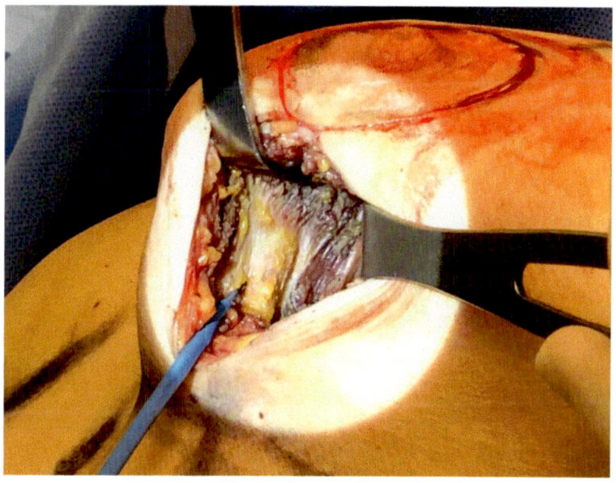

Fig. 6.17 Dissection of pectoralis major staying at least 1 cm above the IMF

The extent of the pocket is completed by defining the medial pectoral border and dividing all of the accessory slips of pectoralis muscle that insert along the ribs, preserving only the main body of the muscle as it inserts along the sternum. Dividing these muscles slips with electrocautery instead of blunt dissection improves postoperative cleavage, weakens the pectoralis muscle action on the implant and maintains hemostasis. This division of the inferior pectoralis muscle just above the IMF during initial pocket dissection creates a level-1 dual plane. Thus, all submuscular pockets where the muscle is released inferiorly are actually dual-plane pockets, as the segment between the caudal edge

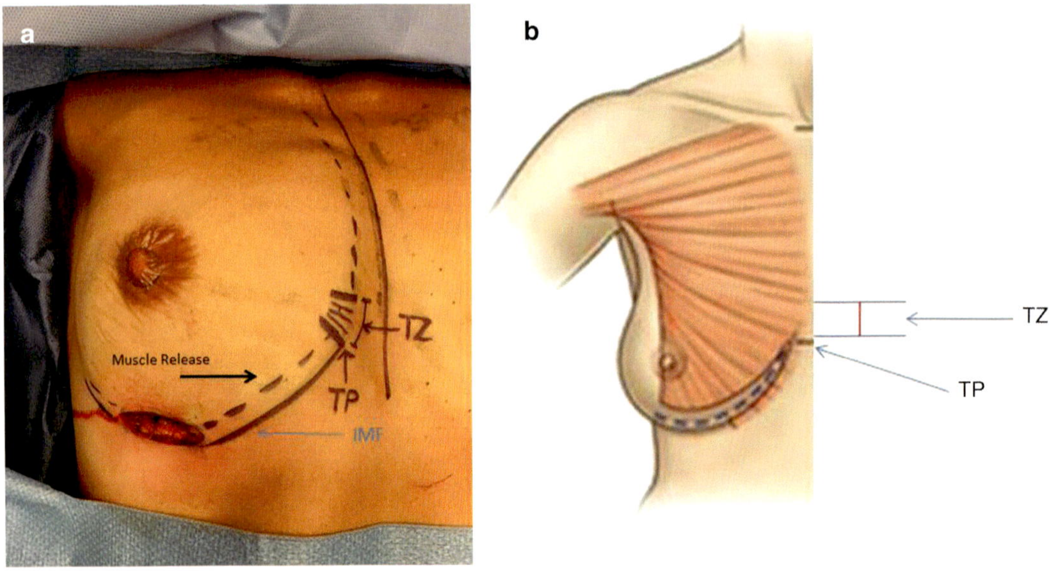

Fig. 6.18 (**a**) TP, is the transition point where the pectoralis major is no longer completely released from costal attachments. The TZ, is the Transition Zone as the pectoralis major is thinned from the TP to the sternum. (**b**) Schematic showing the TP, transition point and TZ, transition zone

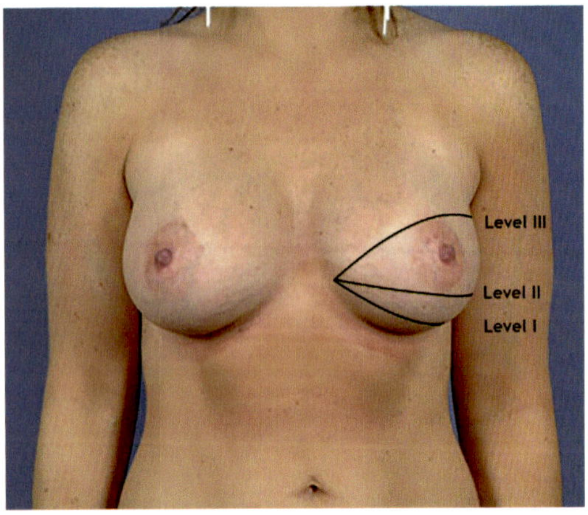

Fig. 6.19 Dual plane types/levels

Table 6.4 Different dual plane type

Dual plane type	Description
Type I	Complete division of the pectoralis major along the IMF
Type II	Same as I plus pectoralis is released from overlying gland and allowed to slide to about the lower border of the areola
Type III	Same as type I plus greater release of the pectoralis from the gland, allowing it to slide to about the upper border of the areola.

of the divided muscle and the inframammary fold is subglandular.

Figure 6.19 shows dual plane types/levels, and Table 6.4 shows different dual plane types/levels.

The level of dual plane required varies, and each surgery can be tailored to provide the optimal level based on soft-tissue requirements and implant selection. The greater the amount of breast parenchyma or breast laxity, the greater the level of dual plane. It is this creation of a lower pole subglandular pocket that allows for an optimal breast-implant interface and soft tissue re-draping. In augmentation mastopexy, the breast-implant relationship is improved with the overlying mastopexy. However, even with a mastopexy, failure to optimize the breast-implant interface during surgery can lead to a waterfall deformity with the breast sliding off the implant.

If IMF lowering is required, it can be more challenging in the submuscular pocket as it is tempting to carry the dissection under the muscle along the chest wall to lower the fold. The dissection along the chest wall at the level of the fold is

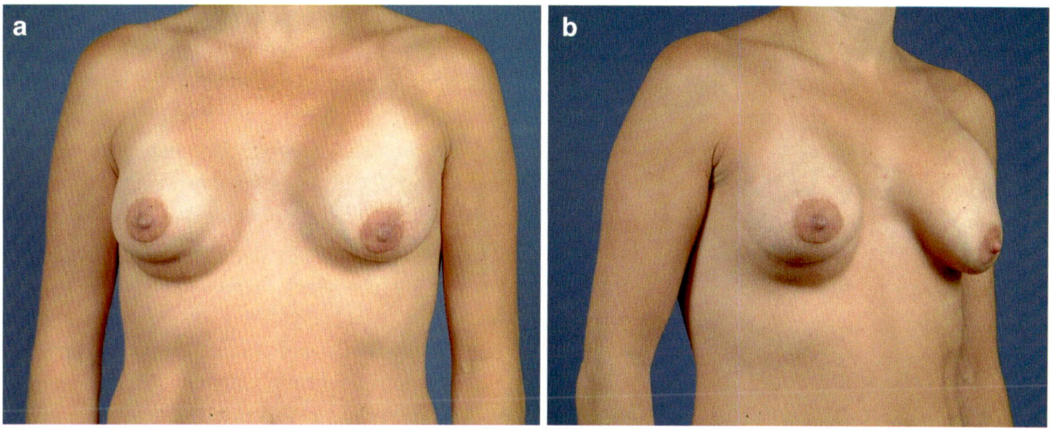

Fig. 6.20 (**a**) AP view of the breast showing a double bubble on the right breast and a waterfall deformity of the left breast. (**b**) Oblique view of the breast showing the double bubble deformity of the right breast and a waterfall deformity of the left breast

deep to the suspensory ligament structures that create the IMF. IMF lowering in the subpectoral pocket requires transitioning into a more superficial subglandular plane above the pectoralis fascia to lower the IMF. Dissection deep to the pectoral fascia will likely result in a lowered fold with persistence of the native fold structure, resulting in a double-bubble deformity.

Figure 6.20a is the AP view of the breast showing a double bubble on the right breast and a waterfall deformity of the left breast.

Figure 6.20b is an oblique view of the breast showing the double bubble deformity of the right breast and a waterfall deformity of the left breast.

This is more likely when dissection begins from above, such as a periareolar or transaxillary approach. Fortunately, when using an IMF incision, the dissection below the native fold begins in the subcutaneous plane until the pectoralis muscle is reached, resulting in appropriate obliteration of the native fold at the correct level.

Subfascial Pocket As you dissect towards the chest wall maintaining a constant upward retraction of the breast tissue the pectoralis major will be exposed with its overlying fascia. Elevation beneath the deep pectoral fascia and overlying breast tissue exposes the pectoral muscle fibers devoid of fascia. The elevation of the pectoralis fascia can start at the IMF and move superiorly or can be elevated with the breast tissue centrally and then dissected superiorly and inferiorly in development of the pocket. Importantly, the inframammary fold is a fusion of the deep fascia attached to the pectoralis and the superficial fascia of the breast. Take care to prevent disruption of the inframammary fold as the inferior edge of the fascia elevated. The inferior extent of the pectoralis fascia is thin and elevation is best carried out with the cut current of the electrocautery. Continued upward retraction of the breast will elevate the fascial plane. The fascia is left attached to the underlying breast tissue and elevated as a single unit. The dissection is carried superiorly, medial and lateral to create the desired pocket. As with any breast augmentation, pocket control is key. Avoid over dissection of your pocket laterally to optimize medial projection of the implant and minimize lateralization of the implant. Subfascial implants have less lateral drift compared to submuscular implants because they lack the lateral action of the forceful pectoralis muscle contraction. As the dissection is carried medially, be aware of the midline to avoid pocket over dissection which could lead to symmastia. The fascia is adherent to the underlying pectoralis muscle as the sternum is approached and will provide some limitation to medial over dissection compared to the subglandular pocket. Importantly, if IMF lowering is needed, the dissection is transitioned into the subglandular pocket as the attachments creating the fold are superficial to the deep pectoral fascia.

Figure 6.21 shows the creation of the subfascial (thin white shiny layer) pocket with overlying breast tissue superiorly, leaving the underlying pectoralis muscle fibers at the base of the pocket.

Subglandular Pocket The elevation of the subglandular pocket is superficial to the pectoralis fascia. As you dissect toward the chest wall a continued upward retraction of the breast will elevate the breast and its thin underlying fascia as a single unit leaving the pectoralis fascia attached to the muscle. The fascia is visualized over the pectoralis muscle as a dull covering obscuring the appearance of the fleshy muscle fibers. The dissection is carried superiorly, medial and lateral to create the desired pocket. The inframammary fold is a fusion of the deep fascia attached to the pectoralis and the superficial fascia of the breast. Take care to prevent disruption of the inframammary fold as the breast is elevated off of the pectoralis fascia. Avoid over dissection of your pocket laterally to optimize medial projection of the implant and minimize lateralization of the implant. Subglandular implants have less lateral drift compared to submuscular implants because they lack the lateral action of the forceful pectoralis muscle contraction. As you carry your dissection medially in the subglandular plane, the midline can quickly be violated due to the lack of sternal muscle attachment that limits dissection in the submuscular plan. Over dissection can lead to medial migration of the implant and the potential for postoperative symmastia. This is especially true when the chest wall is concave or slanting medially, and special caution with limited medial dissection is warranted in these cases. If IMF lowering is indicated, the dissection is more easily accomplished as the subglandular plane dissection inferiorly is in the appropriate plane to lower and obliterate the native fold.

Figure 6.22 shows subglandular pocket dissection superiorly with the underlying pectoralis fascia and muscle.

Implant Placement

Once the pocket is developed, hemostasis is established. Prospective hemostasis with control of any blood staining during the dissection is optimal. The pocket is irrigated with the triple

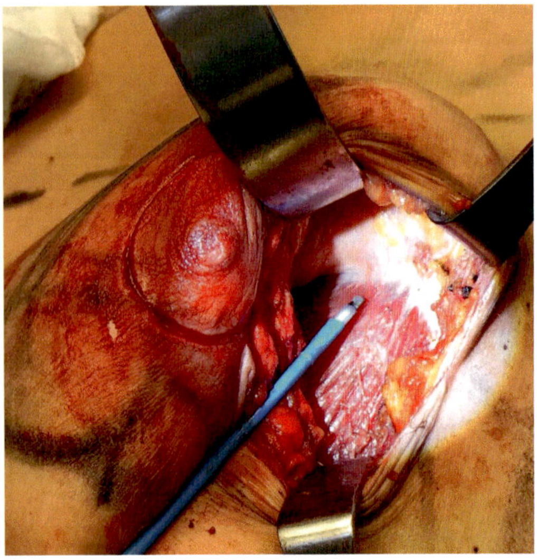

Fig. 6.21 Creation of the subfascial (thin white shiny layer) pocket with overlying breast tissue superiorly, leaving the underlying pectoralis muscle fibers at the base of the pocket

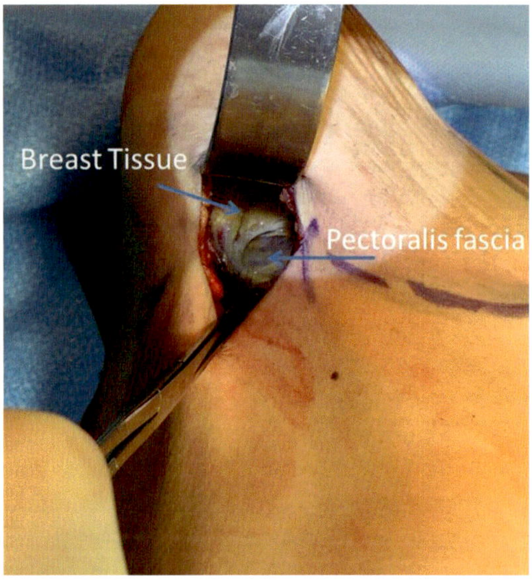

Fig. 6.22 Subglandular pocket dissection superiorly with the underlying pectoralis fascia and muscle

antibiotic solution/betadine solution (1 g of cefazolin sodium, 80 mg gentamycin, 50cc betadine mixed in 500 mL of normal saline) and a final hemostasis check is done. The implants are soaked in the irrigation solution before insertion. Gloves are changed and rinsed with the irrigation solution to remove any residue. The implant is then placed into the pocket with the assistance of an insertion sleeve such as the Keller funnel. The use of the insertion sleeve is even more beneficial in an augmentation mastopexy surgery as the implant is passed through either the circumareolar or vertical incision in the vast majority of patients.

Figure 6.23 shows the use of the Keller funnel to insert implant into the breast pocket.

These access incisions require the implant to pass through the bacteria-laden breast tissue. The insertion sleeve provides a "no-touch" technique which is associated with lower capsular contracture rates [12, 13].

The insertion sleeve is placed deep into the pocket to allow passage with minimal to no contact with the surrounding breast tissue. The opening of the funnel should be cut large enough to allow easy egress of the implant through the funnel. This is easily confirmed by passing the implant with irrigation solution through the funnel prior to insertion. The implant orientation is then confirmed in the funnel, and a maneuver of squeezing the implant through the funnel with pressure exerted on the back of the funnel allows the implant to slip into the breast pocket.

Once the implant is in the pocket, a finger assisted assessment and manipulation of the implant within the pocket is necessary to confirm its proper placement and assure appropriate re-draping of the breast parenchyma over the implant. It is critically important with shaped implants to confirm the orientation marks or tabs are oriented correctly.

Figure 6.24 shows a centrally located white stripe to maintain the vertical orientation of the shaped implant.

This maneuver is especially important with textured devices, round or shaped, as these implants are less mobile and less likely to stretch the pocket and, thus, a distortion or wrinkling of the implant in a tight pocket may be permanent if not resolved before closure. Repeated removal and insertions of the implant should be avoided to minimize implant or incision damage, potential contamination, and pocket over dissection. This is especially

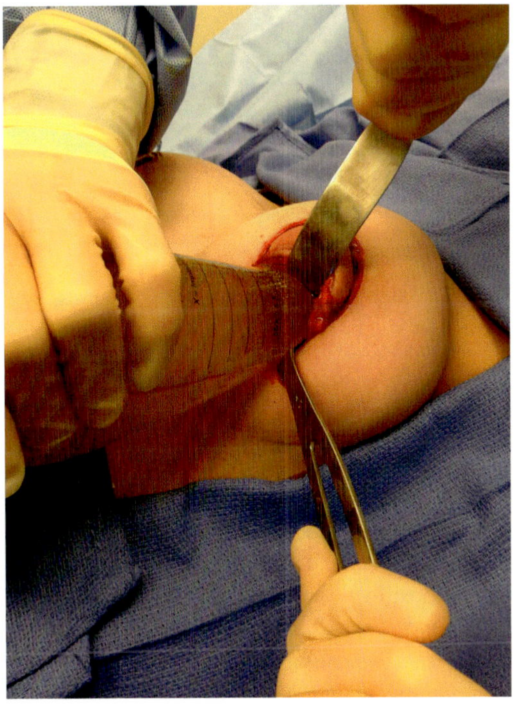

Fig. 6.23 Use of the Keller funnel to insert implant into the breast pocket

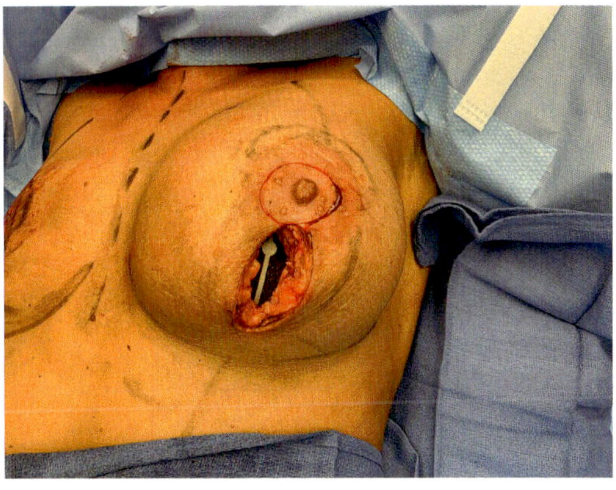

Fig. 6.24 White stripe to maintain the vertical orientation of the shaped implant

important with shaped implants, as a stretched pocket from over manipulation could lead to implant rotation postoperatively.

Tailor-Tacking

Once the implant is in the pocket and oriented appropriately, the final planning of the mastopexy is carried out. Tailor-tacking is a critical step in designing the optimal breast shape. With the circumareolar approach, the areola is stapled to the outer circle and adjusted to create the desired shape prior to de-epithelialization. In the vertical or inverted-T approach, starting usually at what will be the new inferior areola location (6 o'clock position), the medial and lateral vertical limbs are brought together and stapled in a discerning fashion, adjusting by tightening a little more or a little less to create the desired lower pole breast shape, If a vertical approach only, the planned excision tapers down to the fold. The length of the lower pole skin (distance from the inferior areola to IMF) varies based on the size of implant and amount of breast parenchyma that is present. For most augmentation mastopexies, this length is generally 6–8 cm. If this distance is excessive when tailor-tacking, two options exist; expand the circumareolar opening to encompass more of the vertical length (circumvertical approach) or remove a horizontal wedge of skin at the fold to shorten the vertical limb. This often is a small wedge of skin leaving a short horizontal scar (has been referred to as owl's feet) or extended laterally as J-type mastopexy. If the vertical excess is significant, the horizontal wedge excision will create an inverted-T pattern. With the patient in the upright position and the arms extended at 45 degrees, breast shape and symmetry are confirmed. Adjustments are made if necessary until the results are optimal.

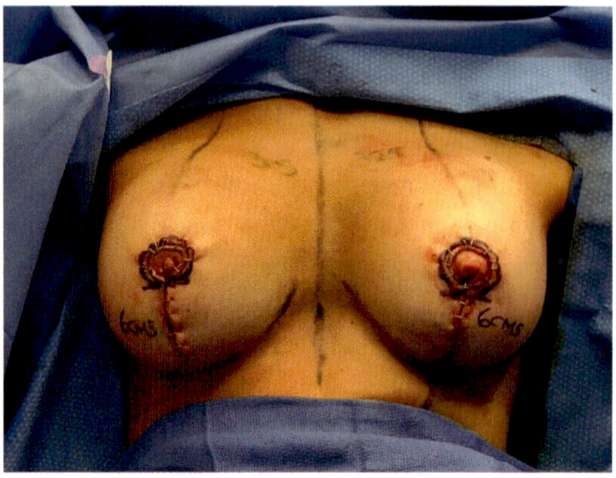

Fig. 6.25 Tailor tacking of the breast. IMF to inferior border of the areola is marked at 6 cm

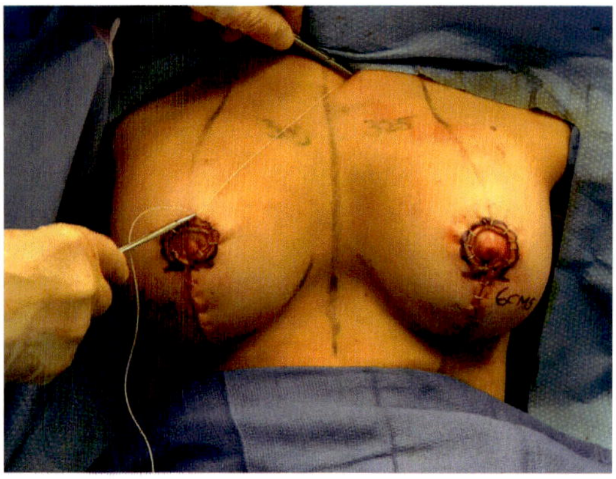

Fig. 6.26 Confirming the NAC placement is symmetrical using the "top-down" approach from sternal notch to top of the areola. Note the "bottom-up" distance of 6 cm confirmed bilaterally

Figure 6.25 shows tailor tacking of the breast. IMF to inferior border of the areola is marked at 6 cm.

Important to mention, once the tacking is complete, a final decision on placement of the NAC must be made. There is flexibility as no skin has been excised at this time. The areolar can be positioned higher or lower to optimize breast shape, placing the NAC centrally along the median of the breast at the point of maximal projection. When considering NAC placement, confirmation can be performed from bottom up, top down or both. "Top down" refers to the distance from the sternal notch to the top of the areola (or nipple) and "bottom up" refers to the distance from the IMF to the inferior areola (or nipple). During tailor-tacking, it is helpful to confirm NAC position and symmetry using both techniques.

Figure 6.26, confirming the NAC placement is symmetrical using the "top-down" approach from sternal notch to top of the areola. Note the "bottom-up" distance of 6 cm confirmed bilaterally.

Once confirmed, the patient is placed supine and the tailor-tacking is marked with methylene blue or permanent marker identifying the planned incision lines.

Breast Flap and Pedicle Dissection

In the circumareolar approach, the area between the areola and outer circle is de-epithelialized. Although an IMF counter-incision is the preferred access for the augmentation, if the periareolar access was used then the deep breast tissue must first be closed with an absorbable 2-0 Vicryl. The dermis is then cauterized for maximal shrinkage.

Figure 6.27, the dermis is cauterized to shrink the tissue and facilitate a tension free closure of the NAC.

The dermis is either left intact or incised just at the periphery to create a small ledge to facilitate closure. A purse-string suture of 3-0 Gortex is placed in a wagon wheel pattern.

Figure 6.28 shows a wagon wheel closure of the NAC with a 3-0 Gortex suture.

In the vertical augmentation mastopexy technique, the superior pedicle is preferred. The incisions are outlined with a scalpel, insuring not to cut deeply into the dermis. The periareolar region is de-epithelialized. The incisions are then made full-thickness through the dermis along all the scored skin. However, in the superior areola the dermis is left intact (from 8 o'clock to 4 o'clock) as the superior dermal pedicle.

As shown in Fig. 6.29, once symmetry is confirmed, tailor-tacked staples are removed, and incisions are demarcated with marking pen around the NAC and vertical limb.

As shown in Fig. 6.30, periareolar and vertical limb are de-epithelialized. Note that the dermis around the NAC is left intact from 8–4 o'clock to maintain NAC perfusion.

The superficial second branch of the IMA courses from the sternum across the breast to enter most commonly just medial to the midline.

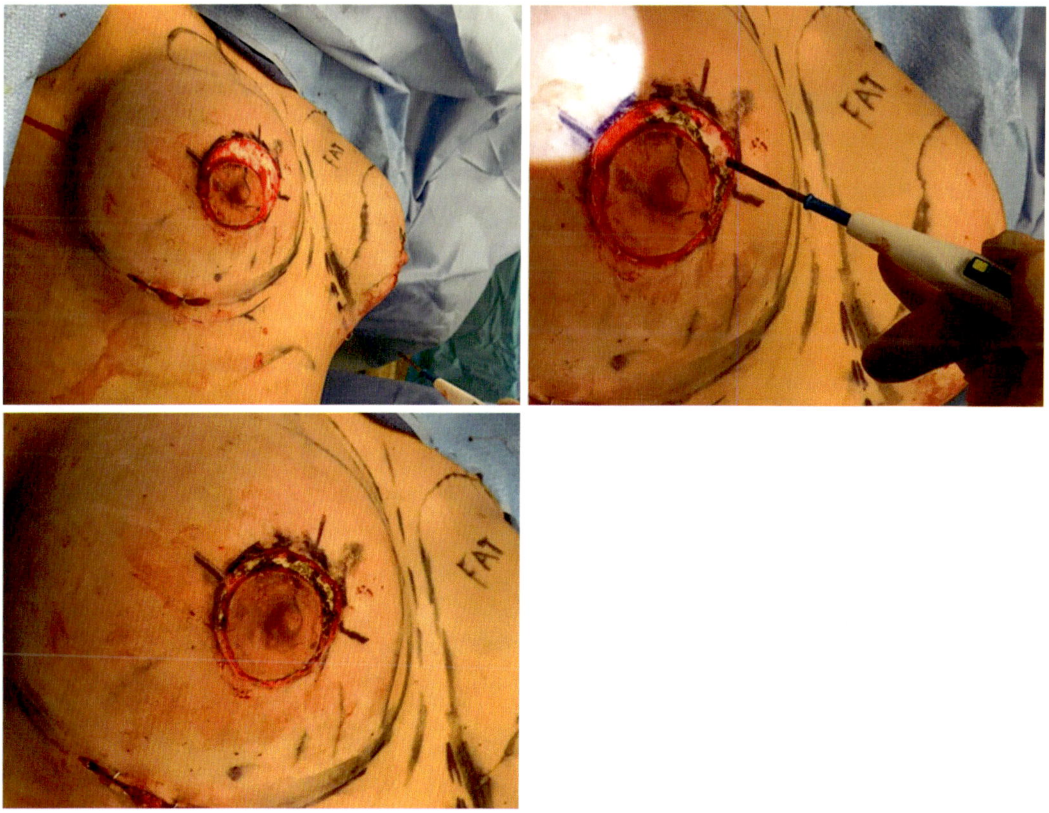

Fig. 6.27 The dermis is cauterized to shrink the tissue and facilitate a tension free closure of the NAC

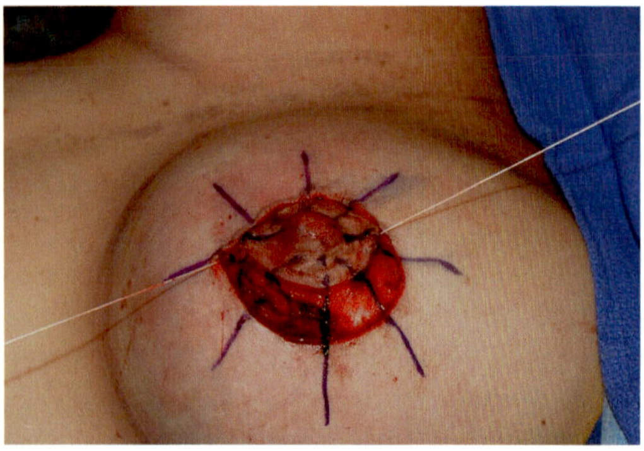

Fig. 6.28 Wagon wheel closure of the NAC with a 3-0 Gortex suture

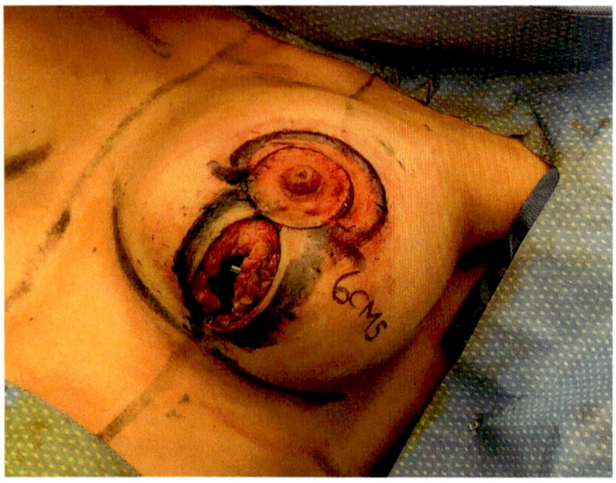

Fig. 6.29 Once symmetry confirmed, tailor-tacked staples removed, and incisions are demarcated with marking pen around the NAC and vertical limb

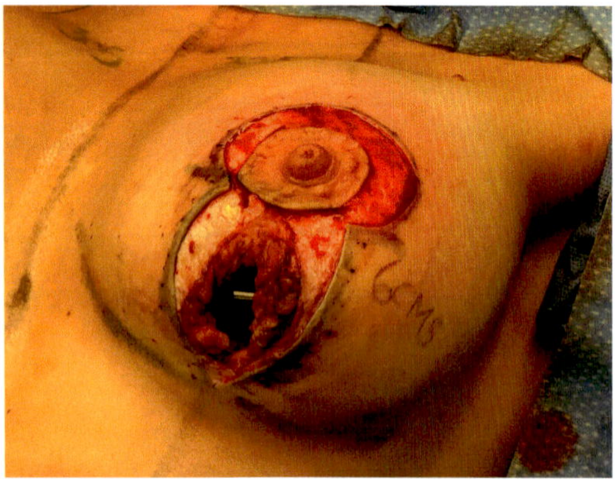

Fig. 6.30 Periareolar and vertical limb are de-epithelialized. Note that the dermis around the NAC is left intact initially and ultimately divided on each side inferiorly but maintaining superiorly from 8–4 o'clock to maintain NAC perfusion

This vessel lies approximate 1–1.5 cm deep, thus protected by the overlying dermis. If the patient is extremely thin, such as in a revision surgery or a patient with paper-thin skin, the vertical skin ± the horizontal skin are de-epithelialized and maintained for additional coverage and support with the mastopexy. However, most patients with ptotic breasts have significant amounts of excess skin and breast tissue in the lower pole. In these patients, de-bulking of the lower pole is probably the single most important step in the procedure to reduce likelihood of recurrent ptosis. Breast flaps along the medial and lateral vertical incisions are initially created, staying approximately 2 cm or greater in thickness. Located centrally is the lower pole segment of breast tissue located from the areola to the IMF within the vertical incisions. This tissue is aggressively de-bulked to reduce lower pole stretch over time with recurrent ptosis. It also reduces the tension on the lower pole mastopexy flap closure. When de-bulking the lower pole, the anterior tissue is removed preserving a posterior lamellae of breast tissue and posterior breast fascia. It is especially important to maintain the "No-Go zone" cuff of breast tissue located above the IMF as this creates the floor for the implant and provides protection for the implant if skin breakdown occurs at the level of the IMF.

Figure 6.31 shows the "No-Go zone" just above IMF to protect the implant.

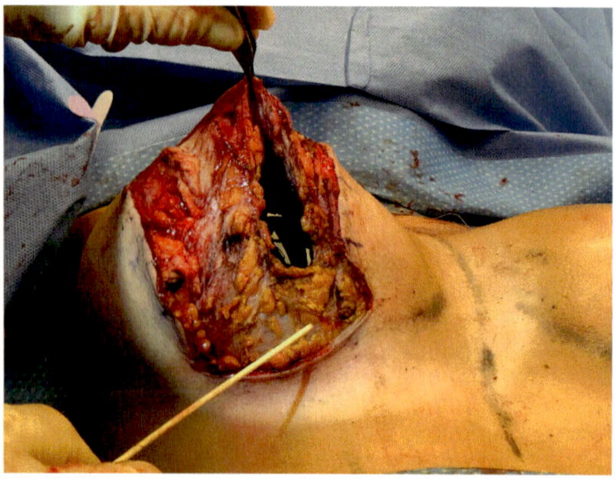

Fig. 6.31 "No-Go zone" just above IMF to protect the implant

Deep Fascial Sling

Once the pedicle has been developed and appropriate skin and breast tissue removed, closure of the breast pocket is performed. However, this step is extremely important to creating a lamellar closure over the implant and developing the shape of the lower pole. As in all mastopexy techniques, controlling the lower pole of the breast through parenchymal shaping and not skin tightening provides increased stability of the results over time. Starting inferiorly, which is just above the "No-Go" cuff of breast tissue, the lateral and medial pillars are brought together at the most posterior aspect of the breast just superficial to the implant with a running 2-0 Vicryl suture. This 2-0 Vicryl running suture carries the closure superiorly towards the NAC, continually tightening the lateral pillar and the medial pillar to create the desired lower pole shape. Therefore, this step is not just closing over the implant, it is parenchymal shaping in a vertical fashion to control overall breast shape and vertical projection. This closure additionally adds an additional layer of closure, protecting the underlying implant.

Figure 6.32a and b shows closure of the posterior lamellae of the implant pocket with a running 2-0 Vicryl suture to provide an additional layer of closure.

Closure

Deep parenchymal sutures of 2-0 vicryl are then placed along the vertical incision bringing the medial and lateral pillars together at the midline.

Figure 6.33 shows closure of medial and lateral breast pillars with 2-0 Vicryl to provide final shape and support of lower breast pole.

All incisions are then closed with interrupted 3-0 PDS dermal sutures. The vertical and horizontal scar are closed with a 4-0 monocryl running subcuticular suture. The areolas are then closed with 3-0 PDS interrupted dermal suture and a simple running 5-0 nylon suture.

Figure 6.34 shows final closure of the breast with patient sitting upright on the operating room table.

Steri-strips are placed over the incision. Contour tape is then placed along the lateral breast border and inframammary fold. The breast are wrapped with a xeroform gauze, Kerlix and ace wrap.

Post-operative Care and Expected Outcomes

The patients are instructed to leave all dressing on for 48 hours. The wraps are then removed, and a sports bra is worn for the following 4 weeks.

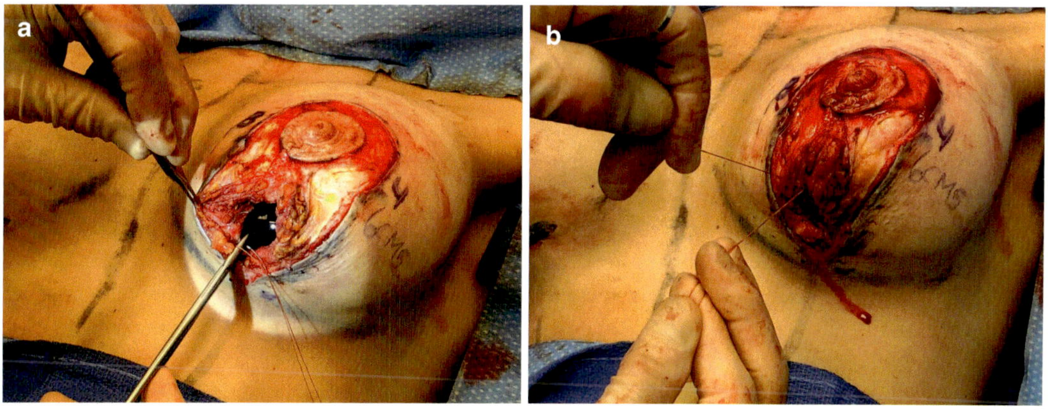

Fig. 6.32 (**a** and **b**) Closure of the posterior lamellae of the implant pocket with a running 2-0 Vicryl suture to provide an additional layer of closure

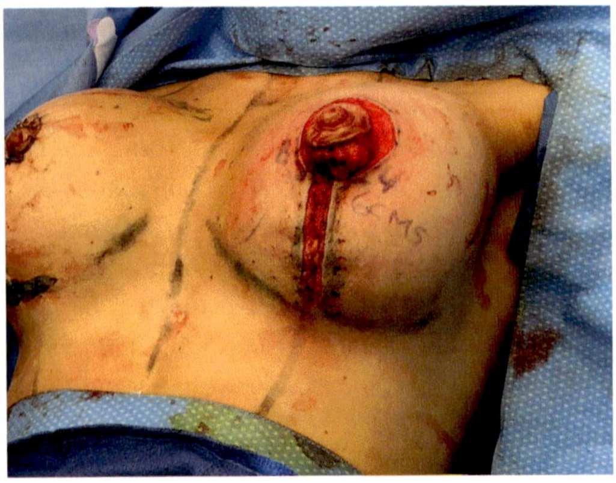

Fig. 6.33 Closure of medial and lateral breast pillars with 2-0 Vicryl to provide final shape and support of lower breast pole

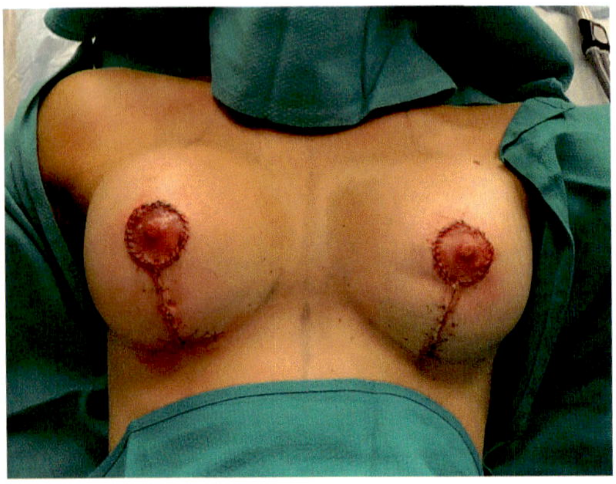

Fig. 6.34 Final closure of the breast with patient sitting upright on the operating room table

Dressing changes with antibiotic ointment and gauze are used over incisions for 1 week. Patients can shower after 48 hours. The contour tape is removed at day 4–7. Nylons around the areolas are removed 6–7 days postoperatively. The subcuticular Monocryls are clipped on the ends as they exit the skin at 2 weeks. Scar management with silicone gel or silicone sheeting is initiated on all patients at 2 weeks. Patients can resume activities of daily living almost immediately. Exercise is usually allowed at 4 weeks with heavy lifting at 6 weeks.

Patients are counseled that they can expect swelling and firmness to develop as her breasts heal. The breasts will continue to soften over time and the breast will relax over the first few months. The results are stable after 6 months, but scars can continue to improve over the first year and some additional relaxation of the breast can continue for even longer.

Complications

The complications in augmentation mastopexy can be considered as tissue-related or implant-related [4, 5]. Two separate procedures are being performed and their associated complications are possible. There are very few significant complications in the early postoperative period. The only significant concern early is ischemia to the nipple-areolar complex or skin flaps. Ischemia may be due to the dissection of the pedicle, but often is secondary to excessive tension on the skin closure and underlying volume under the skin flaps. If recognized immediately, all sutures should be removed to evaluate for improved circulation, improved color, adequate capillary refill and pinprick bleeding. It is important to assure the pedicle is free of tension and not twisted or compromised. Topical nitroglycerin or DMSO (Dimethylsulfoxide) can be used to improved venous outflow. If the closure is too tight due to volume present under the flaps, additional breast volume can be removed, or the implant downsized/removed in an attempt to reduce the closure tension. If any doubt exists, the wound around the NAC should be left unattached and closed the following day if the NAC has clinically improved.

A hematoma usually occurs within the first 24 hours, but a late hematoma at day 10–14 is also occasionally encountered as activity level increases and clots are being resorbed at the end of cauterized vessels. Whereas small amounts of blood within the pocket in a mastopexy without a breast implant is generally less concerning, any blood in the breast pocket around an implant requires exploration and a wash out of the pocket to reduce the risk of capsular contracture postoperatively. Early seromas (less than 1-year postoperative) are more often associated with textured implants and often are treated with aspirations alone. If recalcitrant, exchange to a smooth implant may be required.

Secondary Procedures

Late sequalae include poor scarring, recurrent ptosis, implant malposition, asymmetries, late seromas and capsular contractures. These may require revisional procedures to improve the final aesthetic outcome. Most procedures are delayed at least 6 months or greater to allow for soft tissue remodeling and stabilization of the results. Scars are often the product of excessive tension on the closure and postoperative swelling and can often be improved with scar revisions when the environment for scar maturation is more optimal. An implant malposition requires internal pocket tightening procedures with possible mesh reinforcement. Lower pole stretch deformities and recurrent ptosis are managed similarly with likely the need for a mastopexy revision.

Capsular contracture is the leading cause of implant-related surgery and can be seen early within the first year or may develop years later. For early capsular contractures, non-operative measures are initiated including massage (if a smooth implant), ultrasound therapy (Aspen), Vitamin E, Leukotriene-inhibitor (Montelukast) and possibly a short course of antibiotics. If non-operative management fails, surgical intervention is indicated for Grade 3 and 4 capsular contractures. Treatment includes one or more of the following: a capsulectomy, capsulotomy, implant exchange, pocket exchange, placement of acellular dermal matrix and/or drainage of the breast pocket. In late capsular contractures, it is important to try and solicit any history that may explain its development, such as trauma, dental cleaning, sinus or urinary tract infection or the such. In all late capsular contractures, an implant rupture should also be considered. If treatment mandates surgery, the surgeon should be prepared to exchange the implant if ruptured, although the exchange is often planned already to reduce the incidence of recurrence. If treating the capsular contracture non-operatively, imaging should also be considered to ensure an implant rupture is not present. A late seroma (developing after 1 year) is rare and most associated with textured devices. Although almost always benign, a late seroma is the most common presentation of BIA-ALCL (Breast Implant Associated-Anaplastic Large Cell Lymphoma) and evaluation is mandatory including ultrasound-guided aspiration of the seroma fluid with analysis including testing for CD-30, cell block histology and flow cytometry. Once BIA-ALCL is ruled out, the seroma can be treated like early seromas. If BIA-ALCL is diagnosed, oncologic surgical intervention should be undertaken.

Conclusion

With proper preoperative evaluation and employing accurate surgical techniques, excellent results can be achieved with an augmentation mastopexy. Other than the circumareolar approach, all other augmentation mastopexies are approached as vertical mastopexies based on a superior pedicle blood supply. The pedicle selection and design of the procedure does not refer to the skin excisional pattern, which can range from only a vertical scar to a complete inverted-T pattern. In this technique, any pocket and any implant can be used. Avoidance of recurrent ptosis is a hallmark of a successful procedure. Limiting the size of breast implant and aggressively de-bulking the lower pole breast parenchyma minimize this risk. The fascial sling shaping of the lower pole with a lamellar closure over the implant provides additional support and control of breast shape over time. Although considered challenging by most plastic surgeons, mastery of the techniques outlined in this chapter will provide the best framework for optimizing results, minimizing postoperative complications and insuring high patient satisfaction.

Case Examples

Case 1 34 year old G2P2 female with Grade II ptosis who underwent bilateral Periareolar vertical mastopexy submuscular augmentation with smooth round saline implants; 400cc on the right, 390cc on the left (Fig. 6.35).

Case 2 31 year old female with grade III ptosis after 30lbs weight loss underwent bilateral augmentation periarealor vertical short horizontal mastopexy with textured round moderate profile 305cc silicone implants in the submuscular dual plane pocket (Fig. 6.36).

Case 3 24 year old female with grade III ptosis. Bilateral augmentation periareolar vertical mastopexy with 400cc textured shaped moderate profile silicone implants placed in the submuscular dual plane pocket (Fig. 6.37).

Case 4 34 year old G3P3 female with grade III ptosis underwent bilateral dual plane augmentation full wise (inverted-T) mastopexy with 505cc High profile textured round silicone implants (Fig. 6.38).

Case 5 28 year old female with grade II ptosis underwent bilateral submuscular augmentation periareolar mastopexy with smooth round saline implants filled to 360cc on the right and 320cc on the left (Fig. 6.39).

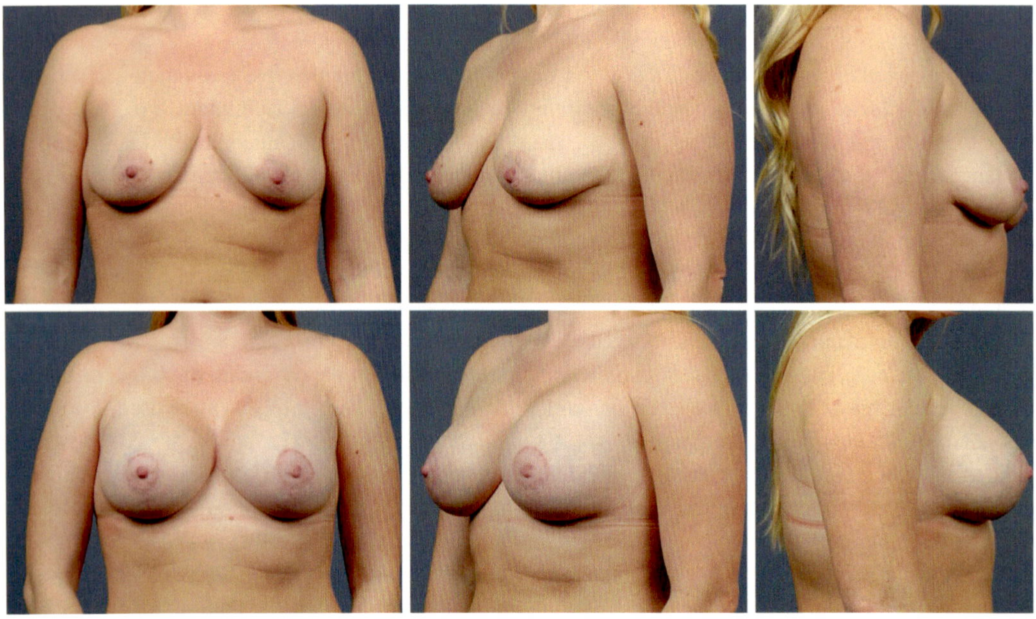

Fig. 6.35 Case example #1

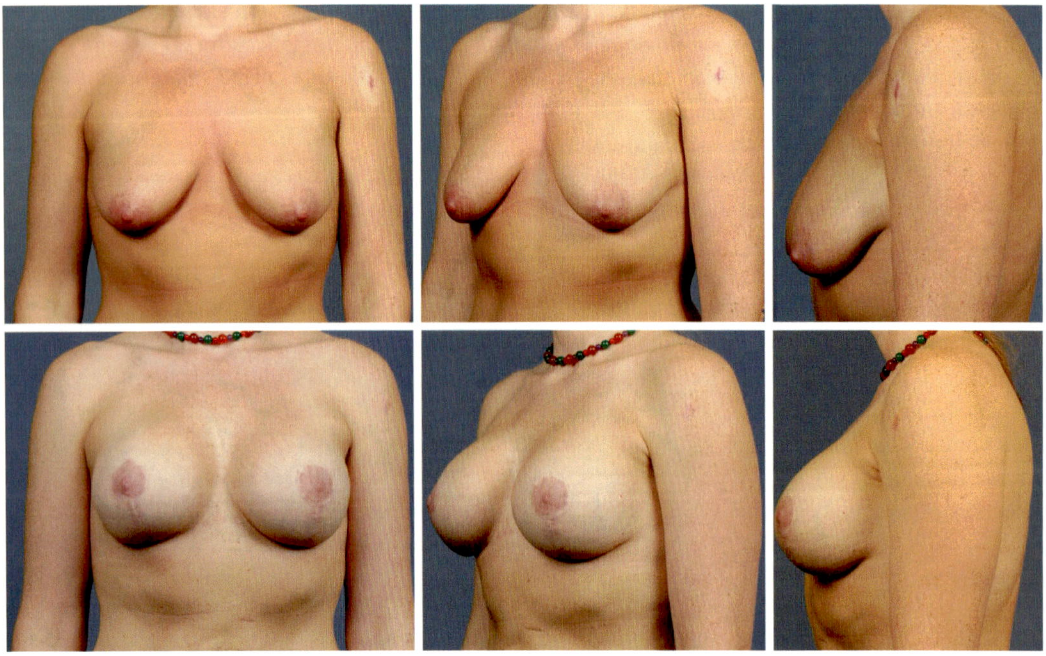

Fig. 6.36 Case example #2

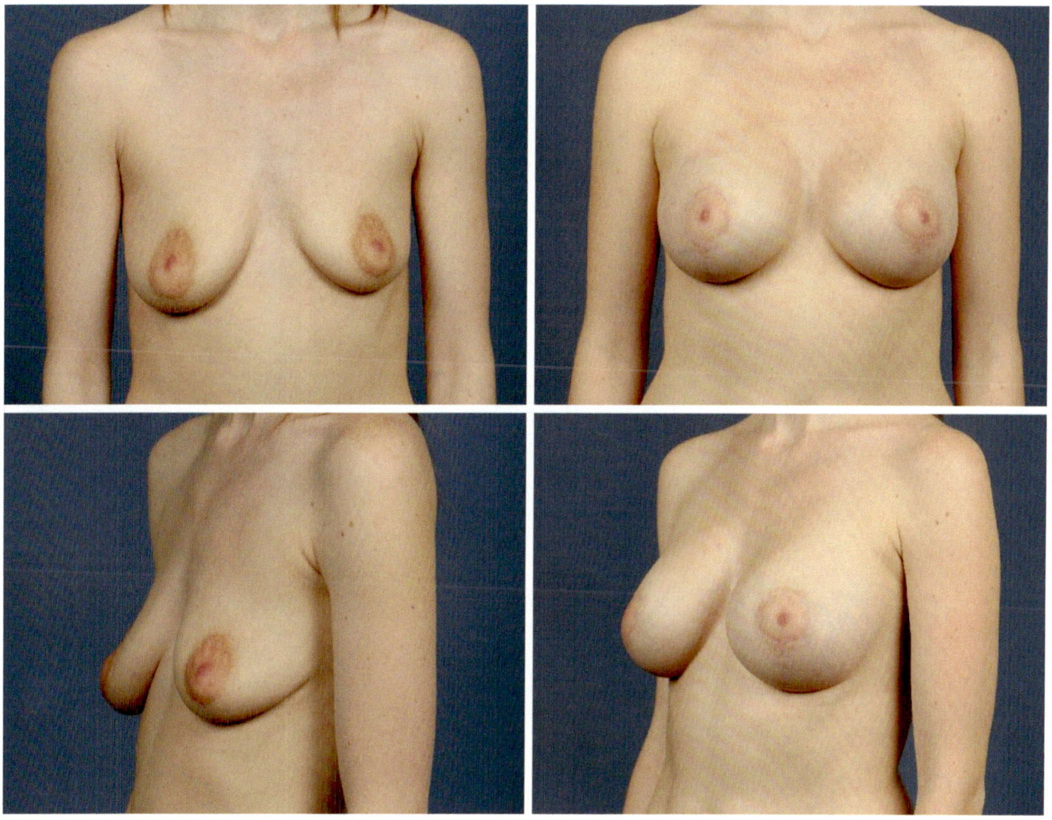

Fig. 6.37 Case example #3

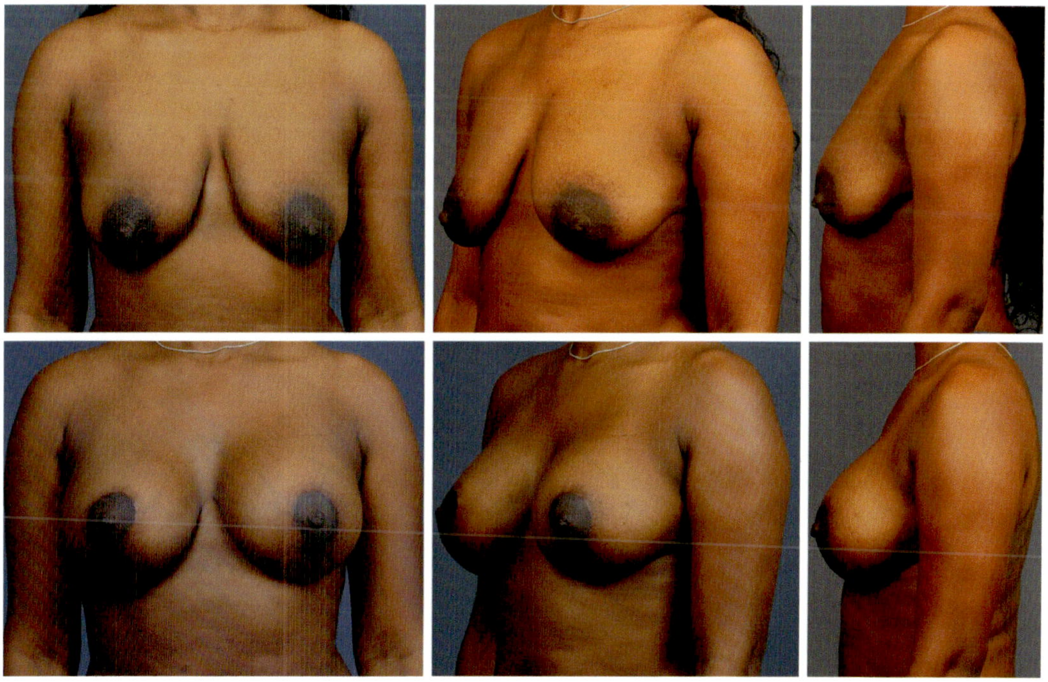

Fig. 6.38 Case example #4

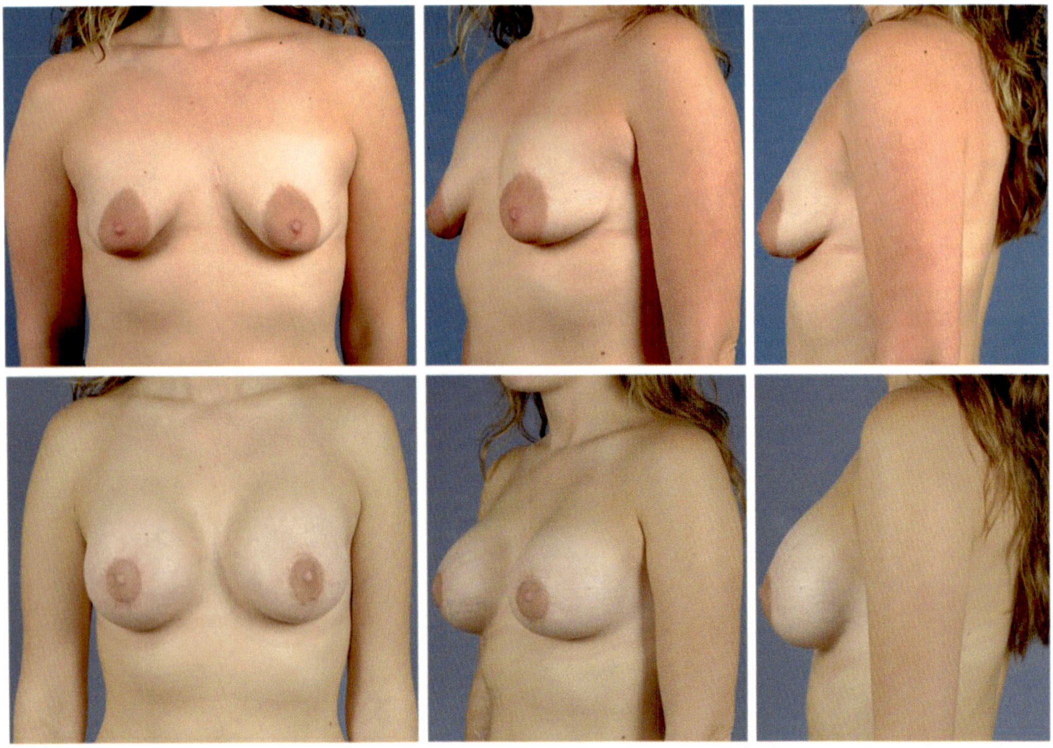

Fig. 6.39 Case example #5

References

1. Hoffman S. Some thoughts on augmentation/mastopexy and medical malpractice. Plast Reconstr Surg. 2004;113:1892–3.
2. Nahai F, Fisher J, Maxwell GP, Mills DC II. Augmentation mastopexy: to stage or not. Aesthet Surg J. 2007;27:297–305.
3. Spears SL. Augmentation mastopexy: "surgeon beware". Plast Reconstr Surg. 2003;112:905–6.
4. Stevens WG, Macias LH, Spring M, et al. One-stage augmentation mastopexy: a review of 1192 simultaneous augmentation and mastopexy procedures in 615 consecutive cases. Aesthet Surg J. 2014;34:723–32.
5. Calobrace MB, Herdt DR, Cothron KJ. Simultaneous augmentation/mastopexy: a retrospective 5-year review of 332 consecutive cases. Plast Reconstr Surg. 2013;131:145–56.
6. Tessone A, Millet E, Weissman O, et al. Evading a surgical pitfall: mastopexy-augmentation made simple. Aesthet Plast Surg. 2011;35:1073–8.
7. Lee MR, Unger JG, Adams WP. The tissue-based triad: a process approach to augmentation mastopexy. Plast Reconstr Surg. 2014;134:215–25.
8. Persoff MM. Mastopexy with expansion-augmentation. Aesthet Surg J. 2003;23:34–9.
9. Hall-Findlay EJ. Breast analysis and clinical concepts. In: Hall-Findlay, editor. Aesthetic breast surgery: concepts and techniques. St. Louis: Quality Medical Publishing, Inc.; 2011.
10. Hall-Findlay EJ. Applied anatomy: key concepts for modern breast surgery. In: Hall-Findlay, editor. Aesthetic breast surgery: concepts and techniques. St. Louis: Quality Medical Publishing, Inc.; 2011.
11. Hall-Findlay EJ. Pedicles in vertical breast reduction and mastopexy. Clin Plast Surg. 2002;29:379–12.
12. Flugstad NA, Pozner JN, Baxter RA, et al. Does implant insertion with a funnel decrease capsular contracture? A preliminary report. Aesthet Surg J. 2016;36:550–6.
13. Mladick RA. "No-touch" submuscular saline breast augmentation technique. Aesthet Plast Surg. 1993;17:183–92.

7 Two-Stage Augmentation Mastopexy

M. Bradley Calobrace, Evan Moore, and Chet Mays

Introduction

To stage or not to stage in augmentation mastopexy continues to be an ongoing discussion among plastic surgeons [1]. Traditionally a two-stage has been the preferred approach as the one-stage approach was believed to have significantly great risk of complications and less predictable long-term results [2–5]. However, surgeons are increasingly employing a one-stage approach in the appropriately selected patients. Recent publications have convincingly demonstrated the combined augmentation mastopexy can be performed safely with good surgical outcomes and high patient satisfaction [6–9]. Some of this is patient driven, as patients prefer one procedure instead of two for obvious reasons including the additional cost and time off work, as well as the natural aversion to additional surgery. Despite this patient preference, it is well-accepted a single stage augmentation mastopexy is one of the more difficult breast procedures due to opposing forces of skin envelope tightening simultaneous with adding more volume and weight to the breast. Thus, not every patient is deemed appropriate for a one-stage procedure [1, 7, 8, 10].

For each patient, an evaluation of the breast is required identifying the unique breast characteristics in regard to tissue quality, soft tissue support, nipple areola complex (NAC) positioning, chest wall anatomy and degree of breast ptosis. This evaluation in combination with assessing the patient's desired outcome, determines the appropriateness of a one-stage or two-stage procedure. A staged procedure is selected if it is believed this approach will produce a more predictable long-term result and/or a resultant lower complication rate, including recurrent ptosis, poor scarring, and/or skin or nipple loss (Fig. 7.1).

This chapter will provide appropriate guidelines for selecting between a one-stage and two-stage augmentation mastopexy. Details of the preoperative planning, surgical approach and postoperative care will be reviewed for a two-stage procedure with an emphasis on the details necessary to achieve optimal outcomes that are predictable and reproducible.

M. B. Calobrace (✉)
Private Practice, CaloAesthetics Plastic Surgery Center, Louisville, KY, USA

Clinical Faculty, University of Louisville, Division of Plastic Surgery, Louisville, KY, USA

Clinical Faculty, University of Kentucky, Division of Plastic Surgery, Lexington, KY, USA
e-mail: drbrad@calobrace.com

E. Moore
Calobrace Aesthetic Surgery Fellowship, Louisville, KY, USA

C. Mays
Private Practice, CaloAesthetics Plastic Surgery Center, Louisville, KY, USA

Clinical Faculty, University of Louisville, Division of Plastic Surgery, Louisville, KY, USA

M. B. Calobrace et al. (eds.), *Augmentation Mastopexy*,
https://doi.org/10.1007/978-3-030-48226-8_7

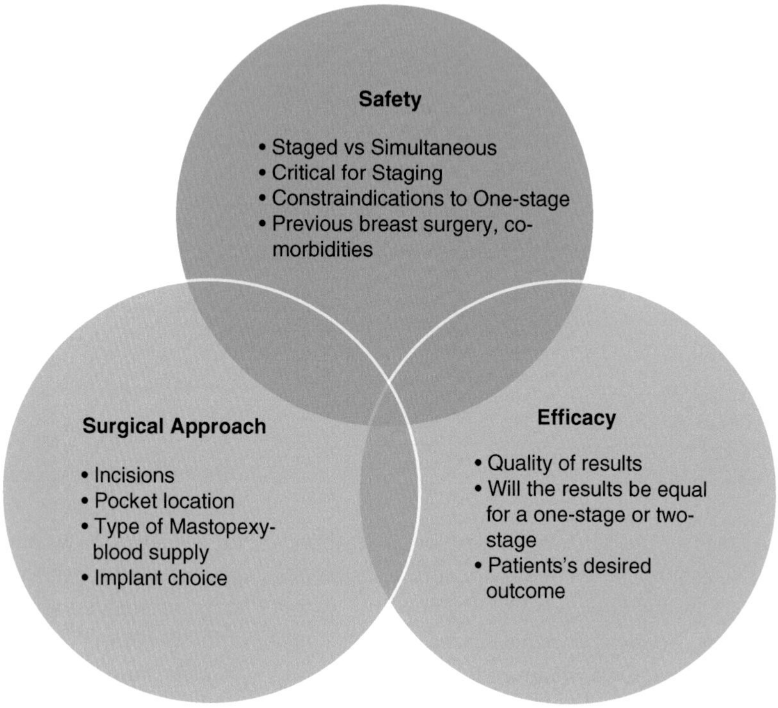

Fig. 7.1 One stage vs Two stage – a balance between the efficacy and safety of a one-stage vs two stage ultimately determined by patient factors, the surgical approach and the desired outcome

Pre-operative Evaluation

Medical history The evaluation preoperatively includes obtaining a patient medical history, performing a focused physical exam, and determining the patient's goals and expectations. Initially, it is important to determine if any previous history of breast pathology, benign or malignant. It is important to determine if any prior breast procedures has been performed including any biopsies, aesthetic or reconstructive procedures, and most importantly any history of breast radiation. This information will aid in identifying the current health and blood supply status of the breast and nipple areolar complex. Obtaining previous medical records can be extremely helpful in determining the breast status and alterations in blood supply from previous procedures that may provide insight into the safety of a simultaneous procedure. A patient with a history of prior breast radiation or aesthetic procedures wanting augmentation mastopexy might be better suited in a two-stage approach due impaired wound healing or worries of vascular supply with a one-stage procedure [11].

A history of blood clots, bleeding disorders, or current use of blood thinning medications should be evaluated. The nicotine status of the patient is also important to establish, including smoking, nicotine gum patches, dips and more recently vaporizers. Smoking impairs wound healing and restricts blood supply and any patient refusing to quit at least 1 month prior to surgery or unable to stop in the time frame of surgery would be best served by staging her augmentation mastopexy [12]. Also pertinent is a history of breast feeding, pregnancies, possible future pregnancies, as well as any significant weight loss or weight gain. This information provides a better understanding of the changes in breast volume and support that may have developed over time. Particularly, massive weight loss patients because their tissue has lost the supportive structure of the breast ligament have a significantly increased risk of postoperative ptosis after a single stage procedure. This increases the risk of postoperative pseudoptosis, or waterfall deformity and this group of patients can often achieve superior results with a staged procedure [13, 14].

Ironically, the patients with large BMIs (BMI >30) without weight loss also have an increased risk of postoperative ptosis due to the heaviness and significant sag of the breast and often do better with a staged procedure [7]. Finally, as related to the medical history, patients with more complicated medical history with associated comorbidities might be best suited for a staged procedure to keep it less complicated with associated decrease operative times and associated risk or anesthesia or wound healing complications.

Physical exam During the breast exam measurements should be taken including the base width, sternal notch to nipple distances, nipple to inframammary fold (IMF) distances at rest and under maximal stretch and the intermammary distance (Fig. 7.2).

The amount of breast ptosis should be noted per the Regnault's classification a based on the relationship of the NAC to the inframammary fold [15]. However, this only provides limitation information in terms of the type of ptosis present and a more thorough evaluation should be documented including the assessment of breast ptosis outlined in Table 7.1.

Breasts that are large pendulous or that have a significant volume requiring a large reduction might be better suited for staged procedures (Fig. 7.3). The relationship of the nipple areola complex (NAC) to the breast mound and inframammary fold should be noted. This will help assess the amount of nipple elevation that may be

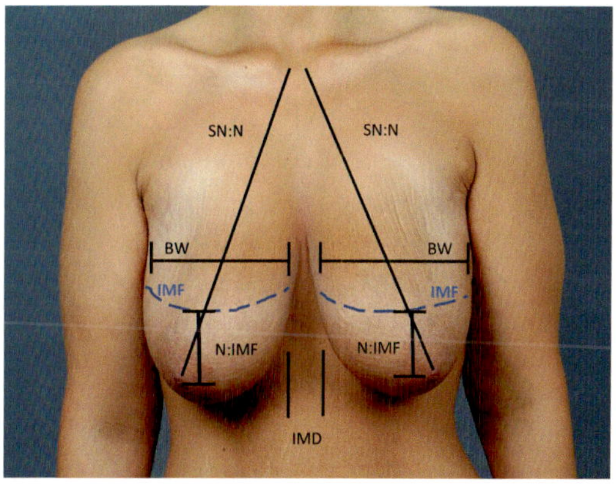

Fig. 7.2 Diagram of preoperative standard measurements

Table 7.1 Assessment of breast ptosis

Relationship of the NAC to the IMF (Regnault's degree of ptosis) **Grade 1**: nipple at the level of the inframammary fold, above the lower contour of the gland **Grade 2:** nipple below the level of the inframammary fold, above the lower contour of the gland **Grade 3:** nipple below the level of the inframammary fold, at the lower contour of the gland
Amount of breast tissue overhanging the fold
Location of the NAC on the breast mound
Amount of vertical excess and horizontal excess
Footprint of the breast on the chest wall – low, medium, high
Quality and quantity of breast parenchyma and skin

required. It is recommended that NAC elevation greater than 5–6 cm is a significant amount of ptosis and would be better staged [7]. The breast compositions should also be evaluated including the quality of breast tissue and skin. Other aspects of the physical exam should focus on the skin thickness and elasticity, the breast fat quantity and location, and the composition and firmness of the breast parenchyma. Asymmetries of the breast should be noted including volume, shape (narrow vs wide), projection and IMF positions. Chest wall contour difference should be noted. All these aspects of the breast will influence the difficulty of the procedure, the final shape of the breast, and ultimately the surgical outcome. Patients with significant asymmetries may best be suited by staging the procedure, performing the mastopexy to make the breast position and volume symmetrical in the first operation, followed by a breast augmentation in the future.

Determining the amount of vertical excess that is present will assist in determining whether a mastopexy is necessary, and if so, what type of mastopexy should be performed. It also can assist in determining the appropriate patients for staging [8]. Patients with similar levels of ptosis can have quite different amounts of vertical excess. To determine the vertical excess (VE), the new nipple position distance to the new inframammary fold is subtracted from the new nipple position and the patient's actual Inframammary fold. It

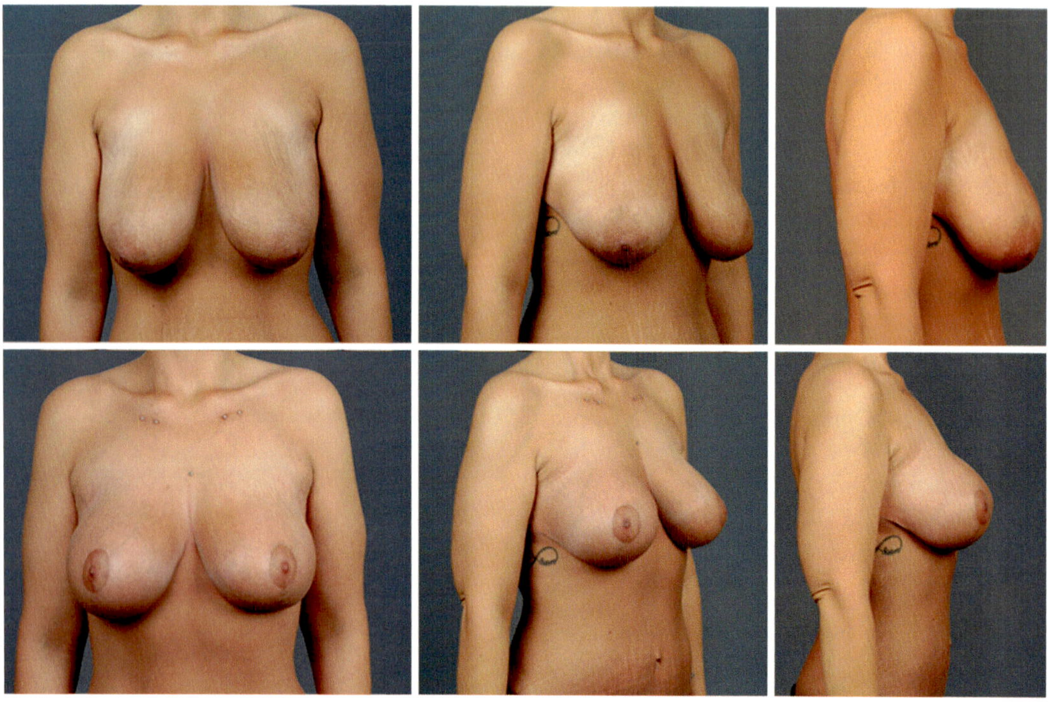

Fig. 7.3 (Above) A large, pendulous breast with poor soft tissue quality and excessive vertical excess. (Below) Postoperative view after undergoing a simultaneous augmentation mastopexy reveals excessive stretching of the mastopexy and loss of upper pole volume. This patient would be more appropriate for a staged procedure

Table 7.2 Vertical excess

Vertical excess (VE)
VE = new nipple to actual IMF – new nipple to new IMF
VE > 6 or 8–10 cm consider staging augmentation mastopexy

has been suggested, patients with vertical excess greater than 8–10 cm should be considered for a two-staged procedure, while others have reported reduced reoperation rates if patients with vertical excess of greater than 6 centimeters are selected for staging (Table 7.2) [7, 8].

Managing Patient Expectations

Managing patient expectations are key to a successful outcome in any procedure and can help aid the surgeon in the decision to combine the two procedures or to separate them. The physician should explain and show what is possible with the patient's breast and chest anatomy. For example, a patient with a small narrow B cup size breast with grade III ptosis might not have good enough quality skin envelope and/or inadequate chest wall dimensions or breast tissue to support an 800 cc implant. In discussing the patient's goals the surgeon can discern the patients desires for having the breasts lifted off of the abdomen back up onto the chest, an enhancement, reduction or similar breast size post-treatment and the degree in which she desires upper pole fullness. Understanding the patient's goals is important to establish a clear line of communication between the surgeon and patient, manage her expectations and plan the approach that has the best chance of achieving her goals. Patients must understand that a single stage augmentation mastopexy has less predictable results with a significant reoperation rate due to issues related to the augmentation and the breast lift [1, 2, 6–8].

It is possible that two separate procedures have a greater potential to allow for more control over the lift and augmentation to obtain a good long-term cosmetic result. For patients desiring significant volumes or upper pole volume, or having unrealistic expectations regarding final breast shape and size, a more predictable outcome may be accomplished with a staged procedure. Patients need to accept the challenges inherent in a single stage procedure with reoperation rates exceeding 20% and unwillingness to accept this would likely be more appropriately selected for a staged procedure. Finally, the patient needs to accept the scars of the mastopexy and the lifelong management and surveillance of breast implants and their associated risks to be acceptable candidates for a one-stage or two-stage procedure.

Managing the patient's expectations throughout the surgical process is critical to successful outcomes and always requires more than one visit or consultation prior to the procedure to reinforce surgical expectations.

One-stage vs Two-stage

The preoperative evaluation provides important insights into the appropriate path to take with the augmentation mastopexy patient, including the history, physical exam and assessment of the patient's expectations. Tables 7.3 and 7.4 summaries these relative indications and considerations for selecting a two-staged augmentation mastopexy vs a one-stage (Tables 7.3 and 7.4).

Additionally, the surgeon should also be self-aware of their own comfort level in performing a single stage augmentation mastopexy. If there is significant discomfort with performing a single stage augmentation mastopexy based on the patient's breast anatomy or the surgeon's experience, it may be preferable to stage the procedures to enhance patient safety and aesthetic outcomes.

Table 7.3 Relative Indications for a staged augmentation mastopexy

Obesity: BMI >30
Large, pendulous breasts – needs volume reduction
Significant breast ptosis – NAC elevation >5–6 cm
Vertical excess >8–10 cm
Unrealistic expectations (patient won't accept reoperation rate > 20%)
Smoker refusing to quit >4 weeks
Previous surgery impacting blood supply

Table 7.4 Additional considerations for a staged augmentation mastopexy

Significant breast asymmetry
Borderline case – May be acceptable for mastopexy or augmentation alone
Previous breast radiation
Large implant volume or "augmented" look desired
Massive weight loss patient
Immunocompromised patient
History of hypertrophic scarring
Multiple medical co-morbidities
Surgeon uncomfortable performing a single stage procedure based on the breast anatomy of the patient or surgeon inexperience

When staging the two procedures, there is no wrong order on which procedure should be performed first, but most surgeons select to perform the mastopexy in the first stage followed by an augmentation in the second stage. Performing the mastopexy first followed by an augmentation also allows for a mastopexy revisions at the time of augmentation. The average timing between the two procedures is usually 6–12 months. In our office we typically wait 6 months to perform the augmentation after mastopexy. Augmentation can be performed first if the patient believes a breast lift may not be necessary. If ultimately a mastopexy is needed, it may be advantageous that expansion has occurred and a capsule formed, putting less stress on the mastopexy postoperatively improving the ultimate outcome.

Surgical Planning

Mastopexy

There are a variety mastopexy designs. The type of mastopexy needed can be determined based on the type and level of ptosis present. In mastopexy design, the goal is to reposition the NAC and the breast itself. In patients who need only NAC elevation, a staged procedure would not be selected and a periareolar augmentation mastopexy would be performed. Likewise, in patients with breast pseudoptosis only where the nipple is in good position above the IMF, a one-stage augmentation would be performed with an augmentation and the vertical excess addressed by a "smile" mastopexy, or IMF resection. Similarly, breast pseudoptosis with good NAC positioning and only vertical and horizontal excess in the lower pole, an augmentation and sailboat mastopexy is performed as a one-stage [10].

The mastopexy for a staged procedure should address repositioning the NAC and managing the vertical excess with repositioning of the breast above the inframammary fold. The preference is to perform the mastopexy through a superior or superomedial pedicle vertical approach [16, 17] (Fig. 7.4). This maximizes the NAC circulation for the staged breast augmentation, as the implant pocket creation does not impact these pedicles as they lie superficial in the breast tissue leading to the NAC. Likewise, in the verical approach, the parenchyma is shaped leaving the volume above and debulking the lower pole, thus providing the best situation for minimizing the chance of pseudoptosis after the staged augmentation. In grade 1 and 2 ptosis with moderate vertical excess, the mastopexy can be performed with a circumvertical or circumvertical with small horizontal wedge. In grade 2–3 breast ptosis with significant horizontal or vertical excess, a vertical approach is accomplished with a inverted-T type skin excision (Fig. 7.5). Only in the most significant types of breast ptosis where a superiorly based pedicle

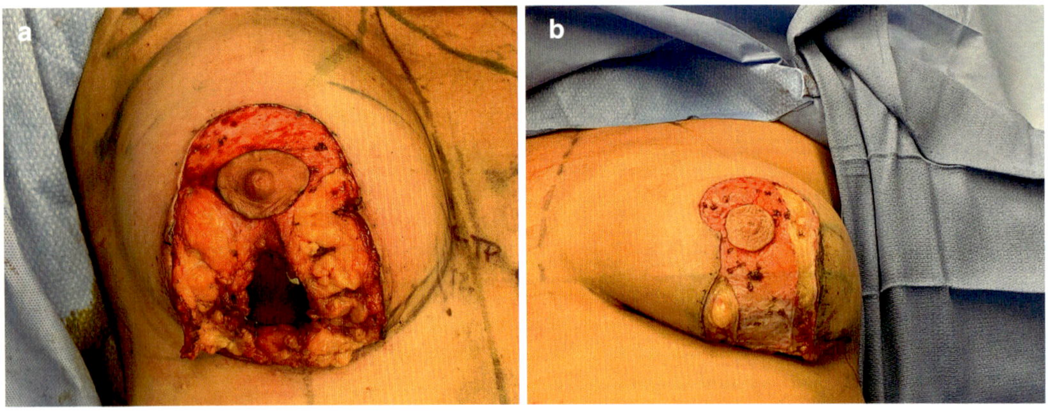

Fig. 7.4 (**a**) Superior Pedicle Design (**b**) Superiomedial Pedicle Design

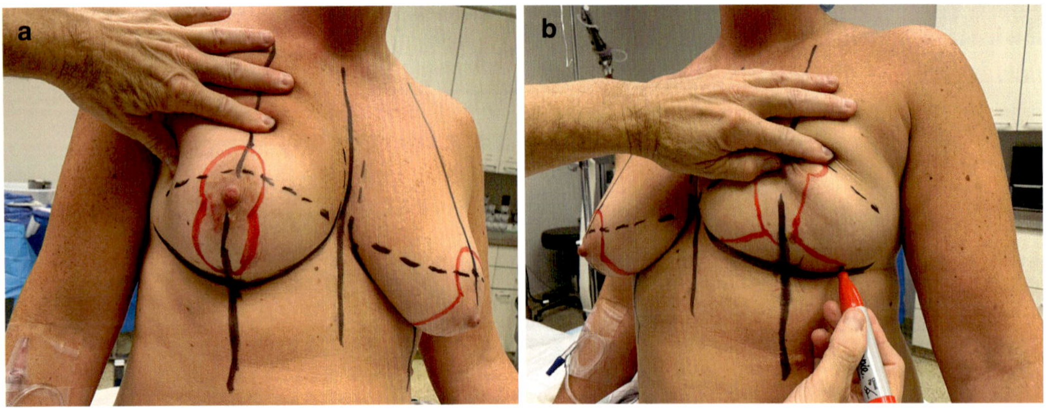

Fig. 7.5 Strategies for skin excision with vertical mastopexies. (**a**) Periareolar Vertical incision (**b**) Periareolar Vertical Short Horizontal Incision to remove vertical excess

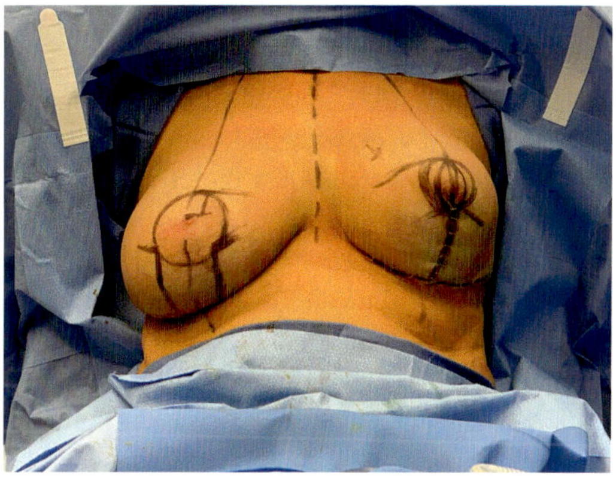

Fig. 7.6 Tailor-tacking the mastopexy design before making incisions

is not possible, a central or inferior pedicle approach is performed with an inverted-T skin wedge. In most mastopexy designs the use of tailor-tacking in the operating room can help confirm and set breast shape desired prior to commitment of the breast markings (Fig. 7.6). Finally, it is important to determine if asymmetry is present and one side requires additional volume or skin removal to produce symmetrical breast. Likewise, a determination on the need for volume reduction is assessed. This is important because when performing the mastopexy without the augmentation, there is no true limitation and any amount of volume reduction can be accomplished.

Augmentation

Implant Selection

In selecting an implant, the breast base width will help guide implant selection along with the desired volume [1]. An optimal breast implant width is determined by the desired breast width (anterior axillary line to 1 cm from the midline of the chest) minus the soft tissue contribution from the native breast using the medial and lateral pinch. Tebbetts' method of implant selection is a more comprehensive method for choosing an implant [18, 19]. If there is some uncertainty about the volume needed operative use of sizers can aid in a finalized decision. The surgeon should choose an implant that can be supported by the new lifted breast and its associated soft tissue characteristics. Certainly, by staging the procedure, the impact of a larger implant will be less than if the larger implant was placed at the same time as the mastopexy. One of the significant advantages of a staged procedure is the ability to more accurately assess the remaining breast volume and shape after the mastopexy and thus more effectively engage the patient to choose the final implant size.

Implant Placement

There are a variety of pockets available to the surgeon for implant placement. Pocket decision is based on the physical exam and lifestyle of the patient. A body builder, for example, may not be the best fit for submuscular placement due to the tendency for animation deformity postoperatively. Whereas a submuscular dual plane is commonly used, patients with at least a 2-centimeter upper pole pinch are considered good candidates also for subglandular or subfascial coverage. In patients with a poor-quality soft tissue envelope such as those seen requiring mastopexies, the submuscular dual plane pocket provides support for the implant and can limit the amount of postoperative stretch of the skin. Additionally, the submuscular pocket is associated with a lower capsular contracture rate [20, 21]. However, the submuscular pocket also can stabilize the implant too much, leading to a waterfall deformity as the loose breast tissue descends off the implant [22, 23].

The subglandular/subfascial pocket however eliminates any animation deformity and allows the implant to more effectively fill out the loose skin envelope without the interference from the muscle. Finally, consideration of the vascular supply is always important as the first stage mastopexy impacts the blood supply. A subglandular/fascial pocket dissection will disrupt pectoralis muscle perforating vessels going to the overlying breast tissue where a submuscular pocket preserves some of these perforating vessels. This may be extremely important if there are concerns as to the type of pedicle performed with the initially mastopexy. Either submuscular or Subglandular/fascial pocket dissection are generally appropriate as staging the procedure and performing the mastopexy initially provides the safest approach to minimize vascular concerns in the second stage augmentation.

Augmentation Incision

The location of the incision is based on the location of the mastopexy scars. The decision should be based on the location that will provide the greatest access and not create new scarring if possible. If a vertical mastopexy was performed, the surgeon can either go through the previous vertical incision or create a new IMF incision and avoid the old scarring. If an IMF incision was part of the mastopexy, that is almost always the first choice. One advantage of the staged mastopexy augmentation is that during the second stage augmentation, the mastopexy can be revised to retighten the skin envelope or revise any unattractive scars and this becomes the access location for the augmentation.

For most patients, the authors prefer mastopexy for the first stage followed by an augmentation in the second stage. One reason is the patient may be perfectly satisfied with her mastopexy and not desire an implant ultimately. Additionally, if the patient fails to follow up for the augmentation, the mastopexy would be better for the ptotic, deflated breast as opposed to an implant with breast tissue hanging over it [10]. The mastopexy performed at the first stage also provides an opportunity to adjust the mastopexy and make any revisions during the augmentation.

Operative Technique

The patient should be marked in an upright position prior to the procedure. The markings are important to establish and confirm operative plans prior to the surgery with both the patient and the surgeon. This is a good time to go over the patient's goals again and reestablish patient expectations of the surgery. The staged plan should be discussed once again to confirm patients understanding of the future surgeries.

Mastopexy

For the first stage mastopexy the patient markings can start by drawing the patient's midline from the sternal notch down the chest to below the inframammary fold (IMF). The breast meridian should be marked in a similar fashion to below the IMF. Mark the IMF on both sides of the breast. The transposition of the patient's breast IMF to the anterior breast can be used to mark the new nipple position (Pitanguy's point). The superior part of the new areola is then marked starting 2 cm above the proposed new nipple position. At this point the rest of the design can be drawn out based on the type of mastopexy. Regardless of the marks, one may select to do tailor tacking at the beginning of the case to get an idea of breast shape based on the patient's anatomy prior to making an incision. Tailor-tacking is critical in a one-stage procedure, placing the implant first and then reassessing and adjusting the mastopexy markings prior to making any incisions (Fig. 7.7). In a mastopexy without implants, it is the surgeon's decision as to the confidence in the markings and whether tailor tacking is helpful (Fig. 7.6). Keep in mind, when tailoring tacking a larger, more ptotic breast, significant volume in the breast may not allow for accurate tailor tacking so the pre-operative markings are critical.

Surgical Technique: The patient is taken to the operating room and placed in the supine position

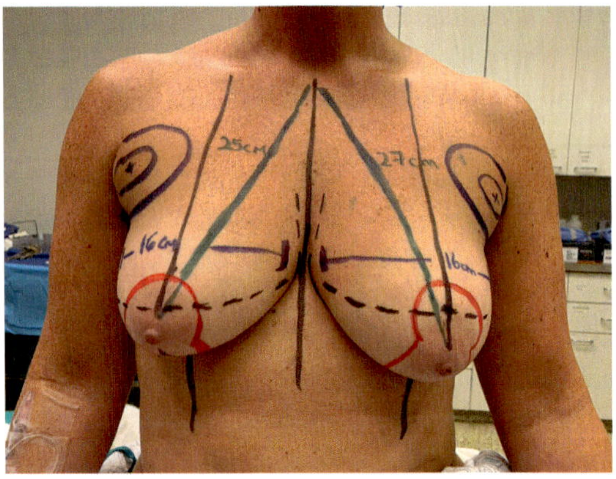

Fig. 7.7 Preoperative markings for the first stage mastopexy

with the arms and placed on arm boards at 45 degrees and securely wrapped to allow the patient to be placed upright during the case for evaluation of the mastopexy (Fig. 7.8). After induction of anesthesia, a local anesthetic field block is performed using a ¼% lidocaine, 1/8% bupivacaine, 1:400,000 epinephrine (Fig. 7.9). Once the field block has been administered, the patient is prepped with Chlorhexidine and draped in a sterile fashion. The markings are then confirmed and reinforced. The areolas are then marked using a 38–45-mm diameter breast cookie cutter and then scored with a 15 blade (Fig. 7.10). If indicated, a stapler is then used to tailor-tack the preoperative breast mastopexy pattern markings. At this point adjustments are made based on the shape of the breast. The final nipple areolar position is then determined and marked with 38–45 mm diameter breast cookie cutter. Methylene blue on a cotton tip is used to outline the preferred shape for the mastopexy. Staples are then removed, and the pattern is then scored with a 15 blade. The mastopexy is then performed based on the type of mastopexy pattern chosen based on the amount of breast ptosis. The superior or superomedial pedicle is de-epithelialized. The medial and lateral pillars are dissected down to the chest wall. The central lower island of breast tissue is either excised or transposed into the subareolar space attached to the superior areola for vascular supply. The remainder of the breast tissue is excised deep on the chest wall, especially laterally to shape the final breast. Hemostasis is assured, pockets irrigated and medial and lateral pillars are brought together with multiple 2-0 Vicryl pillar sutures. The areola to fold distance is generally maintained at 6–8 cm based on the final breast size and any additional vertical length is excised through an horizontal wedge excision.

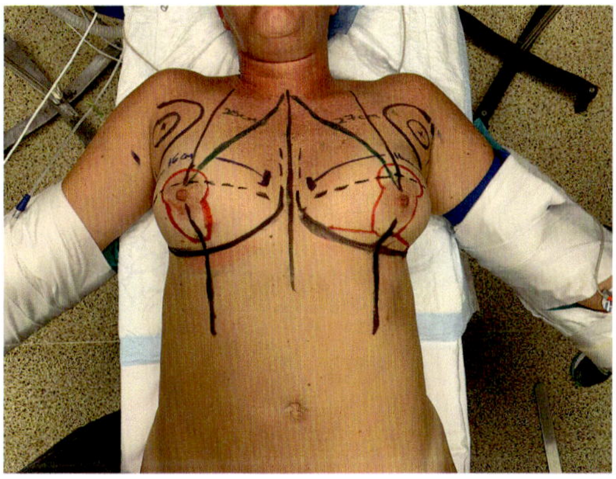

Fig. 7.8 Patient placed in supine position with arms secured at 45 degrees

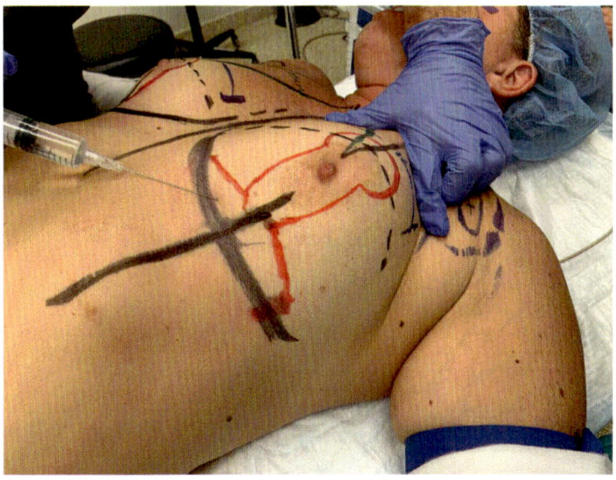

Fig. 7.9 Field block with ¼% lidocaine, 1/8% bupivacaine, 1:400,000 epinephrine

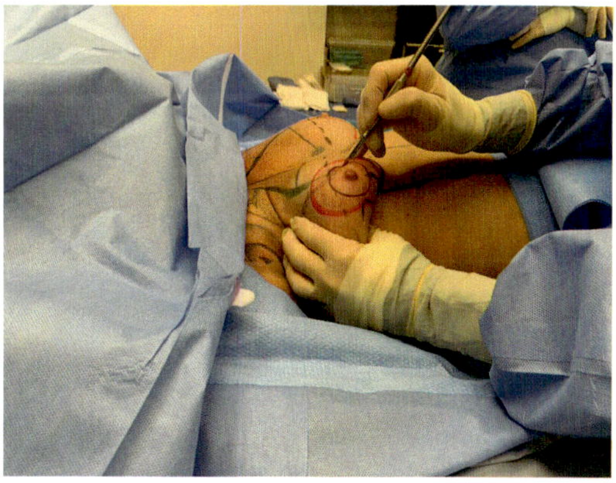

Fig. 7.10 The areolas are marked using a 38–45-mm diameter breast cookie cutter and then scored with a 15 blade

In a vertical mastopexy where a staged augmentation is not planned, the mastopexy may be fashioned with a longer vertical length and the lower pole debulked and the skin allowed to re-drape back onto the abdomen instead of excising it. However, when an augmentation is planned in the future, excision of the vertical excess is preferred to prepare the lower pole for the implant in the future (Fig. 7.11). Certainly, either is appropriate and the will be determined by the patient's anatomy and the surgeon's preference. The remainder of the closure is accomplished with 3-0 PDS interrupted dermal sutures and running subcuticular 4-0 Monocryl sutures along the incisions. The areola is inset with 3-0 PDS dermal sutures and a running 5-0 nylon. The patient is wrapped with xeroform, kerlex and ace wrap for 24 hours followed by a sports bra for 4 weeks.

Second Stage Augmentation

The second stage can be done after 6–12 months following the first procedure depending on the clinical course and the relaxation and softening of the lifted breast. Preoperative planning is ultimately performed as with any other breast augmentation. The significant advantage of the staged procedure is the mastopexy reshapes and lifts the breast, allowing for appropriate sizing of the implant based on the new dimensions of the breast. This likewise allows the patient to more effectively participate in the selection of the implant and ultimate breast size.

In the procedure, preoperative markings are performed including any mastopexy adjustments that may be performed with the augmentation. Local anesthetic is again placed in the

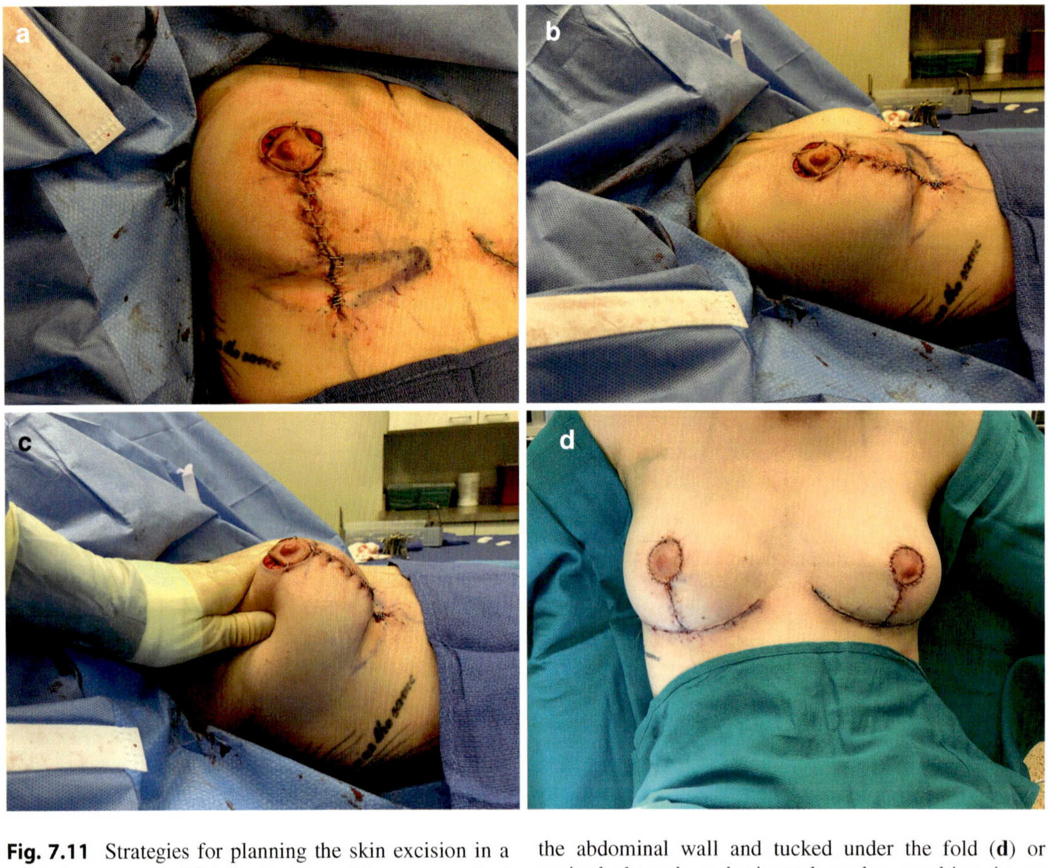

Fig. 7.11 Strategies for planning the skin excision in a vertical mastopexy. (**a**) tailor-tacking with excess vertical length. (**b**, **c**) excess skin can either be re-established onto the abdominal wall and tucked under the fold (**d**) or excised through a horizontal wedge resulting in an inverted-T pattern

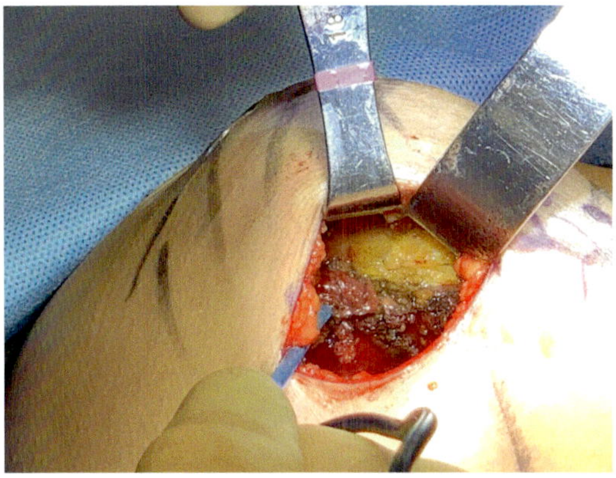

Fig. 7.12 Pocket selection for a staged augmentation include submuscular, subfascial and subglandular. The preferred pocket is a dual-plane submuscular pocket as seen in the image

areas of the planned incisions. The patient is prepped and draped in a similar fashion except nipple shields are placed to improve the sterile field. The preferred incision for placement of the implants will be through the previous mastopexy incisions, either in the vertical scar or along the IMF. If there are to be breast revisions to the augmentation access to pocket dissection through planned revisions is an option to limit further incisions on the breast. If the submuscular pocket is selected, a dual plane technique is performed to allow the implant to expand and lift the lower pole (Fig. 7.12). Pocket development may create more bleeding as there has been previous surgery and dissection in the breast. Meticulous prospective hemostasis is extremely helpful. Sizers can then be placed at this point to confirm implant selection, although generally sizers are reserved for confirmation in significant asymmetry cases. Irrigation is performed with a 50% betadine solution (Fig. 7.13). Gloves are then changed, and the implant is placed using the no touch technique with an insertion device, such as the Keller funnel (Fig. 7.14). The implant pocket is closed using a running 2-0 Vicryl suture. If an IMF incision has been made, or the new fold position is secured with deep bites of the underlying chest/abdominal wall fascia and the superficial fascia. The incision is then closed with 4-0 PDS interrupted dermal sutures and a running 4-0 PDS subcuticular.

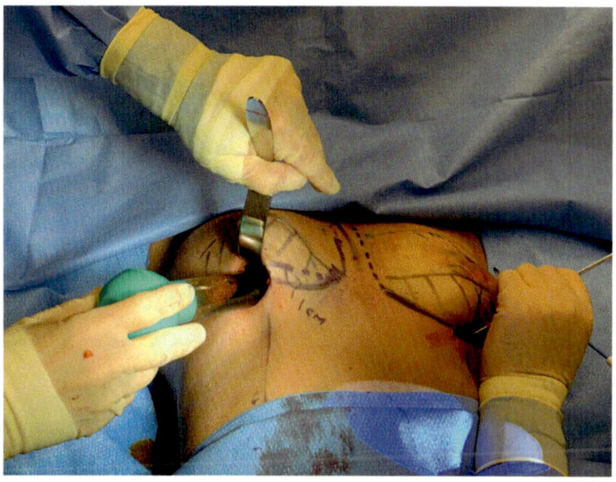

Fig. 7.13 Implant pocket irrigated with a 50% or greater betadyne solution

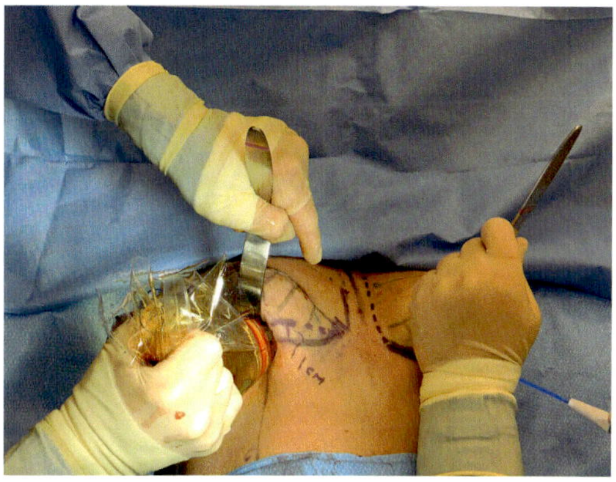

Fig. 7.14 Implant placement with an implant insertion device, such as the Keller funnel, to minimize bacterial contamination especially when the implant is placed through the mastopexy incisions requiring transgression of the implant through the breast tissue

Post-Operative Care

Following the first stage mastopexy procedure, patients have their dressings removed the next day and the NAC and breast flaps evaluated for any vascular compromise. It is important to rule out any hematoma early postoperatively as the unrecognized hematoma can create vascular compromise due to the compression on the breast. Sports bras are then worn for 4 weeks. They are instructed to sleep elevated at 45 degrees for two weeks after surgery. At 2 weeks post operatively, patients are instructed on scar management with silicone-based scar creams (such as Biocorneum) for 3–6 months and sun avoidance for 1 year.

Generally, the second augmentation procedure will be performed 6–12 months following the mastopexy. Patients are wrapped for 24 hours then begin a sports bra for 4 weeks full time and 2 additional weeks at bedtime. They are not to submerge in any type of water for 4 weeks post operatively. Showers may begin 24 hours post-surgery. Patients are instructed to avoid dental work and/or cleanings for 6 months post operatively. If there is a necessity to have dental work, a prescription for antibiotics is provided. Stretching exercises are initiated immediately postoperatively with arm rasies and shoulder rolls. Breast massages protocols are begun usually 4–7 days after the surgery for those with smooth implants. No massage is performed if a textured device is use.

Conclusion

Augmentation mastopexy can be challenging even in the most straightforward cases. Not all patients need or are appropriate for a one stage augmentation mastopexy. Surgeons and patients should be heeding the warning that there can be a trap or an allure of a possibility of a one and done surgery, but both need to understand the challenges inherent in such an undertaking. Patient's with large BMIs (>30), significant breast ptosis, large pendulous breast, notable vertical excess (>8–10 cm) and a patient with unrealistic expectations should be considered for staged procedures. Again, the surgeon needs to keep in mind there are two forces working against each other and when one or both are significant, staging the two procedures may be a safer and more effective option. Clear communication with the patients, understanding their goals and managing expectations sets the stage for a positive outcome no matter what approach is selected.

Case Examples are shown in Figs. 7.15, 7.16, 7.17, and 7.18.

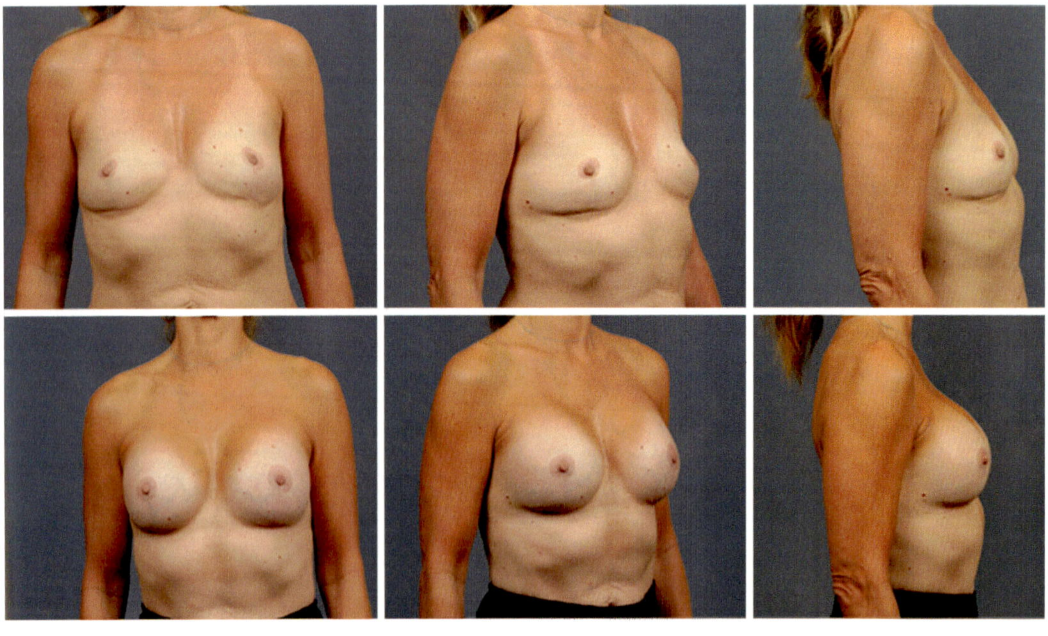

Fig. 7.15 55-year-old G5P4 underwent an explantation and mastopexy 20 years previously resulting in small breasts, lack of upper pole volume and mastopexy scars including inframammary fold irregularities (upper images). She underwent a breast augmentation with a dual plane textured round 385 cc implant and revisions of the vertical and horizontal mastopexy scars (lower images are 1 year postoperative)

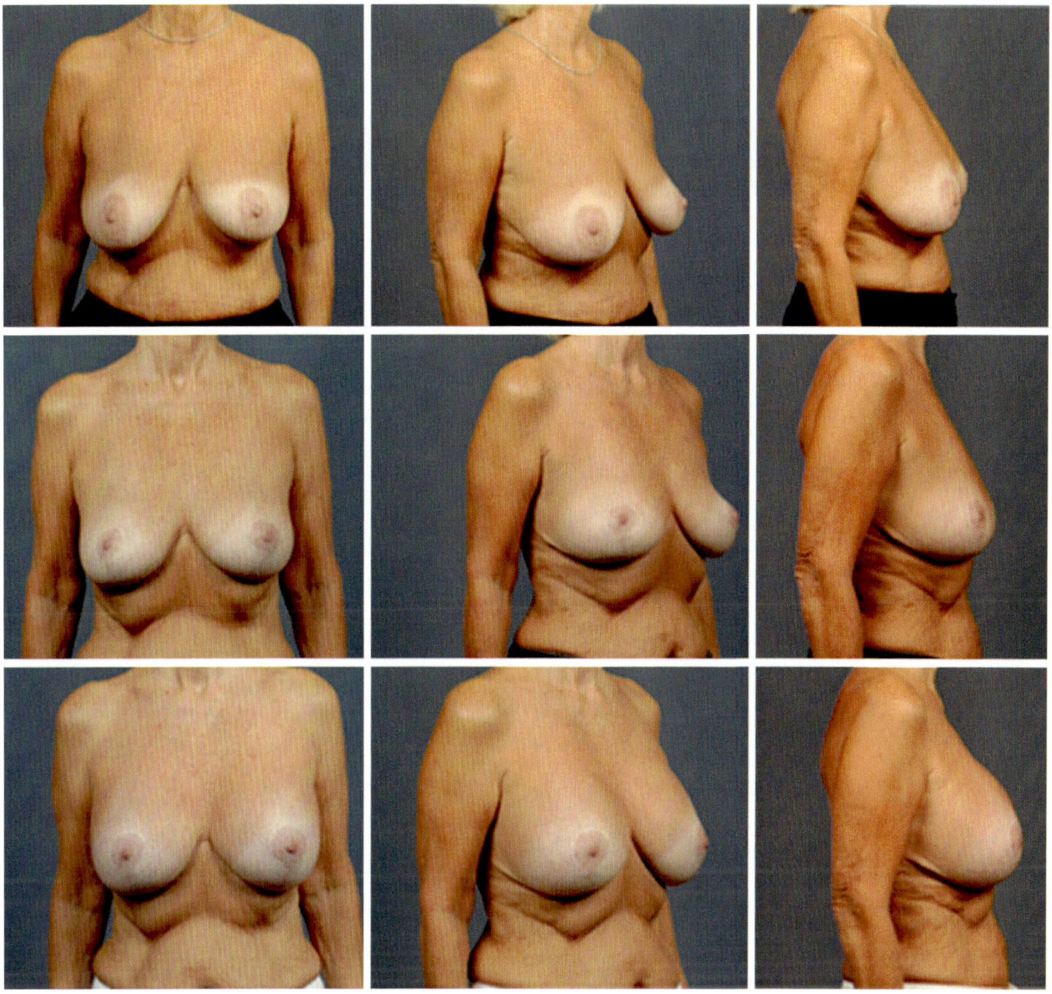

Fig. 7.16 67-year-old G2P2 whom is low-breasted with ptosis (upper images). She underwent stage 1 with a left mastopexy auto-augmentation and a right reduction mastopexy auto-augmentation with axillary liposuction (middle images). 17 months later she underwent stage 2 with 385 cc dual plane breast augmentation with mastopexy revision (lower images – 14 months postoperative)

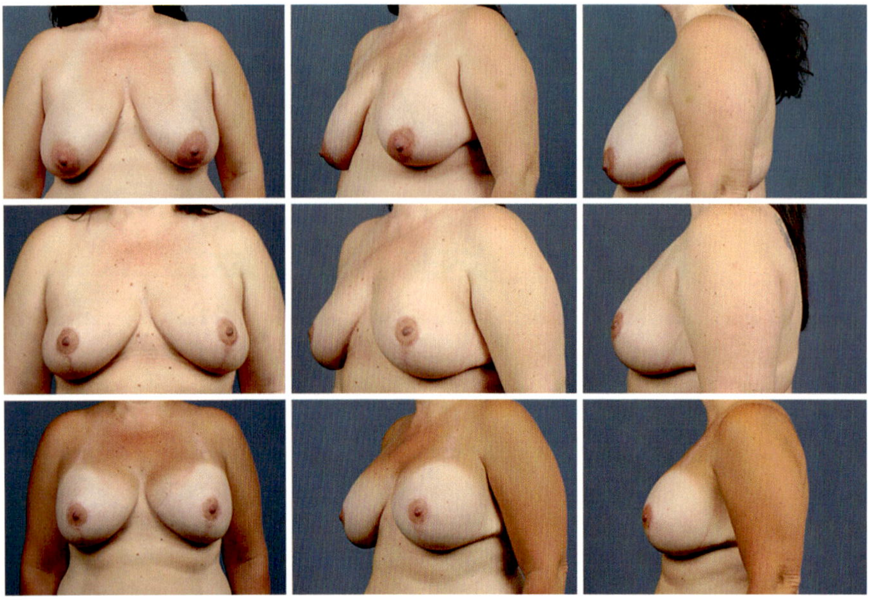

Fig. 7.17 45 year old G3P3 with large, ptotic breasts (upper images). She underwent stage 1 full wise mastopexy reduction with axillary liposuction (middle images – 6 months postoperative). Six months later, she underwent stage 2 dual plane breast augmentation with a 525 cc implant and inframammary fold resection (lower images – 6 months postoperative)

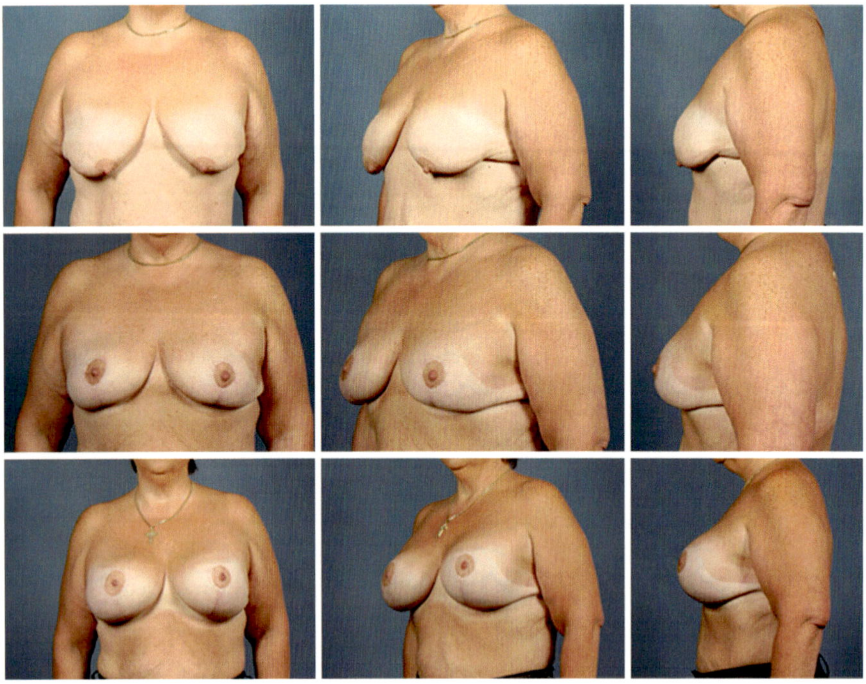

Fig. 7.18 43 year old with breast ptosis and severe volume loss status post gastric banding 10 years prior with a 120 pound weight loss (upper images). She underwent a stage 1 full wise mastopexy with axillary extension (middle images). Stage 2 followed 6 months later with a dual plane smooth round 600 cc high profile augmentation (lower images – 6 months postoperative)

References

1. Nahai F, Fisher J, Maxwell GP, Mills DC II. Augmentation mastopexy: to stage or not. Aesthet Surg J. 2007;27:297–305.
2. Spears SL. Augmentation mastopexy: "surgeon beware". Plast Reconstr Surg. 2003;112:905–6.
3. Hoffman S. Some thoughts on augmentation/mastopexy and medical malpractice. Plast Reconstr Surg. 2004;113:1892–3.
4. Spear SL, Pelletiere CV, Menon N. One-stage augmentation combined with mastopexy: aesthetic results and patient satisfaction. Aesthet Plast Surg. 2004;28:259–67.
5. Spear SL, Boehmler JH, Clemens MW. Augmentation/mastopexy: a 3-year review of a single surgeon's practice. Plast Reconstr Surg. 2006;118:136S–49S,150S–151S.
6. Stevens WG, Macias LH, Spring M, et al. One-stage augmentation mastopexy: a review of 1192 simultaneous augmentation and mastopexy procedures in 615 consecutive cases. Aesthet Surg J. 2014;34:723–32.
7. Calobrace MB, Herdt DR, Cothron KJ. Simultaneous augmentation/mastopexy: a retrospective 5-year review of 332 consecutive cases. Plast Reconstr Surg. 2013;131:145–56.
8. Lee MR, Unger JG, Adams WP. The tissue-based triad: a process approach to augmentation mastopexy. Plast Reconstr Surg. 2014;134:215–25.
9. Khavanin N, Jordan SW, Rambachan A, Kim JYS. A systematic review of single stage augmentation mastopexy. Plast Reconstr Surg. 2014;134:922–31.
10. Hartmann E, Spring MA, Stevens WG. One- and two-stage considerations for augmentation mastopexy. In: Plastic surgery: volume 5: breast fourth edition. Canada; 2018. p. 108–23.
11. Jacobson KL, Johnson MB, Dedhia RD, Niknam-Beinia S, Wong AK. Impaired wound healing after radiation therapy: a systematic review of pathogenesis and treatment. JPRAS Open. 2017;13:92–105.
12. Coon D, Tuffaha S, Christensen J, Bonawitz SC. Plastic surgery and smoking: a prospective analysis of incidence, compliance, and complications. Plast Reconstr Surg. 2013;131(2):385–91.
13. Colwell AS, Driscoll D, Breuing KH. Mastopexy techniques after massive weight loss: an algorithmic approach and review of the literature. Ann Plast Surg. 2009;63(1):28–33.
14. Coombs DM, Srivastava U, Amar D, Rubin JP, Gusenoff JA. The challenges of augmentation mastopexy in the massive weight loss patient: technical considerations. Plast Reconstr Surg. 2017;139(5):1090–9.
15. Regnault P. Breast ptosis. Definition and treatment. Clin Plast Surg. 1976;3:193–203.
16. Lejour M. Vertical mammoplasty for breast reduction and mastopexy. In: Spear SL, editor. Surgery of the breast: principles and art, vol. 73. Philadelphia: Lippincott-Raven; 1998.
17. Hall-Findlay EJ. Pedicles in vertical breast reduction and mastopexy. Clin Plast Surg. 2002;29:379–91.
18. Tebbets JB, Adams WP. Five critical decisions in breast augmentation using five measurements in 5 minutes: the high five decision support process. Plast Reconstr Surg. 2005;116:2005–16.
19. Tebbets JB. A system for breast implant selection based on patient tissue characteristics and implant-soft tissue dynamics. Plast Reconstr Surg. 2002;109(4):1396–409.
20. Headon H, Kasem A. Capsular contracture after breast augmentation: an update for clinical practice. Arch Plast Surg. 2015;42(5):532–43.
21. Calobrace MB, Stevens WG, Capizzi PJ, Cohen R, Godinez T, Beckstrand M. Risk factor analysis for capsular contracture: a 10-year Sientra study using round, smooth, and textured implants for breast augmentation. Plast Reconstr Surg. 2018;141:20S–8S.
22. Calobrace MB, Kaufman DL, Gordon AE, et al. Evolving practices in augmentation operative technique with Sientra HSC round implants. Plast Reconstr Surg. 2014;134(1 Suppl):57S–67S.
23. Calobrace MB. Teaching breast augmentation: a focus on critical intraoperative techniques and decision making to maximize results and minimize revisions. Clin Plast Surg. 2015;42(4):493–504.

Secondary Mastopexy

8

Ziyad S. Hammoudeh and W. Grant Stevens

Introduction

Breast implants produce an expansive force on the breasts while mastopexy tightens the surrounding skin envelope. The safety of performing these procedures simultaneously as a one-stage operation has been questioned as recently as a decade ago due to the potential for complications with these opposing forces in both the primary [1, 2] and secondary [3] setting. Secondary augmentation-mastopexy was referred to as a "recipe for disaster" in the previously augmented breast [3]. Since then numerous articles showing the safety of both primary and secondary augmentation-mastopexy have been published [4–9]. In addition, the safety of primary augmentation-mastopexy has been further validated by several authors [10–14]. However, less has been published about secondary mastopexy-augmentation. The terms "secondary" and "revisional" augmentation-mastopexy lack standard definitions in the literature. We define "secondary" to mean simultaneous augmentation-mastopexy performed on a breast that previously underwent any type of surgery. We define "revisional" as a subcategory of "secondary" augmentation-mastopexy that refers to *immediate* surgical correction of a problem or *late* surgery to improve the results of a previous augmentation-mastopexy. Secondary augmentation-mastopexy has challenges similar to primary augmentation-mastopexy with some additional considerations for achieving optimal outcomes.

Many women that underwent breast augmentation in their twenties or early 30s will develop mammary ptosis following pregnancy or as they age. Some of these patients will have developed capsular contracture and require capsule surgery. Some patients may decide to downsize their implant volume as they get older while others want to exchange from saline or less cohesive silicone implants to highly cohesive silicone implants. These patients may return to their plastic surgeon for exchange of their implants and benefit from a secondary augmentation-mastopexy. In addition, patients may seek to have their implants explanted and prefer to have a mastopexy with autologous volume replacement with fat.

As patients age, the glandular breast parenchyma is replaced by fatty tissue, the volume of the breasts can increase with overall weight gain, skin elasticity decreases producing greater laxity, and the breasts become more ptotic. Particularly with patient preference for smaller implants, downsizing implant volume can result in excessive skin laxity as the skin is

Z. S. Hammoudeh (✉)
Private Practice Marina Plastic Surgery, Marina Plastic Surgery, Marina del Rey, CA, USA

W. Grant Stevens
Private Practice Marina Plastic Surgery, Keck School of Medicine of USC, Division of Plastic Surgery, Marina del Rey, CA, USA

M. B. Calobrace et al. (eds.), *Augmentation Mastopexy*,
https://doi.org/10.1007/978-3-030-48226-8_8

less likely to contract due to the aforementioned factors and require tightening to achieve an optimal breast shape. Similarly, patients may develop recurrent mammary ptosis many years after a primary augmentation-mastopexy and require a secondary augmentation mastopexy. Revisional augmentation-mastopexy would be used in patients that did not achieve a satisfactory result from primary augmentation-mastopexy. For instance, a patient that developed implant malposition or capsular contracture after augmentation-mastopexy requiring pocket adjustment and associated tightening of the skin envelope would be considered a revisional secondary augmentation-mastopexy. Other examples of secondary augmentation-mastopexy include patients that underwent previous breast surgery *without* implants such as mastopexy, breast reduction, lumpectomy, or excisional biopsy and now present for simultaneous augmentation and mastopexy. These patients have undergone alteration in their vascular anatomy with associated scars; therefore, they have the potential for impaired perfusion to the nipple areola complex (NAC) and wound healing problems. They may also have a suboptimal outcome from their primary operation, which makes achieving a satisfactory outcome in a secondary surgery more difficult and the potential need for revision greater. This chapter focuses on indications and preoperative preparation, surgical technique, and outcomes of secondary augmentation-mastopexy to help avoid complications and achieve optimal outcomes. A detailed discussion of implant-related complications associated with augmentation mastopexy and the management is highlighted in the chapter covering complications.

Indications and Preoperative Preparation

Mastopexy Selection

Careful planning is required in patients considering secondary augmentation-mastopexy. Each patient's prior history of breast surgery should be thoroughly evaluated and her pattern of breast scars closely examined. In patients with prior augmentation, the capsules are assessed for capsular contracture. The degree of ptosis is also assessed. Ptosis grades are described according to the Regnault classification (Fig. 8.1). The most ideal mastopexy incision pattern for a secondary augmentation-mastopexy depends on each patient's anatomy following primary breast surgery and their grade of ptosis. Mastopexy skin incisions that can be used include crescent, circumarareolar, circumvertical ("owl"), circumvertical with short horizontal wedge at the inframammary fold ("owl with feet"), Wise, "sailboat," or "smile" (Fig. 8.2).

Cresent or Circumareolar

Patients with Regnault grade I ptosis that require only 1–2 cm of elevation of the NAC with *minimal* laxity of the lower pole of the breast may be candidates for a crescent or circumareolar mastopexy. The crescent technique is effective in patients that have an appropriately sized NAC without surrounding tissue laxity and request a mild NAC elevation. Circumareolar mastopexy tends to flatten the breast rather than the attractive coning effect associated with techniques that utilize a vertical incision. The circumareolar technique has been associated with a higher rate of revision [6]. Figure 8.3 demonstrates the results of a patient that underwent a secondary circumareolar augmentation-mastopexy.

Circumvertical

Patients with Regnault grade II to III ptosis that require >2 cm of elevation of the NAC or patients with grade I ptosis and *substantial* laxity in the lower pole are better treated with a circumvertical pattern. A circumvertical "owl" is planned when the nipple-to-IMF distance is relatively short at approximately 7 cm or less on stretch preoperatively. An "owl with feet" is planned when the nipple-to-IMF distance is >7 cm on stretch; in such cases, the short horizontal wedge ("feet") is typically adjusted on the operating table at the time of closure to shorten the nipple-to-IMF distance to the desired length. The presence of a

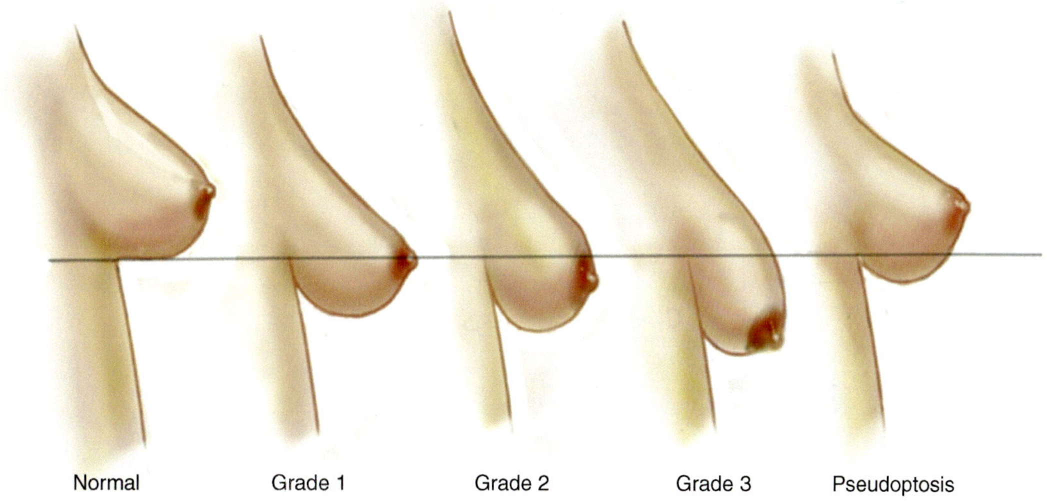

Fig. 8.1 Regnault classification of ptosis. (From Spring et al. [8])

Fig. 8.2 Types of mastopexy incisions. (From Spring et al. [8])

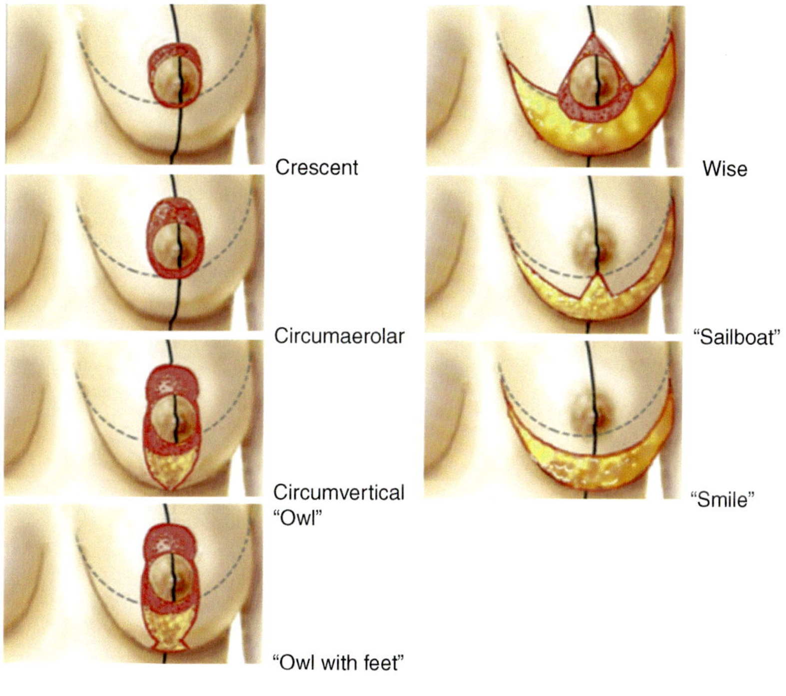

short transverse scar along the inframammary fold is typically well hidden and an inconsequential tradeoff for improved breast shape/dimensions. Figure 8.4 demonstrates the results of a patient with previous augmentation-mastopexy with inverted-T scar that underwent a secondary circumvertical augmentation-mastopexy.

Lower Pole Mastopexy

Many patients that have undergone previous mastopexy alone, augmentation-mastopexy, or breast reduction will have their NAC in an appropriate position superior to the inframammary fold (IMF) with undesired lower pole laxity. The glan-

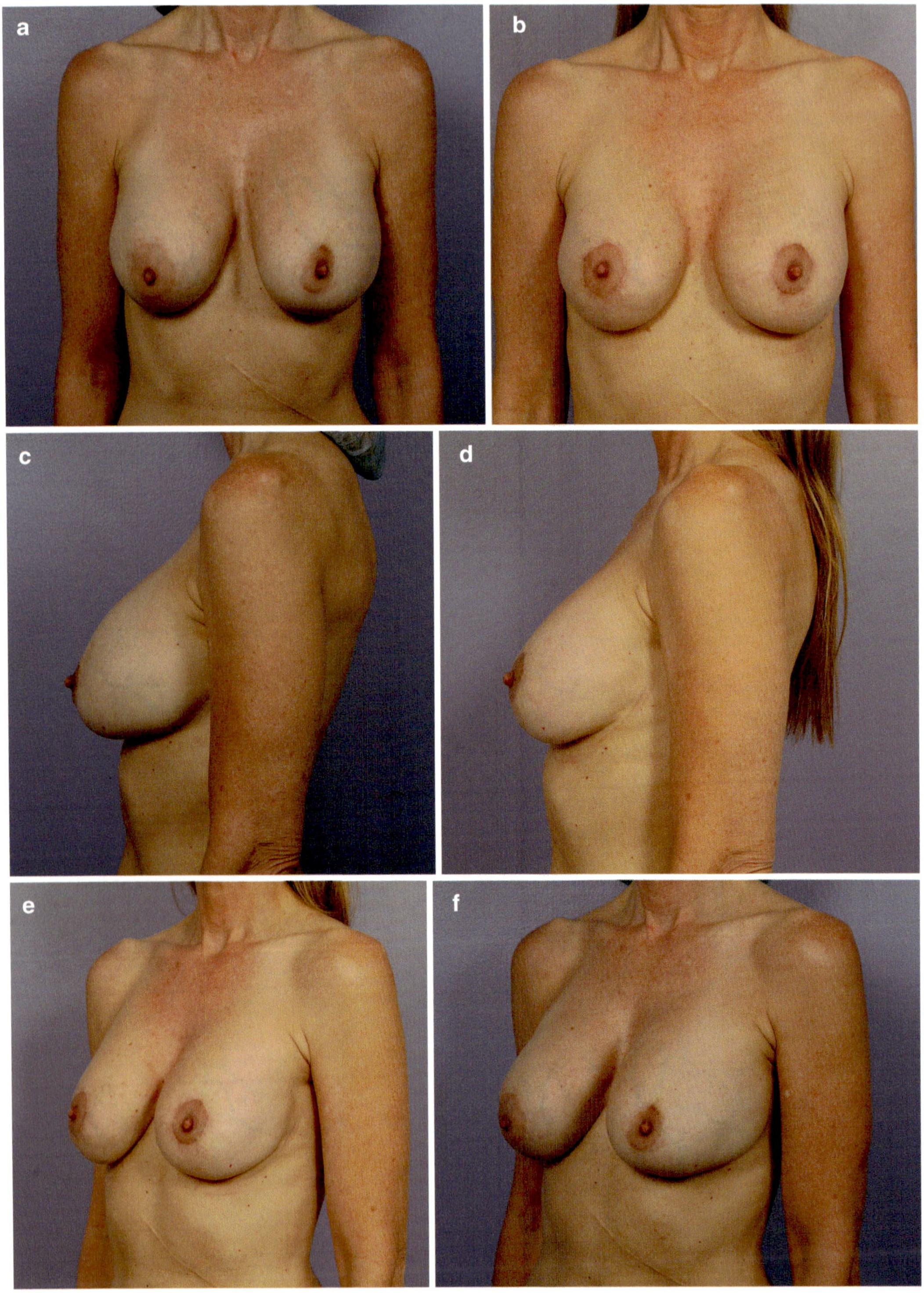

Fig. 8.3 Secondary circumareolar augmentation-mastopexy. This patient had a prior circumareolar augmentation-mastopexy and developed bilateral capsular contractures. During secondary surgery, the previous implants were removed, capsulotomy/capsulectomy performed, 255 cc moderate profile round implants inserted (downsized), and secondary circumareolar mastopexy performed bilaterally. (**a**–**c**) Preoperative. (**d**–**f**) Postoperative 6 months

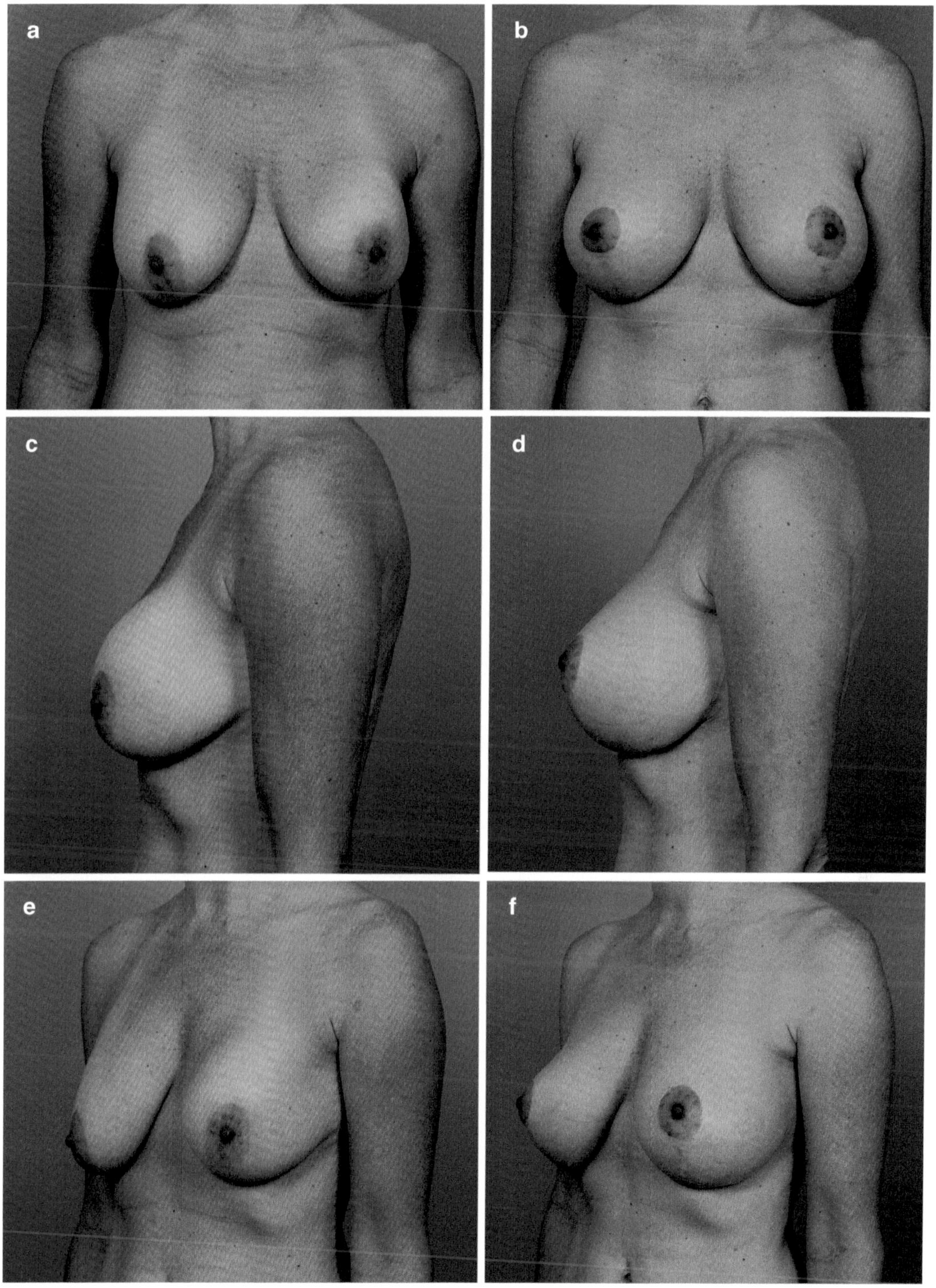

Fig. 8.4 Secondary circumvertical augmentation-mastopexy. This patient had a prior transaxillary subglandular breast augmentation and developed a left capsular contracture. During secondary surgery, the previous implants were removed through a vertical breast incision, left capsulectomy performed, bilateral subglandular to subpectoral pocket change, 507 cc moderate profile round implant inserted on the left (upsized), 469 cc moderate profile round implant inserted on the left (upsized), and circumvertical mastopexy performed bilaterally. (**a–c**) Preoperative. (**d–f**) Postoperative 15 months

dular tissue in the lower pole tends to descend with time while the NAC remains elevated in the position it was placed during the mastopexy or reduction. These patients do not require elevation of the NAC and are better treated with a "smile" or "sailboat" mastopexy. A "smile" mastopexy is effective in patients that have pseudoptosis with a high-riding NAC or long nipple-to-IMF distance (i.e. vertical laxity *without* horizontal laxity). The "smile" mastopexy removes a horizontal wedge of tissue along the IMF to lower the NAC and remove vertical lower pole laxity. A "sailboat" mastopexy is effective in patients with pseudoptosis and laxity in both dimensions (i.e. vertical *plus* horizontal laxity). The "sailboat" mastopexy removes an inverted-T pattern of skin without the circumareolar component. This pattern is very commonly used for secondary augmentation-mastopexy and rarely used for primary augmentation-mastopexy. Figure 8.5 demonstrates the results of a patient that underwent a secondary "smile" augmentation-mastopexy. Figure 8.6 demonstrates the results of a patient that underwent a secondary "sailboat" augmentation-mastopexy.

Symmetry

The breasts are analyzed for the presence of asymmetry, so that symmetry can be improved. Some patients may even need a combination of techniques to address asymmetry. In patients presenting for secondary augmentation-mastopexy that had primary surgery elsewhere, it may be difficult to determine if the need for secondary surgery is due to a planning error from the primary surgery, technical error intraoperatively, or natural progression of breast changes with time.

Patient Assessment Subpectoral vs. Subfascial

In patients with implants, the plane of implant placement should be assessed. Patients should be asked to place both hands on their hips with elbows flexed and push on their hips to flex the pectoralis major muscles. Patients with subpectoral implants may present with requests to correct their animation effect. In some patients with excessive animation deformity, this may be due to inadequate release of the inferomedial attachments of the pectoralis major muscle during the primary surgery. This can be corrected by incising through the capsule and dividing the inferomedial pectoralis muscle fibers at the time of secondary surgery formalizing a dual plane pocket. In other patients with normal but undesired animation, plane change from subpectoral to subfascial may be indicated. The subglandular plane is typically avoided to minimize the risk of capsular contracture development. Caution is advised with plane changes from subpectoral to prepectoral locations during secondary augmentation-mastopexy with thin overlying breast tissue due to the potential for devascularizing the pedicle to the NAC by dividing the thoracoacromial perforators superficial to the pectoralis major muscle. However, prepectoral plane change can be performed in appropriately selected patients that do not require substantial elevation of the NAC, have a satisfactory amount of overlying breast tissue on skin pinch, and are not requesting a large (or substantially larger than current) implant.

Operative Approach

Use of previous incisions, insertion of smaller implants, minimizing dissection during mastopexy, and avoidance of total capsulectomies are safe approaches the surgeon can take to minimize complications. A vertical incision for implant insertion and revision mastopexy is preferred when the patient already has a vertical scar. A vertical incision may also be needed in a patient with prior circumareolar mastopexy in order to achieve the desired breast shape. A superior pedicle technique is also preferred. Some authors have reported thinning and atrophy of the lower breast parenchyma due to the pressure of the implants with gravity in that region [3]. Use of an inferior pedicle is not advisable in such situations for two reasons. First, the blood supply has likely

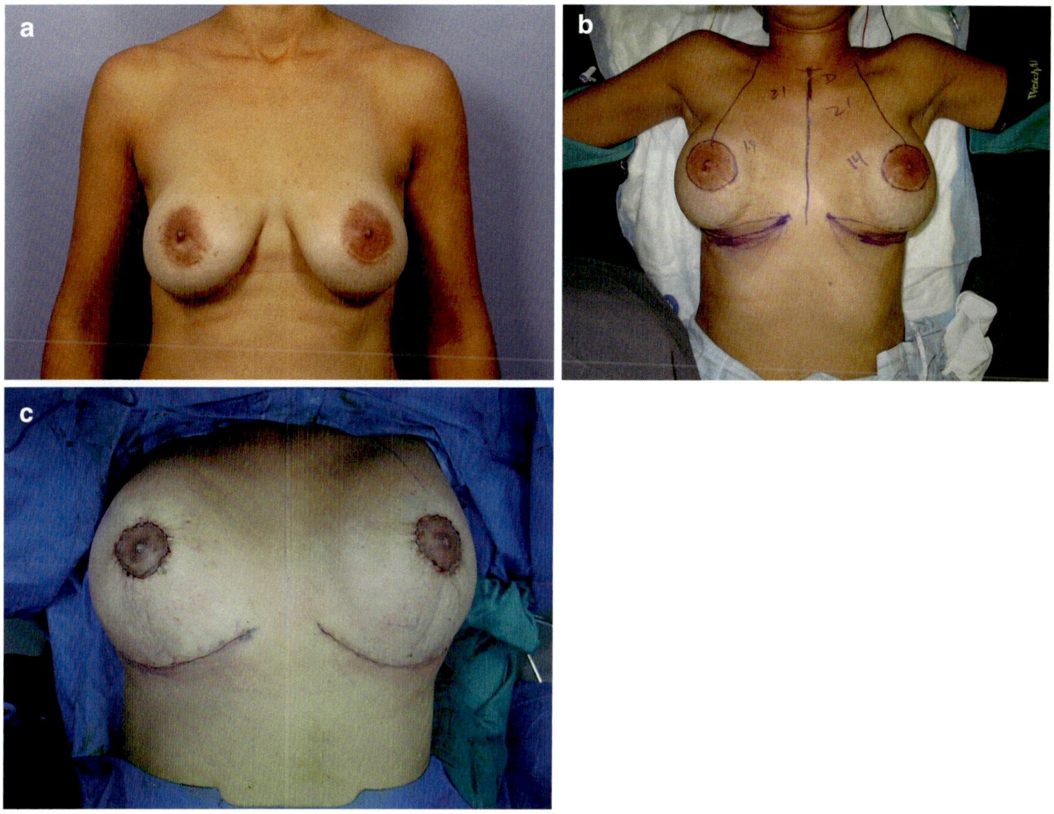

Fig. 8.5 Secondary "smile" augmentation-mastopexy. This patient had a long nipple-to-inframammary fold distance with vertical lower pole laxity with asymmetry of the nipple areola complex. During secondary surgery, "smile" mastopexy was performed via horizontal wedge excision along the inframammary fold and a circumareolar mastopexy to improve symmetry of the nipple areola complex. (**a**) Preoperative. (**b**) Intraoperative markings. (**c**) Postoperative on the operating table

been compromised in the atrophic lower pole tissue and inadequate as a pedicle to the NAC. Second, preservation of lower pole breast tissue to resuspend the NAC has a greater tendency for recurrent lower pole laxity ("bottoming out") and ptosis. The breast parenchyma in the superior pole is more robust with a greater blood supply in the previously augmented patient.

Markings

Markings should be designed for conservative skin resection, particularly when planning to increase the volume of implants. Larger implants can take up some skin laxity, but this is often adequate with the additional need to resect skin via a mastopexy. Smaller implants will take pressure off of the pedicle to the NAC as well as the mastopexy skin flaps. Therefore, downsizing to smaller implants in secondary augmentation-mastopexy is considered relatively safe.

Surgical Technique

Minimizing the amount of dissection during the mastopexy is important to prevent any further devascularization. Some authors have tried to improve the longevity of their mastopexies via autoaugmentation with parenchymal flaps and suspension sutures with circumvertical and Wise pattern techniques [15, 16]. However, these techniques include additional tissue dissection and

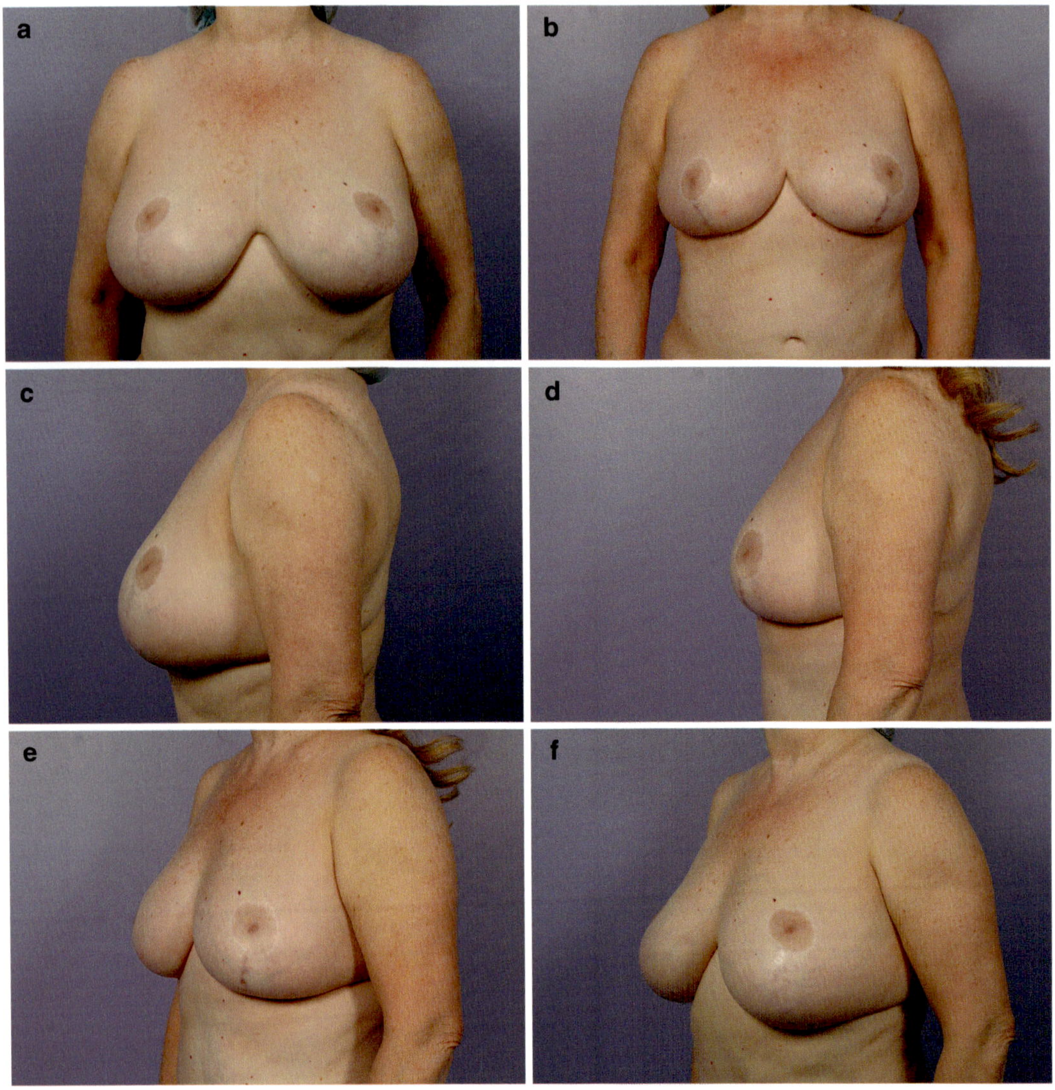

Fig. 8.6 Secondary "sailboat" augmentation-mastopexy. This patient had a primary inverted-T augmentation-mastopexy with implants that were too large for her breast dimensions (455 cc on the right, 435 cc on the left), a long nipple-to-inframammary fold distance, and high-riding nipples bilaterally. During secondary surgery, a "sailboat" pattern of skin was excised to reduce both horizontal and vertical laxity, the previous implants were removed, and 150 cc moderate profile round implants were inserted (downsized) bilaterally. (**a**–**c**) Preoperative. (**d**–**f**) Postoperative 3 months

potential disruption of blood supply to the NAC with increased risk of complications. The effectiveness of these techniques has also been questioned [17]. In addition, many of these patients have such thin tissue that there is minimal tissue available for rearrangement. Therefore, the least aggressive mastopexy to achieve the desired result is preferred. Circumferential undermining of the skin surrounding the deepithelialized skin of a circumareolar mastopexy should also be avoided to maintain as much vascularity as possible when combined with implant/capsule surgery.

The capsule is vascular, so performing a total capsulectomy will remove this bloody supply as well potentially remove some breast parenchyma attached to the capsule. This is especially true in patients that have had augmentation in the subglandular or subfascial plane, as the superior surface of the capsule is in direct communication with the breast parenchyma unlike the subpectoral plane. Prior augmentation in the subpectoral plane has preserved the perforators through the pectoralis major muscle from the thoracoacromial vessels, preserving an additional source of blood supply to the NAC. Some surgeons fear that leaving substantial portions of the capsule in situ leads to seroma formation and inhibits reattachment of breast parenchyma to the underlying chest wall; thus, they recommend roughening the capsule to create a raw surface to promote tissue adhesion and routinely leave suction drains [3]. However, we have not found this to be the case and routinely leave the capsule intact without placement of drains when there is no capsular contracture. Although total capsulectomy is considered the gold standard in managing capsular contracture, a systematic review evaluating management strategies for capsular contracture was not able to show an advantage of capsulectomy compared to open capsulotomy or total compared to partial capsulectomy [18]. However, site-change techniques (e.g. neosubpectoral pocket) were associated with lower capsular contracture recurrence rates, and implant exchange was associated with lower capsular contracture recurrence rates. Likewise, a total capsulectomy cannot be avoided in certain situations such as a capsular mass, calcified capsule or silicone products imbedded in the capsule.

A waterfall ("snoopy") deformity may develop as the lower pole breast parenchyma develops laxity over time and falls caudally off of an implant that remains in the cephalad position in which it was originally placed. This is most commonly associated with a submuscular implant placement. A waterfall deformity can also occur with elevation of the implant due to Baker grade III/IV capsular contracture. In the *absence* of capsular contracture, this waterfall effect is more common with the use of textured implants in the subpectoral plane, as such implants are more resistant to descent with gravity. In such cases, a "smile" or "sailboat" mastopexy may be all that is needed to correct the waterfall deformity without capsule surgery. In the *presence* of capsular contracture, capsule surgery would be required to treat the waterfall deformity. Capsule surgery can include open capsulotomy, capsulectomy, or a neosubpectoral pocket. The neosubpectoral pocket is an effect modality for creating a new pocket while still maintaining the implant in a subpectoral plane without removing the capsule (Fig. 8.7). A neosubpectoral pocket is also an effective approach when substantially downsizing implants (>100 cc) or inserting anatomic implants due to the ability to create a precise pocket with the exact dimensions of the new implant as an alternative to capsulorrhaphies. Capsulorrhaphies are typically less precise than a new pocket and can have visible irregularities from suture placement.

Conclusion

Secondary augmentation-mastopexy can be performed safely with good aesthetic outcomes in appropriately selected patients who have undergone previous breast surgery with or without implants. Various skin design patterns are available depending on each patient's unique anatomy and outcome following primary breast surgery. Tissue-related complications are more common than implant-related complications. Complication rates and revision rates are relatively low with similar results to those reported for primary augmentation-mastopexy. Patients should be informed preoperatively about the potential need for additional surgery. Considering the acceptable complication/revision rate, less economic burden of a single compared to staged surgery, and a single recovery period for a patient that has already undergone one or more prior breast surgeries, performing one-stage secondary augmentation-mastopexy should be strongly considered for patients that meet criteria.

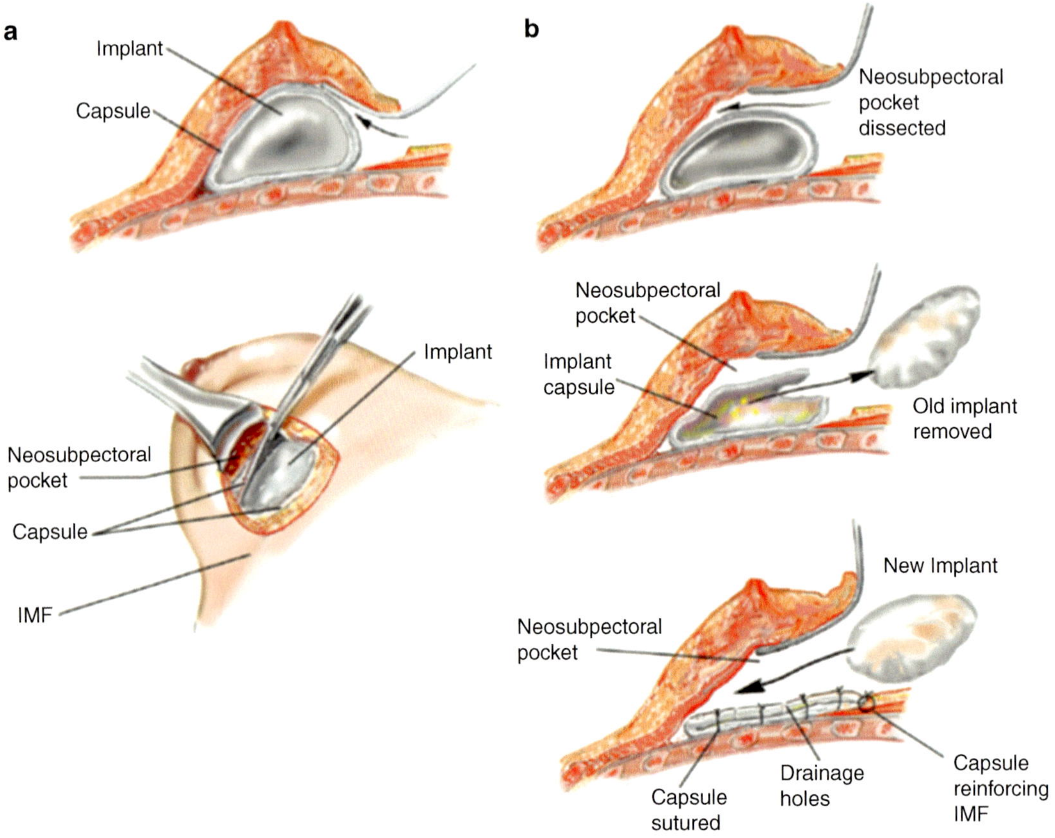

Fig. 8.7 The neosubpectoral pocket. (**a**) The old subpectoral implant is kept in situ, and a plane is created between the superficial surface of the anterior capsule and the deep surface of the pectoralis major muscle. (**b**) After the neosubpectoral pocket has been completely dissected to the dimensions of the new implant, the capsule is incised, and the old implant removed. The old pocket is then closed by suturing the anterior and posterior surfaces of the capsule together, thereby reinforcing the inframammary fold, and the new implant is inserted. (From Spring et al. [8])

References

1. Spear S. Augmentation/mastopexy: "surgeon, beware". Plast Reconstr Surg. 2003;112:905–6, Augmentation/Mastopexy: "Surgeon, Beware".
2. Spear SL. Augmentation/mastopexy: "surgeon, beware". Plast Reconstr Surg. 2006;118(7 Suppl):133S–4S; discussion 135S.
3. Handel N. Secondary mastopexy in the augmented patient: a recipe for disaster. Plast Reconstr Surg. 2006;118:152S–63S; discussion 164S–165S, 166S–167S.
4. Stevens WG, Stoker DA, Freeman ME, Quardt SM, Hirsch EM, Cohen R. Is one-stage breast augmentation with mastopexy safe and effective? A review of 186 primary cases. Aesthet Surg J. 2006;26:674–81.
5. Stevens WG, Freeman ME, Stoker DA, Quardt SM, Cohen R, Hirsch EM. One-stage mastopexy with breast augmentation: a review of 321 patients. Plast Reconstr Surg. 2007;120:1674–9.
6. Stevens WG, Macias LH, Spring M, Stoker DA, Chacon CO, Eberlin SA. One-stage augmentation mastopexy: a review of 1192 simultaneous breast augmentation and mastopexy procedures in 615 consecutive patients. Aesthet Surg J. 2014;34:723–32.
7. Stevens WG, Spring M, Stoker DA, Freeman ME, Cohen R, Quardt SM, Hirsch EM. A review of 100 consecutive secondary augmentation/mastopexies. Aesthet Surg J. 2007;27:485–92.
8. Spring MA, Macias LH, Nadeau M, Stevens WG. Secondary augmentation-mastopexy: indications, preferred practices, and the treatment of complications. Aesthet Surg J. 2014;34:1018–40.
9. Spring MA, Hartmann EC, Stevens WG. Strategies and challenges in simultaneous augmentation mastopexy. Clin Plast Surg. 2015;42:505–18.
10. Calobrace MB, Herdt DR, Cothron KJ. Simultaneous augmentation/mastopexy: a retrospective 5-year review of 332 consecutive cases. Plast Reconstr Surg. 2013;131:145–56.

11. Swanson E. Prospective comparative clinical evaluation of 784 consecutive cases of breast augmentation and vertical mammoplasty, performed individually and in combination. Plast Reconstr Surg. 2013;132:30e–45e.
12. Khavanin N, Jordan SW, Rambachan A, Kim JY. A systematic review of single-stage augmentation-mastopexy. Plast Reconstr Surg. 2014;134:922–31.
13. Doshier LJ, Eagan SL, Shock LA, Henry SL, Colbert SH, Puckett CL. The subtleties of success in simultaneous augmentation-mastopexy. Plast Reconstr Surg. 2016;138:585–92.
14. Qureshi AA, Myckatyn TM, Tenenbaum MM. Mastopexy and mastopexy-augmentation. Aesthet Surg J. 2018;38:374–84.
15. Graf R, Biggs TM. In search of better shape in mastopexy and reduction mammoplasty. Plast Reconstr Surg. 2002;110:309–17.
16. Ritz M, Silfen R, Southwick G. Fascial suspension mastopexy. Plast Reconstr Surg. 2006;117:86–94.
17. Swanson E. A retrospective photometric study of 82 published reports of mastopexy and breast reduction. Plast Reconstr Surg. 2011;128:1282–301.
18. Wan D, Rohrich RJ. Revisiting the management of capsular contracture in breast augmentation: a systematic review. Plast Reconstr Surg. 2016;137:826–41.

9 Simultaneous Short-Scar Mastopexy Augmentation

Simeon Wall Jr., Holly Wall, and Jeffrey R. Claiborne

Introduction

Simultaneous mastopexy augmentation is a challenging procedure. An approach and surgical technique to create consistent, predictable results with a low complication rate has not been well standardized. The inherent difficulty lies in the competing surgical goals and maneuvers – reducing the redundant skin envelope and elevating the breast while concurrently adding volume and weight to the breast. The antagonism between the mastopexy and the augmentation innately creates a degree of complexity that compels some surgeons to tackle the problem in two stages. Or, this complexity forces surgeons to accept less than ideal results or higher than acceptable complications rates. Patients predictably prefer a one stage approach if their goals can be accomplished safely and effectively. Over the years, we have refined our simultaneous mastopexy augmentation technique to reduce scars, maximize consistency, improve surgical efficiency and minimize complications. In this chapter, we evaluate our own experience and outcomes as well as describe the key concepts and steps that allow simultaneous short-scar augmentation mastopexy to be performed safely with predictable results.

Preoperative Planning

In our practice, obesity (BMI > 32) is a relative contraindication and active smoking is an absolute contraindication. Nicotine users are required to stop all nicotine for at least 4 weeks prior to surgery and at least 6 weeks after surgery. A urine cotinine test is performed at the preoperative visit and again on the day of surgery, with a positive result resulting in cancellation of surgery. Obese patients and smokers are more likely to have perioperative complications and are less likely to achieve their desired results [1, 2]. High satisfaction rates with minimal complications are the top priorities, without compromise. All mastopexy augmentations are performed as a one-stage procedure. These patients seek increased upper pole fullness at the desired level of the breast on their chest, altered ratio of upper pole to lower pole breast volume, increased breast projection, elimination of glandular ptosis, and an elevation of the nipple-areolar complex. Mastopexies are performed with a vertical technique using either a

S. Wall Jr.
Private Practice, The Wall Center for Plastic Surgery, Shreveport, LA, USA

UT Southwestern Medical Center, Dallas, TX, USA
e-mail: swalljr@wallcenter.com; info@wallcenter.com

H. Wall
Private Practice, The Wall Center for Plastic Surgery, Shreveport, LA, USA

J. R. Claiborne (✉)
Private Practice, Northshore Plastic Surgery, Mandeville, LA, USA

M. B. Calobrace et al. (eds.), *Augmentation Mastopexy*,
https://doi.org/10.1007/978-3-030-48226-8_9

superior or a superomedial pedicle (rarely a superolateral pedicle but never an inferior pedicle). For patients with marked nipple-to-inframammary fold vertical excess, senior author H.W. uses a short horizontal J-shaped scar extension in the new inframammary fold in less than 10% of cases (senior author S.W.Jr. in less than 2%).

Given the high degree of variability in patient presentation and preference, obtaining certainty of a given patient's desires before the surgery is crucial. The desired final breast size and the desired amount and height of upper pole fullness are the two most important patient-driven aspects of the surgical plan, and any miscommunication between patient and surgeon in this regard can affect patient satisfaction severely. Desired breast size is determined first. As a starting point, patients indicate how many cup sizes they wish to change (increase, decrease, or no change) from their current bra size. Beyond the bra size discussion, we avoid descriptive terminology such as "proportional", "natural", "not too small/big" and other words that tend to mean different things to different people. In contrast, one or more forms of visual simulation are most predictive and helpful in understanding the patient's desires. Viewing pictures of other patients' results helps determine each patient's idea of proportionality and desired size, while also allowing the patient to gain an idea of the scars required. Trying on implants in a bra and shirt in the mirror, or utilizing three-dimensional simulations (Canfield Vectra, Divina), can also be helpful in selected patients. Patients also need to understand why avoiding overly large breasts is important for long-term results and the avoidance of another lift. Armed with the agreed upon final breast size, the desired level and amount of upper pole fullness is simulated in a standing, arms relaxed position, in front of a full-length mirror, with the torso fully exposed. The surgeon pushes up on the core of the breast, similar to how a push-up bra elevates the core of the breast into the upper pole. The height of the top of the desired breast is demonstrated and shown at multiple levels in order to give the patient a realistic representation of reasonable, or unreasonable, upper pole height. In most patients, maximum upper pole height is at, or within 1 cm below, the vertical level of the manubrium, and in our patient population, about 80–90% of patients choose their anatomically dictated level of maximum upper pole fullness. An understanding by the patient of the limits of upper pole fullness on her chest is mandatory before proceeding. When using bra size change for preoperative sizing, it is important to realize that a large portion of the implant's volume will be sitting in the empty superior pole of the breast and will not be accounted for within the bra itself, leaving some patients with the perception that their breasts are not as large as they thought they would be. The uncounted upper pole implant volume should be accounted for preoperatively for accurate sizing. In an isolated mastopexy, the patient will lose breast volume and decrease in cup size [3, 4]. As an illustration of these concepts, if a patient wants to stay about the same cup size but increase upper pole fullness, an implant is needed that allows the breast to fill out the area of the bra appropriately, and also provides the unaccounted-for volume for the upper pole fullness that will not be counted in most bras. To increase a full cup size, the augmentation-mastopexy patient who will lose some volume with the mastopexy requires a somewhat larger implant relative to the augmentation patient desiring a one cup size increase, also considering that the upper to lower pole balance of volume is typically much higher in the mastopexy augmentation patient. These generalities aside, individual patients can have highly variable starting breast volume and parenchymal distribution that may alter how these concepts are applied.

Markings

Nipple Position and Mosque Design Preoperative markings are performed with the patient standing and surgeon sitting. Careful attention is paid to scoliosis, leg-length discrepancy, shoulder height and chest wall irregularities. These asymmetries are pointed out to the patient. Reference lines are drawn in the midline chest, each desired breast meridian, and the existing inframammary folds. Inframammary fold height discrepancy is marked on the chest midline. The desired breast meridian line corrects for asymmetries and horizontal nipple displacement, and does not necessarily transect the preoperative nipple. Correcting medially, laterally, or asymmetrically displaced nipples are important components in creating the proper breast balance and new nipple location.

Correctly marking the new vertical nipple position is the most challenging step. Most patients require elevation of the entire footprint of the breast on the chest, which affects the new nipple position significantly. The new, elevated position of the IMF is determined by pushing up on the IMF, feeling for the amount of IMF laxity and simultaneously determining the new inferior breast border. The inferior breast border is best visualized by the confluence of the breast meridian, the elevated IMF that is being pushed up, and the level of the medial breast border at the IMF, keeping in mind the desired footprint of the new breast mound. The new nipple location is then typically marked 2 cm higher than the level of the new IMF, with some variability for the base diameter and projection of the implant to be used, and the amount of coning of the native breast. For reference, the new nipple location is typically marked 3–5 cm higher than our markings for a vertical breast reduction or mastopexy on a given patient. Over the years, as our desire and ability to elevate the footprint of the breast has become axiomatic, we have become very comfortable with planning the new nipple location somewhat higher than what has been typically described. This higher nipple location corresponds well to the typical elevation of the entire breast footprint of about 2–3 cm with our mastopexy augmentation technique. We agree wholeheartedly with Stevens' statement that the hardest problem to fix is a nipple that is placed too high, but that the most common problem is a nipple that is placed too low (G. Stevens, personal communication, 2012). Next, a mosque-dome pattern is drawn. Senior author H.W. freehand draws the mosque-dome pattern. Senior author S.W.Jr. has a more mathematical approach. For the key points of the mosque design from this nipple position, a mark is made 2 cm up, 3–4.5 cm down, and 2.5–3 cm laterally (Figs. 9.1, 9.2 and 9.3). This pattern will provide a mosque circumference of 13.5–16.5 cm. The drop down of the mosque will be on the longer end of the range (4.5 cm) for patients with more vertical excess and ptosis. Similarly, the lateral points will be wider (3–4 cm) for patients with larger base diameters. Gathering some of the vertical and horizontal skin excess at the areolar inset allows a relative shortening of

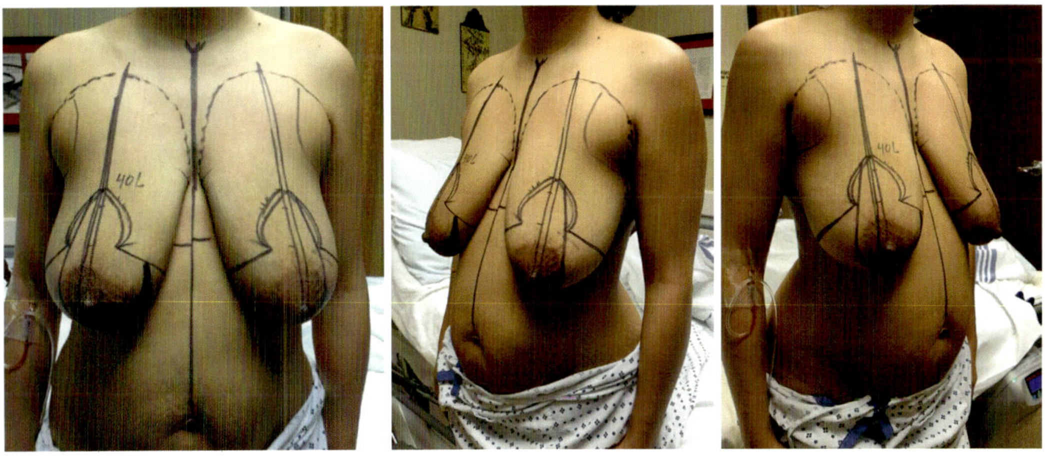

Figs. 9.1, 9.2 and 9.3 Standard preoperative markings for augmentation mastopexy, Case 1. (©Simeon Wall Jr)

the vertical closure, which can minimize any skin redundancy that can be left at the IMF at the end of the procedure (thereby preventing the need for a longer scar).

Pedicle Choice and Inferior Pole Skin Excess For patients who need nipple elevation of less than <6 cm, a superior pedicle is chosen. The superior pedicle is robust, and the mastopexy is quicker and easier. If the nipple needs to be elevated more than 6 cm and the preoperative areola is completely below the mosque-dome markings, a superomedial pedicle is preferred. When moving the nipple position greater distances, the superior pedicle must compress or fold on itself which can make the inset cumbersome [5–7]. The pedicle compression can also generate high tension and turgor and cause venous obstruction [5–7]. With the superomedial pedicle, the nipple rotates into position and does not require as much pedicle compression. The limits of a superior pedicle can be expanded in patients with lax tissues (i.e. weight loss patients) because their tissues are more malleable and will generate less tissue turgor during pedicle compression and nipple inset. Along the same lines, patients with very dense, stiff, fibrous breast tissue will not tolerate the compression of a superior pedicle and these patients will more readily kink their superior pedicles with distances greater than 6 cm.

To mark the vertical limbs, the width of the skin resection beneath the NAC is defined by displacing the breast medially and laterally along the marked breast meridian. The skin excision pattern stops 1.5–6 cm (average 2.5 cm) above the IMF, and the vertical pillar height is marked at 6–9 cm (average 7 cm). A medial and lateral triangle of parenchyma inferior to the bottom of the pillars is then marked for excision (breast parenchyma excision, not skin excision).

One marking option: Large augmentations reduce the horizontal skin excess and there is a learning curve on exactly how hard to medially and laterally displace the breast pillar markings preoperatively. In superior pedicle cases with senior author H.W., she determines the width of the skin resection with medial and lateral displacement intraoperatively after the augmentation has been completed on the table supine – therefore only the mosque marking needs to be completed preoperatively. As a personal preference for H.W., waiting until after the augmentation has been completed adds more certainty and allows her to ensure that the correct amount of skin and parenchyma will be excised, and to make subtle adjustments to the nipple height if needed. As noted by the surgical fellows, this technique is also easier to learn.

To design the superomedial pedicle, plan the pedicle base to capture the 2nd – 3rd internal mammary perforator. The pedicle begins superiorly 1 cm lateral to the breast meridian and extends halfway down the medial vertical limb (typically 3.5–4.5 cm). Over the last several years, we have shifted this pedicle base more superiorly to help capture the 2nd internal mammary perforator, which often lies in the breast meridian and is highly reliable and robust [8, 9]. As an added bonus, this slightly more superior base position of a superomedial compared with a medial pedicle makes it easier for the pedicle to reach superiorly, avoiding any tension on the most inferior part of the medial pedicle. In very ptotic breasts, a medial pedicle can tether the areola to the inferior aspect of the medial pillar making it difficult for superior positioning into the mosque.

Finally, lateral breast and axillary lipodystrophy is marked for SAFELipo. The lipodystrophy can be an isolated area of the superior-anterior axilla, but often includes the entire lateral chest wall and posterior axilla. Addressing these areas of lipodystrophy helps shape the lateral breast, improve the femininity of the chest, and harmonize the overall female silhouette.

Intraoperative Technique (Mastopexy First Technique)

Both senior authors perform the augmentation mastopexy very similarly, but they sequence the surgery differently – S.W.Jr. performs the mastopexy first while H.W. starts with the augmentation. To begin with the mastopexy, the surgeon must be willing to commit to the preoperative markings and nipple position.

For vasoconstriction, breast tumescent solution consisting of 1 L of Lactated Ringer's, 10 ccs of 1% lidocaine, and 2 mg of epinephrine is used. The skin to be incised and the entire area of the pedicle are hyper-infiltrated using a 25 gauge needle. The inferior Wise-pattern wedge of parenchyma inferior to the pillars is infiltrated with a blunt cannula attached to a 60 cc Luer Lock syringe. The area of infiltration extends several centimeters below the IMF, many times extending to the upper abdomen, with 60–180 cc's used on each breast's inframammary and submammary area. Additional infiltration is usually added to the axilla and lateral chest in preparation for SAFELipo when indicated. Simultaneous Separation and Tumescence is utilized for these peripheral areas [10].

Lower Pole Release Skin flaps are elevated to the thickness of mastectomy flaps over the inferior parenchymal wedges (inferior to the pillars) using curved Mayo scissors and counter-tension (this is the skin which would typically be excised with a Wise-pattern excision). This 0.5–1 cm thick flap extends 1–2 cm inferior to the native inframammary fold. The release of this skin flap from the underlying parenchyma and retaining fascial bands and extension past the native IMF is a critical step that allows the creation of a new IMF positioned higher on the chest, accompanied by skin decruitment onto the abdomen to minimize the vertical skin excess. This maneuver helps prevent the need for a horizontal skin excision, fosters skin retraction postoperatively, redrapes some of the vertical excess onto the abdomen and lays the foundation for the development of a new, higher postoperative IMF with a smooth lower pole.

Pillar Sculpting and NAC Inset The circumareolar and pedicle skin is deepithelialized after marking the areolas on tension with 34–38 mm cookie-cutters (rarely as large as 42 mm). The breast pillars are developed with a scalpel to make clean, perpendicular cuts through the parenchyma. The wedge of tissue between the pillars is excised, careful to preserve the deep breast fascia which will serve as a critical layer to isolate and support the implant. The NAC is inset into the mosque with eight deep dermal 4-0 monocryl and then a running subcuticular 4-0 PDS circumareolar blocking suture with the suture ends buried and tied to one another to prevent areola spread. After the NAC is in position and prior to pillar sutures, the augmentation portion of the case is performed.

Augmentation Working between and caudal to the pillars, and at the same subcutaneous entry height as an inframammary breast augmentation approach, the submuscular pocket is developed using a short horizontal (2–3 cm) fascial incision. We elevate the IMF and breast parenchyma footprint in nearly all cases, so the implant pocket needs to be centered behind this elevated level. It is important that the entry tunnel to the subpectoral pocket is in the breast meridian or slightly medial to the breast meridian – entering laterally predisposes the patient to bottoming out by weakening this critically important inferolateral buttress. Mastopexy patients already have an attenuated fascial support network which predisposes the breast tissue and breast implants to falling down-and-out, so we respect and preserve this inferolateral quadrant. From within the pocket visualizing the posterior surface of the pectoralis major muscle, we release the pectoralis inframammary origin medial to our fascial access site. During this release, it is important to (1) preserve the anterior muscular fascia to keep this pocket sealed from the mastopexy, and (2) do not transect the muscle directly off the ribs – leave a 1.5–3 cm cuff of muscle on the ribs. Smooth, round silicone implants are used in the overwhelming majority of cases. After pocket irrigation and deposition of 0.25% Marcaine into the pocket, the implants are placed using a sterile implant funnel. The submuscular pocket is closed with 2-0 PDS to keep the implant isolated from the parenchyma and mastopexy.

Lateral Breast Sculpting If the patient requires SAFELipo of the axilla or lateral chest wall, this is performed prior to placing the implant. Access is through the open mastopexy, and the cannulas should not violate the submuscular implant pocket. Angled cannulas and medial traction of the breast by an assistant simplifies navigation into the areas of lipodystrophy and avoidance of critical axillary structures. The principles of SAFELipo will ensure a smooth and well-defined transition from the lateral chest to the breast.

Vertical Pillar Closure The breast pillars are closed with 2-0 PDS – usually 3–5 deep pillar sutures are needed to effectively cone the breast and shape the lower pole. It is critical that these sutures are placed in the same manner on both breasts, or in the desired compensatory manner for asymmetry cases, and started from the bottom up, given that the vertical pillar closure effectively sets the height of the new, elevated IMF. This closure also sets the length of the new lower pole of the breast. Ideally, after the deep pillar sutures are placed, the dermis will already be aligned and without a gap. Occasionally though, a few more 2-0 PDS pillar sutures are needed to narrow the gap and some 3-0 monocryl deep dermal sutures are placed to better align the dermis. Importantly, the weight of the parenchyma and closure tension should rest entirely on the deep pillar 2-0 PDS sutures.

Breast Tissue Equalization After the pillars are closed and the implants are secured, mastopexy patients often are left with a horizontal fold of tissue at the interface of the new, elevated IMF, the old IMF, and the chest wall immediately below the old IMF. One option is to excise this tissue with a Wise-pattern horizontal skin excision. However, these scars can be reduced or eliminated using breast tissue equalization (BTE). The skin folds and irregularities below the new IMF are the result of (1) tethering fascial bands and inframammary ligaments, (2) tissue and adipose thickness disparities between the breast and chest, and (3) excess lower pole breast skin. The lower pole release maneuver performed at the start of each case treats the tethering fascial bands and inframammary ligaments. To treat the tissue thickness disparity and excess skin, the concepts of SAFELipo are employed in the form of BTE. Using a 4 or 5 mm exploded Wall Cage cannula without suction, the tissues inferior to the new IMF are manually separated and equalized. In the same way that SAFELipo's Fat Equalization corrects contour deformities, the entire area is equalized – the tissue becomes more pliable, thickness differences are corrected, and skin excess is widely redraped, or decruited, inferiorly onto the abdomen. By relaxing the entire fascial infrastructure of the old IMF and equalizing the tissue disparities, the new lifted breast can establish a new IMF and the old IMF will blend seamlessly with the surrounding tissues. A J-shaped scar extension laterally into the new IMF is used if there is a persistent IMF irregularity or if the vertical scar is so long that it could extend onto the chest (senior authors H.W. and S.W.Jr. find this necessary in less than 10% and 2% of cases respectively).

Final Closure After BTE, the vertical lower pole incision is closed with running 3-0 intracuticular monocryl suture. A 4 mm gap is left at the inferior end of the closure for an unsecured ¼ inch Penrose drain to sit into the dead space associated with old IMF. The Penrose drain encourages the passive drainage of any remaining IMF fluid overnight and collapses the dead space. Given that the implant pocket is entirely and completely isolated from the mastopexy, there is no concern for cross-contamination. A small crescent cut-out of gauze-lined ½″ Reston (3M, St. Paul, MN) foam is placed over the old IMF (and any axillary areas of SAFELipo) and a soft compression Microfoam (3M, St. Paul, MN) tape bandage is placed over the breasts and the equalized areas. The patient removes the tape bandage and embedded Penrose drains on postop day one. A supportive bra and foam are worn for the first 5 days postop to ensure that the lower pole transition settles smoothly, followed by an underwire bra around the clock for the first year after surgery.

Anatomic Challenges

Dense Breast Tissue Patients with dense breast tissue seem to have the benefit that their breasts will hold up well over time, but the tissue is not very pliable intraoperatively which creates its own challenges. The goal is to have the sculpted breast tissue seamlessly transition to the implant to create a unified breast mound. However, in a patient with dense fibrous breasts, the unyielding tissue fosters high closure tension as well as a "breast on a breast" appearance in the superior pole. To reduce inset tension, additional parenchyma should be released or even resected, if necessary, from the periphery of the mosque to make room for the pedicle and to allow better redraping of parenchyma over the implant. The deep surface of the pedicle can be safely trimmed as needed, preserving the superficial 3 cm which contains the critical vasculature [9, 11]. Failure to reduce the tension can lead to poor scarring, wound dehiscence and venous compromise. Despite these simple maneuvers, the rigidity of the tissue can still leave a residual "breast on a breast" deformity. Although this deformity softens over time postoperatively, it does not always completely correct itself. If needed, we vertically score the deep parenchyma of the superior pole to increase tissue compliance (similar to lower pole parenchymal scoring for a tuberous breast deformity). Also, tissue equalization with an exploded tip cannula can be performed. Using a 4–5 mm exploded tip (Wall Cage) cannula without suction, the upper pole is equalized throughout the parenchyma to reduce the rigidity of the tissue and increase the compliance of the breast. In cases where the parenchyma is too dense to allow for proper equalization, manual scoring is employed. There is no additional risk to the perfusion of the superior pedicle based on the principles of SAFELipo and the superficial course of the vasculature.

Low, Medially Displaced NAC The patient with a low, medially displaced NAC is particularly challenging. As previously discussed, it is preferable to move a very ptotic NAC with the rotational movement of a superomedial pedicle rather than a superior pedicle. However, when the NAC is medially displaced, it shortens the rotation arm and arc length of the superomedial pedicle. The NAC is tethered to the medial limb. Usually this translates to an inability of the medial corner of the mosque to transpose around the NAC for closure. For mild cases of medially displacement, the medial corner of the mosque can be elevated at the dermal-parenchymal junction for 1–3 cm to allow for transposition and closure of the mosque. However, when the NAC is markedly displaced medially, we recommend a superolateral pedicle. The one caveat to a superolateral pedicle is that since the blood supply is not as robust, and that it is not as consistently superficial compared to the superomedial pedicle [9, 11], we do not employ or recommend aggressive debulking to the deep surface of a lateral pedicle. Instead, when required, SAFELipo should be utilized.

Our Experience

Over the 10-year time period between 2005 and 2015, the two senior surgeons (S.W.Jr. and H.W.) performed 1217 one-stage augmentation mastopexy procedures – 1044 (86%) were primary breast cases and 173 (14%) were secondary cases (*see* Table 9.1, *operative data*). The average length of follow-up was 39 months (4–141 months). The average patient age at the time of surgery was 36 years (14–73). Average BMI was 23.9 kg/m^2 (17–33). Prior history of nicotine use was present in 29% of patients. The average implant size was 383 cc (170–1000). There were no cases of major nipple necrosis but one case of partial nipple necrosis. There were no cases of emergent reoperation, hematoma, implant loss, implant exposure or major wound dehiscence.

The overall revision rate was 4.8% (58 patients). Patients who had undergone prior breast surgery were statistically more likely to require a revision compared with patients who had virgin breast tissue (10.4% vs 3.8%, $p = 0.0005$). The revision rate for S.W.Jr. and H.W. was 4.0% and 5.2% respectively. Although the two senior surgeons sequence the surgery differently (S.W.Jr. performs the mastopexy first and H.W. performs the augmentation first), there was no significant difference in their revision rates ($p = 0.35$). On average, revision surgeries were performed at 23.4 months postop (range, 1–90) (*see* Fig. 9.4, *timing of revision surgery*). 28% of the revisions were performed more than 2 years after the original surgery and 16% were performed more than 6 years later. If we shorten our length of follow-up to 1 year, our revision

Table 9.1 Operative data

No. of patients	1217
Primary cases	1044 (86%)
Secondary cases	173 (14%)
Operative revisions	58 (4.8%)
Revisions from primary breast cases	40 (3.8%)
Revisions from secondary breast cases	18 (10.4%)
Time lag for revision surgery, months	23.4 (1–90)
Age, years	36 (14–73)
BMI, kg/m^2	23.9 (17–33)
Prior history of nicotine use	29%
Length follow-up, months	38.6 (4–141)
Implant type	
Silicone	43%
Saline	57%
Implant size, cc	383 (170–1000)

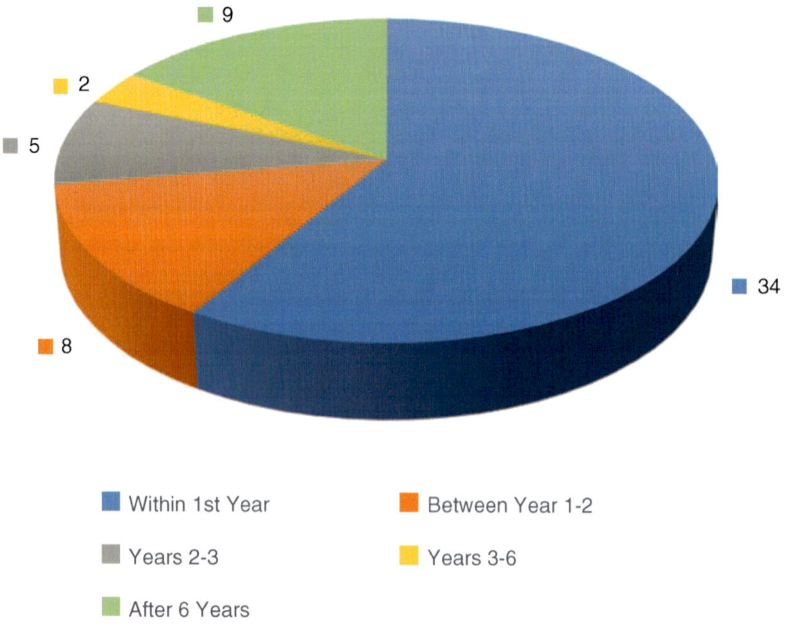

Fig. 9.4 Timing of revision surgery postoperatively. (©Simeon Wall Jr)

rate drops in half: from 4.8% to 2.5%. Of the 58 revision cases, 90% were purely implant or implant-pocket related (*See* Figs. 9.5 and 9.6 *and Table 9.2, indication for revision*).

Discussion and Literature Review

Rejuvenation of the aging breast has dramatically grown in popularity over the last decade. Based on survey data from the American Society for Aesthetic Plastic Surgery (ASAPS), breast lifts are up 649% from 1997 to 2015, while the average increase for other aesthetic procedures is 94% [12]. Based on 2017 survey data, breast augmentation is the most popular surgical procedure for women and breast lift is third [13]. At the same time, patients want aesthetic correction with as little surgery as needed, as indicated by the growing popularity of nonsurgical procedures [12]. Specifically, patients have a desire and expectation for a full upper pole at the desired height of the breast on their chest.

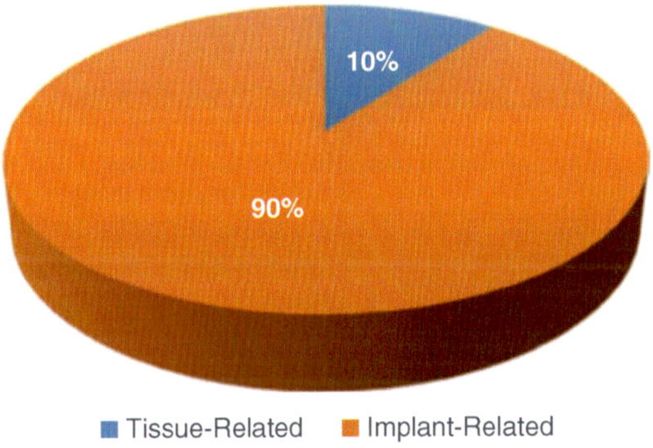

Fig. 9.5 Primary indication for revision. (©Simeon Wall Jr)

The safety and predictability of single-stage augmentation mastopexy has been scrutinized extensively [14–20]. Proponents of staging the surgery have two main arguments – staging will (1) improve results by simplifying the surgery technically by reducing the number of moving parts, and (2) reduce complications since the two components fundamentally oppose one another (volumizing the breast while reducing the skin envelope). However, our experience is in agreement with a growing body of research indicating that with proper planning and technique, a one-stage procedure can be highly reliable and rewarding [3, 20–30]. Swanson and Calobrace et al. independently demonstrated that although a single stage augmentation mastopexy may have a measured reoperation rate higher than that of either procedure performed alone, the revision rate of combining the procedures was less than additive [3, 27].

To reduce the morbidity of a single stage procedure, steps should be taken to isolate the two surgical components and prevent them from competing with one another. We deliberately dissect high submuscular pockets, place our implants unnaturally high initially while preserving the pectoralis major fascia, and securely close the

Fig. 9.6 Revision procedures. (©Simeon Wall Jr)

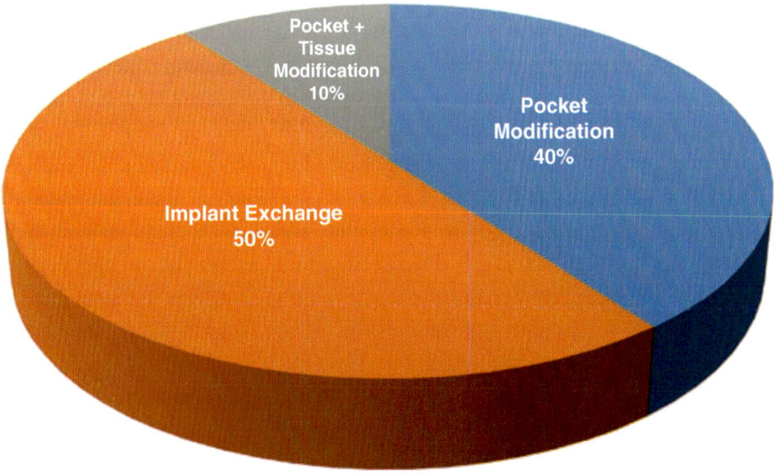

Table 9.2 Indication for revision

No. of patients	Indication for revision	Surgery performed	Timing of revision (Avg months postop)	Notes
18	Implant malposition	Capsulotomy and/or capsulhorraphy	8.6	
16	Implant upsize	Implant exchange	25.2	Average size change was 392–544 cc
8	Implant failure/ deflation	Implant exchange	37.1	
3	Capsular contracture	Capsulectomy, pocket revision	11.3	
3	Breast volume loss	Revision aug-masto	40.7	Postoperatively, all 3 patients lost more than 25 lb
2	Implant malposition with tissue asymmetry	Capsule modification with mastopexy	12	
2	Implant malposition and implant upsize	Implant exchange, capsule modification	51	
3	Implant downsize	Implant exchange, mastopexy	50.5	Average size change was 317–227 cc
1	Implant malposition with tissue laxity	Revision aug-masto	78	Patient was exercising 6.5 years postop and had a sudden implant pocket tear and malposition
1	Implant deflation due to threatened NAC	Implant exchange	11	Patient began smoking POD 0. NAC was threatened. Surgeon delfated implants POD 1
1	Implant upsize, NAC partial loss	Implant exchange, NAC scar revision	7	A massive weight loss patient with a prior history of smoking

fascia to isolate the subpectoral pocket from the mastopexy dissection. This ensures that our implant is completely protected from the mastopexy, situated cephalad and physically isolated, and does not compete with pillar and mastopexy closure. With this approach, implant exposure is prevented even if a wound develops. By using subpectoral smooth implants, the implants reliably drop into position over several weeks or months postoperatively once the mastopexy has already healed.

The long-term stability of the augmented and lifted breast should be critically examined with a goal of building patients for life. Research methodology needs to account for the postoperative changes in breast shape during the first year and final assessments of results should not be made prematurely. Eder et al. demonstrated that with an isolated subpectoral breast augmentation, the volume and shape of the breast did not stabilize until around 6 months postoperatively [31]. Quan et al. performed sequential 3D imaging after short scar breast reductions and verified that breast ptosis does not stabilize until the end of the first postoperative year [32]. Eder et al. evaluated breast morphology after inverted T-scar and vertical scar reduction mammoplasty and demonstrated that breast shape does not stabilize until after 6–9 months postoperatively [33]. In our experience, it is incomplete and cursory to evaluate augmentation-mastopexy results without long-term follow-up to critically assess how tissue and implant dynamics change over time. Our average length of follow-up in this study was 39 months.

Breast rejuvenation should be considered a marathon, not a sprint. A recent systematic review of single stage augmentation mastopexy revealed that of the 23 studies that met inclusion criteria, only 8 studies (35%) had an average patient follow-up of at least 1 year [34]. The majority of published data on complication rates and revision rates is based on studies with patients that have not even made it to their 1 year follow-up [34]. A critical assessment of an augmentation mastopexy result cannot be made in the first few months postoperatively. Additionally, if a patient has breast ptosis at 12 months postoperatively with stable weight, this should be classified as a failure of the original surgery and incomplete correction, not recurrent ptosis as it is defined within some methodology. Khavanin et al. demonstrated that when a minimum mean follow-up of 1 year is applied to the bulk of data available, the augmentation mastopexy reoperation rate increases dramatically – from 10.7% to 16.1% [34]. Shorter patient follow-up gives a premature assessment of results and also a misleading revision rate. If we shorten our length of follow-up to 1 year, our revision rate drops in half: from 4.8% to 2.5%. In our study, ten patients required revisions more than 5 years postoperatively, and of those revisions, 80% were to electively change implant sizing or to correct a ruptured implant. This demonstrates that this technique holds up well over time because these revisions at more than 5 years out are not related to ptosis, tissue dynamics or implant pockets.

Our revision rate of 4.8% compares favorably to other published series of single stage augmentation mastopexy (Table 9.3, *study comparisons*). However, use caution when making comparisons between case series because there is significant methodology variability. The vast majority of our revisions, 90%, were primarily implant-related rather than tissue-related. However, other published series have found a greater relative percentage of tissue-related complications. This is likely technique dependent. Our technique places the implant 2–5 cm higher than ideal intraoperatively to make the mastopexy technically easier with less chance of breakdown postoperatively. We believe this strategy lowers our tissue-related complication rate and risk of infection. However, this strategy comes at the risk of implants remaining too high. Of our 58 revision surgeries, 18 (31%) were isolated capsulotomies for one implant remaining too high. These operative corrections were performed at an average of

Table 9.3 Indications for reoperation for recent reports of single-stage augmentation mastopexy

Reference	No. of patients	Length of study in years	Revision rate (%)	Average followup in months (range)	Implant-related (%)	Tissue-related (%)
Wall et al. [10]	1217	10	4.8	39 (4–141)	4.4	0.7
Messa and Messa 2019 [35]	1131	10.6	14.7	43 (4–121)	6.9	7.9
Stevens et al. 2014 [29]	615	19.3	16.9	17 (1–151)	9.8	7.1
Calobrace et al. 2013 [27]	332	5	23.2	18 (12–72)	9.9	13.3
Sanniec and Adams 2019 [20]	251	11	3.6	16.9 (1.5–120)		
Swanson 2013 [3]	146	10	20.5	8 (0.2–46)	7.5	17.8
Castello et al. 2014 [36]	107	5	12.1	15 (3–29)	7.5	6.5
Doshier et al. 2016 [30][a]	106	10	12.4[a]	16 (1.5–67)		
Seify et al. 2010 [37]	88	3.5	6.8	15 (1–33)		
Beale et al. 2014 [28]	83	8	19.3	38	10.2	9.1
Tessone et al. 2011 [25]	60	6	10.0	–	3.3	6.7

Some patients had both implant-related and tissue-related indications for revision surgery

[a]In the original publication, revision rate was calculated as a percentage of operative breasts rather than patients. So true revision rate is much higher than 12.4

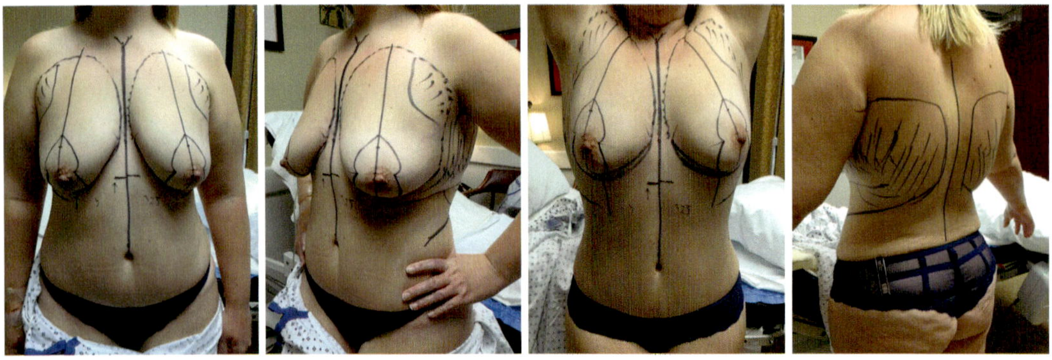

Fig. 9.7 Case 1, Markings for augmentation mastopexy with SAFELipo and breast tissue equalization of the axilla and breast borders. (©Simeon Wall Jr)

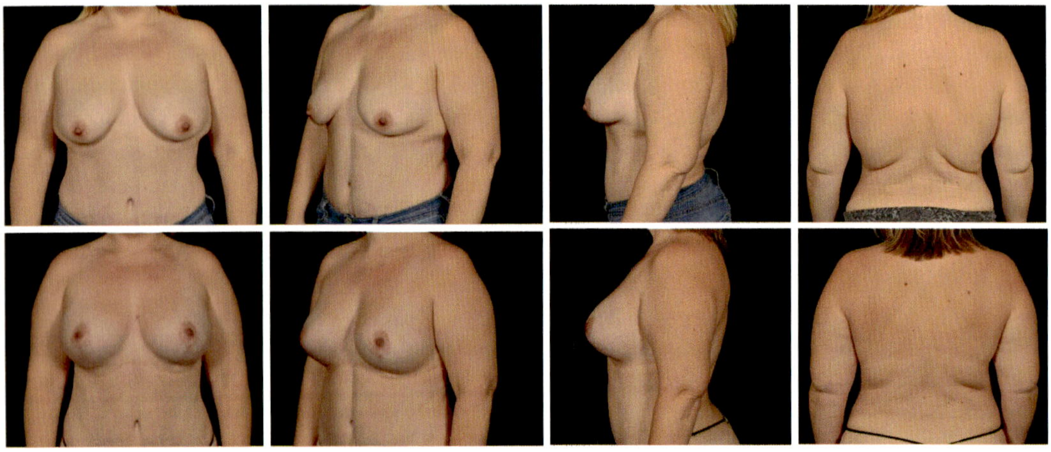

Fig. 9.8 Case 1: Before and 1 year after photo. Note the improvement in the lateral ches t on AP view

8.6 months postoperatively. This is a trade-off we are willing to accept. A capsulotomy to drop an implant one centimeter is relatively quick and easy compared with other potential problems.

Despite the availability of liposuction as an adjunctive mammoplasty technique since its description by Teimourian et al. in 1985, a survey in 2002 by Rohrich et al. showed that the majority of surgeons used liposuction on 10 percent or fewer of their breast reductions [38, 39]. We have found SAFE liposuction to be an indispensable tool in the majority of augmentation mastopexy cases, and breast tissue equalization (BTE) in all of them. Breast tissue equalization and SAFELipo are powerful techniques to naturally define the breast borders, accentuate chest wall femininity and eliminate lipodystrophy (Case 1, Figs. 9.7 and 9.8). The multistep approach minimizes the risk of breast contour deformities which has plagued traditional liposuction [40]. Breast tissue equalization ensures that the transition areas are smooth and natural by (1) eliminating dramatic changes in tissue thickness, (2) widely distributing skin excess, and (3) softening any tethering fibrous adhesions. It also is a critical maneuver for allowing elevation of the breast footprint without leaving deformities associated with the old IMF. We have found breast tissue equalization to be particularly useful in the dense fibrous breast patient to soften the rigidity of the tissue. Lejour in 1994 noted a similar experience with breast liposuction stating "after liposuction, the breast is softer, more pliable, and easier to shape. This altered consistency is especially helpful when the areola is elevated on a long pedicle." [41]

Reducing mammoplasty scar burden on the breast has been a perpetual goal over the last century [42–45]. While breast shape takes priority over scars, inverted T scars can be unsightly, misplaced, diminish perfusion and increase the risk for delayed wound healing. With breast tissue equalization and SAFELipo at the IMF, a scar extension in the IMF is required less than 10% of the time (H.W.) or less than 2% of the time (S.W.Jr.). This technique works by widely separating and equalizing the entire IMF area. This weakens the tethering fascial bands, corrects for tissue thickness differences, distributes skin excess onto the abdomen and importantly, induces skin contraction postoperatively. We find this concept useful in all surgeries at transition areas to eliminate dog ears and irregularities.

For severely ptotic breasts with long pedicles, the superomedial pedicle can be safely trimmed and reduced in bulk to decrease closure tension and aid with NAC elevation and inset. For arterial preservation, le Roux showed that at the NAC boundary, the mean arterial depth was 10.3 mm (standard deviation (SD): 2.5) and 3 cm from NAC the mean depth was 14.2 mm (SD 4.6) [11]. Critical veins run in the superficial 5 mm [11]. Therefore, superomedial pedicles can be safely trimmed to 3 cm thickness if needed.

For patients with mild breast ptosis wanting an augmentation, we have a low threshold to recommend a simultaneous mastopexy. When the NAC is at the level of the IMF, we agree that these patients *can* be treated with an isolated augmentation. However, the better question is *should* an isolated augmentation be performed and will adding a mastopexy give a better long-term result. Adding a "footprint elevating" mastopexy allows (1) higher implant position (improved cleavage and full upper pole at the desired position), and (2) an elevated breast footprint (more youthful breast with longevity). Augmenting a slightly ptotic breast provides more volume that looks great in clothes. But unsupported, the breast can look lower and heavier, and actually more matronly. The slightly ptotic appearance can be exacerbated – the perceived notch to nipple distance is elongated. Adding volume but sacrificing overall breast shape and chest wall aesthetics is usually not a good trade-off, especially once they have settled. This absolutely comes down to patient preference. This discussion can be tough because instinctively women do not want a mastopexy. Usually after we show patients photos and have a full discussion, most of these patients elect for a simultaneous mastopexy because long-term breast position and shape is their number one priority over scars.

This study was limited in its acquisition of only reoperative cases that required the operating room. Although very rare, we did not gather data for patients that may have had minor complications that required a small procedure postoperatively in clinic (i.e. seroma aspiration). The goal of the study was to assess the incidence of treatment failure with one formal surgery.

Case Studies 2-5 are shown in Figs. 9.9, 9.10, 9.11, and 9.12.

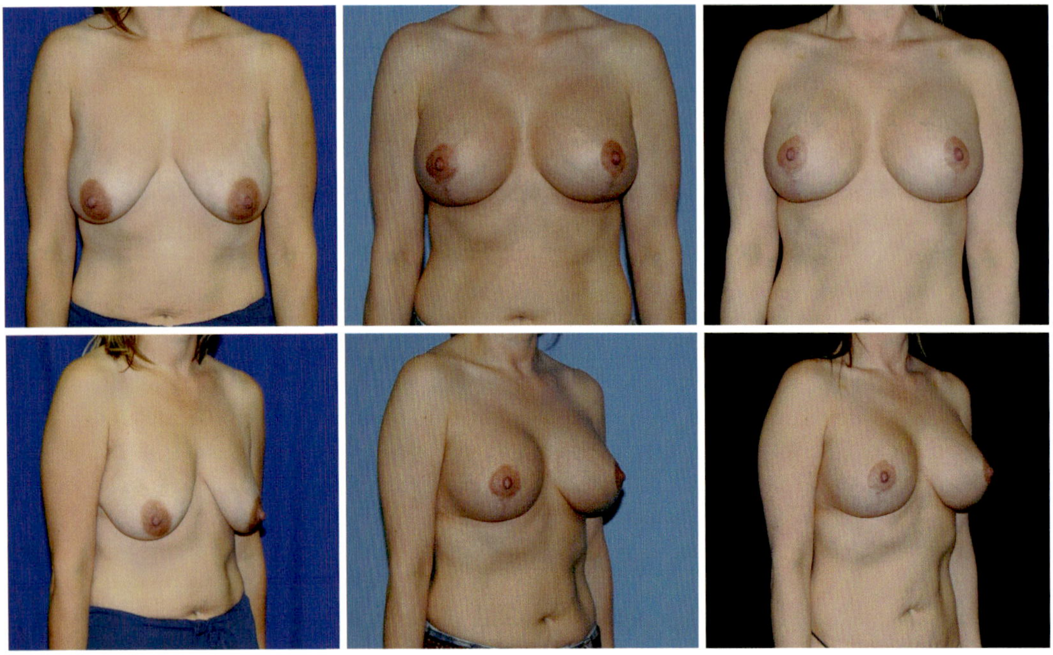

Fig. 9.9 Case 2: Short-Sec augmentation mastopexy. Before, one year and 4 year postoperative results

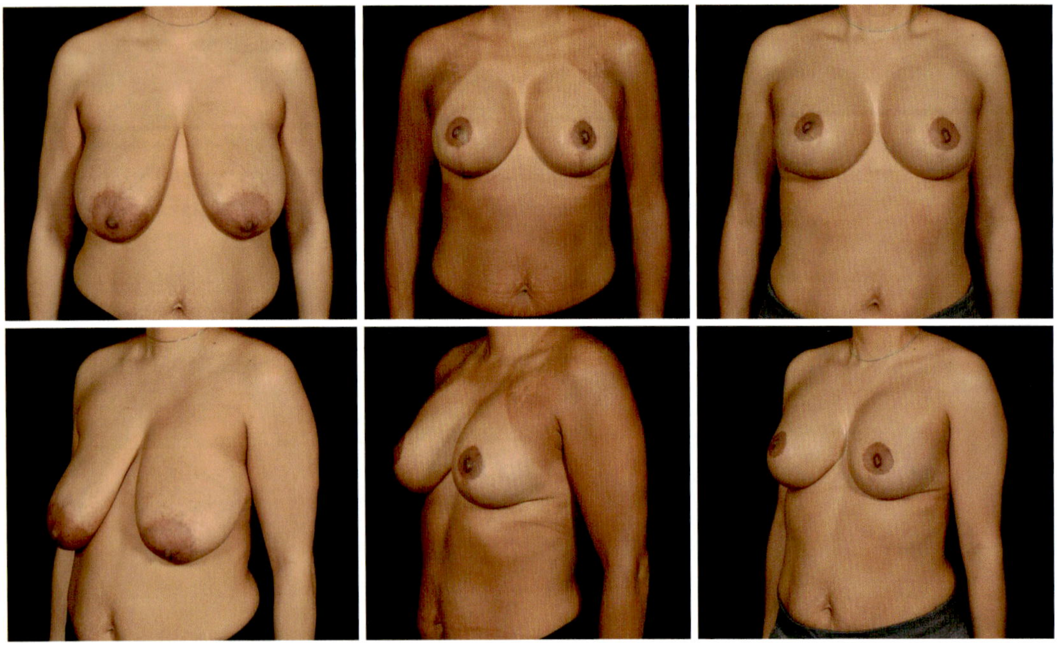

Fig. 9.10 Case 3: Short-Sec augmentation mastopexy. Before, one year and 5 year postoperative results

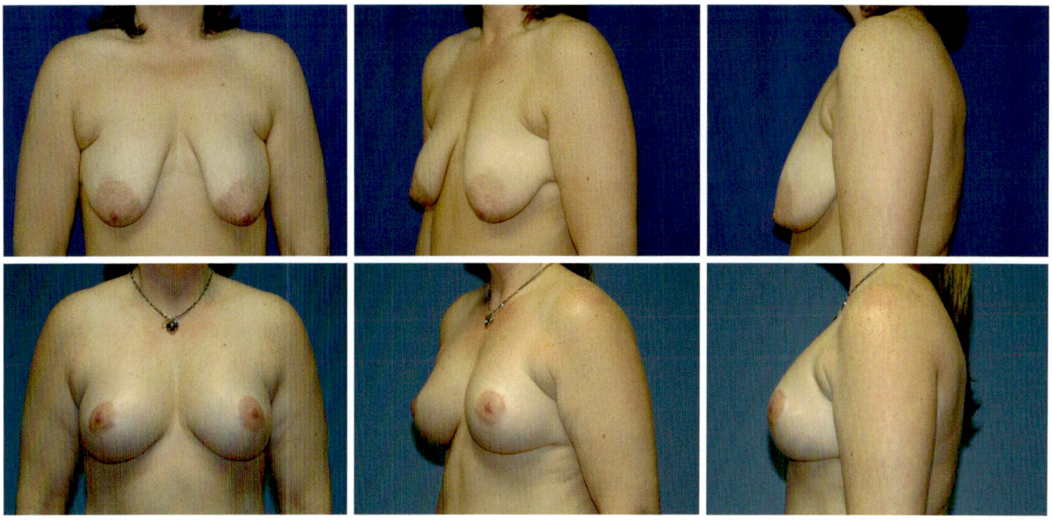

Fig. 9.11 Case 4: Short-Sec augmentation mastopexy. Before and 6 months postoperative results

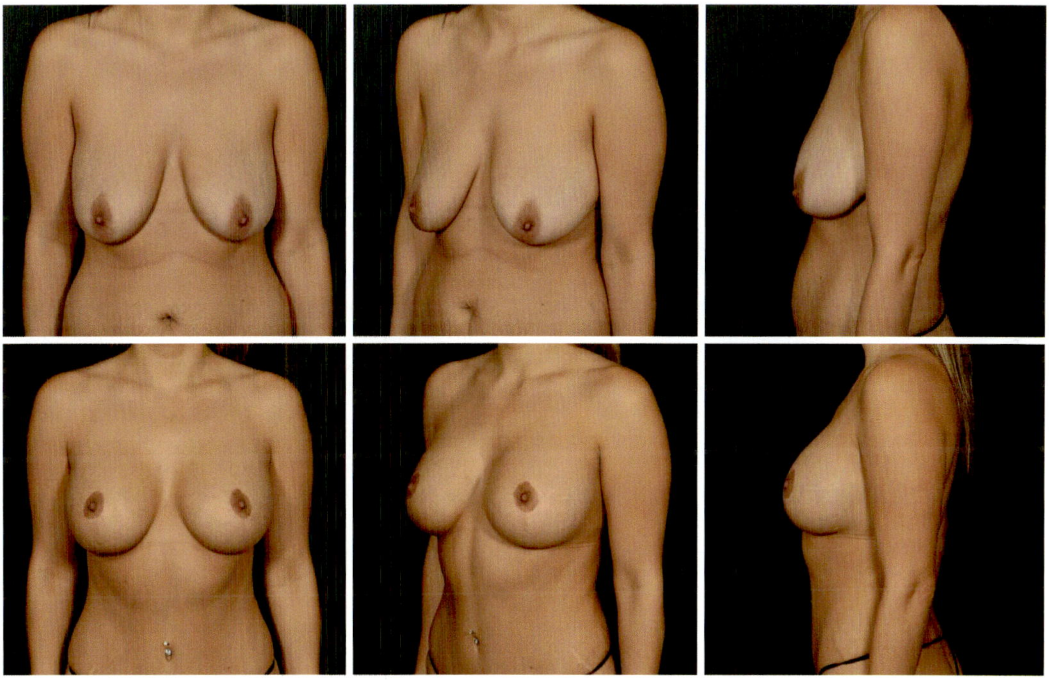

Fig. 9.12 Case 5: Short-Sec augmentation mastopexy. Before and 2 years postoperative results

Conclusion

The purpose of the study was to demonstrate to the reader our technique for single stage augmentation mastopexy to simplify the surgery. The strategies reported have helped the senior authors maximize consistency and minimize complications and can hopefully serve as an educational reference.

References

1. Theocharidis V, Katsaros I, Sgouromallis E, Serifis N, Boikou V, Tasigiorgos S, Kokosis G, Economopoulos KP. Current evidence on the role of smoking in plastic surgery elective procedures: a systematic review and meta-analysis. J Plast Reconstr Aesthet Surg. 2018;71(5):624–36.
2. Sieffert MR, Fox JP, Abbott LE, Johnson RM. Obesity is associated with increased health care charges in patients undergoing outpatient plastic surgery. Plast Reconstr Surg. 2015;135(5):1396–404.
3. Swanson E. Prospective comparative clinical evaluation of 784 consecutive cases of breast augmentation and vertical mammaplasty, performed individually and in combination. Plast Reconstr Surg. 2013;132(1):30e–45e.
4. Weichman K, Doft M, Matarasso A. The impact of mastopexy on brassiere cup size. Plast Reconstr Surg. 2014;134(1):34e–40e.
5. Lassus C. The Lassus vertical technique. Aesthet Surg J. 2011;31(8):897–913.
6. Lassus C. A 30-year experience with vertical mammaplasty. Plast Reconstr Surg. 1996;97(2):373–80.
7. Lista F, Austin RE, Singh Y, Ahmad J. Vertical scar reduction mammaplasty. Plast Reconstr Surg. 2015;136(1):23–5.
8. Carr BW, Bishop WE, Anson BJ. Mammary arteries. Q BullNorthwest U Med School. 1942;16:150–4.
9. van Deventer PV, Graewe FR. The blood supply of the breast revisited. Plast Reconstr Surg. 2016;137(5):1388–97.
10. Wall SH Jr, Del Vecchio D. Expansion Vibration Lipofilling (EVL) – concepts and applications of a new paradigm in large volume fat transplantation. Presented at the American Society for Aesthetic Plastic Surgery Annual Meeting, San Diego, CA, May 2017.
11. Michelle le Roux C, Kiil BJ, Pan WR, Rozen WM, Ashton MW. Preserving the neurovascular supply in the Hall-Findlay superomedial pedicle breast reduction: an anatomical study. J Plast Reconstr Aesthet Surg. 2010;63(4):655–62.
12. American Society for Aesthetic Plastic Surgery. Cosmetic surgery national data bank statistics 2015. http://www.surgery.org/sites/default/files/ASAPS-Stats2015.pdf . Accessed 25 Mar 2019.
13. American Society for Aesthetic Plastic Surgery. Cosmetic surgery national data bank statistics 2017. https://surgery.org/sites/default/files/ASAPS-Stats2017.pdf. Accessed 25 Mar 2019.
14. Spear SL. Augmentation/mastopexy: surgeon beware. Plast Reconstr Surg. 2003;112:905–6.
15. Hoffman S. Some thoughts on augmentation/mastopexy and medical malpractice. Plast Reconstr Surg. 2004;113:1892–3.
16. Nahai F, Fisher J, Maxwell PG, Mills DC II. Augmentation mastopexy: to stage or not. Aesthetic Surg J. 2007;27:297–305.
17. Spear SL, Boehmler JH, Clemens MW. Augmentation/mastopexy: a 3-year review of a single surgeon's practice. Plast Reconstr Surg. 2006;118:136S–47S; discussion 148S–149S, 150S–151S
18. Spear SL, Giese SY. Simultaneous breast augmentation and mastopexy. Aesthet Surg J. 2000;20:155–63.
19. Spear SL, Pelletiere CV, Menon N. One-stage augmentation combined with mastopexy: aesthetic results and patient satisfaction. Aesthet Plast Surg. 2004;28:259–67.
20. Sanniec K, Adams WP Jr. The tissue-based triad in augmentation mastopexy: single-stage technical refinements. Aesthet Surg J. 2019;39(12): 1331–4.
21. Gallent IM, Pons MR, Drever M. Vertical scar mastopexy with an implant. Aesthet Plast Surg. 2003;27:406–10.
22. Karnes J, Morrison W, Salisbury M, Schaeferle M, Beckham P, Ersek RA. Simultaneous breast augmentation and lift. Aesthet Plast Surg. 2000;24:148–54.
23. Stevens WG, Freeman EM, Stoker DA, Quardt SM, Cohen R, Hirsch EM. One-stage mastopexy with breast augmentation: a review of 321 patients. Plast Reconstr Surg. 2007;120:1674–9.
24. Stevens WG, Stoker DA, Freeman ME, Quardt SM, Hirsch EM, Cohen R. Is one-stage breast augmentation with mastopexy safe and effective? A review of 186 primary cases. Aesthet Surg J. 2006;26:674–81.
25. Tessone A, Millet E, Weissman O, et al. Evading a surgical pitfall: mastopexy–augmentation made simple. Aesthet Plast Surg. 2011;35:1073–8.
26. Persoff MM. Mastopexy with expansion-augmentation. Aesthet Surg J. 2003;23:34–9.
27. Calobrace MB, Herdt DR, Cothron KJ. Simultaneous augmentation/mastopexy: a retrospective 5-year review of 332 consecutive cases. Plast Reconstr Surg. 2013;131(1):145–56.
28. Beale EW, Ramanadham S, Harrison B, Rasko Y, Armijo B, Rohrich RJ. Achieving predictability in augmentation mastopexy. Plast Reconstr Surg. 2014;133(3):284e–92e.
29. Stevens WG, Macias LH, Spring M, Stoker DA, Chacón CO, Eberlin SA. One-stage augmentation mastopexy: a review of 1192 simultaneous breast augmentation and mastopexy procedures in 615 consecutive patients. Aesthet Surg J. 2014;34(5):723–32.

30. Doshier LJ, Eagan SL, Shock LA, Henry SL, Colbert SH, Puckett CL. The subtleties of success in simultaneous augmentation-Mastopexy. Plast Reconstr Surg. 2016;138(3):585–92.
31. Eder M, v Waldenfels F, Sichtermann M, Schuster T, Papadopulos NA, Machens HG, Biemer E, Kovacs L. Three-dimensional evaluation of breast contour and volume changes following subpectoral augmentation mammaplasty over 6 months. J Plast Reconstr Aesthet Surg. 2011;64(9):1152–60.
32. Quan M, Fadl A, Small K, Tepper O, Kumar N, Choi M, Karp N. Defining pseudoptosis (bottoming out) 3 years after short-scar medial pedicle breast reduction. Aesthet Plast Surg. 2011;35(3):357–64.
33. Eder M, Klöppel M, Müller D, Papadopulos NA, Machens HG, Kovacs L. 3-D analysis of breast morphology changes after inverted T-scar and vertical-scar reduction mammaplasty over 12 months. J Plast Reconstr Aesthet Surg. 2013;66(6):776–86.
34. Khavanin N, Jordan SW, Rambachan A, Kim JY. A systematic review of single-stage augmentation-mastopexy. Plast Reconstr Surg. 2014;134(5):922–31.
35. Messa CA, Messa CA. One-stage augmentation mastopexy: a retrospective ten-year review of 2183 consecutive procedures. Aesthet Surg J. 2019;39(12):1352–67. https://doi.org/10.1093/asj/sjz143.
36. Castello MF, Silvestri A, Nicoli F, Dashti T, Han S, Grassetti L, Torresetti M, Perdanasari AT, Zhang YX, Di Benedetto G, Lazzeri D. Augmentation mammoplasty/mastopexy: lessons learned from 107 aesthetic cases. Aesthet Plast Surg. 2014;38(5):896–907.
37. Seify H, Ismail K, Evans G. Primary augmentation/mastopexy using large implants: is it a safe technique? A 4-year single surgeon review. Plast Reconstr Surg. 2010;126(4):67.
38. Teimourian B, Massac E Jr, Wiegering CE. Reduction suction mammaplasty and suction lipectomy as an adjunct to breast surgery. Aesthet Plast Surg. 1985;9:97–100.
39. Rohrich RJ, Gosman AA, Brown SA, Tonadapu P, Foster B. Current preferences for breast reduction techniques: a survey of board-certified plastic surgeons 2002. Plast Reconstr Surg. 2004;114:1724–33; discussion 1734–1736
40. Wall SH Jr, Lee MR. Separation, aspiration, and fat equalization: SAFE liposuction concepts for comprehensive body contouring. Plast Reconstr Surg. 2016;138(6):1192–201.
41. Lejour M. Vertical mammaplasty and liposuction of the breast. Plast Reconstr Surg. 1994;94(1):100–14.
42. Lötsch F. Uberhangebrustplastik. Zentralbl Chir. 1921;50:1241.
43. Dartigues L. Procedè de mastopexie par incision et resection cutanèes verticales subareolaires. Bull Mem Soc Chir Paris. 1924;24:897–913.
44. Arie G. Una nueva tecnica de mastoplastia. Rev Latinoam Cir Plast. 1957;3:23.
45. Lassus C. Possibilités et limites de la chirurgie plastique de la silhouette féminine. Hopital. 1969;801:575–85.

Circumareolar Augmentation Mastopexy

10

Robert Cohen

Introduction

Circumareolar (also known as periareolar) mastopexy is an extremely useful breast surgery technique that can be combined with augmentation mammaplasty in order to correct a number of aesthetic issues [1]. This technique can shift the areolar position on the breast mound, tighten a loose skin envelope around an implant framework, reduce the diameter of an excessively large areola, and can compress an over projecting (tuberous) breast [2]. In addition to its ability to correct a number of surgical problems, one of the main attributes desirable to patients is the avoidance of a vertical breast scar.

Despite its many uses, this technique has garnered a reputation in some plastic surgery circles as a somewhat unreliable or suboptimal option due to issues with scar spread, wound healing issues and distortion of the breast shape [3]. When inappropriately applied, the circumareolar mastopexy certainly can cause any of these issues. However, many of these complications stem from misuse of the technique or poor patient selection. For the very reason that many patients are attracted to this option due to the lack of a vertical scar, well-meaning surgeons can be tempted to offer this "less invasive" procedure in situations where it may not be the best choice, leading to patient dissatisfaction [4–6].

The goal of this chapter is to re-introduce this versatile and safe procedure by demonstrating specifically when and how to use this technique in order to expand the range of options available to improve breast aesthetics.

Physics of the Circumareolar Mastopexy Technique

Understanding the shape of the breast and dynamics of the soft tissue and how it will react to periareolar skin resection is critical in understanding when and how to use the circumareolar mastopexy technique [7]. The first principle the surgeon must understand is that this is an inherently compressive technique. Unlike a vertical mastopexy, which increases breast projection due to narrowing the skin of the lower pole, circumareolar tightening will flatten the breast centrally as more and more tissue is resected. What this means is that this technique is excellent for over-projected or "pointy" breasts, but it is a poor choice for breasts needing more projection such as those with more severe grade 2 or grade 3 ptosis, or glandular ptosis [8]. In these situations, well-meaning surgeons that want to accommodate their patient's wish for minimal scarring may unfortunately exacerbate the flattened or

R. Cohen (✉)
Beverly Hills Center, Beverly Hills, CA, USA

Scottsdale Center for Plastic Surgery, Paradise Valley, AZ, USA

M. B. Calobrace et al. (eds.), *Augmentation Mastopexy*, https://doi.org/10.1007/978-3-030-48226-8_10

droopy breast shape with the periareolar skin resection.

Figure 10.1a, b shows that by adding implants to expand the breast footprint, and using a circumareolar mastopexy to compress the skin and herniated breast tissue, a tuberous breast is converted into a round breast.

The second dynamic that needs to be understood is the fact that lateral breast forces are stronger than vertical breast forces, thus a concentric circle will be pulled into a horizontally oriented oval once the skin resection is completed. To counteract these forces, it is imperative that the vertical height of the outer incision is longer than its width (usually by approximately 1 cm). The inner incision, which comprises the new cut edge of the areola, is not susceptible to these forces and is therefore created as a true circle with a cookie cutter in the same fashion as is performed with a standard mastopexy or breast reduction.

Figure 10.2a–d shows pre and postoperative photos of a breast augmentation and left unilateral circumareolar mastopexy to improve breast symmetry. In this case, early in the author's practice, concentric circles were used instead of a vertically oriented oval. Although the overall result is good, note the horizontally oriented oval shape of the left areola which could have been avoided with more vertical skin resection.

The third dynamic is related to skin thickness and elasticity. With increasing skin thickness and elasticity comes increased outward force on the skin. Looser and less elastic skin will have weaker forces. Because of this, a larger degree of skin resection can be performed in patients with weaker skin with a low risk of excessive areolar spread or scar hypertrophy. This principle can be verified simply by manually tightening the skin around the areola to simulate the skin resection once an implant is in place. Patients with thin, less elastic skin will be much easier to tighten in this fashion compared to the opposite subset of patients. This can also be a useful technique to judge the appropriate size of the outer skin resection during surgery.

Figure 10.3a–c shows a patient with very thin skin and poor elasticity. In this case it is possible

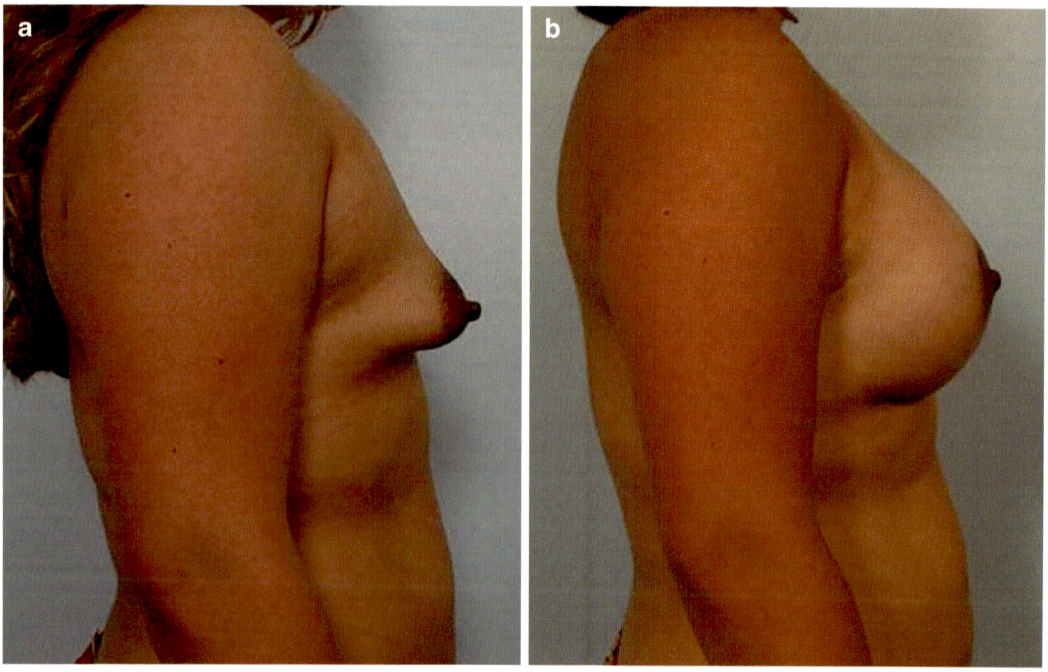

Fig. 10.1 (**a**, **b**) By adding implants to expand the breast footprint, and using a circumareolar mastopexy to compress the skin and herniated breast tissue, a tuberous breast is converted into a round breast

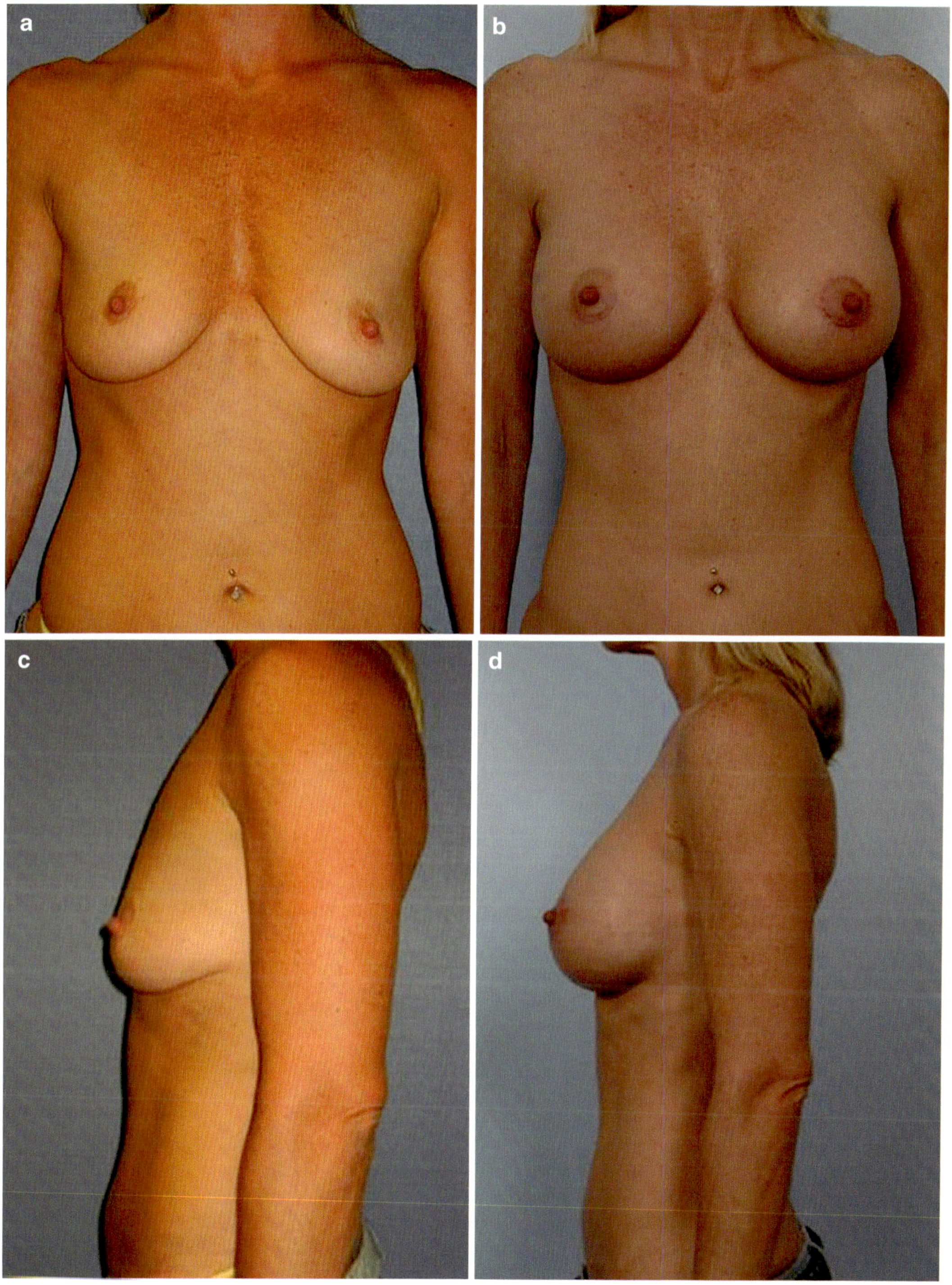

Fig. 10.2 (**a–d**) Pre and postoperative photos of a breast augmentation and left unilateral circumareolar mastopexy to improve breast symmetry. In this case, early in the author's practice, concentric circles were used instead of a vertically oriented oval. Although the overall result is good, note the horizontally oriented oval shape of the left areola which could have been avoided with more vertical skin resection

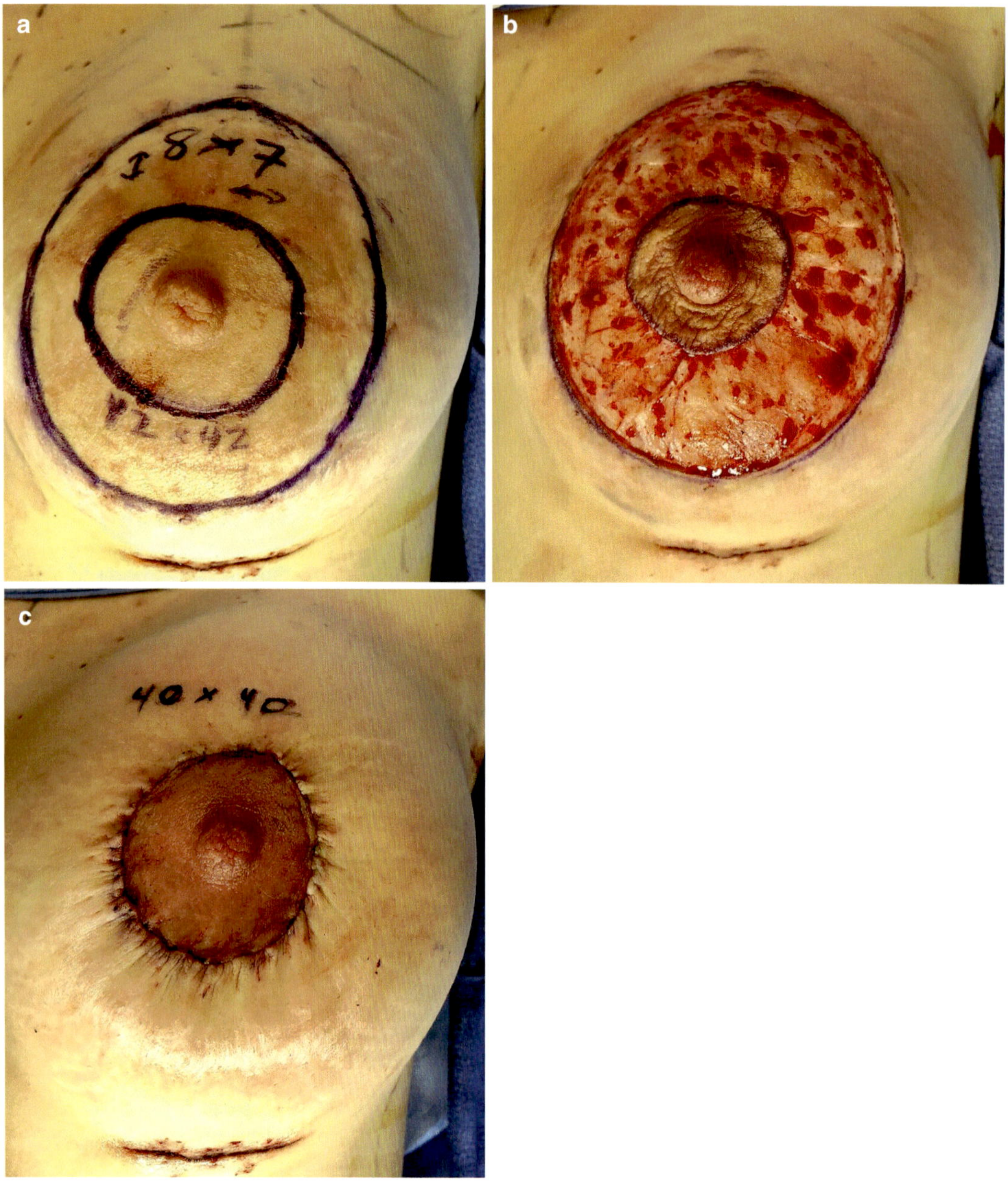

Fig. 10.3 (**a–c**) In this patient with very thin skin and poor elasticity, it is possible to reduce a very large natural areola from approximately 7 by 7 cm to 4 by 4 cm with an oval resection pattern of 8 cm high by 7 cm wide. This very aggressive skin resection is only possible due to the patients weak tissues which were tested by manually pinching and tailor tacking prior to incisions. Note the large degree of skin resection with minimal skin distortion. The dermis is left intact to preserve the subdermal plexus. It is extremely important to understand that in a patient with tighter or more elastic skin, this large a resection would result in disaster with a flattened breast, distorted areola and spread scar. The technique used for this closure is described later in this chapter

to reduce a very large natural areola from approximately 7 by 7 cm to 4 by 4 cm with an oval resection pattern of 8 cm high by 7 cm wide. This very aggressive skin resection is only possible due to the patients weak tissues which were tested by manually pinching and tailor tacking prior to incisions. Note the large degree of skin resection with minimal skin distortion. The dermis is left intact to preserve the subdermal plexus. It is *extremely* important to understand that in a patient with tighter or more elastic skin, this large a resection would result in disaster with a flattened breast, distorted areola and spread scar. The technique used for this closure is described later in this chapter.

Blood Supply

Many techniques have been demonstrated in how to perform a circumareolar mastopexy, some of which involve partially or completely dissecting through the dermis with the possible addition of skin undermining [9–12]. This disrupts the subdermal plexus blood supply, putting the areola at higher risk for congestion or necrosis in patients with very thin subcutaneous tissues (for example, in patients with longstanding capsular contractures in need of revision). As will be demonstrated in the techniques portion of this chapter, the author will show how the entire dermis can be maintained intact, therefore protecting the subdermal plexus and allowing a circumareolar mastopexy even in extremely compromised breasts.

Uses for Circumareolar Mastopexy Part 1 – Areolar Reduction

The simplest indication for circumareolar mastopexy is an oversized areola. In this situation, the diameter of the areola is larger than the patient desires, and the excess areolar tissue can be removed by removing a donut of outer areolar skin. The skin of the areola is very thin and has the potential to heal with a very fine scar, but because of this skin thinness, it is also prone to scar spread if excess tension is applied. The more aggressive the areolar reduction, the more outward tension is placed on the areolar incision creating a higher chance for suboptimal scarring. As noted earlier, the tighter the breast skin, the more caution needs to be exerted in the degree of tissue resection. After augmentation, if the areolar skin is fairly taut, it may be better to avoid the technique altogether. In patients with loose skin, a more extensive resection can be performed safely.

Figure 10.4a–d shows a patient starting with aesthetically oversized areolas and undersized implants and for whom a revision surgery with larger implants is planned. As the areolas would likely stretch even larger with the increase in implant size, a circumareolar mastopexy is performed to moderately reduce and stabilize the areolar diameters.

Uses for Circumareolar Mastopexy Part 2 – Areolar Repositioning

Many patients prior to breast augmentation will have undesirable nipple areolar complex (NAC) positions on the breast mound. Most commonly the NAC are in too low of a position, but they can also be excessively high, medial or lateral in their location. In some cases there is a different NAC location issue on each breast (for example, one can be too high while the other is too low). By offsetting the outer oval pattern in the desired direction of NAC movement, the NAC can be shifted to improve its position on the breast mound. Once again, skin tightness is a factor, and with looser skin, a greater degree of movement is possible. In general, a maximum of approximately 2.5 cm of movement can be expected, but this will vary depending on skin laxity.

In the patient in Fig. 10.5a–d superior elevation of the areolas was desired for an improved aesthetic outcome. Approximately 1–1.5 cm of elevation was achieved by offsetting the skin resection above the areolas with additional NAC centralization coming from expansion of the lower portion of the breast.

Figure 10.6a–e shows how the design of the outer oval pattern relative to the nipple areolar complex (NAC) will determine the movement of the NAC relative to the breast mound. (a) Centered resection results in skin tightening without areolar movement. Offsetting will result in superior (b), inferior (c), superomedial (d) or medial (e) movement. The surgeon can apply differential resections in cases of asymmetry.

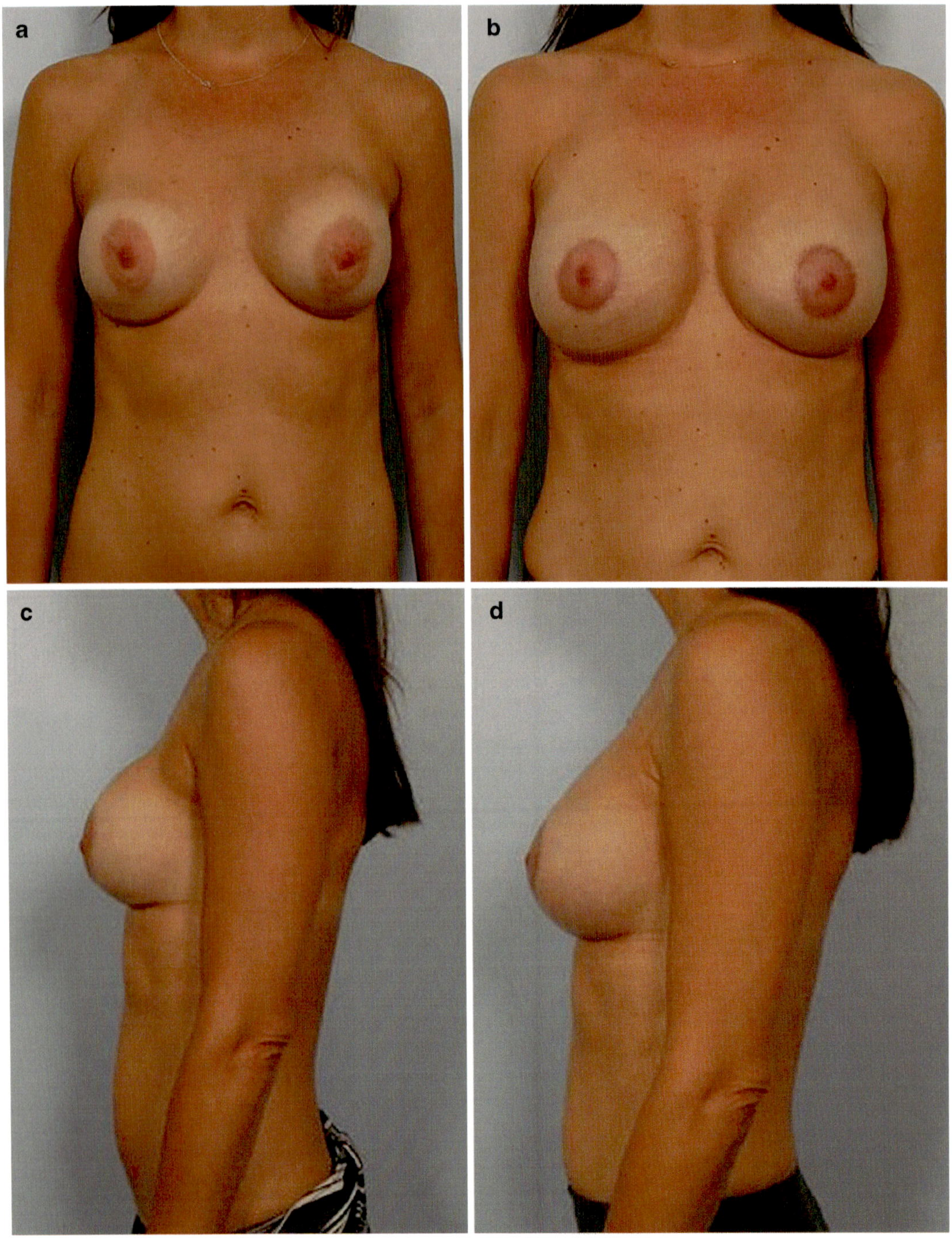

Fig. 10.4 (**a**–**d**) In this patient starting with aesthetically oversized areolas and undersized implants, a revision surgery with larger implants is planned. As the areolas would likely stretch even larger with the increase in implant size, a circumareolar mastopexy is performed to moderately reduce and stabilize the areolar diameters

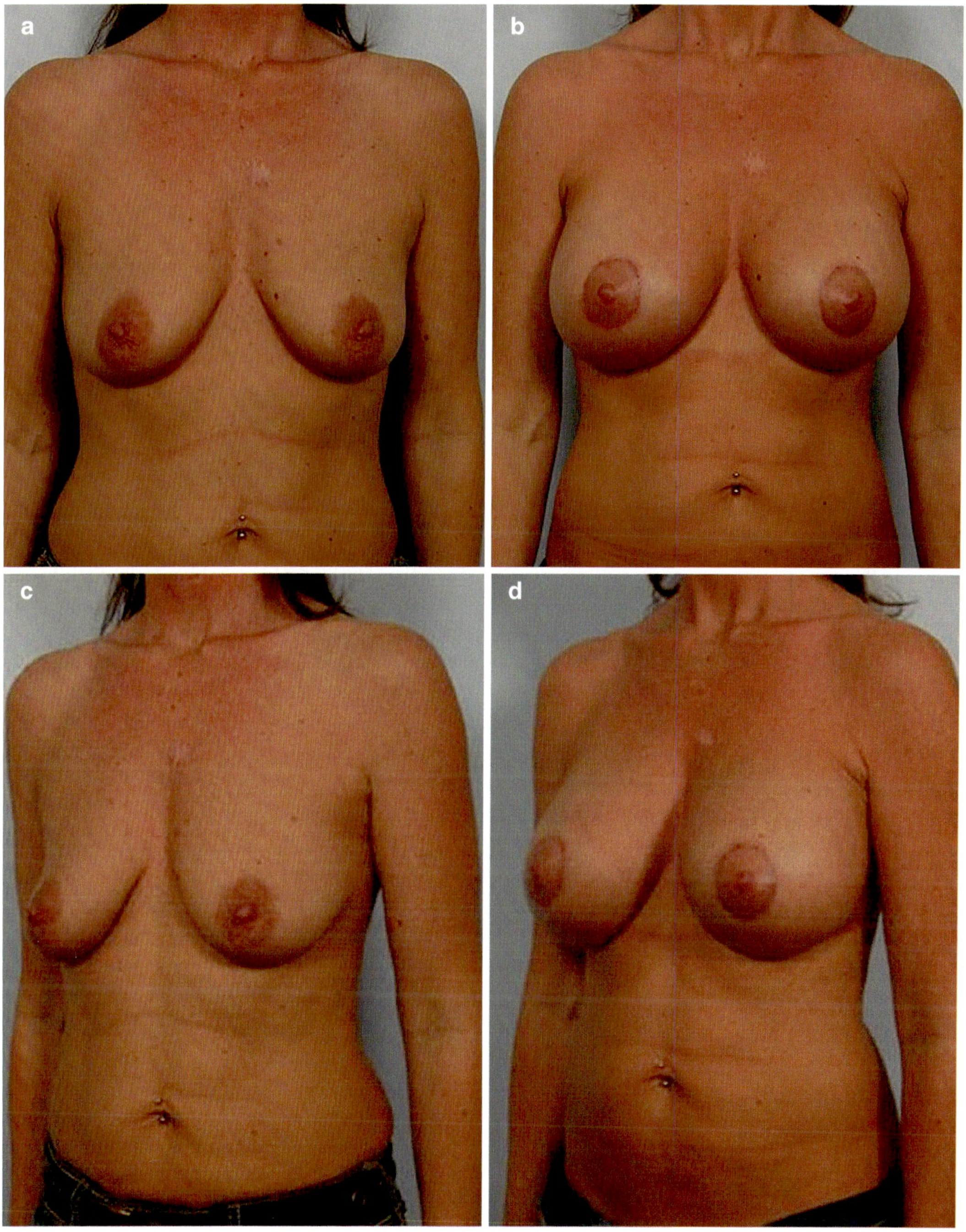

Fig. 10.5 (**a–d**) In this patient, superior elevation of the areolas was desired for an improved aesthetic outcome. Approximately 1–1.5 cm of elevation was achieved by offsetting the skin resection above the areolas with additional NAC centralization coming from expansion of the lower portion of the breast

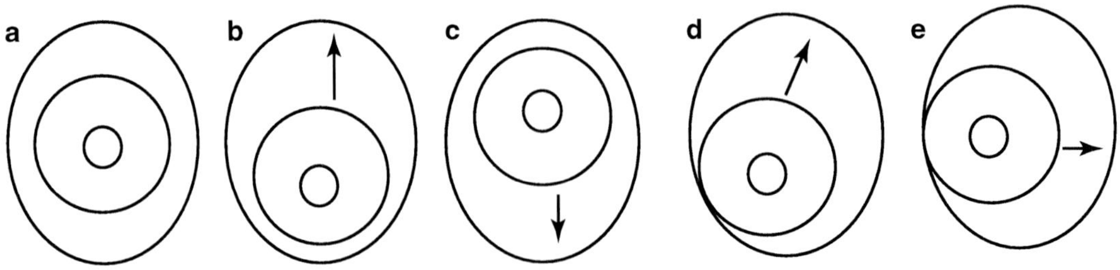

Fig. 10.6 (**a**–**e**) The design of the outer oval patern relative to the nipple areolar complex (NAC) will determine the movement of the NAC relative to the breast mound. (**a**) Centered resection results in skin tightening without areolar movement. Offsetting will result in superior (**b**), inferior (**c**), superomedial (**d**) or medial (**e**) movement. The surgeon can apply differential resections in cases of asymmetry

Figure 10.7a–d shows augmentation mammaplasty with differential circumareolar mastopexy patterns (superomedial movement of the right NAC and mildly inferomedial movement of the left) allows for better postoperative symmetry in this patient.

Uses for Circumareolar Mastopexy Part 3 – Lax Breast Skin/Mild Ptosis

There are a number of patients that present with relative skin laxity and/or mild ptosis that are not severe enough for a full vertical or inverted-T scar mastopexy, but are also too loose to be ideally corrected simply with an augmentation mastopexy. In these cases, a circumareolar mastopexy can complement the volumetric improvement provided by implants [13]. The implants themselves will fill much of the skin envelope and provide projection, while the circumareolar mastopexy serves to cinch the skin tighter on the implant framework. The "cinching" action can also be useful in reducing a double bubble appearance as it redistributes the soft tissue more effectively around the implant. In gray area cases, such as moderate grade 2 ptosis, where it is unclear whether the circumareolar mastopexy will be sufficient, the patient should be consented for a full mastopexy as a backup plan during surgery.

Figure 10.8a–d shows how circumareolar mastopexy in combination with augmentation is used to elevate the NAC and tighten the breast skin while avoiding a vertical breast scar. An abdominoplasty was performed simultaneously.

Figure 10.9a–e shows complex revision surgery (a) (b) preoperatively, (c) (d) 6 months postoperatively and (e) 4 years postoperatively. The previous surgeon had underestimated the complexity of correcting tuberous breasts resulting in a double bubble and tissue clustering behind the areolas. In addition to lower pocket tightening, acellular dermal matrix reinforcement, implant exchange and internal tissue scoring, a circumareolar mastopexy was performed bilaterally in order to tighten the breast skin and reduce the double bubble appearance. Note the stability of the circumareolar repair over time with minimal recurrence of the double bubble.

Figure 10.10a–e shows (a) (b) Preoperative photos of a patient with severe post-pregnancy involution and ptosis; (c) Overzealous application of the circumareolar mastopexy by the author early in his career which resulted in a suboptimal improvement; and (d) (e) Conversion to a vertical mastopexy which corrected the residual ptosis.

Uses for Circumareolar Mastopexy Part 4 – Tuberous Breasts

1. Perhaps the most ideal anatomical indication for the circumareolar mastopexy technique is the tuberous breast. A tuberous breast is notable for a constricted lower pole, a high inframmamary fold, a wide intermammary distance, and a low set/oversized areola with herniated breast tissue. Each of these issues is improved with the dynamics of the implant placement in combination with a circumareolar mastopexy.

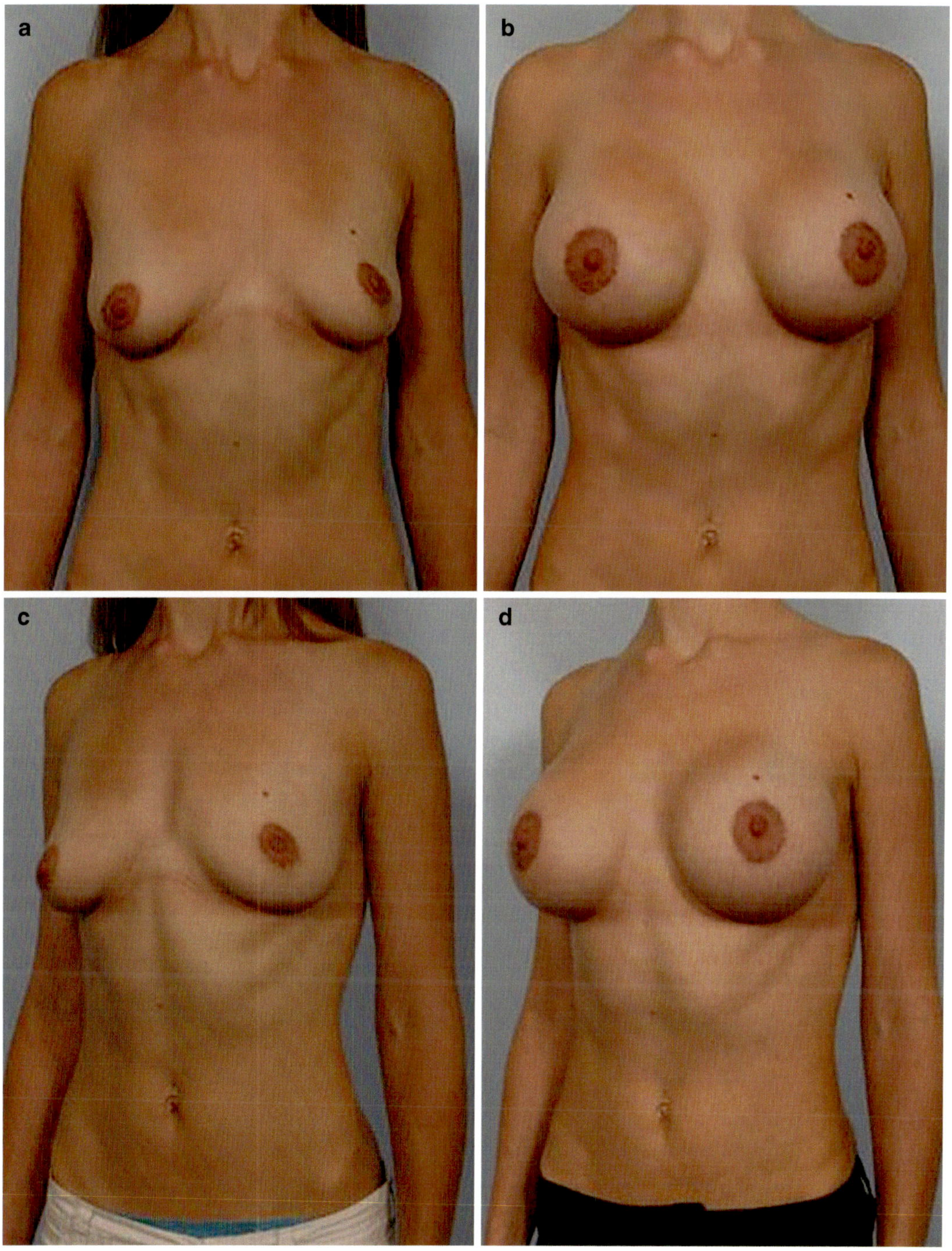

Fig. 10.7 (**a–d**) For this breast augmentation, with proper planning and differential circumareolar mastopexy pattern designs (superomedial movement of the right NAC and mildly inferomedial movement of the left NAC), ultimate symmetry with regards to areolar size and position on each breast mound is achieved

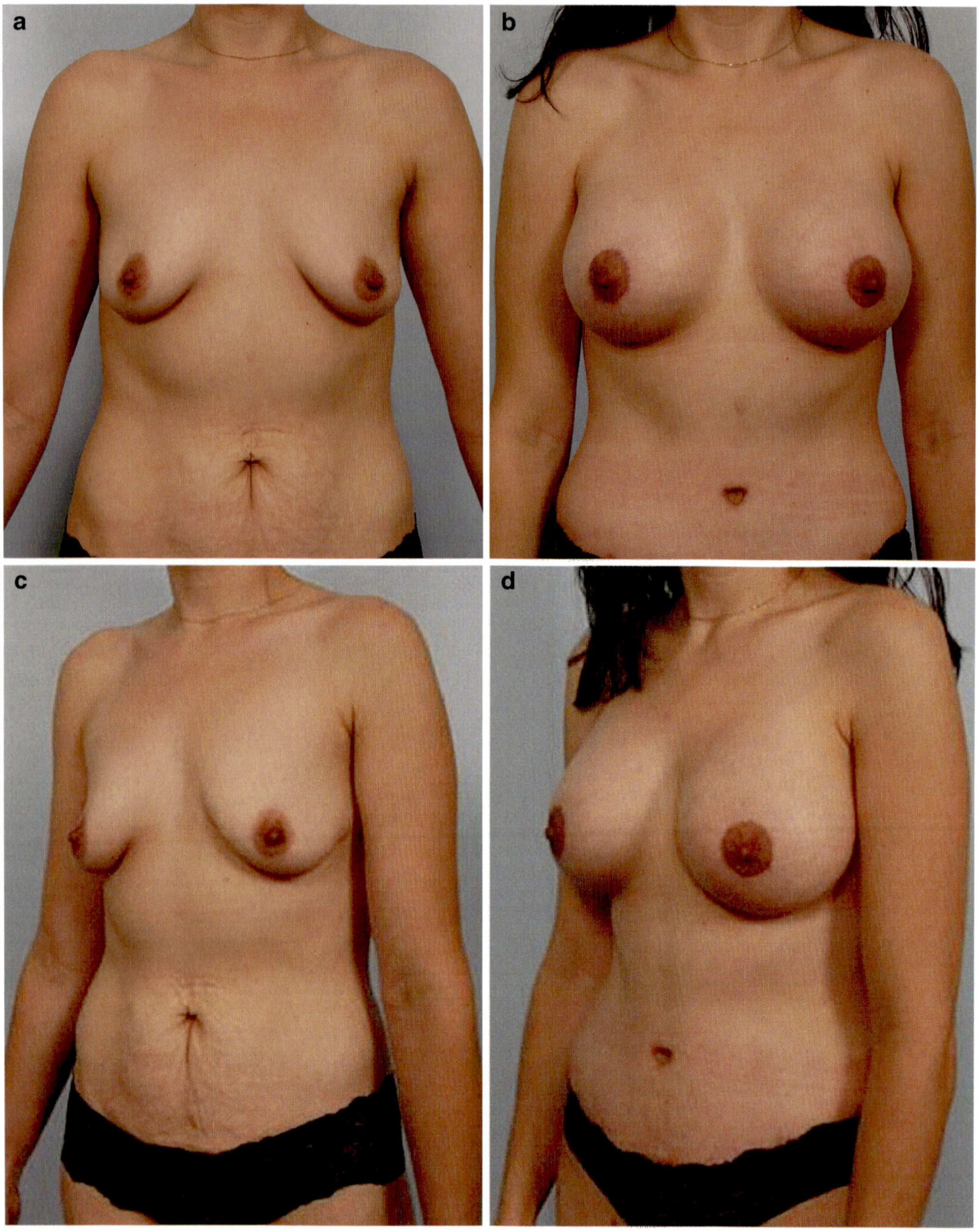

Fig. 10.8 (**a–d**) Circumareolar mastopexy in combination with augmentation is used to elevate the NAC and tighten the breast skin while avoiding a vertical breast scar. An abdominoplasty was performed simultaneously

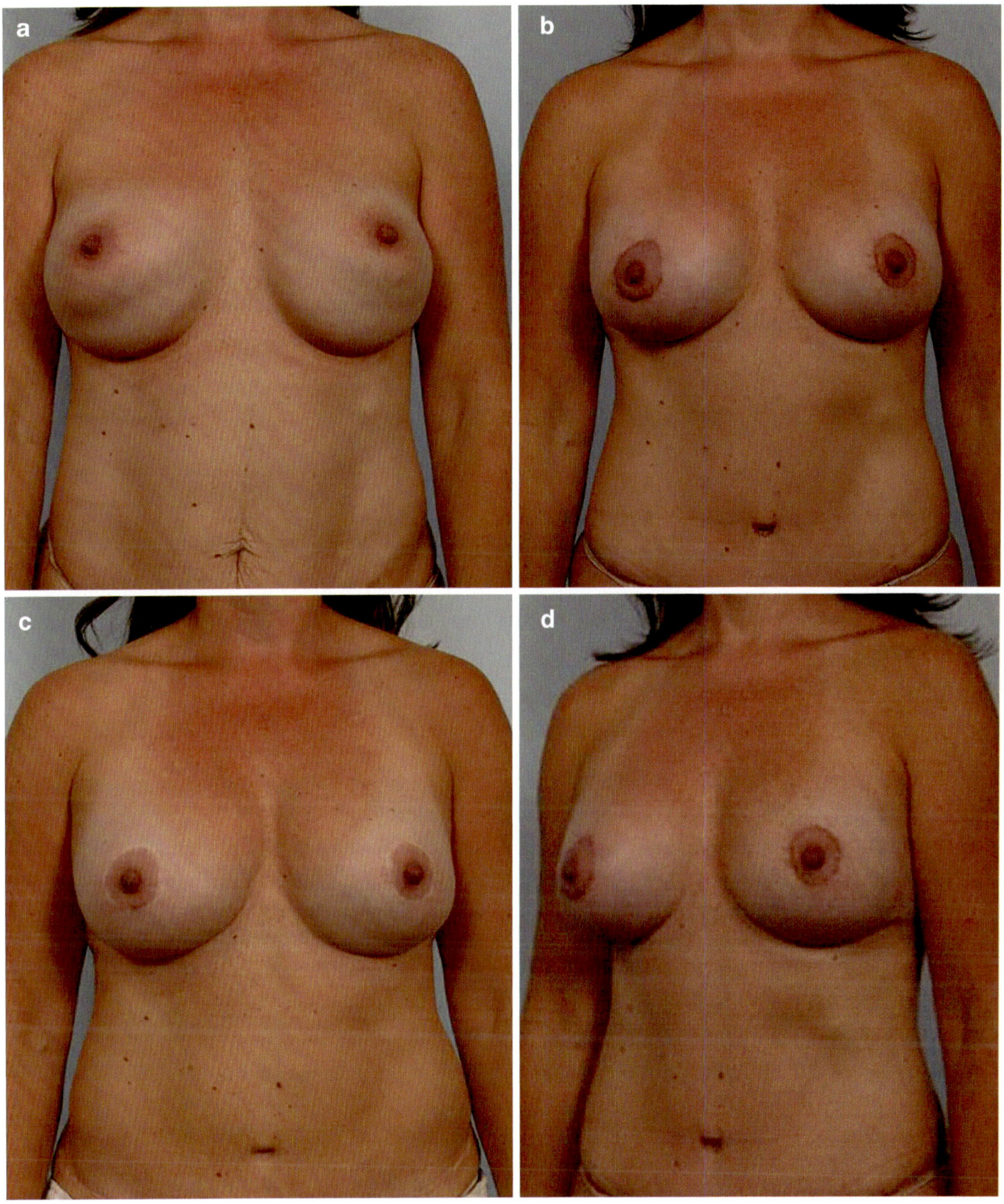

Fig. 10.9 (**a**–**e**) Complex revision surgery (**a**, **b**) preoperatively, (**c**, **d**) 6 months postoperatively and (**e**) 4 years postoperatively. The previous surgeon had underestimated the complexity of correcting tuberous breasts resulting in a double bubble and tissue clustering behind the areolas. In addition to lower pocket tightening, acellular dermal matrix reinforcement, implant exchange and internal tissue scoring, a circumareolar mastopexy was performed bilaterally in order to tighten the breast skin and reduce the double bubble appearance. Note the stability of the circumareolar repair over time with minimal recurrence of the double bubble

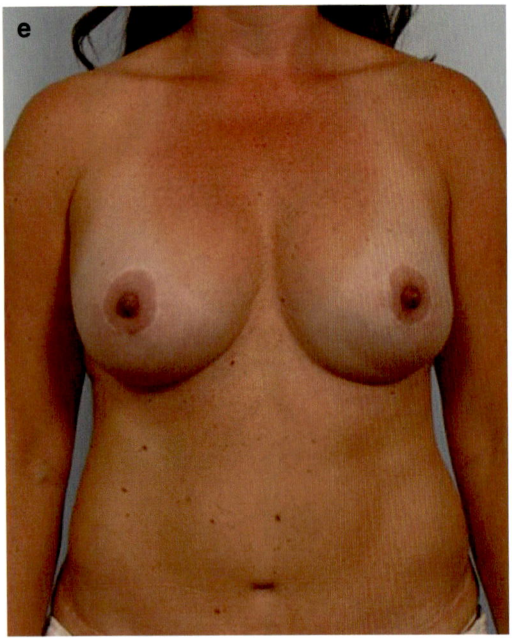

Fig. 10.9 (continued)

The high, constricted pole often creates a double bubble appearance when the inframmamary fold is lowered and the implant is placed. This is softened or eliminated as the skin is pulled tighter on the breast implant framework with a circumareolar mastopexy. The same blending effect occurs medially as the wide intermammary distance is narrowed with implants and the skin tightened. Oversized areolas are reduced in size, and the protruding tissue and conical shape of the breast is compressed into a rounder and more aesthetic shape. Finally, expansion of the tight breast is not hindered since this mastopexy avoids any skin resection or tightening in the lower pole.

Figure 10.11a–f shows preoperative and postoperative photos after augmentation mammoplasty with lower pole tissue scoring and circumareolar mastopexies to correct tuberous breasts. Note that despite the significant forces on the incision from the implant, the scar still heals without significant hypertrophy.

Figure 10.12a–f shows another example of tuberous breast correction with breast augmentation, circumareolar mastopexies and internal tissue scoring.

Markings for Circumareolar Mastopexy

As compared to a standard vertical or inverted-T scar mastopexy, the circumareolar mastopexy markings are simpler, however close attention for symmetry and a safe degree of skin resection is still important. Markings are made with a sizer or final implant in place for maximum accuracy.

Preoperatively, the breast meridian lines are marked and the inframammary folds are transposed onto the breast. After this, 5 cm intervals are drawn on the meridian lines to ensure that the distance from the sternal notch to each mark is even from side to side. Having multiple marks will help if some of the marks are washed off during surgery and will allow for even nipple placement even if the patient shifts under the drapes during the procedure.

Figure 10.13 shows a patient with mildly constricted and ptotic breasts, with the right side being larger and more severe than the left. The midline and breast meridians are marked with a 2 cm "no touch" zone on the sternum. Next, the inframammary fold marks are transposed onto the breasts. In this patient the left nipple was at the fold, whereas the right transposed fold is seen as the lowest horizontal mark. These two points are measured from the sternal notch to ensure they are equidistant, then 5 cm intervals are drawn up the meridians. In this case, the axillary fat collections are also marked for liposuction.

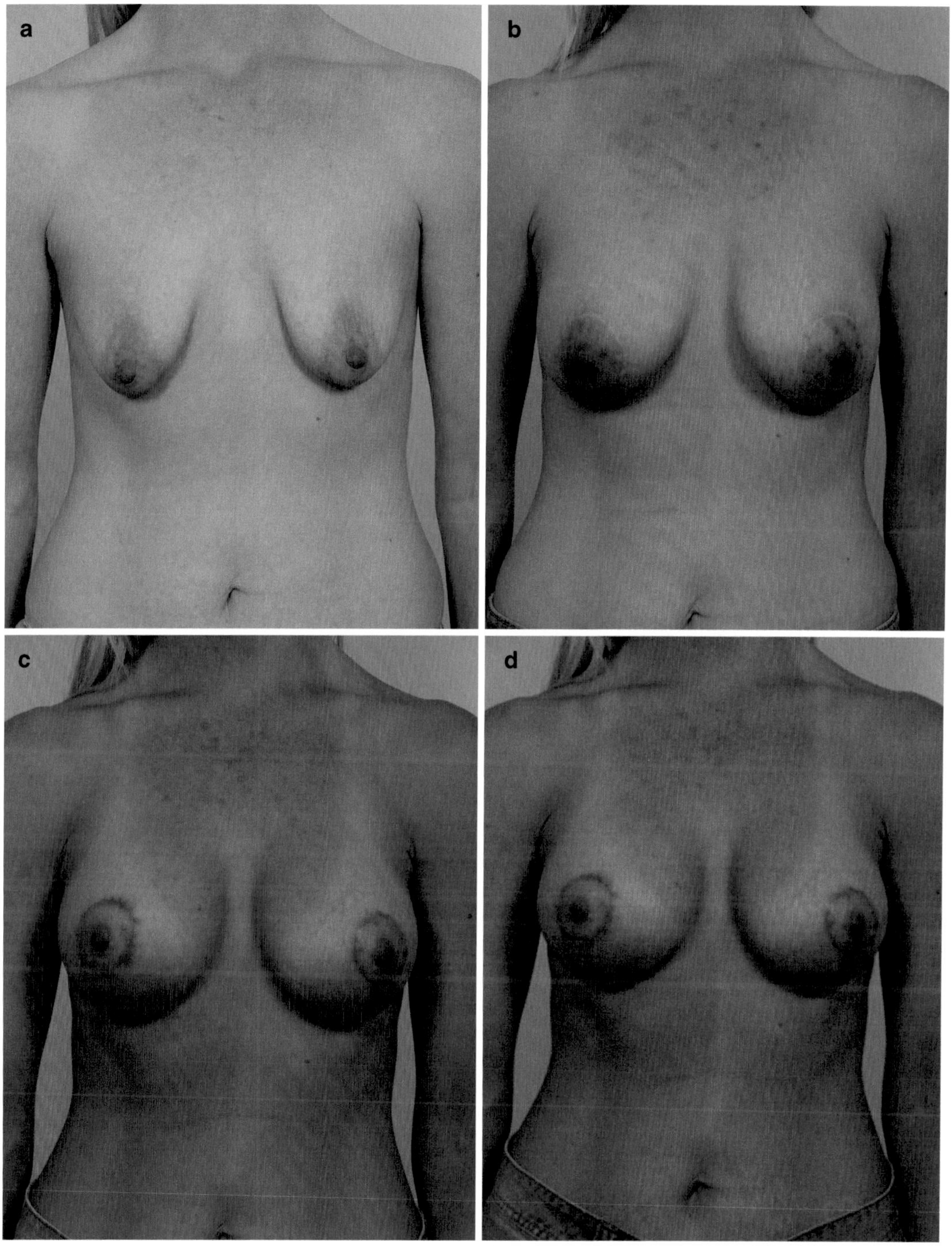

Fig. 10.10 (**a**) Preoperative photo of a patient with severe post-pregnancy involution and ptosis. (**b**) Overzealous application of the circumareolar mastopexy by the author early in his career which resulted in a suboptimal improvement. (**c**, **d**) Conversion to a vertical mastopexy which corrected the residual ptosis.

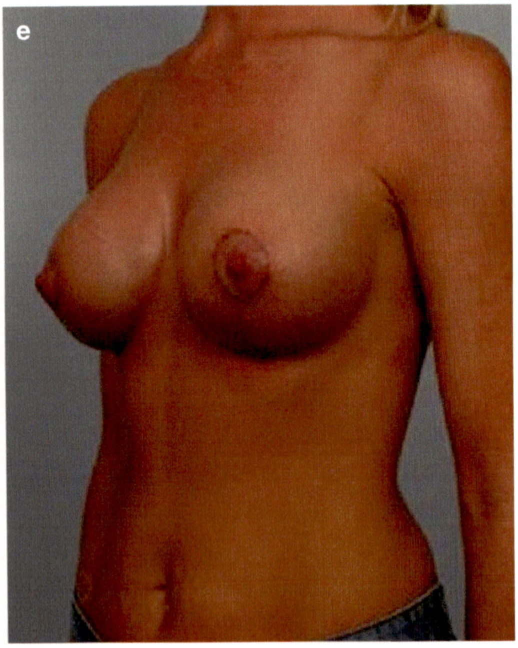

Fig. 10.10 (continued)

The key measurements for the circumareolar mastopexy are the distance from the bottom of the resection pattern to the inframammary fold (usually 6–7 cm), and from the upper border of the resection pattern to the sternal notch. Regardless of the starting points of the NAC on the breast mound, these measurements should ideally be even to ensure symmetry at the end of the procedure (Fig. 10.14).

Figure 10.14 shows how on table markings will be based on measurements as well as empirical skin pinch testing. In this example, the patient has asymmetrically located nipples. Regardless of the nipple position, the distance from one of the reference marks to the top of the resection (measurement X) should be the same. Additionally, the distance from the bottom of the resection to the inframammary fold on stretch (measurement Y) should also be the same. The length of measurement Y is generally 6–7 cm in most patients.

As stated earlier, the pattern should be drawn with the vertical height of resection approximately 1 cm longer than the width to end up with a circular areola. In more modest resections, a 0.5 cm differential is often sufficient. The areola itself is marked with a cookie cutter, usually in the 38–42 mm range. Keep in mind that herniated areolas require a smaller cookie cutter as some of the excess skin will protrude into the cookie cutter itself. Once markings are completed, the skin is pinched manually to ensure that an appropriate amount of resection was drawn. If it requires a significant amount of force to pull the skin to its final desired position, a more conservative marking can be redrawn. Alternatively, a surgical stapler can be used to temporarily tack the tissues prior to making incisions.

Circumareolar Mastopexy Technique

Many techniques for circumareolar mastopexy have been described by excellent surgeons, and a comprehensive discussion on this topic is beyond the scope of this chapter [14–16]. What will be presented is the author's technique which combines many aspects of previously mentioned surgeon's ideas into a safe, reliable procedure with minimal impact on blood supply even in breasts compromised by tissue thinning and stretch deformities.

After markings are made, they are incised with a #15 blade scalpel and the skin within the

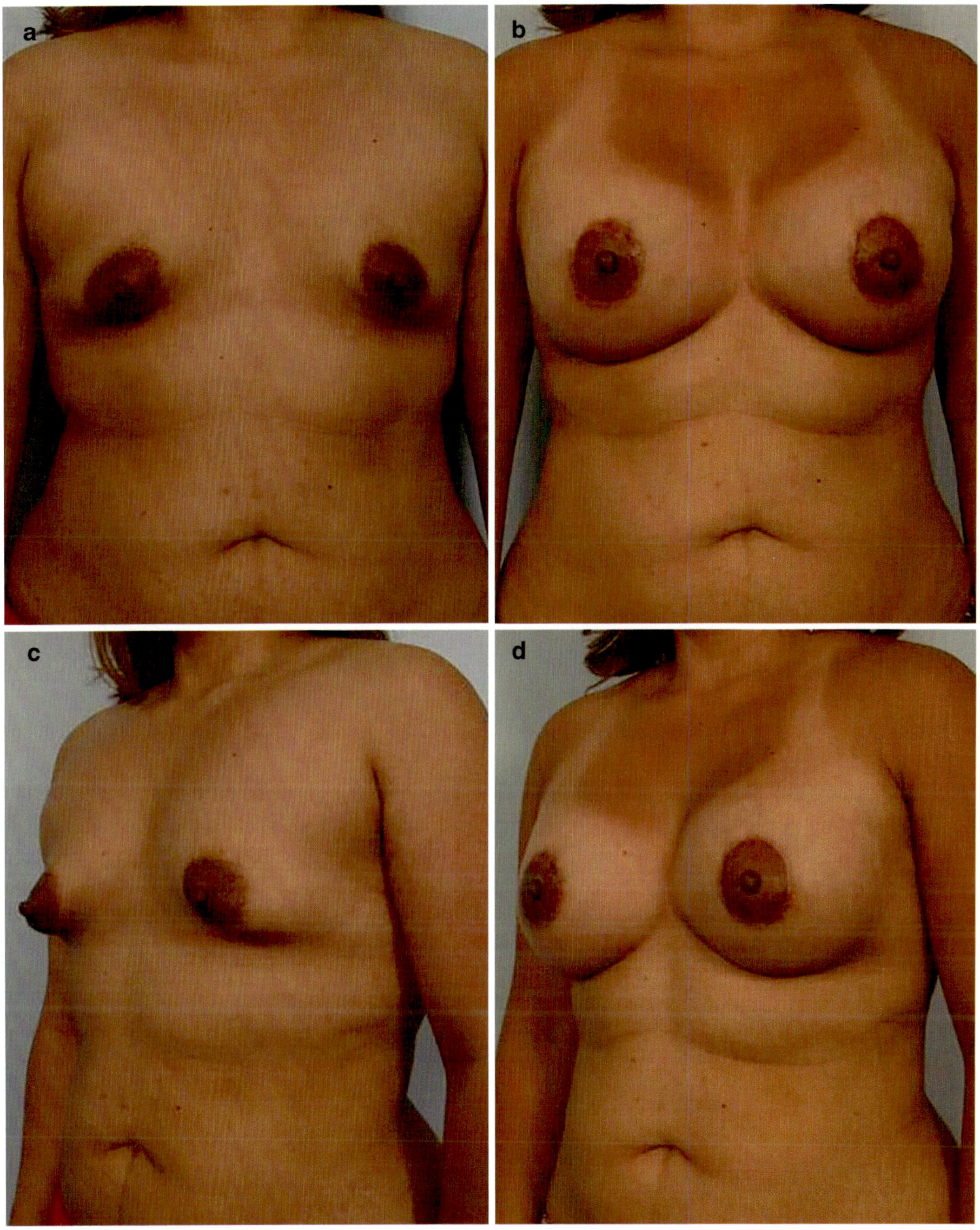

Fig. 10.11 (**a–f**) Preoperative and postoperative photos after augmentation mammoplasty with lower pole tissue scoring and circumareolar mastopexies to correct tuberous breasts. Note that despite the significant forces on the incision from the implant, the scar still heals without significant hypertrophy

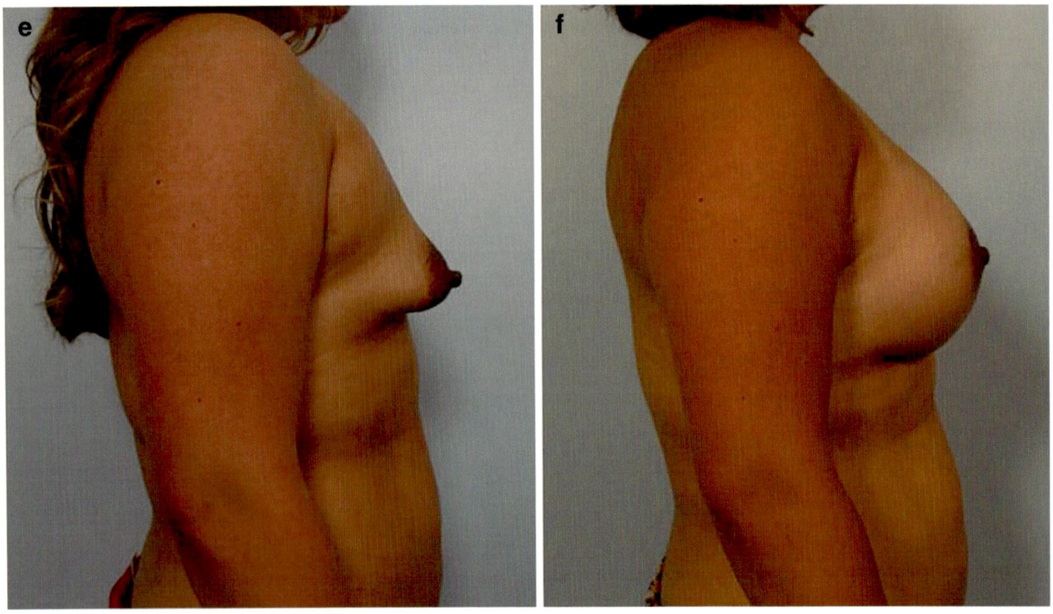

Fig. 10.11 (continued)

pattern is deepithelialized with a #10 blade scalpel. Electrocautery on a setting of 30–40 (based on a Valley Lab Force FX or equivalent device) is then used to cauterize the surface layer of the dermis, which simultaneously stops bleeding and shrinks the dermis significantly. The skin should be pinched into a lax state by the surgeon's non-dominant hand during the cauterization to allow for maximum dermal shrinkage. This maneuver alone can reduce the outer diameter by 1 or more centimeters, starting the process of skin tightening even before suture placement. Although this might seem like a dangerous maneuver with regards to the subdermal plexus, the blood supply can be confirmed by nicking the deep dermis with a scalpel. The author has performed well over 500 circumareolar mastopexy procedures in this way, including some patients with very compromised (<4-mm subcutaneous tissue) breasts, without a single partial or complete areolar loss.

Once the cautery phase is completed, a small opening in the dermis is made at the 6:00 position with the cautery, and a 3.0 PDS suture is tied with the knot buried under the dermis. The PDS is then used in running whip-stitch fashion to imbricate the dermis circumferentially to take much of the tension off the skin and set the areola up for the next layer of suturing. Minimal bunching or pleating should be seen at the end of this part of the procedure, and the diameter should be within 5 mm of the final goal size. If the edge of the repair is not perfectly circular at this point, a cookie cutter can be used to further refine the shape of the outer incision.

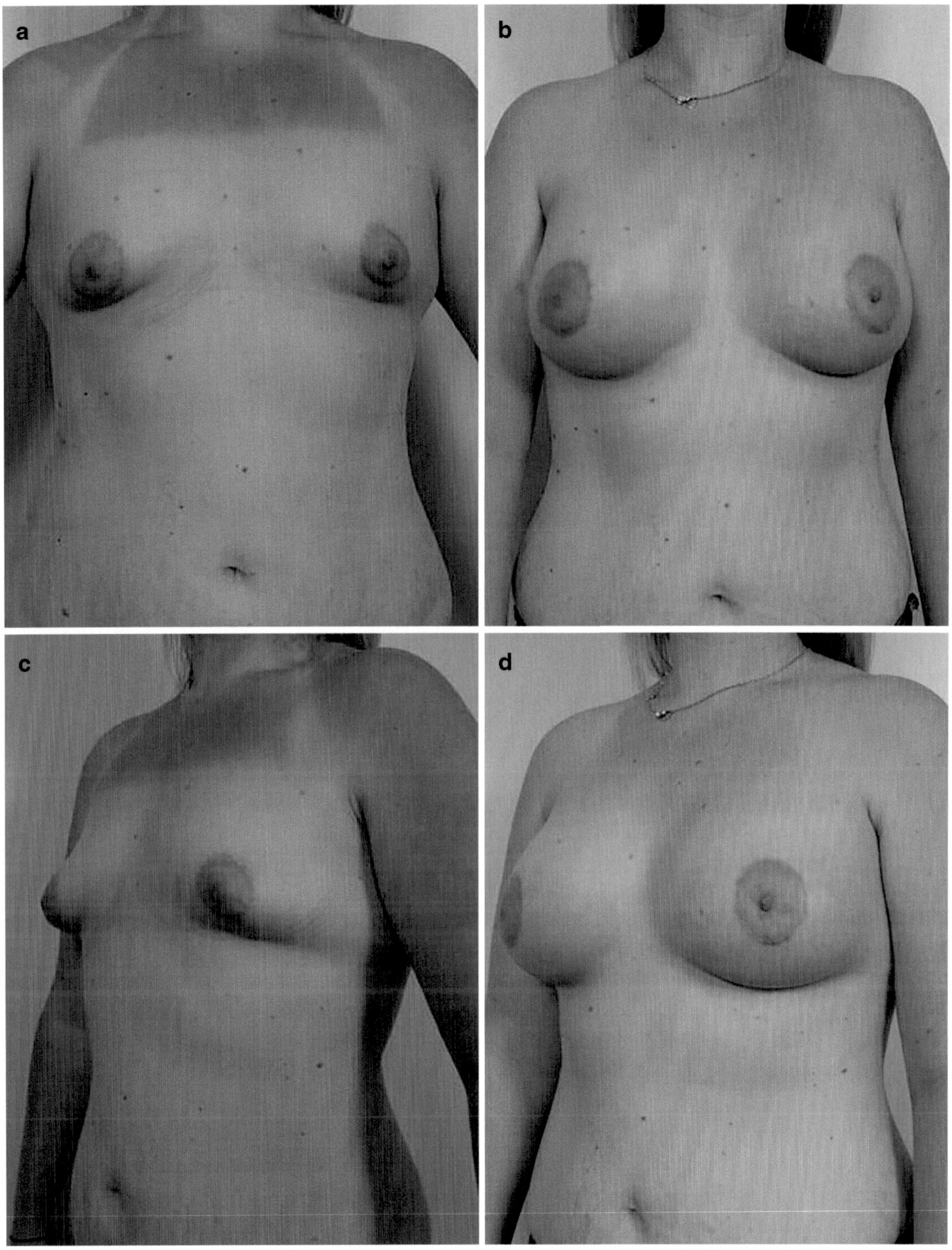

Fig. 10.12 (a–f) Another example of tuberous breast correction with breast augmentation, circumareolar mastopexies and internal tissue scoring

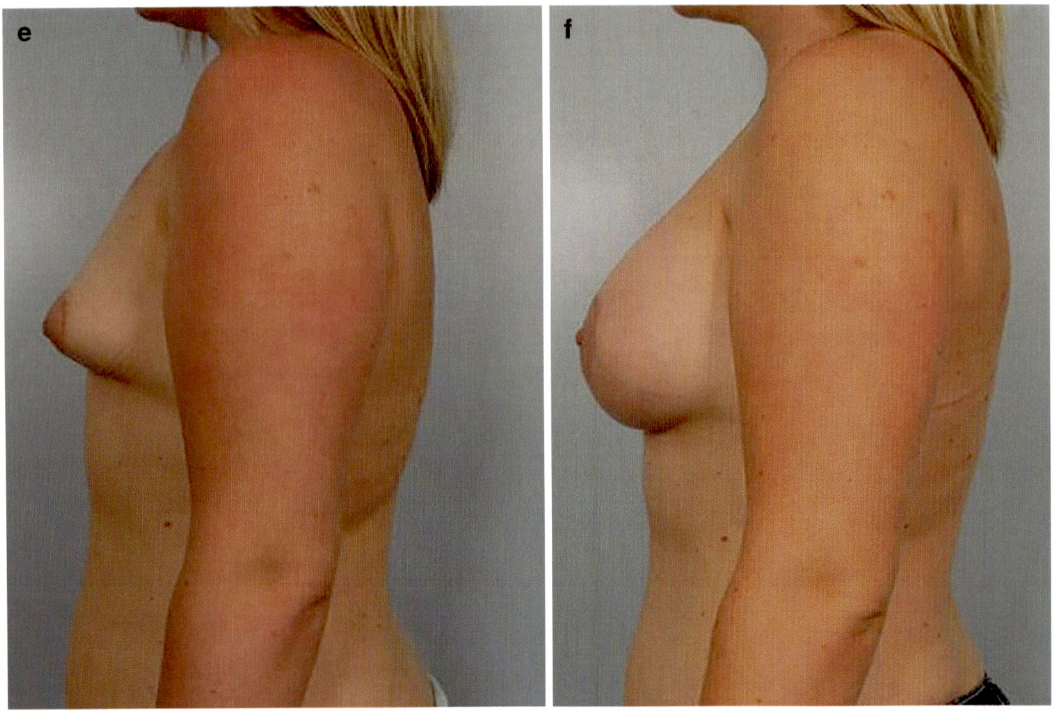

Fig. 10.12 (continued)

Next, a 3–0 prolene suture is started at the 12:00 position, and run in a "deep subcuticular" fashion circumferentially and tied again as a purse string suture. Because of the previously placed PDS, very little tightening should be needed and the areolar diameter should now be within 1–3 mm of the final size. This suture is used more to stabilize and reinforce the PDS closure, rather than to create much tightening. The prolene is tied with 7 throws, the tails are completely cut from the knot, and the knot dunked under the imbricated layers of dermis with smooth forceps. If this knot is not completely set under the dermis, there is a higher chance that it will be palpable or protrude through the skin at some point.

Finally, the skin is closed with 4–0 monocryl in true subcuticular fashion to create a smooth and watertight closure, and 0.25% marcaine with or without epinephrine can be injected for postoperative analgesia. Once the closure is completed, it should have minimal irregularities. Despite 3 layers of closure there will only be 3 staggered knots which will minimize the risk of suture spitting. The incisions are then dressed with benzoin and Steristrips.

Figure 10.15a–h shows the technique for author's circumareolar mastopexy applied to a patient that needed areolar elevation for symmetry and skin tightening to soften a mild double bubble apparent in the upright position (not seen in the supine position). Please note the vertical and horizontal measurements with each phase marked on the breast. (a) Areola is marked on stretch with a 38 mm cookie cutter and the outer vertically oriented oval skin resection is marked as well. (b) The skin is scored with a #15 blade scalpel. (c) The skin is deepithelialized with a #10 blade scalpel. (d) The dermis is cauterized while pinched manually to create a laxity that

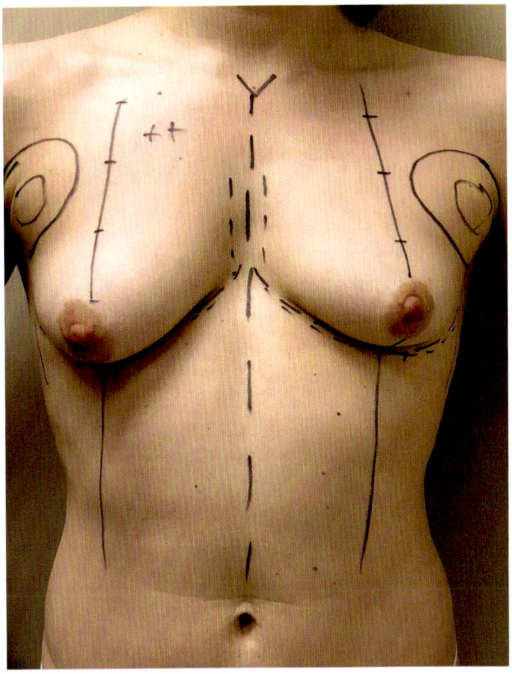

Fig. 10.13 This is a patient with mildly constricted and ptotic breasts, with the right side being larger and more severe than the left. The midline and breast meridians are marked with a 2 cm "no touch" zone on the sternum. Next, the inframammary fold marks are transposed onto the breasts. In this patient the left nipple was at the fold, whereas the right transposed fold is seen as the lowest horizontal mark. These two points are measured from the sternal notch to ensure they are equidistant, then 5 cm intervals are drawn up the meridians. In Fig. 10.14- On table markings will be based on measurements as well as empirical skin pinch testing. In this example, the patient has asymmetrically located nipples. Regardless of the nipple position, the distance from one of the reference marks to the top of the resection (measurement X) should be the same. Additionally, the distance from the bottom of the resection to the inframammary fold on stretch (measurement Y) should also be the same. The length of measurement Y is generally 6–7 cm in most patients. This case, the axillary fat collections are also marked for liposuction

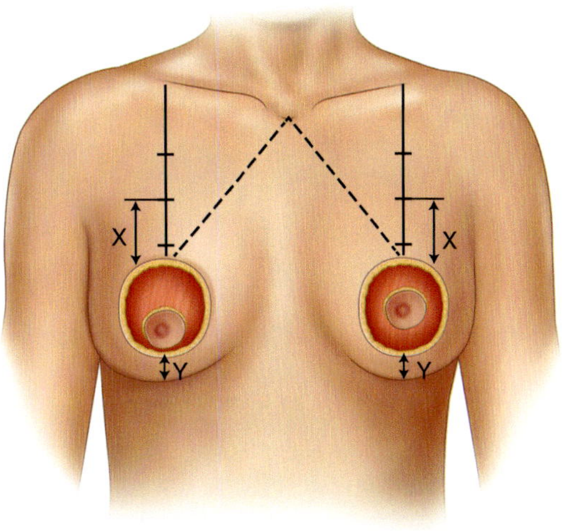

Fig. 10.14 Regardless of nipple position on the breast mound, if the skin resection patterns for the circumareolar mastopexy are designed with even distances from the upper border of the resection to the sternal notch ("X" based on 5cm crosshatch markings as described earlier in the chapter), and from the lower border of the resection pattern to the inframammary folds "Y", the ultimate areolar position should be symmetrical

will allow for maximum shrinkage. Note that this reduced the areolar diameter by 1 cm without suturing. (e) A small nick is made in the dermis with cautery and a 3.0 PDS tied as a buried knot at the 6:00 position. This suture is used to imbricate the dermis in running fashion, which has been partially completed at this point. (f) 3.0 PDS layer is completed and the diameter has now been reduced further and stabilized. (g) 3.0 Prolene is started at the 12:00 position and run as a "deep subcuticular" suture and tied, resulting in further areolar reduction. The knot is buried deeply to avoid palpability or suture spitting. (h) The skin is closed with a 4.0 monocryl in running subcuticular fashion.

Postoperative Management

Postoperative care for the circumareolar mastopexy itself is relatively simple. Pain is usually well controlled and short lived. Some patients will report a sensation of mild skin burning for a day or two after surgery. Nipple sensation is rarely affected as the level of dissection is very superficial and should have minimal impact on sensory nerves. As an aside, future breast feeding will also be unaffected by this surgery as no milk ducts are divided during surgery. Steri strips are removed approximately 1 week after surgery and scar care (topical silicone or silicone sheeting) is started 2–3 weeks postoperatively.

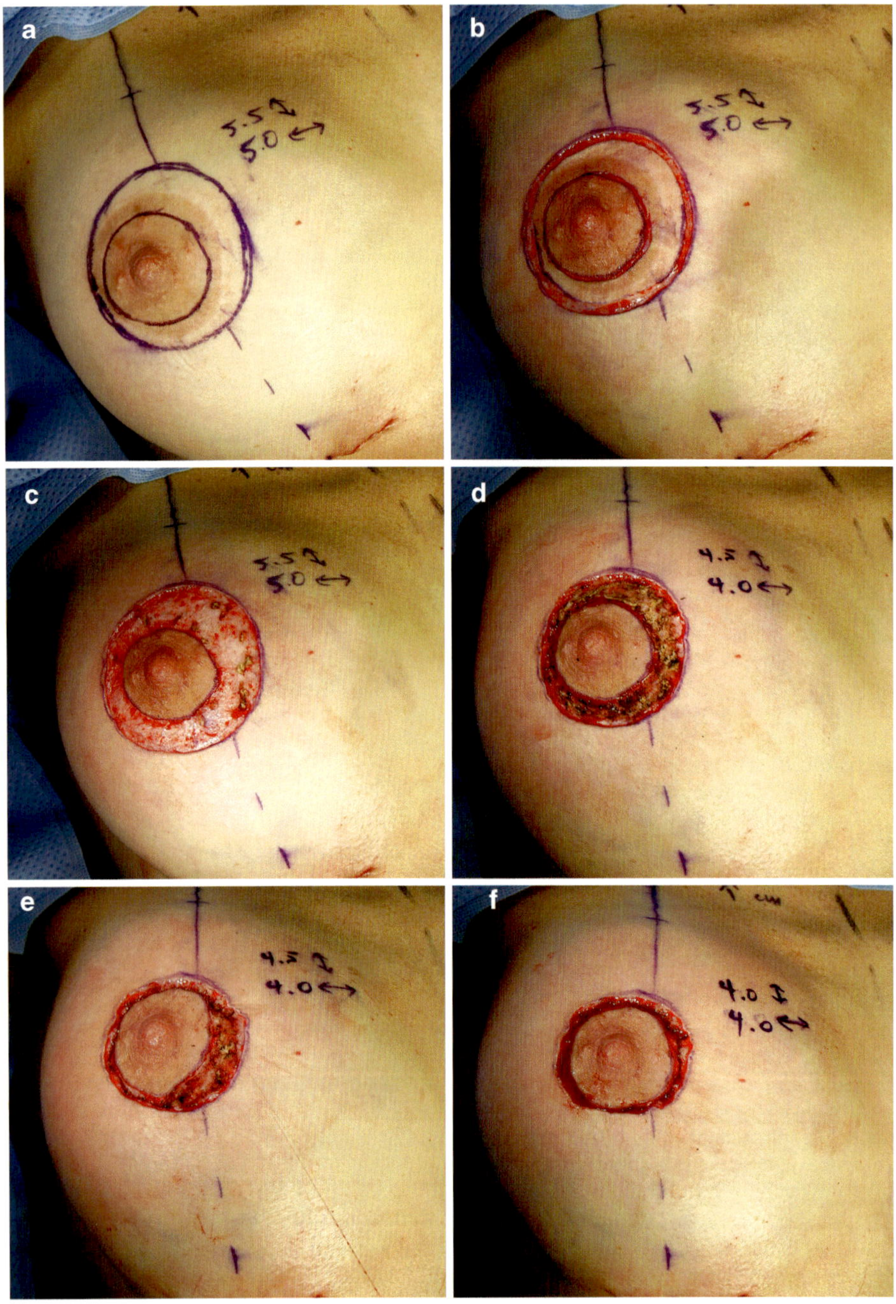

Fig. 10.15 (**a**–**h**) Technique for author's circumareolar mastopexy applied to a patient that needed areolar elevation for symmetry and skin tightening to soften a mild double bubble apparent in the upright position (not seen in the supine position). Please note the vertical and horizontal measurements with each phase marked on the breast. (**a**) Areola is marked on stretch with a 38 mm cookie cutter and the outer vertically oriented oval skin resection is marked as well. (**b**) The skin is scored with a #15 blade scalpel. (**c**) The skin is deepithelialized with a #10 blade scalpel. (**d**) The dermis is cauterized while pinched manually to create a laxity that will allow for maximum shrinkage. Note that this reduced the areolar diameter by 1 cm without suturing. (**e**) A small nick is made in the dermis with cautery and a 3.0 PDS tied as a buried knot at the 6:00 position. This suture is used to imbricate the dermis in running fashion, which has been partially completed at this point. (**f**) 3.0 PDS layer is completed and the diameter has now been reduced further and stabilized. (**g**) 3.0 Prolene is started at the 12:00 position and run as a "deep subcuticular" suture and tied, resulting in further areolar reduction. The knot is buried deeply to avoid palpability or suture spitting. (**h**) The skin is closed with a 4.0 monocryl in running subcuticular fashion

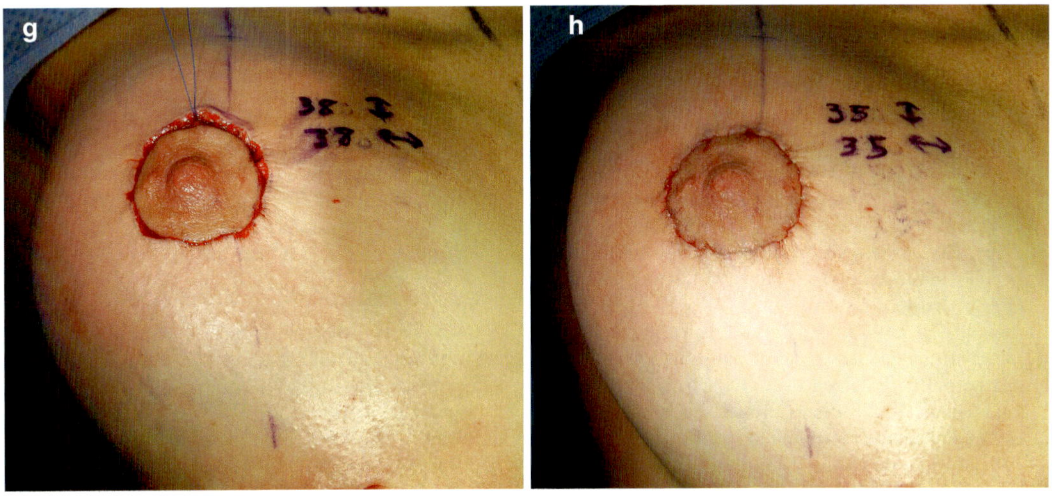

Fig. 10.15 (continued)

Complications

Very few serious complications will be seen with the technique described above, and most complications are minor and related to scarring or wound healing. Hypertrophic scarring is always possible, although rare, and patients must understand that this is a possibility. Wound dehiscence can occur, but with multilayered suturing this is an even rarer event. Minor infections can occur but are easily treated with antibiotics. More serious aesthetic complications such as severe areolar spread or a flattened appearance to the breast are generally avoided during the planning and execution of the skin resection. Performing simultaneous augmentation and mastopexy has been shown to be safe, but the surgeon should also be prepared to perform revision surgery when indicated if complications arise [17, 18].

Conclusion

As demonstrated by this chapter, the circumareolar mastopexy can be a versatile technique with scars that are generally well tolerated by patients. Proper understanding and application of the technique is the key to achieving predictable and safe results. For surgeons unfamiliar with this technique, starting with smaller, less aggressive resections for milder cases would be a reasonable approach, with gradual expansion into more significant applications as one becomes more comfortable with the procedure's dynamics.

Acknowledgements I would like to thank Margaret Zheng for her help with the formatting and technical layout of this chapter.

References

1. Davison SP, Spear SL. Simultaneous breast augmentation with periareolar mastopexy. Semin Plast Surg. 2004;18:189–202.
2. Spear SL, Venturi ML. Augmentation with periareolar mastopexy. In: Spear SL, editor. Surgery of the breast: principles and art, vol. 2. 2nd ed. Philadelphia: Lippincott Williams & Wilkins; 2006. p. 1393–402.
3. Baran CN, Peker F, Ortak T, et al. Unsatisfactory results of periareolar mastopexy with or without augmentation and reduction mammoplasty: enlarged areola with flattened nipple. Aesthet Plast Surg. 2001;25:286–9.
4. Hoffman S. Some thoughts on augmentation/mastopexy and medical malpractice. Plast Reconstr Surg. 2004;113:1892–3.
5. Reisman NR. Chapter 6: Medico-legal issues in plastic surgery. In: Neligan PC, editor. Plastic Surgery, vol. 1. 3rd ed. Seattle, Washington: Elsevier; 2013. p. 92–103.

6. Spear SL. Augmentation/mastopexy: surgeon, beware. Plast Reconstr Surg. 2003;112:905–6.
7. Gruber RP, Jones HW Jr. The "donut" mastopexy: indications and complications. Plast Reconstr Surg. 1980;65(1):34–8.
8. Grolleau JL, Lanfrey E, Lavigne B, Chavoin JP, Costagliola M. Breast base anomalies: treatment strategy for tuberous breasts, minor deformities, and asymmetry. Plast Reconstr Surg. 1999;104:2040–8.
9. Spear SL, Davison SP. Breast augmentation with periareolar mastopexy. Oper Tech Plast Reconstr Surg. 2000;7:131–6.
10. Benelli L. A new periareolar mammaplasty: the "round block" technique. Aesthet Plast Surg. 1990;14:93–100.
11. Gasperoni C, Salgarello M, Gargani G. Experience and technical refinements in the "donut" mastopexy with augmentation mammaplasty. Aesthet Plast Surg. 1988;12:111–4.
12. de la Fuente A, Martin del Yerro JL. Periareolar mastopexy with mammary implants. Aesthetic Plast Surg. 1992;16:337–41.
13. Elliott LF. Circumareolar mastopexy with augmentation. Clin Plast Surg. 2002;29:337–47.
14. Spear S, Giese SY, Ducic I. Concentric mastopexy revisited. Plast Reconst Surg. 2001;107:1294–9.
15. Hammond DC, Khuthaila DK, Kim J. The interlocking Gore-Tex suture for control of areolar diameter and shape. Plast Reconstr Surg. 2007;119:804–9.
16. Benelli LC. Periareolar benelli mastopexy and reduction. In: Spear SL, editor. Surgery of the Breast: Principles and Art. Philadelphia: Lippincott-Raven; 1998. p. 685.
17. Spear SL, Low M, Ducic I. Revision augmentation mastopexy: indications, operations, and outcomes. Ann Plast Surg. 2003;51:540–6.
18. Calobrace MB, Herdt DR, Cothron KJ. Simultaneous augmentation/mastopexy: a retrospective 5-year review of 332 consecutive cases. Plast Reconstr Surg. 2013;131:145–56.

Tuberous Breast Correction

11

M. Bradley Calobrace, Louis P. Bucky, Chet Mays, and James M. Smartt Jr.

Introduction

Originally described by Rees and Aston in 1976, tuberous breast is a rare deformity affecting young women unilaterally and bilaterally [1]. Possessing a variety of characteristic abnormalities of the breast base with a wide array of clinical manifestations has been referred to by many names, including tuberous breast, constricted breast, lower pole hypoplasia, snoopy breasts, and herniated or domed nipples [2–4]. These terms all describe varying degrees of the same clinical deformity with a wide variety of surgical techniques for their correction.

M. B. Calobrace (✉)
Private Practice, CaloAesthetics Plastic Surgery Center, Louisville, KY, USA

Clinical Faculty, University of Louisville, Division of Plastic Surgery, Louisville, KY, USA

Clinical Faculty, University of Kentucky, Division of Plastic Surgery, Lexington, KY, USA
e-mail: drbrad@calobrace.com

L. P. Bucky
Private Practice, Bucky Plastic Surgery, Clinical Faculty, University of Pennsylvania School of Medicine, Division of Plastic Surgery, Philadelphia, PA, USA

C. Mays
Private Practice, CaloAesthetics Plastic Surgery Center, Louisville, KY, USA

Clinical Faculty, University of Louisville, Division of Plastic Surgery, Louisville, KY, USA

J. M. Smartt Jr.
Bucky Plastic Surgery, Philadelphia, PA, USA

The etiology of this syndrome has been the subject of much controversy, but the most plausible identifies some abnormality in the superficial fascia layer creating strong adherence of the skin to the underlying muscle or the presence of an abnormal constricting fibrous rings due to thickening of this fascia. This abnormality restricts the normal development and natural expansion of the developing breast, thus creating protrusion of the developing breast through the unrestricted nipple areolar complex where superficial fascia is not present [3, 5, 6]. Commonly referred to as tuberous breast deformity today, the clinical presentation consists of one or more findings including; hypoplasia, constricted lower breast parenchyma and skin envelope, superiorly malpositioned inframammary fold, pseudoherniation and/or hypertrophy of the nipple areolar complex and often quite significant asymmetries.

Correction of the deformity requires first recognizing the congenital deformity and understanding the particular anatomic anomalies that are part of each case, which may vary significantly and consist of only part of the characteristics or may constitute all aspects of the deformity. Once identified, a surgical plan must consist of employing specific surgical techniques to address each of the abnormalities. Failure to recognize and develop an appropriate plan will undoubtedly lead to less than satisfactory results and predispose the patient to sequalae such as double-bubble, superiorly or inferiorly malpositioned implants, misshaped breasts, inadequately corrected lower pole constriction or nipple areolar

M. B. Calobrace et al. (eds.), *Augmentation Mastopexy*,
https://doi.org/10.1007/978-3-030-48226-8_11

herniations, and/or implant visibility. In this chapter, we will focus on the identification and classification of the particular tuberous deformities with a focus on the surgical corrective techniques employed utilizing implants, mastopexies and/or fat grafting to achieve optimal outcomes in what many consider the most challenging breast cases faced by the plastic surgeon.

Anatomy and Classification

The etiology of tuberous breast deformity is not completely understood. Although considerations to a phylogenic relapse or failure of tissue differentiation in a limited zone of the fetal thorax have been proposed, it seems that quite possibly it may be simply abnormalities in the superficial fascial system in the lower pole of the breast and/or weakness in the periareolar supporting tissue [2]. Grolleau suggested a stronger than normal attachment of the dermis and muscle in the lower pole that the developing breast is unable to expand [5]. More recent theories have proposed fibrous rings of superficial fascia inhibiting expansion and possibly weakened tissue in the periareolar region allowing herniation of the expanding breast into the areola [3, 6].

Considering these theories, the anatomic characteristics of the tuberous breast include an investing layer of superficial fascia that envelopes the breast beneath it and the deep fascia which lies on the muscle deep to the breast. The superficial fascia consisting of thickened rings that in some way develop and constrict the normal expansion of the lower pole. Additionally, this thickened fascia is absent at the area of the areola, allowing the breast to expand vertically into the space creating a tuberous appearance with areolar enlargement and pseudoherniation. This abnormal development creates a myriad of clinical findings that are highly suggestive of tuberous breast development, including hypoplasia, constricted lower breast parenchyma and skin envelope, superiorly malpositioned inframammary fold, pseudoherniation and/or hypertrophy of the nipple areolar complex and often quite significant asymmetries. Table 11.1: Fig. 11.1a, b, illustrates many of the clinical findings typical in a tuberous breast deformity.

A classification system was described my Von Heimberg based on the deficiencies in the lower quadrants of the breast and subareolar regions [2] (Table 11.2; Fig. 11.2).

Table 11.1 Findings seen in tuberous breast deformity

Breast hypoplasia
Constricted lower breast parenchyma and skin envelope
Superiorly malpositioned inframammary fold
Pseudoherniation and/or hypertrophy of NAC

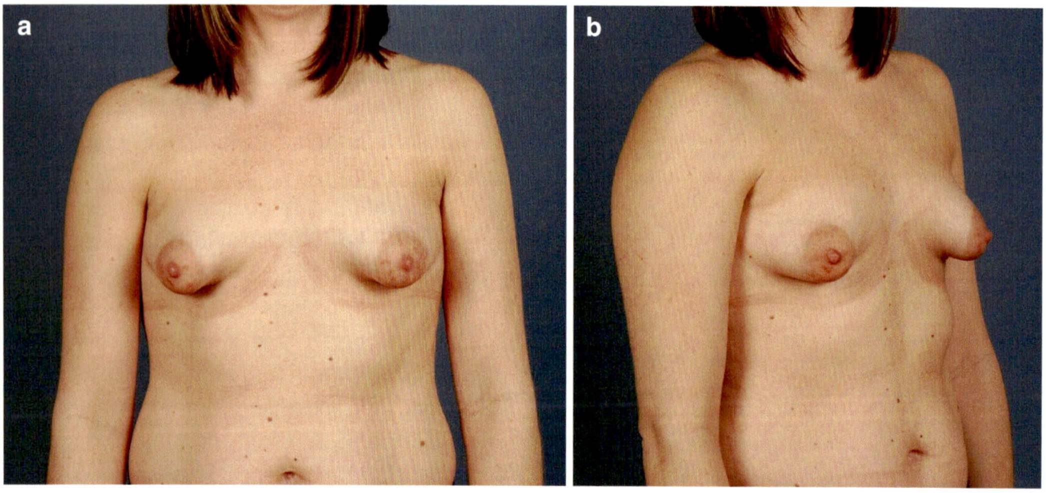

Fig. 11.1 (**a**, **b**) A patient with the four tuberous breast findings; hypoplastic breast, constricted lower breast parenchyma and skin envelope, superiorly malpositioned inframammary fold, and pseudoherniation of the NAC

Table 11.2 Von Heimburg classification of tuberous breast

Type I	Hypoplasia of lower medial quadrant
Type II	Hypoplasia of the lower medial and lateral quadrants, sufficient skin in the subareolar region
Type III	Hypoplasia of the lower medial and lateral quadrants, deficiency of skin in the subareolar region
Type IV	Severe breast constriction, minimal breast base

More recently, a classification system based on the degree of areolar herniation has been described, defined as the ratio between the amount of forward projection of the areola divided by the areolar diameter, known as the Northwood Index. [7] Whereas a normal breast has an average 0.19, an index 0.40 or greater is considered to be a tuberous breast (Table 11.3).

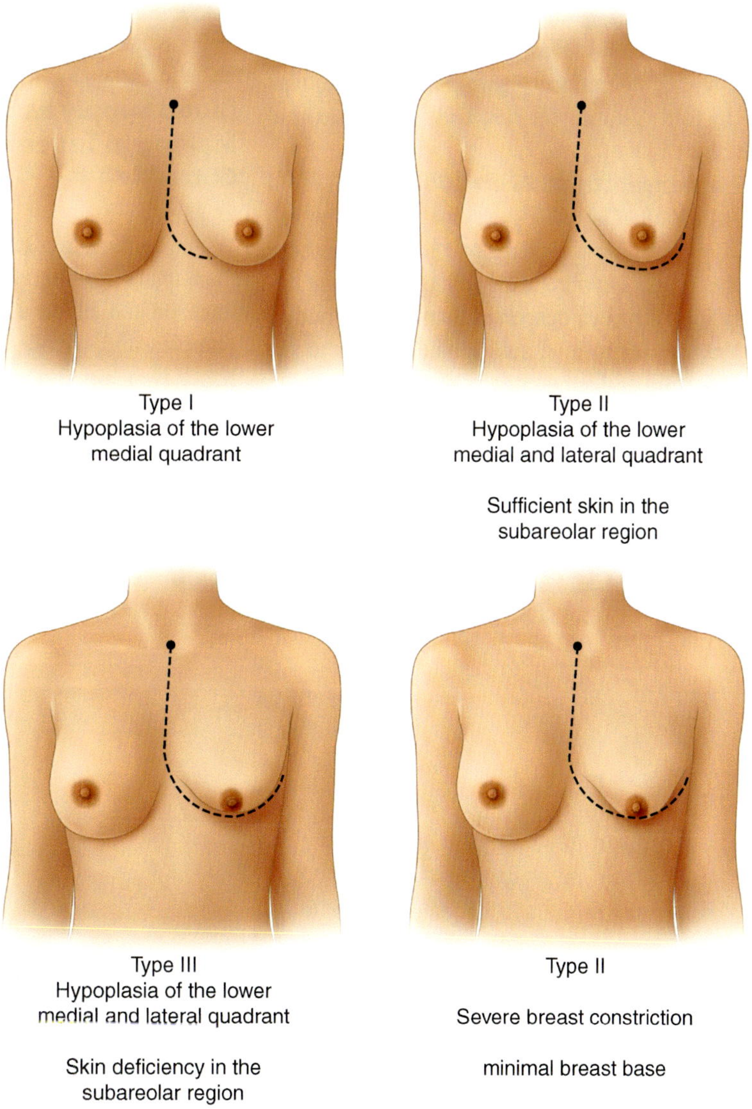

Fig. 11.2 Von Heimburg classification of tuberous breast

Pre-operative Evaluation

The most important aspect is to identify the tuberous breast deformity, understands its congenital nature and the challenges facing optimal correction. Whereas classification systems can be helpful in understanding and describing the severity of the deformity, clinically a thorough physical exam and documentation of findings will provide the best understanding of the deformity. Surgical correction will then be planned to address the attributes present in the breast.

The evaluation should begin with a breast exam with breast measurements including the base width, sternal notch to nipple distance, nipple to fold distance (at rest and under maximal stretch).

The degree of tightness in the lower pole should be assessed. The IMF expansion test, which involves grasping the breast and rotating the base of the breast outward expanding the inframammary fold, has been described by the senior author as a maneuver to give some indication as to the true location and adherence of the IMF and lower pole expansion potential [8] (Fig. 11.3a, b).

Table 11.3 Degree of areolar herniation determined by the Northwood Index

Northwood Index =	Projection of areola / areola diameter

This will assist in determining the ease or difficulty in lowering the lower pole and expanding the base of the breast (See Table 11.4).

Assessment should also include evaluation of the skin thickness and elasticity, the quantity and distribution of subcutaneous fat, the composition and firmness of the breast parenchyma, the integrity of the Cooper's ligaments, the nature and position of the underlying musculature and the shape and slope of the underlying chest wall. All of these aspects of the breast composition influence the shape of the breast and ultimately the outcome after tuberous breast correction.

Blood Supply as It Impacts Decision Making in Tuberous Deformity Correction

When correcting a tuberous breast, many of the maneuvers required and the impact this might have on the blood supply to the nipple areolar complex and surrounding breast skin. The breast has a rich blood supply from multiple sources, including the internal mammary artery perforators, the lateral thoracic arteries, the thoracoacromial and the anteriolateral and anteriomedial intercostal perforators. All aspects of the planned surgical maneuvers, including breast augmentation (Implant selection, pocket selection), paren-

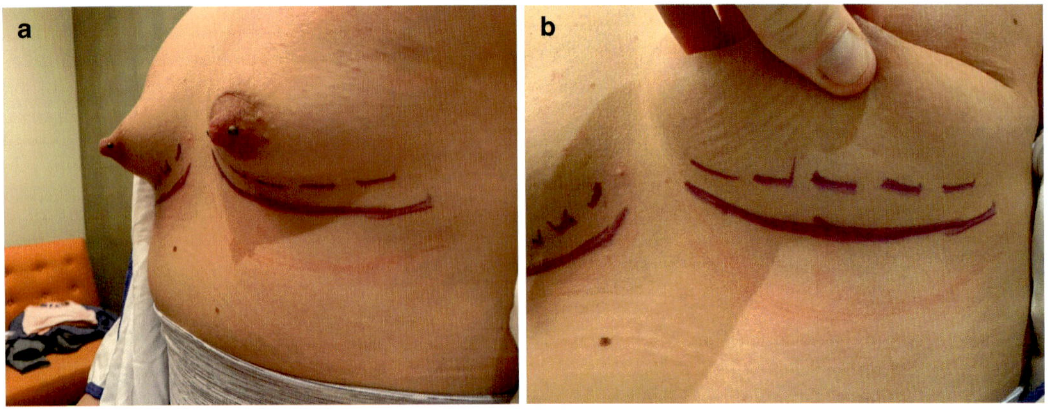

Fig. 11.3 (**a**) Dotted line represents the current constricted lower breast parenchyma and superiorly malpositioned IMF. The solid line represents the new planned IMF (**b**) The IMF expansion test reveals the ability of the lower pole to expand from the current IMF (dotted line) to the new IMF (solid line)

chymal scoring or rearrangement, fat grafting and especially a mastopexy (and the extent of skin undermining) all impact the blood supply to the NAC and breast skin flaps [9] (Fig. 11.4).

To insure the most reliable blood supply to the NAC and skin flaps, consideration must always be given to the effect on the blood supply. The subpectoral pocket maintains the musculocutaneous perforators (unless an extensive dual plane is performed) and is less likely to interfere with the blood supply compared to a subglandular/subfascial pocket. Likewise, larger implants placed in any pocket, but especially the subglandular/subfascial pocket that results in undue tension on the mastopexy closure can also create vascular compromise to the NAC or overlying skin flaps, resulting in skin or NAC necrosis. This is especially relevant in the tuberous breast, as the skin tightness of the lower pole significantly constricts the implant, creating significant forces on the overlying breast. A mastopexy can reduce vascularity, especially if significant skin undermining is performed. Parenchymal and subareolar scoring and thinning can impair circulation. Therefore, when planning the surgical procedure, great care must be taken to respect the vascularity and ensure that decision making always includes the safety of the maneuvers being performed simultaneously. Table 11.5:

It may be necessary to stage the procedures in some way if vascular compromise is of significant concern when performed simultaneously.

Table 11.4 Analysis of the tuberous breast

Degree of hypoplasia of the breast
Assess asymmetries (volume, fold, areolar size, pseudoherniation, etc.)
Width of areola (areolar enlargement) and degree of pseudoherniation
SN-N distance at rest and under maximal stretch
IMF expansion test – tightness of lower pole and IMF

Patient Expectations

In planning the operative approach in tuberous breast deformity, it cannot be overstated how important patient education is in managing expectation in these challenging cases. These patients most often come to a consultation requesting a breast augmentation, but when asked are aware that their breasts are misshapen or have never

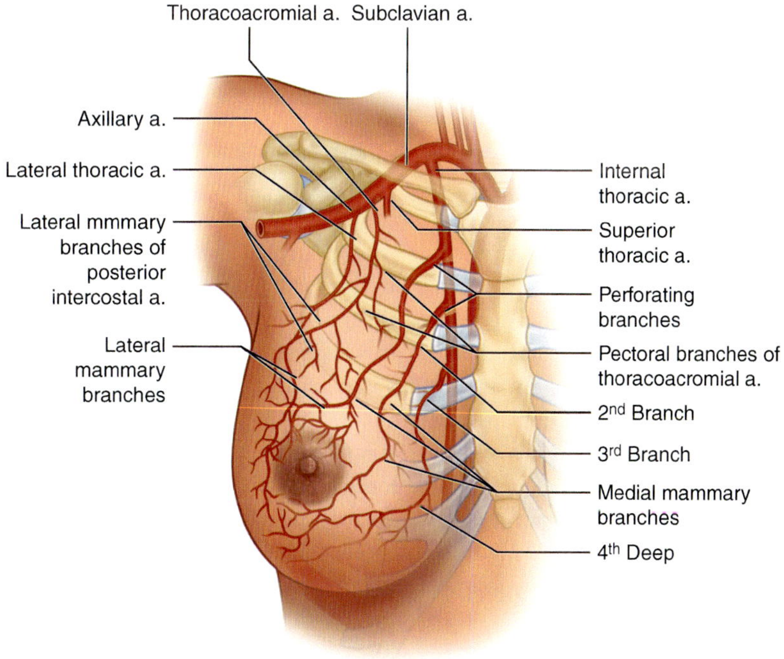

Fig. 11.4 Blood supply of the breast illustrating the 2nd, 3rd, and 4th branch of the internal mammary artery that supplies the varies pedicles to the NAC

Table 11.5 Maneuvers performed during tuberous breast correction impacting blood supply

Pocket decision: Subglandular or subfascial
Implant choice
Mastopexy with skin flap undermining
Parenchymal scoring

looked "normal". These patients, however, are often unaware of just how much of a challenge full correction of their tuberous deformity may be. Patients often are unaware of the challenges faced with correction of significantly hypoplastic breast with significant asymmetries, extremely tight lower pole skin envelope, a very narrow breast base width, wide intermammary distance, short nipple to fold distance, and protruding enlarged areolas. The results of tuberous breast surgery are not the same as a standard breast augmentation in most patients. Patients should be educated on their specific clinical findings, with a frank discussion not only about the anticipated results, but also the limitations of the procedure. These patients will more likely postoperatively to have more scarring, implant visibility or palpability, stria development, persistence of the original inframammary fold, persistence of areolar protrusions and potential for some residual asymmetries. The unique challenges need to be understood by the patient, with an understanding that a revision may be necessary to achieve the final outcome.

Treatment Goals

The clinical presentation varies widely from only some minor elements that resemble tuberous breast findings to the most severe, asymmetric breast with extremely constricted, narrow breast base, elongated, projecting breast with associated areolar pseudoherniation. In determining the planned surgical approach to the deformity, it is helpful to first start by identifying the components of this syndrome that are present in the patient. The surgical approach should be comprehensive and address as many of the following components as needed to optimize results. In general, correction should address three major components: correction of the constricted skin and breast tissue in the breast base, correction of the areolar hypertrophy and pseudoherniation and correction of asymmetries. There are many maneuvers to correct these elements, employing the ones which are appropriate for the particular deformity. Table 11.6 lists some of the techniques utilized, which we discussed in more detail in this chapter.

Table 11.6 Treatment goals in tuberous breast deformity

Correction of the constricted breast Lower pole through vertical and horizontal scoring
Expansion of lower pole with implant, tissue expander or fat
Mastopexy to improve nipple position on implant or correct ptosis
Lowering of IMF and obliteration of old IMF
Correction of asymmetries
Correction of hypoplasia
Correction of areolar hypertrophy and pseudo-herniation

Surgical Approach

There have been a multitude of techniques developed in an attempt to correct the significant deformities seen in tuberous breast deformity. These have included many variations of internal glandular reshaping techniques to address the lower pole deficiencies. These have involved transposing subareolar parenchymal tissue either based anteriorly off the areola or posteriorly off the chest wall transposed down into the lower pole to address the constricted breast [10–12]. Although the senior author has used these techniques in a few select cases, the vast majority of cases can be successfully treated with an implant-based approach or more recently a fat grafting approach, with or without an implant. The focus of this book is on the application of augmentation (implants or fat) used in conjunction with mastopexies and other ancillary techniques to achieve successful outcomes in a one-stage procedure.

Implant-Based Correction of the Tuberous Breast

Correction of the Constricted Breast Base A successful outcome in the correction of tuberous breast deformity is most affected by the ability to adequately expanded the constricted breast base. This can be extremely challenging in the most severe cases, and if inadequate, results in an abnormal shaped breast with inframammary fold abnormalities or malpositioned breast implant. The effective expansion of the lower pole is accomplished often with a combination of techniques. One maneuver often used is a release of the constriction bands of the breast base through scoring of the lower pole tissue. When lifted off the muscle, the posterior surface of the breast tissue between the NAC and IMF is visualized. This can be accessed through a periareolar or a newly planned Inframammary incision. It is important to remember if making and inframammary incision, the location of the new IMF must be determined based on implant size and the incision and placed in that location. The incision should not be made in the original IMF as it generally positioned too high and will ultimately be obliterated in the correction. The posterior breast tissue is then scored vertically and horizontal in the lower pole, creating a checkerboard-like appearance to the tissue (Figs. 11.5 and 11.6).

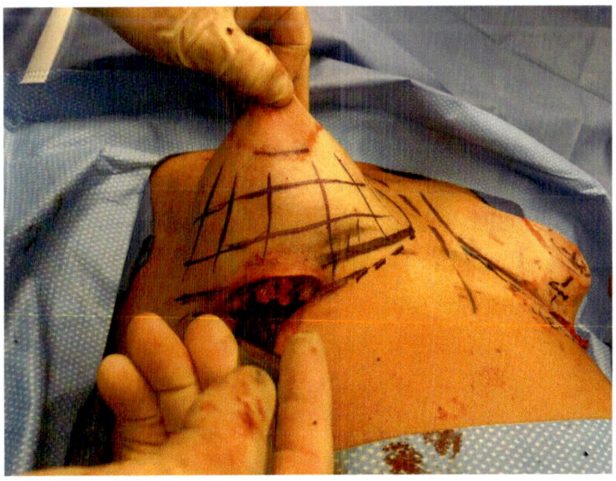

Fig. 11.5 vertical and horizontal markings on the lower pole of the breast represent anticipated areas of tissue scoring to allow expansion of the lower pole of the breast

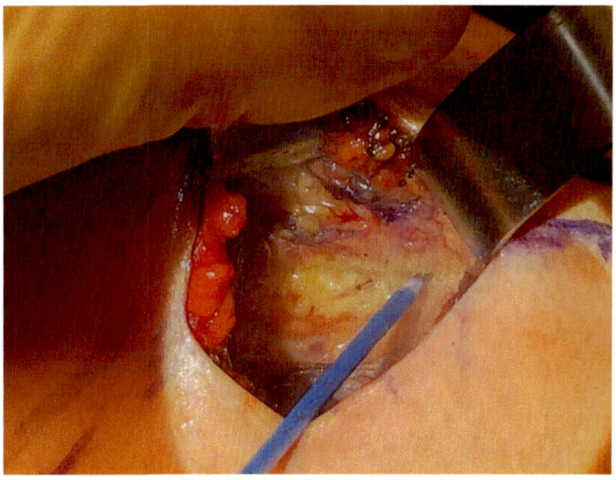

Fig. 11.6 Scoring of the constricted tissue with electrocautery to allow lower pole expansion

The depth of division varies, but in general is deep enough to allow maximal expansion but without creating deformity visible on the surface of the breast. This can require scoring all the way to the dermis. The original inframammary fold can be assessed and scoring accomplished to help disrupt and obliterate it as much as possible.

Breast Augmentation Expansion of the constricted lower pole and volumization of the hypoplastic breast is most often accomplished through breast augmentation. The implant creates an expanding force to the extent the soft tissue and skin will allow. In the most severe cases, where expansion of the lower pole and obliteration of the old fold are deemed to be unsuccessful despite aggressive scoring of the lower pole, consideration should be given to placement of a tissue expander and accomplishing the correction in two stages. The vast majority of cases, however, can be successfully treated in one stage with placement of breast implants.

The decision on which incision to utilize is selected to allow for exposure and scoring of breasts, minimize scarring, allow for removal of skin with necessary and surgeon preference. When a periareolar mastopexy is planned, the implant can be placed through the periareolar approach, eliminating an additional scar. Additionally, the location of the new fold when lowered does not need to be predetermined and can be lowered incrementally through the peri-

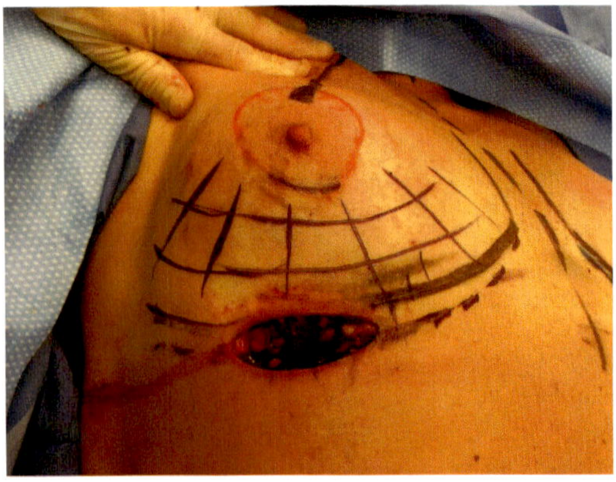

Fig. 11.7 IMF counter incision used for pocket dissection, lower pole expansion and implant insertion in periareolar augmentation mastopexy

areolar incision. However, the periareolar approach is not perfect and can create lower pole deformities and unstable inframammary folds postoperatively. The IMF incision has become the preferred approach even when performing a periareolar mastopexy (Fig. 11.7).

Using the IMF incision, the entire lower pole can be completely visualized, including the parenchyma located between the areola and the original IMF, as well as the skin and subcutaneous tissue between the original IMF and the new IMF. Visualization is improved for parenchymal scoring and the adequacy of IMF obliteration can be assessed as it transitions from the breast to the lower pole subcutaneous tissue. The IMF incision also allows the surgeon to stabilize the new inframammary fold after it has been lowered, as discussed below. One additional benefit that can be helpful is the ability to separate the augmentation pocket from the mastopexy incisions. Thus, no matter the extent of scoring or periareolar techniques are performed to address the deformity, the implant pocket is separate and not at risk if there is a wound healing issue.

The implant pocket selection is based on the ability to maximally expand the tight, constricted breast and yet provide adequate soft-tissue coverage over the implant to avoid visibility, palpability and wrinkling. In patients with adequate soft tissue with a upper pole pinch of 2 cm or greater, the preferred pocket is subglandular to allow maximal expansion of the tight lower pole tissue. If the patient has inadequate coverage (less than 2 cm of upper pole pinch) and a submuscular pocket it preferred, then a dual plane 2 or 3 submuscular pocket is preferred. The dual plane 3 creates a pocket that has muscle coverage from the upper NAC complex and above, leaving everything subareolar and in the lower pole completely subglandular. Both the subglandular pocket and dual plane 3 pocket allow access to the lower pole tissue and subareolar space for scoring of the constriction bands and maximal expansion of the lower pole. Because the advantages of placing in the implant subglandular are so great, some surgeons will even elect to utilize the subglandular pocket in tuberous breast deformity in all patients and simply fat graft the breasts of those patients with inadequate upper pole volume (less than 2 cm of pinch) to improve coverage and minimize wrinkling postoperatively. The subfascial pocket can provide additional support in the upper pole and may be utilized in these cases, but the lower half of the breast still requires a subglandular pocket as the fascia restricts complete expansion and is basically destroyed with the scoring of the constriction bands (Fig. 11.8a–c).

The decision on implant selection is multifactorial, but in general, limiting the size of the implant is prudent. Tissue-based planning proves very beneficial in determining the appropriately sized implant based on the soft tissue characteristics. The most common mistake is to try and place an oversized implant into the very tight tuberous breast pocket. The skin and tight lower pole have a maximal capacity for expansion, and when exceeded, breast deformity occurs. A larger implant also requires greater IMF lowering. The result of placing an oversized implant into a lower pole that will not accommodate its size is an implant that lies too high in the pocket (superior malposition) or stretches below the fold (inferior malposition) with the native fold visible (double bubble) (Fig. 11.9).

Additional implant attributes can contribute to improved lower pole expansion and stability of the improvement.

Smooth Implants Smooth implants have been the most common implant utilized in the United States for breast augmentation, both saline and silicone. With increased scrutiny and limited access to textured implants, smooth devices or nanotextured devices are now increasingly used also around the world. Smooth implants allow for excellent expansion of the tight lower pole and due to the non-adherence, the implants continue to stretch the lower pole for the first few months after the augmentation until the capsule has fully formed. Smooth Implants with increased cohesiveness have some advantages in tuberous breast augmentation. The increased cohesiveness provides more stability to the implant and resists deformation from the tight skin envelope. The implants with increased cohesiveness will maintain the shape and projection to a greater extent compared to a less cohesive gel implant. These implants are also less likely to have rippling and wrinkling, a concern with aggressive scoring and subglandular implant position. Thus, **smooth round implants** with a more cohesive gel are the implant of choice in our practice when treating tuberous breast (Fig. 11.10).

Textured Implants Although textured implants have come under increased scrutiny recently and the future availability has not been fully realized, it is worth discussing some of their merits. Of course, there are many types of textures and the success of employing a textured device and the risk associated with its use varies based upon the type of texture. However, textured implants have occasionally proven beneficial in the tuberous breast patient. The stability created by the textured device assists

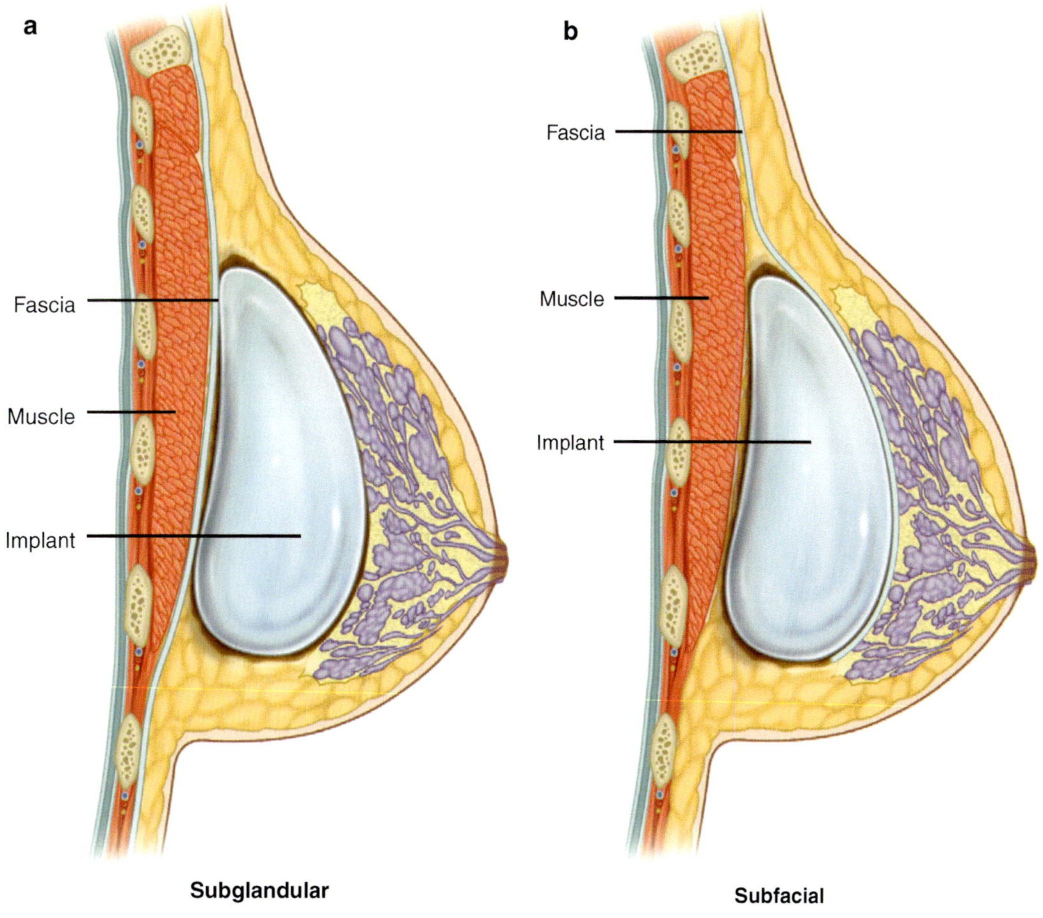

Fig. 11.8 Different implant pocket locations. (**a**) Subglandular. (**b**) subfascial (**c**) submuscular

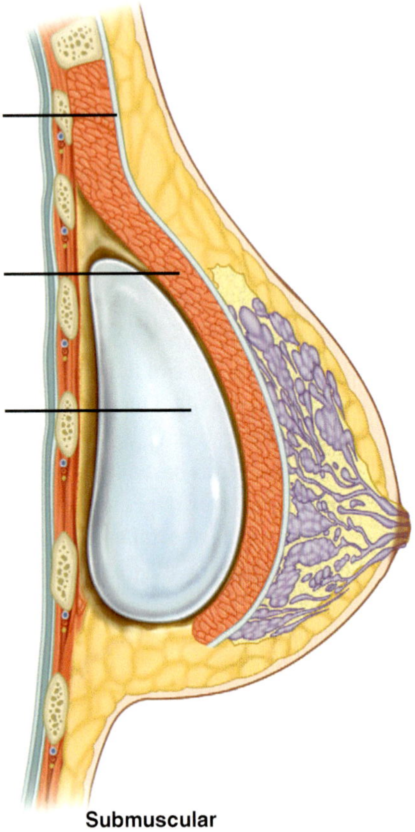

Fig. 11.8 (continued)

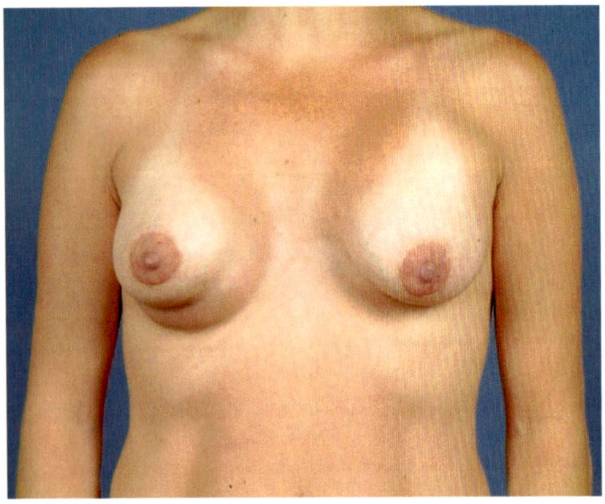

Fig. 11.9 Double bubble of the patient's right breast and high-riding implant with waterfall deformity from under-expansion of the left breast

in holding the implant in the lower pole and resists moving cephalad from the forces of the tight lower pole. Each manufacturer has unique textures and it is important to use the texture that will provide adequate stability. The textured implants can also be helpful in stabilizing the position of the lowered inframammary fold. The lowered fold has been made inherently unstable due to the disruption and lowering and textured devices have limited downward stretch on the new inframammary fold compared to smooth implants. All shaped implants are textured as well, thus allowing placement of different shapes and sizes of implants to optimize results. Finally, there is compelling data that demonstrates that textured implants reduce the capsular contracture rate, especially in the subglandular pocket. This is relevant as the preferred pocket is subglandular in tuberous breast augmentation (Fig. 11.11).

Shaped Implants Shaped implants, which are textured and more cohesive, carry all these attributes already mentioned. Additionally, shaped implants are created to provide a point of maximal projection that is lower. This can be extremely beneficial in these patients with high inframammary folds and constricted lower poles. Extra volume is distributed in the lower poles of the implant, exactly where the tissue is tight and deficient in the tuberous deformity. The shaped implants are also helpful in accommodating a variety of chest morphologies which can be beneficial. These implants can "shape" the breast and hold the tight soft tissue in the desired position rather than the tight tissue deform the implant. This improves the control of the augmentation (Fig. 11.12).

Saline Implants Although currently used much less often than in the past, saline implants have a place in the correction of tuberous breast patients. One aspect relates to the FDA-approval of silicone includes patients 22 years of age and older. Tuberous breast patients are often younger than 22 years of age at time of correction. In the author's opinion, due to the congenital nature and challenges faced in correction, the use of silicone implants if deemed advantageous is clearly appropriate and defensible. But saline implants may be a good alternative in certain tuberous patients. In some ways, saline implants provide a type of lower pole tissue expansion over time not always

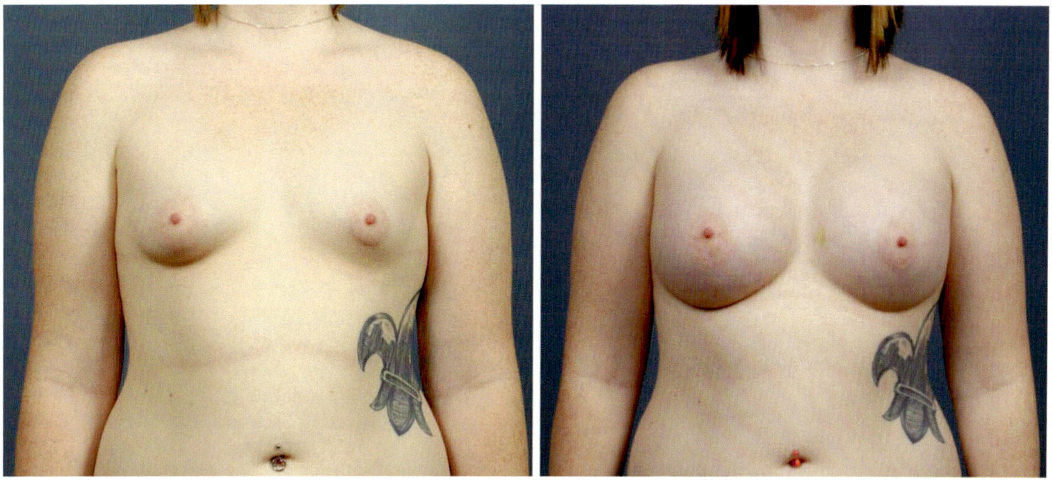

Fig. 11.10 22-year-old female underwent bilateral submuscular augmentation mammoplasty with smooth round 492 cc cohesive silicone implants with inframammary fold lowering and lower pole expansion

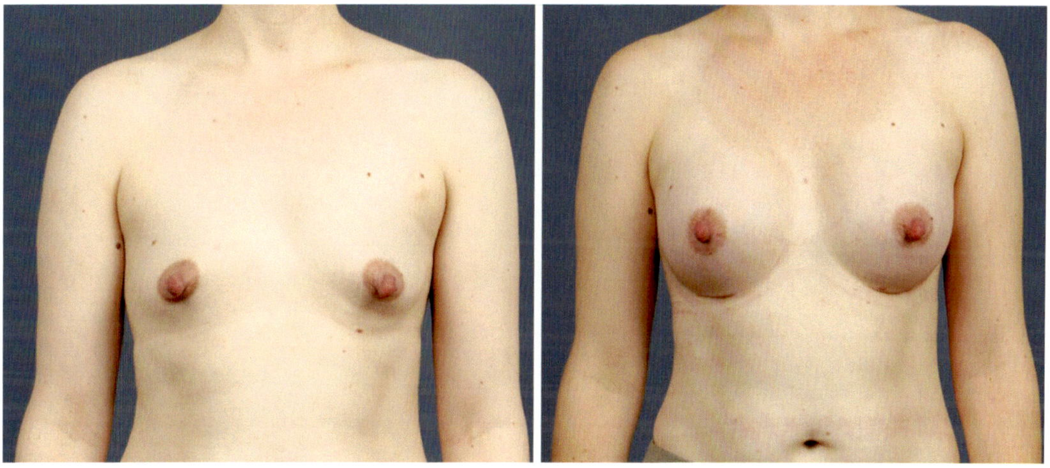

Fig. 11.11 32-year-old female underwent bilateral submuscular breast augmentation with moderate profile textured round silicone implants. She has a 305 cc implant on the right and 285 cc implant on the left

seen with softer silicone implants. So, if a patient is extremely tight and a tissue expander may be in consideration, a saline implant can provide similar expansion over time and may allow correction in one stage. It is the negative sequela of a saline implant, increased lower pole stretch over time compared to silicone, that can be used as an advantage in the tight tuberous breast. The challenge is in determining and controlling the amount of expansion, which makes the results somewhat less predictable. In patients in whom the old inframammary fold is still visible at completion of the surgery, this extra expansion of saline implants improves the appearance over the first 6 months. This may not be the case in more stable implants. Undoubtedly, a significant downside of saline implants is the potential for implant visibility and wrinkling as the soft tissue is often thinned extensively for expansion. It is prudent to discuss with the patient, and possibly parents, the possibility to use of a saline implant instead of a tissue expander but that additional correction may be necessary postoperatively. A tissue expander does allow slower expansion and control, and thus the sur-

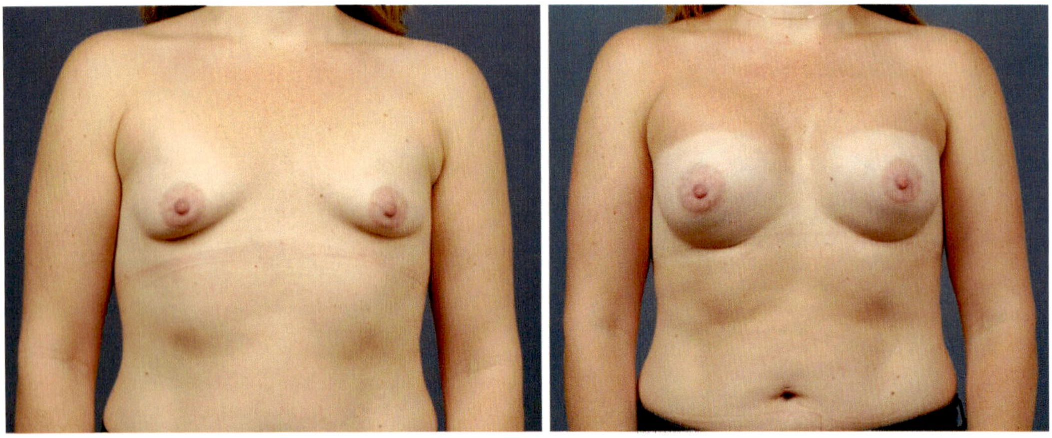

Fig. 11.12 39-year-old female underwent submuscular breast augmentation with anatomic shaped textured 350 cc silicone implants

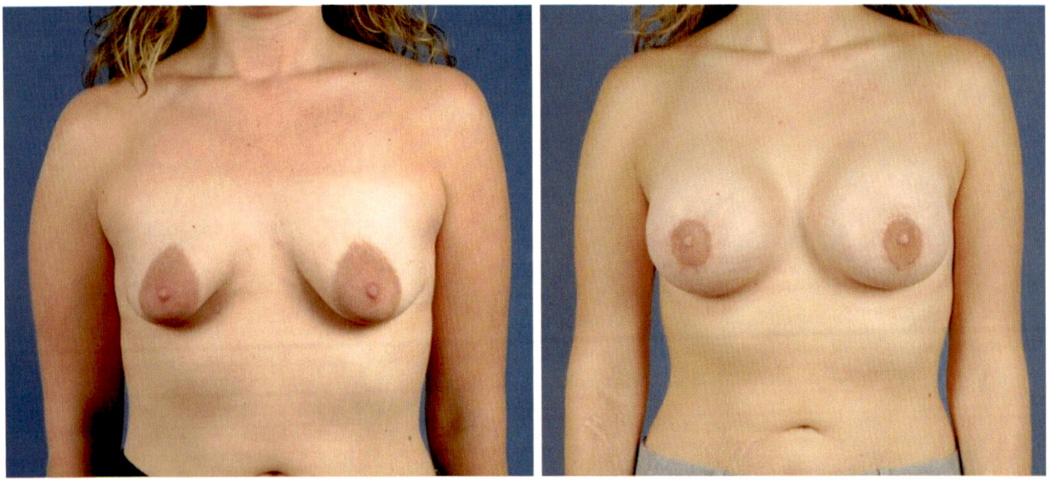

Fig. 11.13 29-year-old female underwent periareolar augmentation mastopexy with smooth round mentor saline 300 cc filled to 360 cc on the right and 320 on the left

geon must weigh the benefits of each and decide the optimal approach for each patient (Fig. 11.13).

Lowering and Controlling the Inframammary Fold Almost all tuberous breast deformities have a superiorly malpositioned inframammary fold that will require lowering to accommodate a breast implant and create a balanced look between the nipple position and the inframammary fold. When utilizing the inframammary incision, the new position will need to be pre-determined based on the size and dimensions of the implant in order to know where to appropriately make the incision. This new location of the IMF scar is related to the length of skin needed from the NAC to the IMF to allow for the implant and have the new IMF scar land at the base of the implant and the NAC centered on the breast mound. There are many ways to calculate this, but the senior has found to methods extremely helpful.

One technique is based on determining the location of the nipple after augmentation (the Stockholm point described by Per Heden, MD), and then determining the location of the implant centered over that new point [13]. Of course, one must decide how much of the implant is desired above and below the new nipple position. There have been some new reports that when using round implants, 45% of the implant above the nipple and 55% below the nipple is the most aesthetically pleasing, but there may be difference based on surgeon or patient preference, as well as difference when using shaped vs round implants [14].

This is accomplished by having the patient raise their arms up over their head, and the position the nipple takes in this position is marked on the chest (the Stockholm point). Based on the height of the implant, the implant position is planned to provide the desired volume above and below that point, and the distance of the new nipple position down to the fold marks the new inframammary fold position. For example, if an implant with a 12 cm height is used and a 50:50 ratio is preferred for implant positioning, then the new fold position would be marked 6 cm (50% of the 12 cm height) below the Stockholm point (Fig. 11.14).

The senior author has found a more simplified technique extremely useful and accurate. This does not base IMF positioning on implant placement, it is based on the amount of skin needed from the nipple to the IMF to accommodate the implant. The formula is shown in Table 11.7.

Using the formula above we use the following guideline we can place our optimal nipple to IMF distance based on certain implant parameters (Table 11.8).

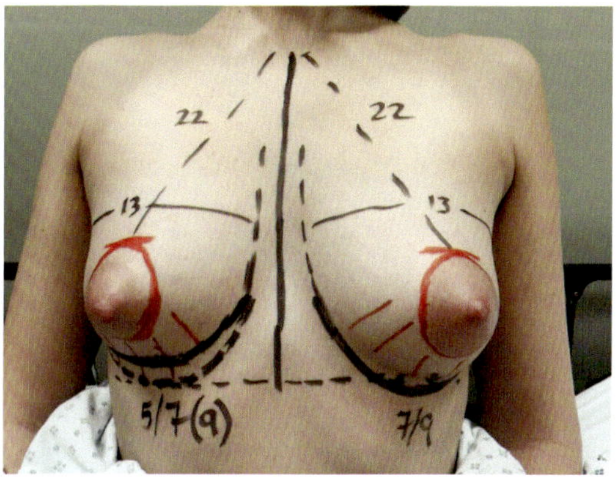

Fig. 11.14 Red periareolar markings indicate PA mastopexy. Vertical red lines indicate planned radial scoring of the constricted lower pole breast tissue. The right breast IMF higher and more constricted. Right breast, black dotted line indicates location of new lowered IMF compared to the left inframammary fold

Table 11.7 Counter Inframammary fold (IMF) incision shown in relation to the periarolar incision. Cross hatched purple lines between the periareolar and IMF incision represent parenchymal scoring to allow lower pole expansion

Optimal N-IMF distance = ½ implant projection + ½ implant height

Table 11.8 Optimal nipple to IMF distance based on implant base diameter and volume

Optimal N-IMF distance (cm)	Base diameter (cm)	Volume (cc)
7	11	200
8	12	300
9	13	400

cm centimeters

It is important to remember that these two calculations are not referring to the same distance. The Stockholm point technique determines how much of the height of the implant will need to be below the new nipple position, and the fold is marked on the chest wall. The formula above determines the amount of skin required on maximal stretch, and the new fold is marked at that position. It can be very helpful and reassuring in challenging tuberous breast cases requiring significant IMF lowering to determine the new IMF position using both techniques.

Once the distance is determined, the inframammary incision is made at this new predetermined location and the augmentation and scoring are performed through this access. The repositioning of the inframammary fold however creates an unstable fold structure that is at risk of bottoming out over time. A significant advantage of the inframammary approach compared to the periareolar approach is the ability to accurately and effectively control the fold position during closure of the incision. The maneuver is accomplished by securing the caudal edge of the Scarpe's fascia present on the lower incisional edge to the underlying deep fascial structures with an absorbable suture such as 2-0 Vicryl. This suturing is usually done by simply incorporating the superficial fascia and deep fascia on the inferior skin edge and then closing to Scarpe's fascia on the upper skin edge (Fig. 11.15).

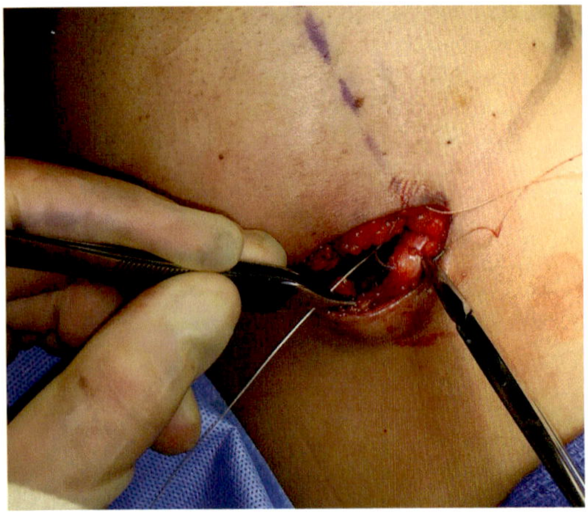

Fig. 11.15 2-0 Vicryl used to lock the IMF fold. A cusp of superficial and deep fascia on the inferior skin edge is closed to a cusp of superficial fascia on the upper skin edge

Correction of Areolar Hypertrophy and Pseudoherniation Correction of the areolar deformities with or without lifting the NAC is critical to creating a natural appearing breast. The planned excisional technique is based on the NAC position and the amount of skin excess or ptosis present. The most common mastopexy technique is the circumareolar mastopexy or occasionally a circumvertical. The circumareolar component of both of these procedures addresses many aspects of the areolar deformity; such as reduction in the areolar diameter, reduction in the protrusion of the overprojection and pseudoherniation of the areolar tissue, widening of the breast base, and suture control of the resultant areola diameter. The technique involves placement of a permanent 3-0 Gortex suture around the areola in a wagon-wheel purse string fashion with minimal dermal release. Dermal cauterization is also helpful to allow shrinkage of the dermis and reduction of the areolar diameter prior to purse string closure. The areola is then inset with 3-0 PDS interrupted dermal sutures and a running 5-0 nylon suture (Figs. 11.16, 11.17, and 11.18).

The circumareolar approach can probably not elevate the NAC more than 2 cm in most cases, especially with a tight lower pole skin

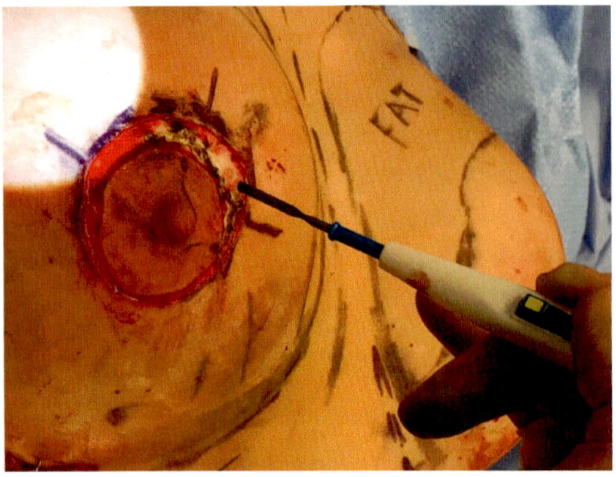

Fig. 11.16 Cauterization of the Periareolar dermis to provide shrinkage prior to final closure

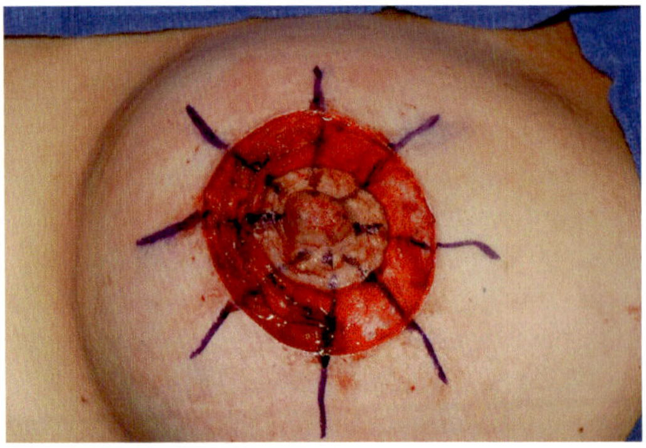

Fig. 11.17 Markings of the NAC where the wagon-wheel purse string suture will be inserted to insure proper alignment

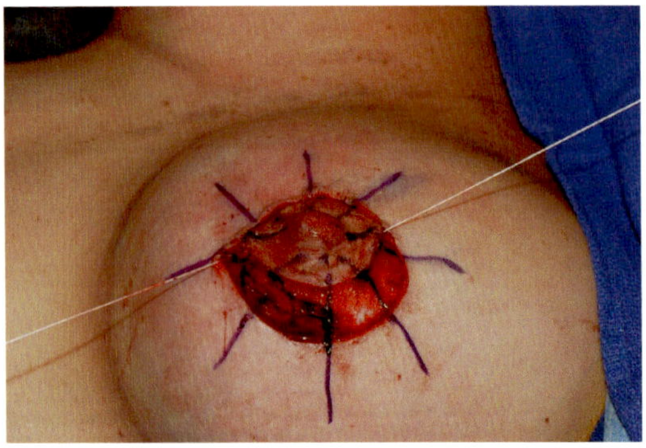

Fig. 11.18 Picture showing the wagon wheel purse string closure of the NAC with a 3-0 Gore-Tex suture

envelope. Thus, other than the 1–2 cm of NAC elevation, any remaining improvement in NAC position in relationship to the breast mound will require IMF lowering to achieve. In less severe case with less constriction and some ptosis present, a cirumvertical mastopexy may be appropriate. This technique can allow much more significant elevation of the NAC compared to a circumareolar approach, and can may be helpful when enough tissue is present in the lower pole to utilize this technique. This can reduce or eliminate the need for IMF lowering (Fig. 11.19).

Correction of Asymmetries When symmetrical tuberous breast deformities are present, treating each side with the same technique can provide the best chance at a symmetrical outcome. Unfortunately, the vast majority of these patients have some degree of asymmetry, sometimes quite significantly. A patient with a hypoplastic, constricted tuberous breast on one side and a large ptotic breast on the opposite side is quite common. In most of these cases, the larger breast has many tuberous characteristics, such as a high inframammary fold with a constricted base and ptosis over the high fold. Treatment of the larger breast usually includes either a mastopexy or reduction trying to recreate the look of the lower pole and nipple positioning achieved on the hypoplastic side. It is helpful to do these procedures simultaneously in the initial procedure to provide the best chance for symmetry. If an additional proce-

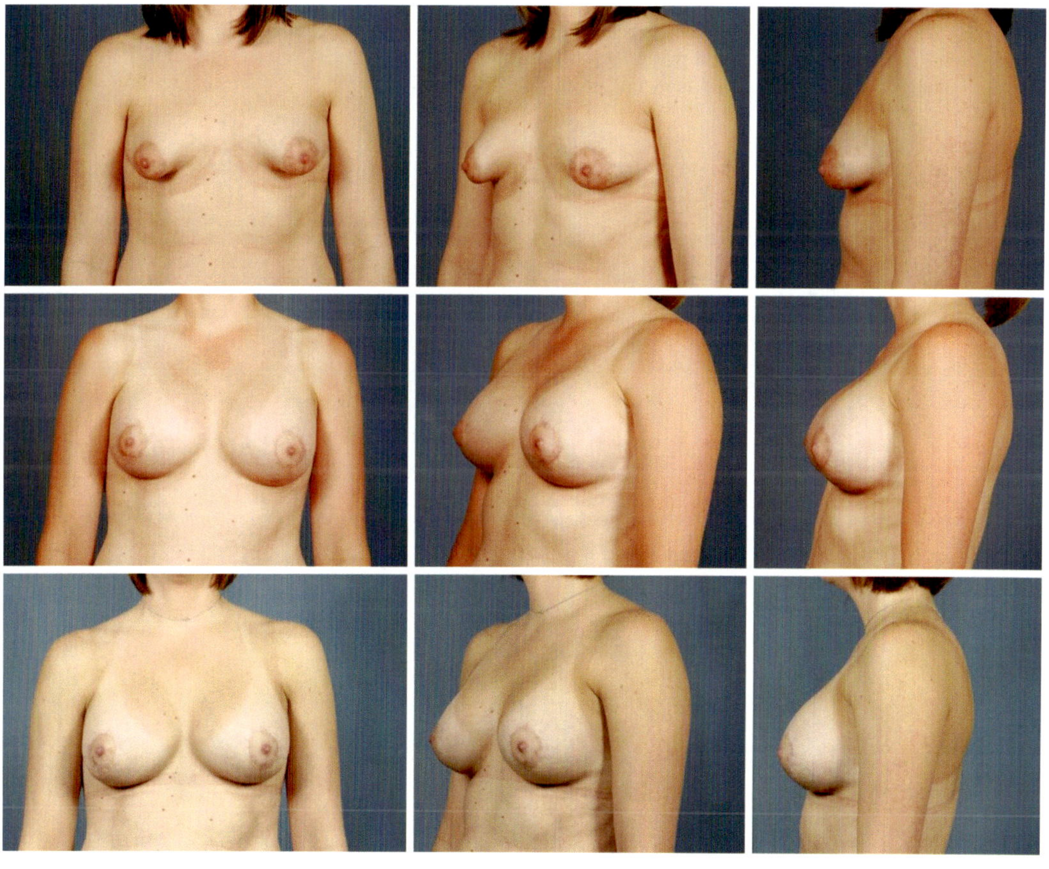

Fig. 11.19 34-year-old female underwent periareolar augmentation mastopexy with Gore-Tex suture and round silicone moderate plus 375 cc implants. Post op results shown at 1 year and 3 years

dure is required to improve the outcome, the revision will be simplified by having the two breasts much closer in shape and size for the subsequent surgery. When approaching these patients, the more hypoplastic breast is treated first followed by the opposite side to create symmetry to the initial side (Figs. 11.20, 11.21, 11.22 and 11.23).

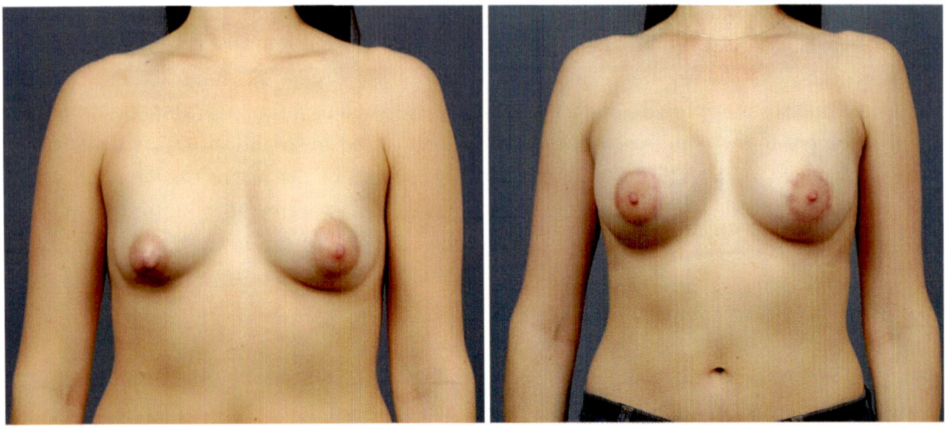

Fig. 11.20 24-year-old female with asymmetry underwent bilateral periareolar augmentation mastopexy with Gore-Tex suture. Left side with round moderate profile textured 295 cc silicone implant. Right side with round high profile textured 385 cc silicone implant

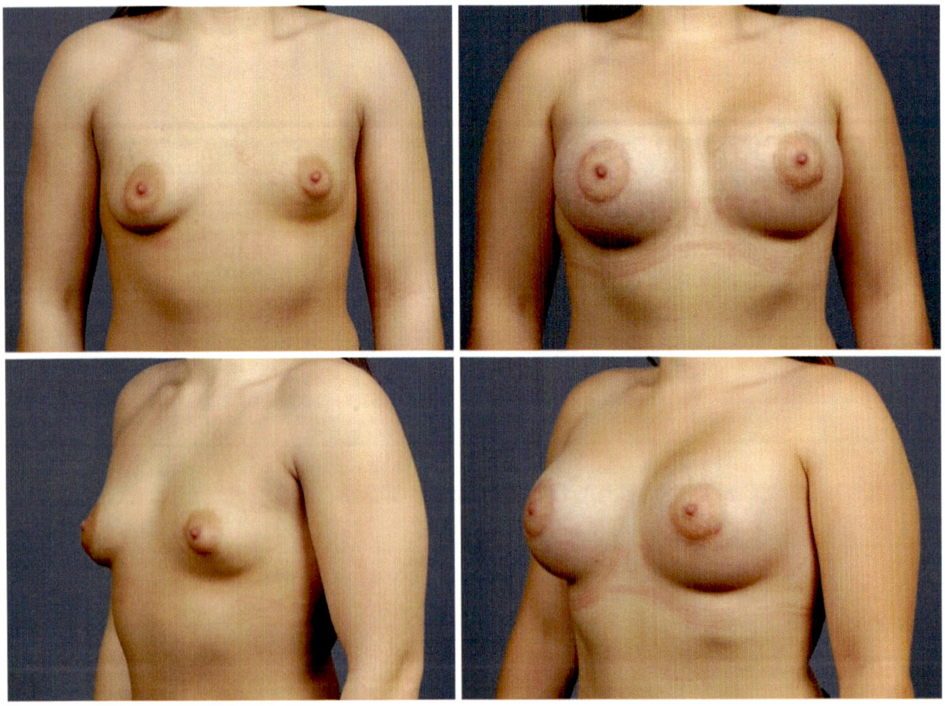

Fig. 11.21 22-year-old female with breast and chest wall asymmetry underwent Bilateral Periareolar augmentation mastopexy and unilateral fat grafting. On the right side a 440 cc high profile textured round implant was used. On the Left, a 385 cc moderate profile round textured silicone implant was used with needle band release and 75 cc of fat grafting to the lower pole

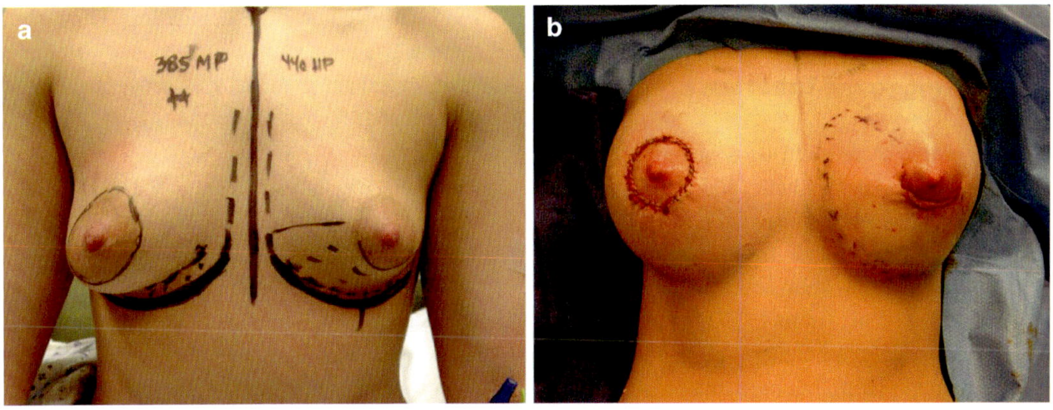

Fig. 11.22 (**a**, **b**) pre-operative markings and the on-table result of the patient from Fig. 11.21. The right breast inframammary fold was lowered and 75 cc of fat was injected into the left breast lower pole

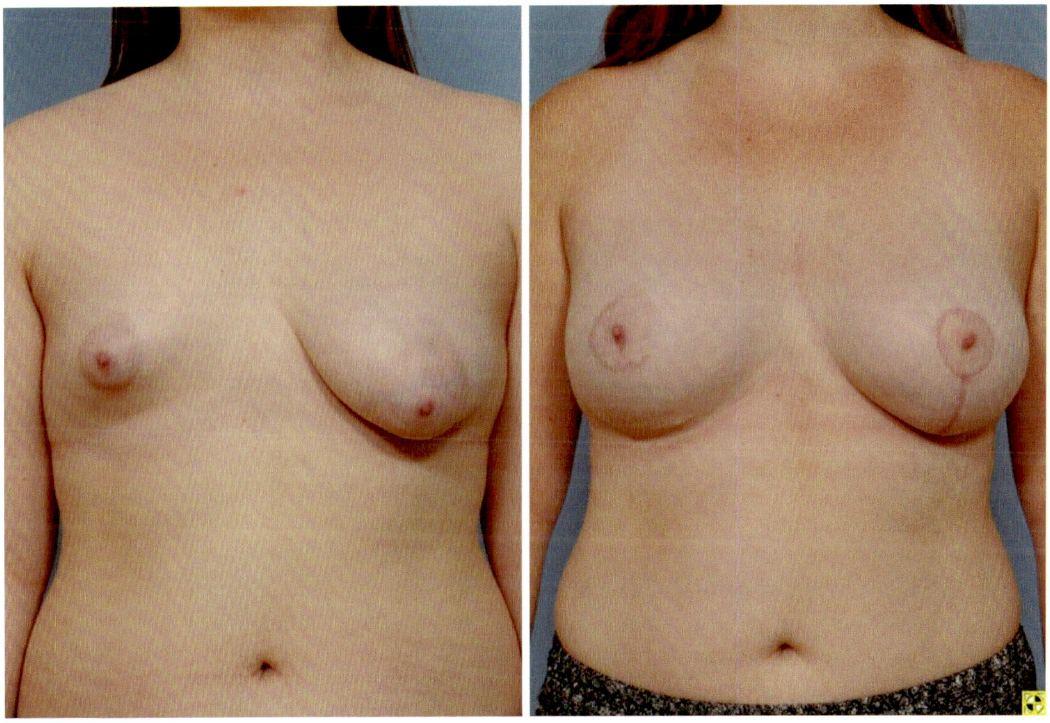

Fig. 11.23 20-year-old female with asymmetry and tubular breast underwent bilateral breast Augmentation, right periareolar mastopexy with autologous fat grafting and left periareolar vertical mastopexy. Right side 375 cc round moderate plus silicone with 185 cc of autologous fat transfer. Left side with a 205 cc low profile silicone implant and periareolar mastopexy

Preoperative counseling is important as perfect symmetry postoperatively is extremely challenging to achieve. Even if perfectly symmetric at the end of the procedure, the unpredictable nature of the soft tissue envelopes often leads to asymmetric results as the breast stretch and relax. Patients are reminded that the breasts will often end up being more like "sisters" and less like "twins".

Fat-based Correction

Fat Grafting to the Tuberous Breast

The innovation of fat grafting to the breast has had a major impact on aesthetic and reconstructive breast surgery [15–18]. The characteristics of the tuberous breast place it in the center of the spectrum of deformities seen in both cosmetic and reconstructive breast surgery. The tuberous breast is deficient in breast parenchyma in the vertical and horizontal planes, but particularly in the inferior pole of the breast. The deformity also presents with some degree of herniation of the nipple areolar complex. Most importantly, as has been mentioned previously, the tuberous breast is varied in its clinical presentation—with a spectrum of deformities which render each patient unique in their reconstructive requirements. It is exactly this varied presentation which makes fat-based correction (with or without the use of implants) such an effective modality in the tuberous breast. The ability to place fat right where you need it the most gives fat grafting the tremendous advantage over straight forward volume augmentation with implants. When placement of autologous fat is coupled with the appropriate release of the constricting elements of the deformity, the results attained can be nearly anatomic in their correction.

Volume restoration within the tuberous breast must be considered in the context of each patient's particular deformity. Generally speaking, the goal is to find a method of reconstruction that supplies overall volume restoration and treats the specific quadrants of volume deficit or constriction, with the minimum number of surgical interventions. There are three general categories for utilizing fat with tuberous breast deformity:

1. **Composite augmentation**: those patients that require use of an implant to achieve core volume with fat placed where breast needs it the most
2. **Fat Grafting with Needle Band Release**: Those who can be treated with fat grafting alone with the release of particular areas of constriction
3. **Fat Grafting with Pre-expansion**: Those that require pre-expansion of the breast envelope with staged fat grafting, this process requires the use of an expansile device, i.e. BRAVA

Composite Augmentation with Breast Implants and Fat Grafting

Composite augmentation with fat grafting is an incredibly versatile modality that is useful in a large percentage of patients (roughly 70%). In these cases, an implant supplies core volume, yet fat grafting and the techniques associated with fat grafting, such as needle band release of the inferior pole and periareolar rings can make significant improvements in breast shape. In most cases, these maneuvers are combined with mastopexy to reposition the nipple areolar complex in an appropriate position, while also releasing elements of constriction via the incisions provided by a periareolar or vertical mastopexy incision.

Historically, the choice of implant selection in the tubular breast is limited by the constricted nature of the breast in both the vertical and horizontal planes—with obvious attention to the sometimes severely constricted inferior pole. The deformity is sometimes accompanied by a severe deficit of glandular tissue in inferior pole. Furthermore, the distance from inframammary fold to nipple is quite short. Without manipulation of this distance, the choice of breast implant is obviously limited with regard to base width and overall volume. Whether or not combined with a mastopexy, the resulting breast mound is generally neither of sufficient size nor appropriate shape.

Many of these challenges are overcome using composite approach utilizing a narrower implant for core volume, with the addition of fat to the periphery of the breast to attain optimal shape. This gives the appearance of a wider implant and can augment the regions that specifically require more volume. Again, when combined with a periareolar or vertical mastopexy, optimal breast shape and location and appearance of the nipple areolar complex can be achieved (Figs. 11.24, 11.25 and 11.26).

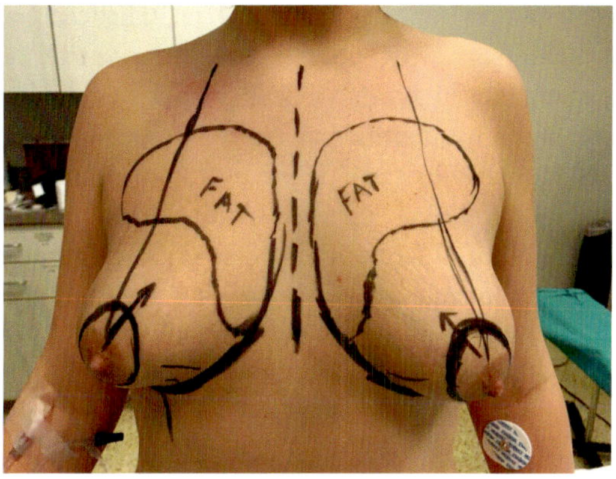

Fig. 11.24 Pre-operative markings of a composite augmentation peri-areolar mastopexy. Upper pole and medial cleavage of the breast marked for autologous fat transfer. The vertical lines in the lower pole of the breast represent areas of radial scoring to release the constriction

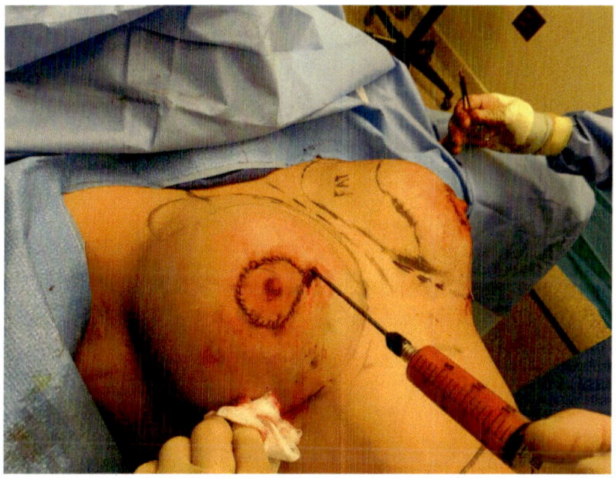

Fig. 11.25 Autologous fat injection into the patient from Fig. 11.24 with a 20 cc syringe and 2 mm cannula

Lipofilling for Volume Augmentation Combined with Needle Band Release

The technique of lipofilling of the tuberous breast has been addressed by authors in the past [19–22]. It is important to first discuss the role that needle band release, or the creation of small vascularized potential spaces play in appropriate fat grafting of the breast. Mere injection of autologous fat into the adolescent or young adult breast can be met with significant frustration. Graft take is affected by not only the viability of the fat itself, but the vascular network in which the fat is placed. Ideally, autologous fat will provide the best volume correction if the micro aliquots of fat are able to take within small well vascularized spaces that still maintain a controlled (albeit small) domain. In this setting, the large devascularized spaces that are created using some traditional forms of radial scoring are not well suited to this purpose. Using the technique of needle band release, the constricting elements of the tuberous breast deformity can be adequately treated, without the creation of large devascularized spaces in which grafted fat will create "lakes" with poor graft take and the increased likelihood of complications like fat necrosis and cyst formation.

The authors have found the technique of needle band release (NBR) provides for the creation of increased surface area and appropriately shaped and vascularized potential spaces in which to then graft autologous fat. In the author's experience,

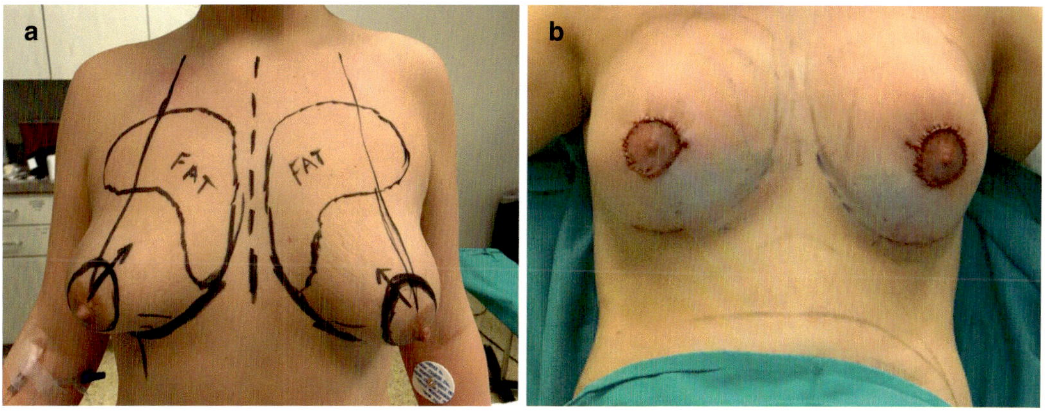

Fig. 11.26 (**a**) Pre-op photo and (**b**) immediate on-table result after composite augmentation mastopexy

fat grafting combined with NBR can enhance the shape by removing or releasing the constrictions of the inferior pole of the breast and passively filling the potential space created in this new region. Furthermore, the NBR technique is ideal for releasing the constricting ring associated with the areolar deformity in the tubular breast, without using radical radial scoring techniques that are often associated with unnecessary incisions or soft tissue deformities (Fig. 11.27).

Fat Grafting Requiring the Use of an External Pre-expansion Device

The use of the BRAVA device has been addressed in earlier publications which documented the reliability of the technique when applied to breast reconstruction [15]. We have found that this form of breast reconstruction is effective when the patient desires only the use of autologous fat as a method of volume augmentation. The technique provides for larger volumes of fat than can be grafted using NBR alone. Furthermore, the technique is useful as areas of constriction within the breast can be identified as the pre-expansion process moves forward. Ultimately, as expansion nears completion, an ideal potential space and tissue bed for large volume fat grafting is produced. The technique is, however, not without its drawbacks. The vast majority of patients find the device cumbersome to wear, is universally uncomfortable, and relatively time consuming when compared with intraoperative autologous fat transfer. As such, the authors reserve this modality for cases of severe tuberous breast deformity in patients adamantly opposed to the use of breast prostheses (Fig. 11.28). Unfortuantely, the BRAVA system has become less available recently and it is hopefully that it or a similar device will ultimately emerge to assist in the most challenging tuberus breast cases benefiting from correction with fat grafting.

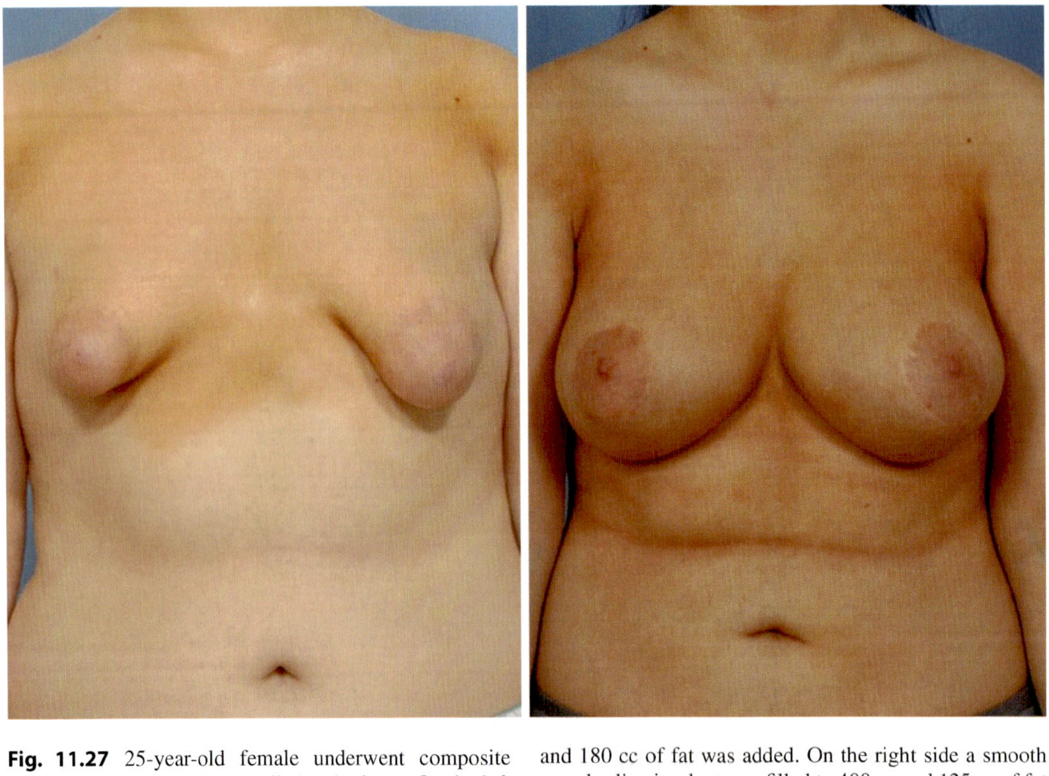

Fig. 11.27 25-year-old female underwent composite breast augmentation with needle band release. On the left side a smooth round saline implant was filled to 370 cc and 180 cc of fat was added. On the right side a smooth round saline implant was filled to 400 cc and 125 cc of fat was grafted

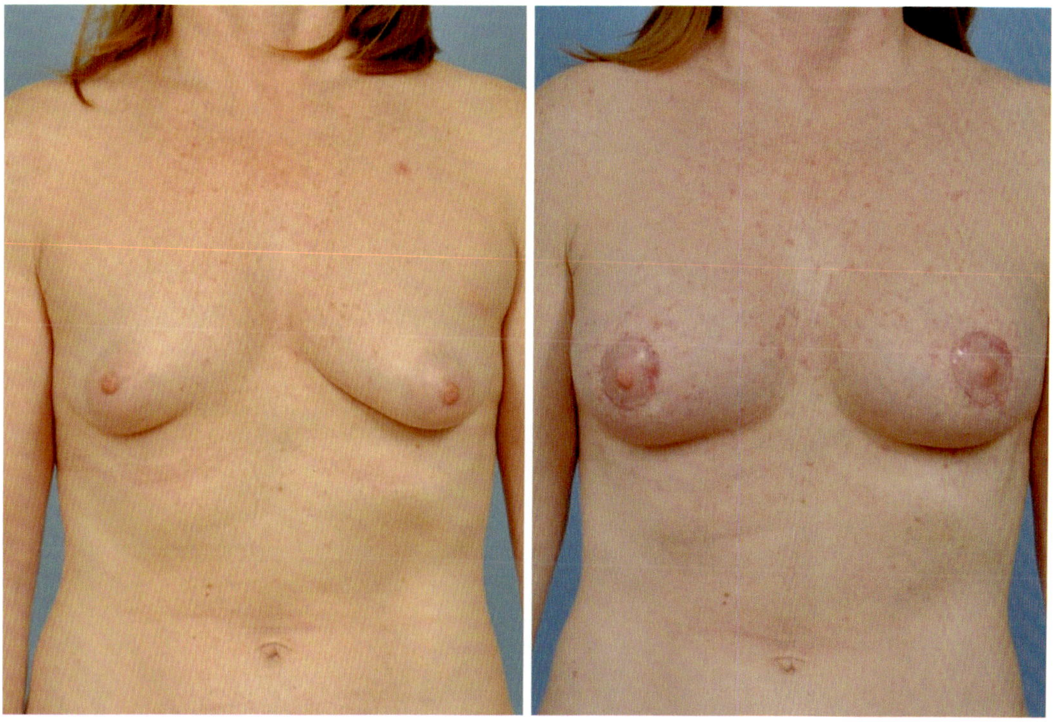

Fig. 11.28 36-year-old female underwent pre-expansion with the BRAVA system then bilateral periareolar mastopexy with large volume fat grafting. On the left side 480 cc of fat was added and on the right side 460 cc of fat was grafted

Complications

The risk of complications or unwanted sequalae is particularly significant in tuberous breast correction as the challenges are great and preoperative asymmetry is the norm. The complications that are associated with breast augmentation, mastopexies and fat grafting are similar in the tuberous breast patients. The management of the enlarged areola can lead to postoperative sequelae, such as areolar widening, hypertrophic scarring, persistent pseudoherniation and flattening of the breast (Fig. 11.29).

The wagon-wheel purse string technique has significantly reduced these issues, and revision of the areolar deformity adequately addresses these issues in most cases.

One complication particularly unique to a severe tuberous deformity is related to the persistence of the old inframammary fold creating a double-bubble deformity (Fig. 11.30).

These can be challenging to treat and have often required reoperation with additional constriction band scoring, expansion and/or glandular redistribution. More recently, fat grafting with needle release of the persistent fold has become the treatment of choice. This can be very effective in obliterating the residual fold structure. These patients' breasts are also extremely hypoplastic and the expansion and band releases can create implant visibility and wrinkling postoperatively. This is primarily managed with fat grafting, is an extremely successful technique for adding much needed additional coverage over the implants.

Additionally, under-expansion of the lower pole or placement of an oversized implant can lead to superior malposition of the implant. This is managed with either additional lower pole

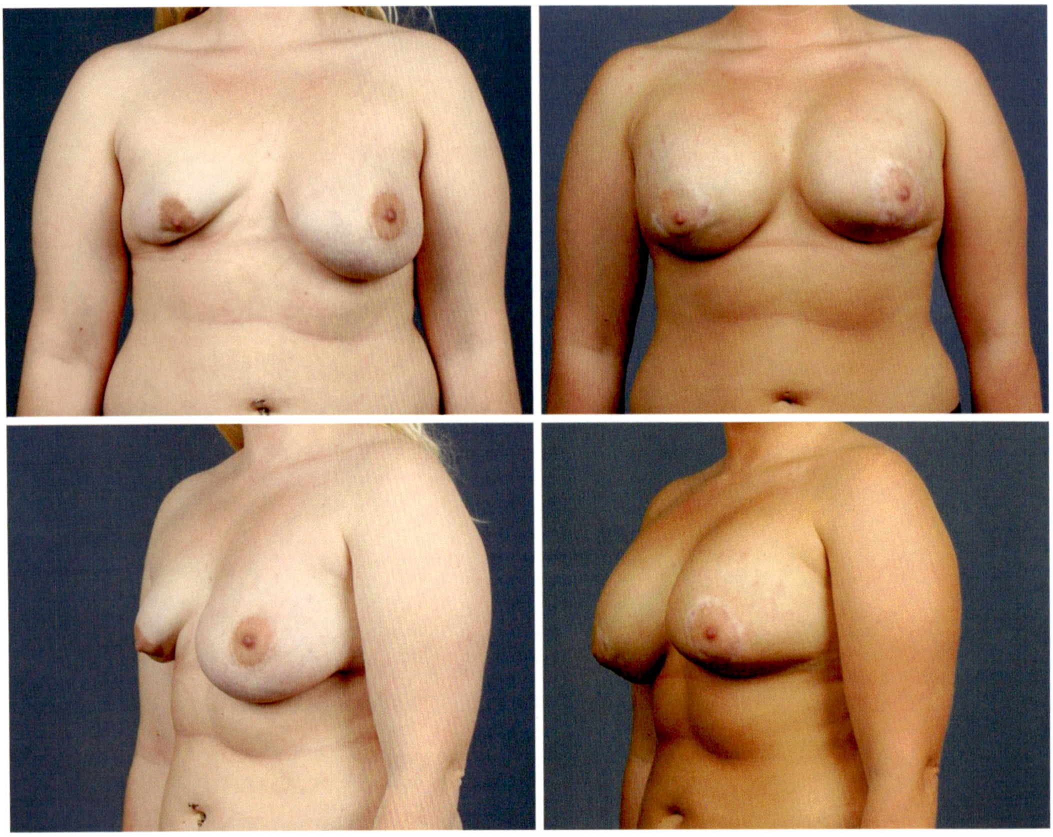

Fig. 11.29 Post-operative sequelae; hypertrophic scarring of the periareolar incision with high riding implants, double bubbles and lower pole contour irregularities

release and expansion or downsizing of the implant. Over dissection of lower pole, placement of the new IMF too low, not securing the new IMF location or placement of a large implant creating lower pole stretch, can lead to inferior malposition of the implant. This usually requires a capsulorraphy to elevate the fold, possible creation of a new pocket (neosubpectoral pocket) and possible excision of some lower pole excess skin (Fig. 11.31).

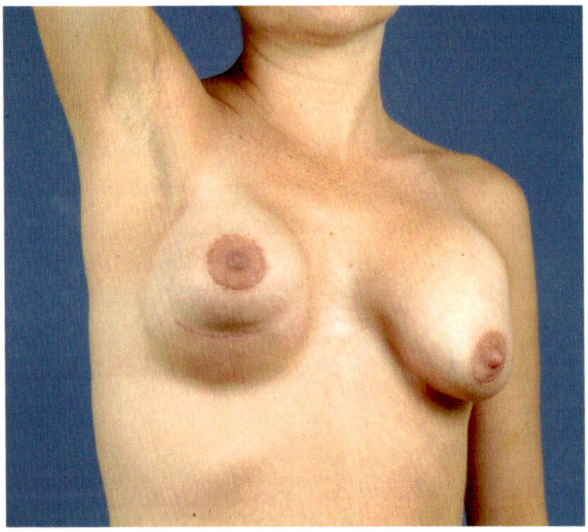

Fig. 11.30 Double bubble of the patient's right breast and a waterfall deformity of the left breast

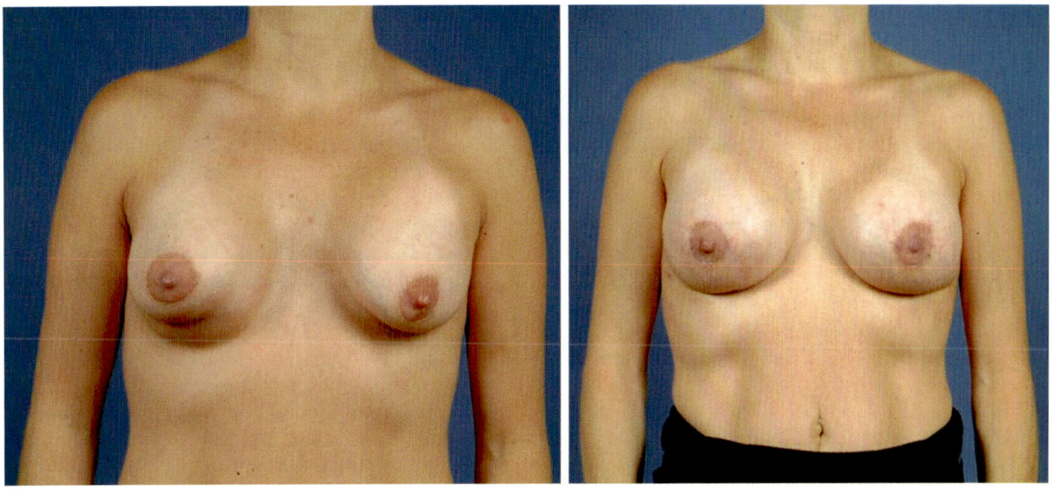

Fig. 11.31 Before and after photo. Correction of right breast double bubble deformity with a partial capsulectomy, right inferior suture capsulorrhaphy, and a neosubpectoral pocket creation with implant exchange

Conclusion

With proper preoperative evaluation and the utilization of the appropriate surgical technique, excellent results can be achieved in the treatment of tuberous breast deformities. The keys to success involve the diagnosis of the deformity by recognizing the presence of breast hypoplasia, constricted lower breast parenchyma and skin envelope, superiorly malpositioned inframammary fold, pseudoherniation and or hypertrophy of the NAC (nipple areolar complex). Once the diagnosis is made then the treatment plan can address the cause of the deformity with a variety of techniques. The insertion of implants can improve the lower pole constriction and improve breast hypoplasia. Treating the NAC deformity with various mastopexy techniques can improve the aesthetics of the breast by making the areola smaller and lifting the breast mound over the core projection of the implant. Finally, fat grafting can be utilized to increase volume and provide shape to the tuberous breast. Addressing these problems associated with the deformity and providing the appropriate surgical treatment will improve the overall aesthetics of the breast.

References

1. Rees T, Aston S. The tuberous breast. Clin Plast Surg. 1976;3:339–47.
2. von Heimburg D, Exner K, Kruft S, Lemperle G. The tuberous breast deformity: classification and treatment. Br J Plast Surg. 1996;49(6):339–45.
3. Mandrekas AD, Zambacos GJ. Aesthetic reconstruction of the tuberous breast deformity: a 10-year experience. Aesthet Surg J. 2010;30(5):680–92.
4. Teimourian B, Adham MN. Surgical correction of the tuberous breast. Ann Plast Surg. 1983;10(3):190–3.
5. Grolleau J, Lanfrey E. Breast base anomalies: treatment strategy for tuberous breasts, minor deformities, and asymmetry. Plast Reconstr Surg. 1999;104(7):2040–8.
6. Spears SL, Eilley S, Robb G, et al. Surgery of the breast. 3rd ed. Philadelphia: Wolters Kluwer Health/Lippincott Williams and Wilkins; 2010.
7. Pacifico P, Cagli B, Tenna S, et al. The tuberous breast revisited. J Plast Reconstr Aesthet Surg. 2007;60:455–64.
8. Calobrace MB. Teaching breast augmentation: a focus on critical intraoperative techniques and decision making to maximize results and minimize revisions. Clin Plastic Surg. 2015;42:493–504.
9. Hall-Findlay EJ. Applied anatomy: key concepts for modern breast surgery. In: Hall-Findlay E, editor. Aesthetic breast surgery: concepts and techniques. New York: Thieme Publishers New York.
10. Ribeiro L, Accorsi AJ, Rocha RB. Tubular breasts. In: Bucky LP, Mottura AA, editors. Aesthetic breast surgery. Philadelphia: Saunders Elsevier; 2009.

11. Ribeiro L, Accorsi A, Argencio V. Tuberous breast syndrome. Aesthet Surg J. 2005;29(6):398–402.
12. Serra-Rennom JM, Munoz-Olmo J, Serra-Mestre JM. Treatment of grade 3 tuberous breasts with Puckett's technique (modified) and fat grafting to correct the constricting ring. Aesthet Plast Surg. 2011;35:773–81.
13. Szemerey IB, Bajusz H, Heden P. Preoperative planning. In: Szemerey IB, editor. Augmentation mammoplasty with anatomical implants. Budapest: Mediburg Klinika Kft; 2008. p. 32–8.
14. Mallucci P, Brandford OA. Shapes, projections and variations if breast aesthetic ideals: the definition of breast beauty, analysis, and surgical practice. Clin Plastic Surg. 2015;42:451–64.
15. Del Vecchio DA, Bucky LP. Breast augmentation using preexpansion and autologous fat transplantation: a clinical radiographic study. Plast Reconstr Surg. 2011;127(6):2441–50.
16. Kanchwala SK, et al. Autologous fat grafting to the reconstructed breast: the management of acquired contour deformities. Plast Reconstr Surg. 2009;124(2):409–18.
17. Katzel EB, Bucky LP. Fat grafting to the breast: clinical applications and outcomes for reconstructive surgery. Plast Reconstr Surg. 2017;140(5S Advances in Breast Reconstruction):69S–76S.
18. Stark RY, et al. Utilizing large volume fat grafting in breast reconstruction after nipple sparing mastectomies. Gland Surg. 2018;7(3):337–46.
19. Brault N, et al. Correction of tuberous breast deformity: a retrospective study comparing lipofilling versus breast implant augmentation. J Plast Reconstr Aesthet Surg. 2017;70(5):585–95.
20. Claudio Silva-Vergara C, Fontdevila J, Weshahy O. Fat grafting technique, a paradigm shift in the treatment of tuberous breast. World J Plast Surg. 2018;7(1):72–7.
21. Delay E, Sinna R, Ho Quoc C. Tuberous breast correction by fat grafting. Aesthet Surg J. 2013;33(4):522–8.
22. Derder M, et al. The use of lipofilling to treat congenital hypoplastic breast anomalies: preliminary experiences. Ann Plast Surg. 2014;73(4):371–7.

12 Augmentation Mastopexy with Breast Asymmetry

Michael R. Schwartz

Introduction

Breast asymmetry has been described as early as 1841 when Poland described the eponymous syndrome of chest wall deformity that can include musculoskeletal, breast and nipple malformations [1]. While most patients have some asymmetry of the breast, there can be significant differences in size, shape and position in some patients requiring unique thought and approach to achieve satisfying aesthetic and symmetry goals for the patient and surgeon [2]. Breast symmetry can have a significant psychological effects [3]

Anatomy and Evaluation

Evaluation of the patient with asymmetry should include a full examination with attention to the breast, nipple, and chest wall; all with consideration of the patient's aesthetic goals. Each of these can contribute to the patient's presentation and effect the approach to its correction [4].

M. R. Schwartz (✉)
Private Practice, Westlake Village, CA, USA
e-mail: doc@drschwartz.com

Breast

The breast should be evaluated for its footprint on the chest wall. This includes the base diameter on each side, the breast shape, and the overall breast volume. Hall-Findlay [5] described the assessment of the key breast dimensions. The surgeon must assess the breast differences discussed to create a plan to effect change toward symmetry. This includes the evaluation of all four breast borders, and the shape of each breast. (Table 12.1)

The volume of the breast can be assessed by three dimensional imaging [6, 7]. The use of a volumetric sizing system allows the patient and surgeon to assess both the patient's volume asymmetry, and aesthetic goals. (The difference in sizers used on each side to achieve the patients desired look) (Fig. 12.1).

The breast footprint includes the evaluation of each breast border, as well as its location on the chest wall.

Nipple

The nipple should be evaluated for position, shape, and diameter. Nipple position should include the measurement of Nipple to IMF distance on stretch (N-IMF), Sternal Notch to Nipple distance (SN-N), and midline to nipple distance (M-N). Nipple shape should include

M. B. Calobrace et al. (eds.), *Augmentation Mastopexy*,
https://doi.org/10.1007/978-3-030-48226-8_12

projection, herniation, and symmetry. Finally, nipple diameter should be noted on each side [8].

Chest Wall

The shape and symmetry of each patients chest wall should be evaluated. This includes the chest cavity itself, pectoral muscle, and axillary fullness (Fig. 12.2).

The chest cavity should be assessed for overall shape [9]. This includes pectus deformities of either prominence or hollowing, upper chest fullness, asymmetry of chest cavity prominence, lateral slope, and vertical slope. Pectus excavatum can contribute significantly to both pre and post op asymmetry. Often it is limited to one side of the chest. In these patients, great attention to implant projection and surface are required to achieve stable symmetry. Smooth walled implants tend to "roll" downhill medially and will fail to maintain stable shape or projection. Synmastia is a common post-operative complication.

Table 12.1 Steps in the evaluation of Breast Asymmetry

1. Patient goals
2. Size discrepancy
3. Location of upper breast border
4. Location of lower breast border (IMF)
5. Locations of medial and lateral Borders (base diameter)
6. Shape including nipple
7. Nipple position symmetry
(a) Vertical
(b) Horizontal
8. Nipple size

Adapted from Hall-Findley

Patients with Pectus Carinatum often have wide set breast and nipple position. Again a smooth walled device may fall significantly laterally over time to increase this appearance post-operatively. In addition, sizer volumes may underestimate the required implant size as the lateralization of implants post op decreases the effective projection required to satisfy the patients aesthetic goals.

Patients with a full upper chest cavity often have significant early ptosis at presentation. This is due to the down hill fall of natural breast tissue, which will likely be repeated post operatively. These patients need counseling on appropriate expectations for their final result, as they will not maintain a high breast position. In addition, in the authors opinion textured devices are contraindicated as they will most likely result in a waterfall deformity long term.

Three dimensional imaging can also be used to evaluate the differences in projection of the chest wall on each side. This can be used to select

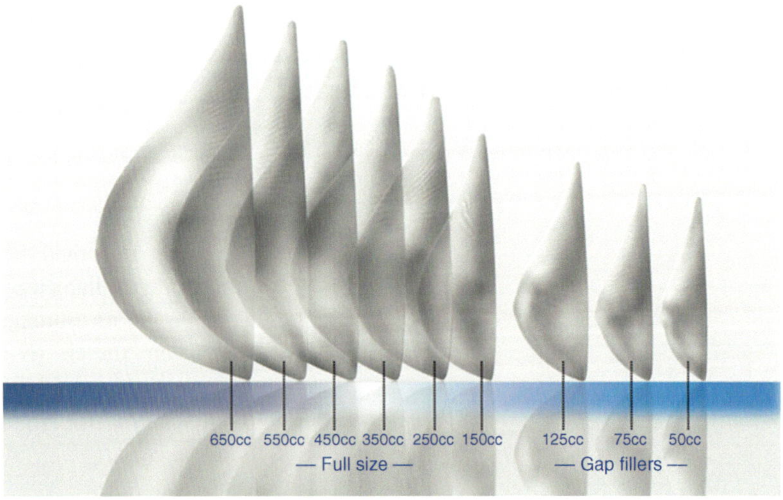

Fig. 12.1 Volumetric sizing system for evaluation of Patient desired size and symmetry

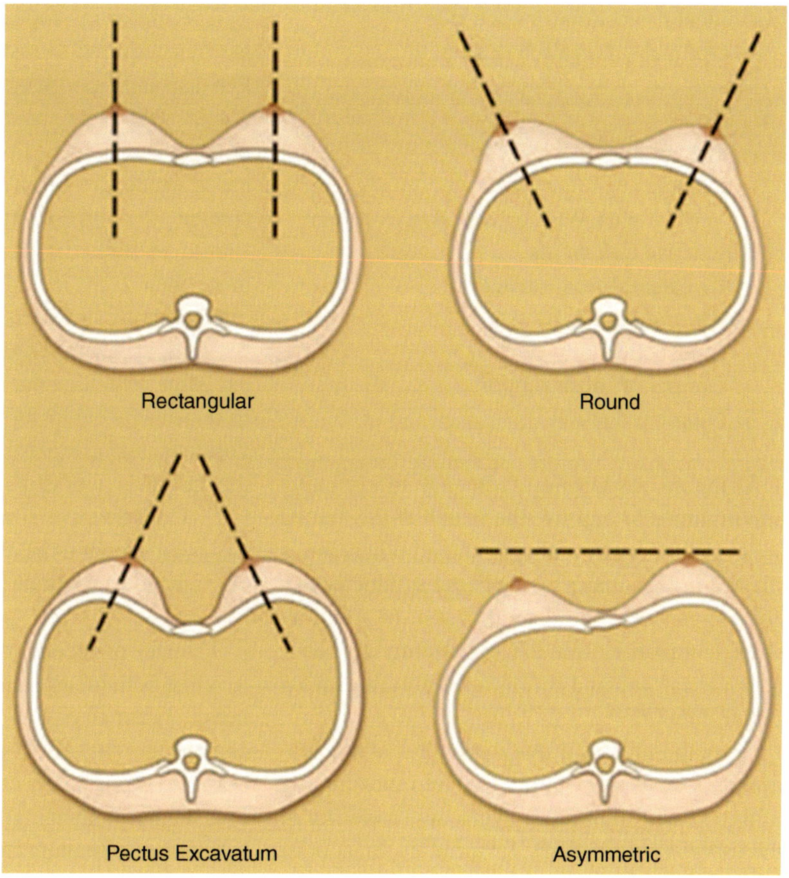

Fig. 12.2 Evaluation of Chest wall shape (Schwartz 2017)

the appropriate implant projection for each side of the chest to improve symmetry. Different volume and projection implants can be used on each side, with similar base diameters to create a better visual match to the breasts [7].

Finally assessing the patients axillary breast, fat and muscle tissue can allow selection of an appropriately shaped device to prevent exaggeration of this area. Taller shaped implants can be turned to avoid the axillary fullness, or lower height devices can be used to avoid over-filling the upper chest [8].

Treatment Modalities

The patient goals should be discussed to include:

- Size goals – Is either breast the appropriate size, and if so which?
- Shape goals – Does the patient desire a more natural, or augmented look?
- Implant tolerance – Will the patient accept an implant to correct her asymmetry?
- Scar tolerance – Will the patient accept mastopexy scars to correct her asymmetry?

It is important for both patient and surgeon to understand that symmetry is best achieved and maintained when both breasts are treated as similarly as possible. It is difficult to achieve long term symmetry with an implant in only one breast.

Once these areas have been discussed, the surgeon can utilize any combination of the following modalities and considerations to achieve a more aesthetically pleasing and symmetric breast:

- Augmentation with asymmetric Implants
  - Shaped vs Round implants
  - Smooth vs Textured

  - Ideal projection for each side
  - Optimal fill for each device
- Mastopexy
  - None
  - Peri-areolar
  - Vertical
  - Vertical with Wise pattern skin excision
- Adjunctive treatments
  - Unilateral breast reduction
  - Fat grafting
  - Liposuction
  - Dermal or Mesh support
  - Nipple reduction

Using an implant for symmetry offers many opportunities to improve the match of the treated breast. While many authors contend otherwise, a shaped implant may provide better symmetry to a non-augmented contralateral breast. In addition, shaped implants offer the opportunity to better match chest wall and soft tissue deformities from side to side [9].

Smooth implants provide excellent augmentation in patients who do not require repositioning of the breast footprint (ie aggressive lowering of the Inframammary fold). Textured implants offer more stability in patients with pitched chest wall in any direction, and in preventing long term implant malposition when aggressive breast reshaping is required [10].

Implants with differing projection and similar base diameter can correct asymmetry of breast volume and projection while giving the appearance of a more symmetric overall shape and breast base [11].

Finally implants with more optimal fill, and/or more cohesive gel may hold a better shape in the face of peri-areolar mastopexy, which causes flattening of the breast shape initially [7].

The use of mastopexy in achieving symmetry is often required to reshape one or both breasts. Peri-areolar mastopexy should be used to control nipple shape and position, but in the authors opinion is usually not powerful enough as a skin based procedure to effectively lift the breast, or change the breast footprint. This technique should be limited to repositioning the nipple no more than 2 cm in order to avoid nipple deformity, scarring or excessive stretch.

Vertical mastopexy, with any pattern of skin excision, provides the power of tissue excision to remove ptotic lower pole tissue, match breast volumes, and elevate the IMF. This technique is the author's workhorse for breast asymmetry [12]. Conservative simultaneous augmentation has been shown to be a safe and effective means of correcting breast volume and shape [13–15].

Primary or secondary fat grafting can be used to refine both breast shape, and volume to achieve better symmetry. Fat grafting can effectively change the shape and position of all the breast borders. Liposuction can be used to narrow the breast base diameter, and to create a more attractive shape, especially in the lateral breast border.

Case Examples

Figure 12.3 shows a 37 year old patient with breast and Chest wall Asymmetry.

Figure 12.4 shows a 34 year old with asymmetry of volume and ptosis.

Figure 12.5 shows a 29 year old patient with asymmetry of volume, nipple position and enlarged nipple diameter.

Figure 12.6 shows a 18 year old patient with volume, shape, and nipple asymmetry.

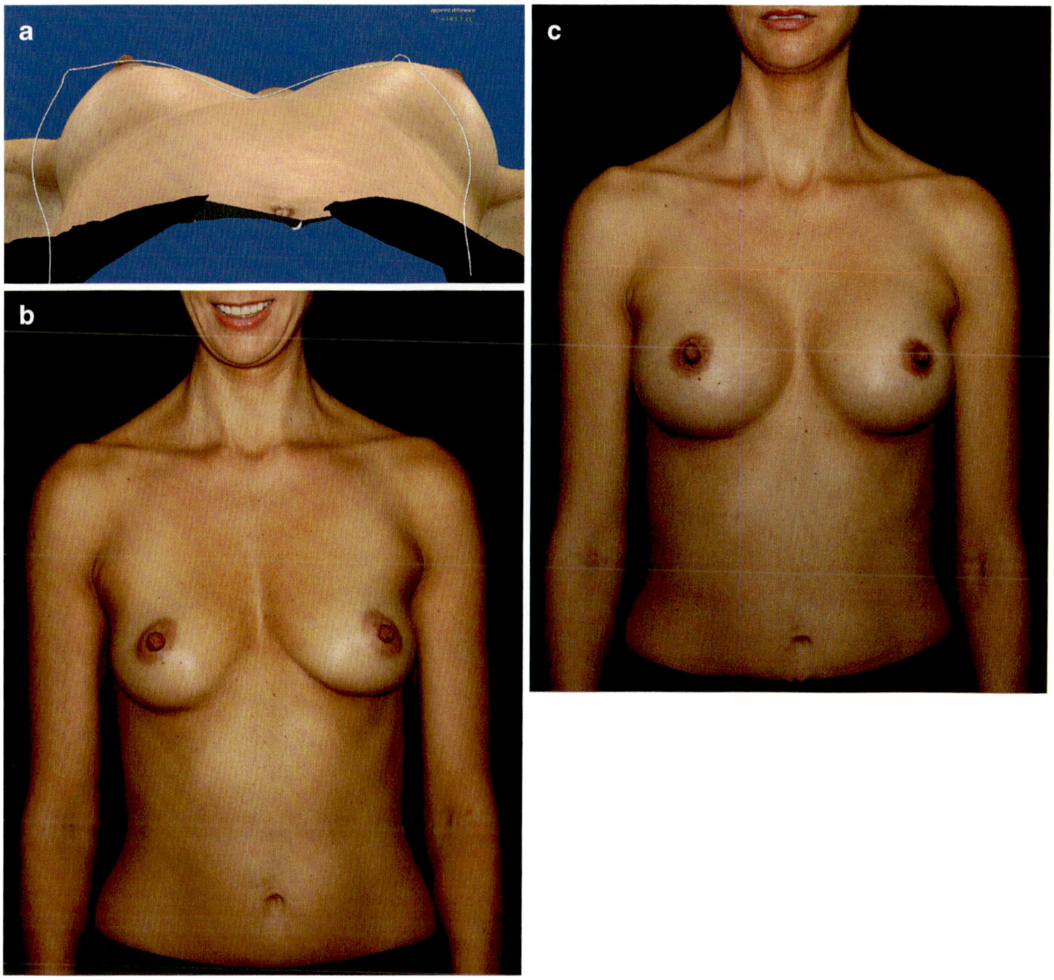

Fig. 12.3 37 year old patient with breast and Chest wall Asymmetry. (**a**) is a supine 3-D image showing volume and chest wall asymmetry. (**b**) shows pre-operative AP View. (**c**) shows 6-month Post operative views (Left breast – Allergan Style 115,222 cc, Right Breast – Allergan Style 410 MM 320 cc)

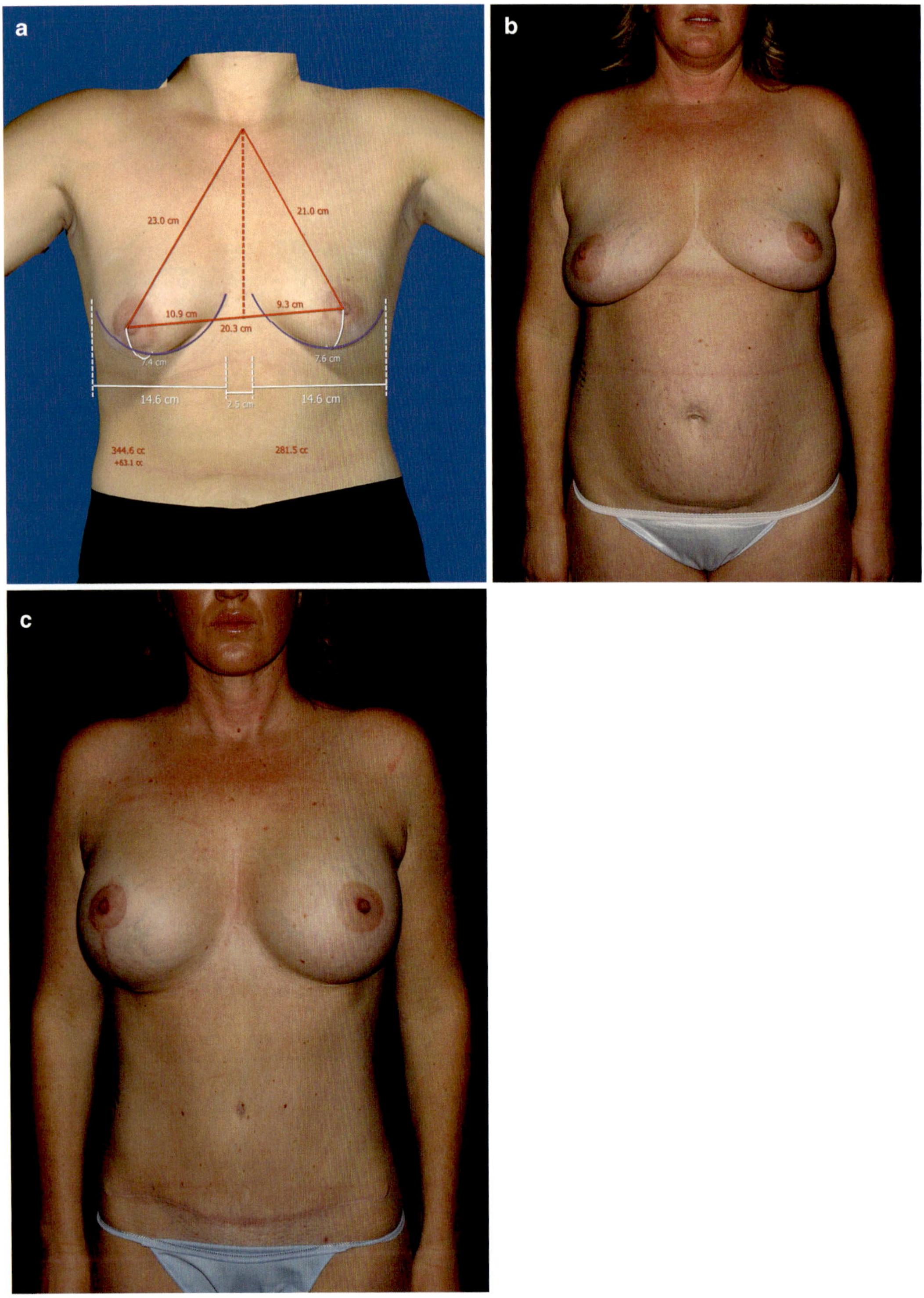

Fig. 12.4 Thirty-four year old with asymmetry of volume and ptosis. (**a**) Pre- op 3-D image. (**b**) Pre-op AP view. (**c**) Post op AP view. Patient underwent right augmentation with vertical mastopexy. Eighty-seven grams of breast tissue was removed. Left breast augmentation alone. Sientra 415 cc Round High Profile Textured Implants

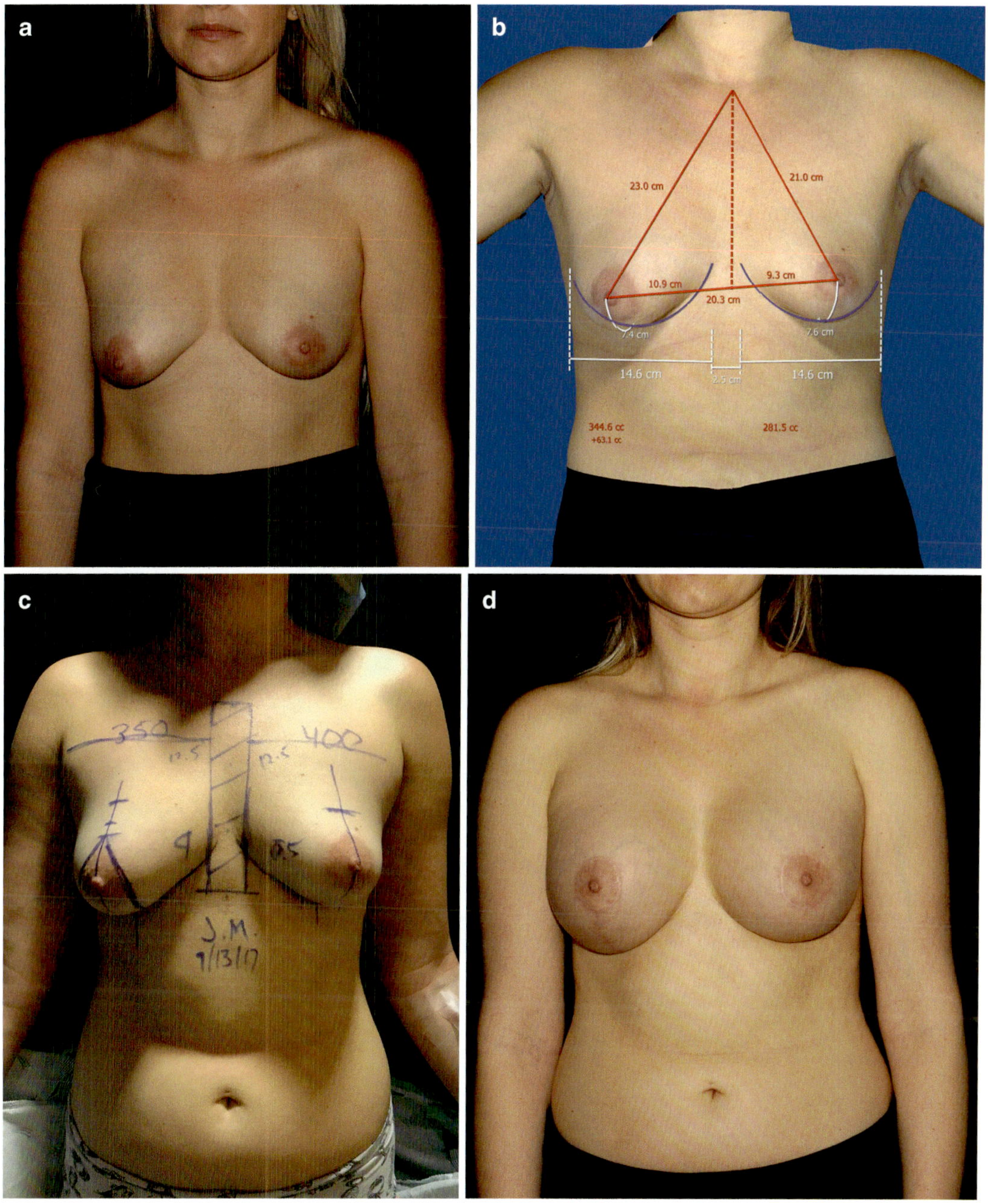

Fig. 12.5 A 29 year old patient with asymmetry of volume, nipple position and enlarged nipple diameter. (**a**) shows pre-op AP. (**b**) shows pre-operative volume and nipple asymmetry with Vectra imaging. (**c**) shows pre-op Markings. (**d**) shows six-month post op AP. The patient underwent Right Vertical mastopexy with removal 50 grams of breast tissue (Left Peri-areolar mastopexy. Sientra 415 cc Moderate Smooth implant both sides). Each breast was treated differently due to the difference in breast size and degree of ptosis. Differential tissue removal allows symmetric implants to create similar breast footprints

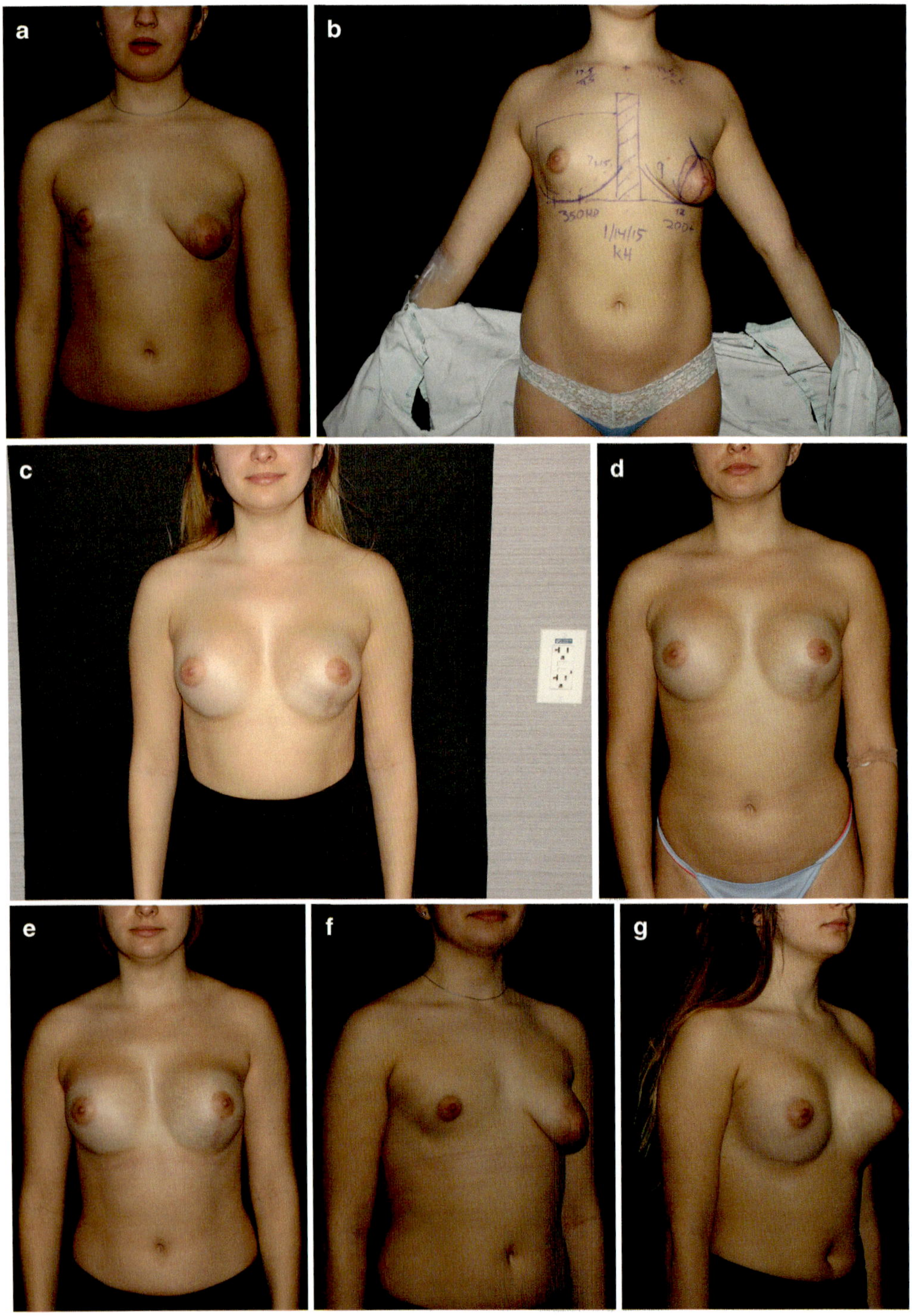

Fig. 12.6 Eighteen year old patient Volume, shape, and nipple asymmetry. (**a**) Pre op AP. (**b**) Pre operative Markings. (**c**) Six months Post op. (**d**) Three years post op. (**e**) 6 months post op Fat grafting to left breast. (**f**) Pre-op Oblique. (**g**) Six month post op Oblique. (**h**) Three year post op oblique. (**i**) Six month post fat graft Oblique. Surgery 1. Right Breast augmentation Sientra Round textured 350 cc High Profile. Left breast Vertical Mastopexy with removal of 53 grams of breast tissue, Sientra Round Textured 255 cc Moderate Profile

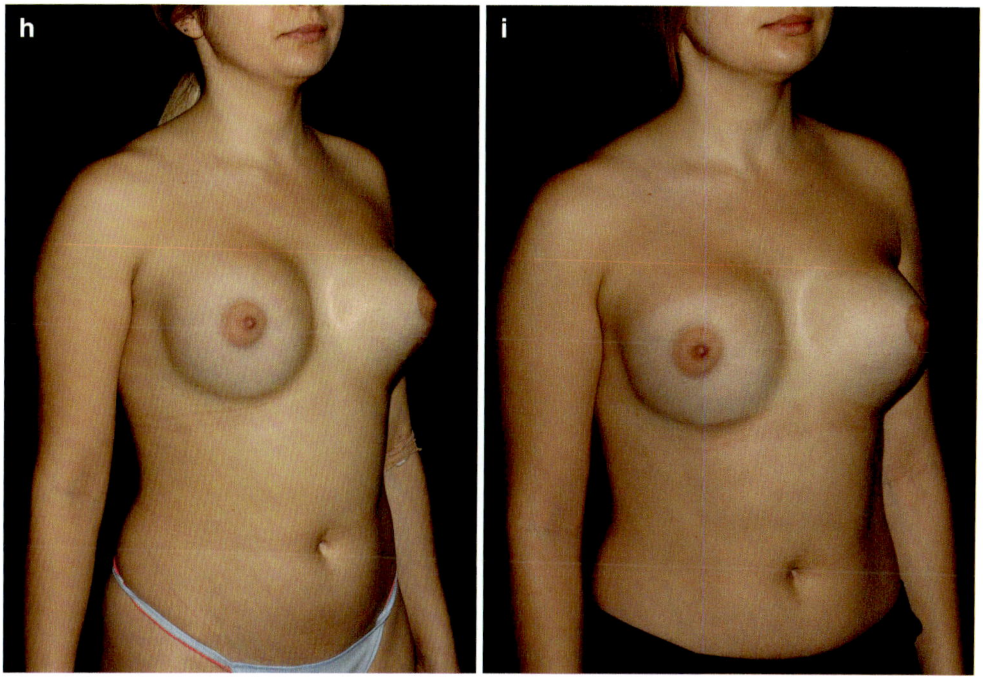

Fig. 12.6 (continued)

Bibliography

1. Poland A. Deficiency of the pectoral muscles. Guy's Hosp Rep. 1841;6:191.
2. Rohrich RJ, Hartley W, Brown S. Incidence of breast and chest wall asymmetry in breast augmentation: a retrospective analysis of 100 patients. Plast Reconstr Surg. 2003;111(4):1513–9.
3. Labow BI, et al. Psychological impact of breast asymmetry on adolescents: a prospective cohort study. Plast Reconstr Surg. 2014;134:1116.
4. Martinovic ME, Blanchet NP. BFACE: a framework for evaluating breast aesthetics. Plast Reconstr Surg. 2017;140:287e.
5. Hall-Findlay EJ. The three breast dimensions: analysis and effecting change. Plast Reconstr Surg. 2010;125(6):1632–42.
6. Roostaeian J, Adams WP. Three-dimensional imaging for breast augmentation: is this technology providing accurate simulations? Aesthetic Surg J. 2014;34(6):857–75.
7. Donfrancesco A, Montemurro P, Heden P. Three-dimensional simulated images in breast augmentation surgery: an investigation of patients' satisfaction and the correlation between prediction and actual outcome. Plast Reconstr Surg. 2013;132:810–22.
8. Schwartz M. Algorithm and techniques for using Sientra's silicone gel shaped implants in primary and revision breast augmentation. Plast Reconstr Surg. 2014;134:18S–27S.
9. Schwartz M. Evidence-based medicine: breast augmentation. Plast Reconstr Surg. 2017;140:109e.
10. Heden P, Montemurro P, et al. Anatomical and round breast implants: how to select and indications for use. Plast Reconstr Surg. 2015;136:263–72.
11. Caplin DA. Indications for the use of MemoryShape breast implants in aesthetic and reconstructive breast surgery: long-term clinical outcomes of shaped versus round silicone breast implants. Plast Reconstr Surg. 2014;134:27S–37S.
12. Calobrace MB. Reply: Simultaneous augmentation/mastopexy: a retrospective 5-year review of 332 consecutive cases. Plast Reconstr Surg. 2013;132:311e.
13. Stevens WG. One-stage mastopexy with breast augmentation: a review of 321 patients. Plast Reconstr Surg. 2007;120:1674–9.
14. Kim JYS, et al. A systematic review of single-stage augmentation-Mastopexy. Plast Reconstr Surg. 2014;134:922.
15. Pickett CL, et al. The subtleties of success in simultaeous augmentation-mastopexy. Plast Reconstr Surg. 2016;138:585.

Maintaining Upper Pole Fullness: Auto-augmentation Mastopexy with Soft Tissue Support Matrix and Lipofilling

13

Kamakshi R. Zeidler and R. Laurence Berkowitz

Introduction

The use of mastopexy has increased dramatically over the last 20 years; in 2019, mastopexy was the 7th most commonly performed cosmetic surgery in the US [1]. Desired outcomes of mastopexy include enhanced breast projection, corrected ptosis, prevention of bottoming out, minimal scarring, and durable upper-pole fullness. Consistently providing and maintaining optimal breast shape, particularly upper-pole fullness, is the greatest challenge in mastopexy procedures. Furthermore, many patients desire an aesthetic result without the use of implants.

A number of approaches to mastopexy have been described, including various skin incisions (eg, inverted-T, vertical, periareolar) and methods of rearranging breast dermis and/or parenchyma. Common approaches include the use of autologous tissues (eg, dermal shaping and flap-based auto-augmentation or "auto-implant" techniques), combined mastopexy/implant-based augmentation, and the use of biologically compatible meshes and soft tissue support matrices to maintain breast shape [2–11]. Auto-augmentation mastopexy is an evolving option for patients who want improved breast shape without the use of an implant. This technique can correct ptosis, while increasing the projection and apparent volume of the breast, and provides a more durable result with less tension on scars compared to dermal reshaping [12].

In the 1970s, Ribeiro et al. first described a technique using an inferior dermaglandular pedicle, which was pulled superiorly beneath the nipple-areola complex (NAC) during reduction mammaplasty [2]. The technique obviated the need for an implant by moving tissue from an area with excess mass, under the central parenchyma, and to an area that is often loose and empty, thereby providing improved upper-pole fullness and good vascularization of the lower portion of the breast. This inferiorly based dermaglandular flap derives vascular supply from the fourth, fifth, and sixth intercostal perforators of the internal mammary artery, allowing for greater lateral and medial reshaping than superior-based flaps, which have a superficial vascular supply [13, 14].

Despite the widespread use of the Ribeiro technique and its variations, surgeons noted a risk for bottoming out and a lack of fullness in the upper pole that developed over months following surgery. In 2000, Graf et al. reported an adaptation of the Ribeiro technique, in which the de-epithelialized dermaglandular flap is passed under a loop of pectoralis muscle (Figs. 13.1 and 13.2) [3]. The nipple remains attached to a superior pedicle and is inset once the medial and lateral breast columns are closed caudal to and on top of the affixed flap. This pectoralis sling, along

K. R. Zeidler (✉) · R. L. Berkowitz
Aesthetx, Campbell, CA, USA
e-mail: drz@aesthetx.com

M. B. Calobrace et al. (eds.), *Augmentation Mastopexy*,
https://doi.org/10.1007/978-3-030-48226-8_13

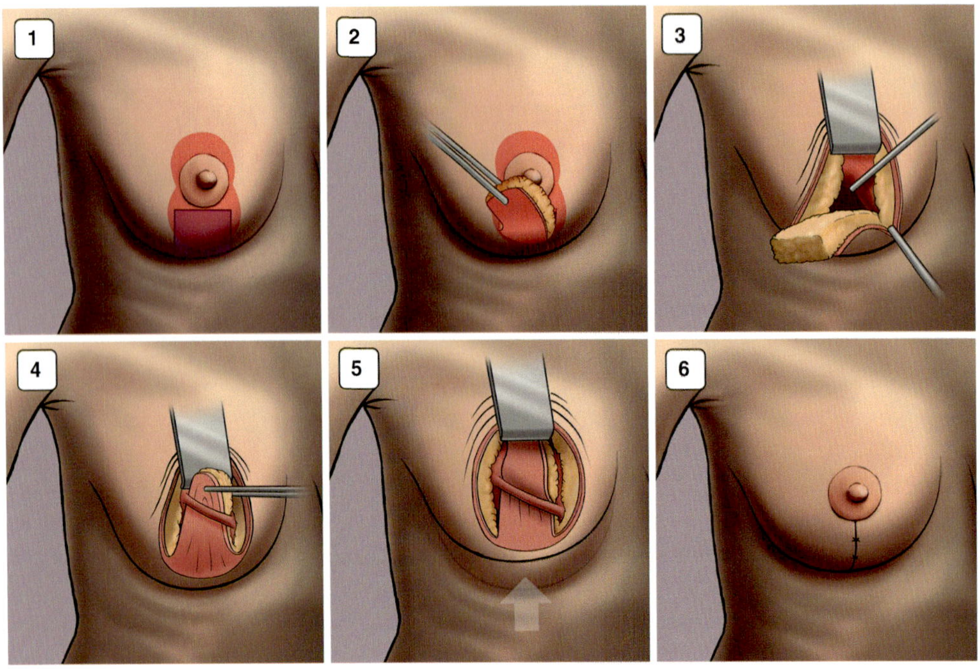

Fig. 13.1 Auto-augmentation mastopexy with pectoralis muscle sling. This demonstrates the Graf adaptation of the Ribeiro technique. (1) A vertical skin pattern is de-epithelialized (2). An inferiorly based chest wall dermaglandular flap is fashioned and separated from the surrounding medial and lateral breast pillars (3). The flap is folded caudally to show separation from surrounding tissue while the superior breast tissue is elevated off the pectoralis muscle fascia (4). A pectoralis sling is created from the pectoralis muscle and the autoaugmentation segment is passed under this muscle sling (5). The autoaugmentation segment is held in place with the pectoralis muscle sling in a more elevated position (6). The medial and lateral breast pillars are sutured together and the vertical incision is closed

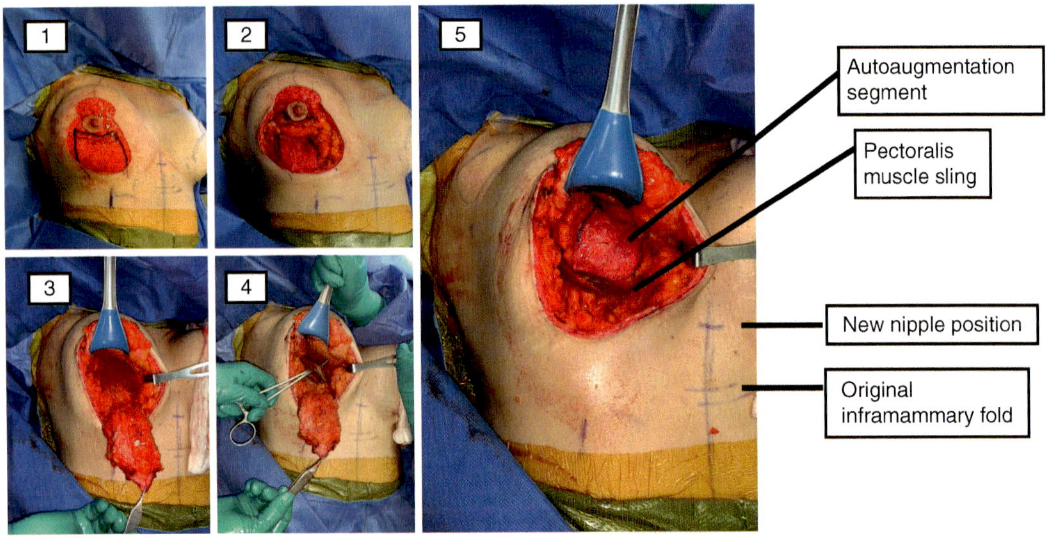

Fig. 13.2 Auto-augmentation mastopexy with pectoralis muscle sling. This demonstrates the steps illustrated in Fig. 13.1 (1). A vertical pattern skin reduction is de-epithelialized (2). An inferiorly based chest wall dermaglandular flap is fashioned and separated from the surrounding medial and lateral breast pillars (3). The flap is folded caudally (4). A pectoralis sling is created and the autoagmentation segment is passed under this loop of pectoralis muscle (5). The autoagmentation segment is held in place with the pectoralis muscle sling in a more elevated position. Note that the bulk of the tissue sits in the top pole of the breast, higher than the marked new nipple position. Also note that this elevation also raises the inframammary fold

with tacking sutures between the flap dermis and the pectoralis fascia, holds this flap in place under the NAC, preventing bottoming out and maintaining upper-pole fullness.

In the same timeframe, surgeons have developed techniques utilizing prosthetic mesh and soft tissue support matrix materials to create and maintain the desired breast shape [15–18]. In the 1990s, for example, Goes et al. reported a technique using synthetic mesh to improve long-term maintenance of breast shape [15, 19]. In these techniques, synthetic mesh acts as a form of connective tissue, providing breast support, particularly in the lower pole.

Even with these advanced techniques, optimizing breast projection and upper-pole fullness and preventing bottoming out have remained challenging with auto-augmentation strategies [20]. In particular, most variations of the Graf technique have limited utility in cases with very dense breast tissue that is difficult to slip behind the loop of pectoralis muscle or when the pectoralis muscle is too high to hold the breast tissue in place.

To further increase the durability of upper pole fullness following mastopexy, the author developed a modification of the Graf technique using synthetic (GalaFLEX®; Galatea Surgical, Lexington, MA) or biologic (Strattice™; Allergan, Inc., Dublin, Ireland) soft tissue support matrix ("matrix"). This three-part technique includes separating an inferiorly based dermaglandular flap, securing this flap to the pectoralis major muscle with a belt of synthetic or biologic matrix, and lipofilling to maintain upper pole stability and fullness.

Surgical Markings for Auto-augmentation Breast Lift

A vertical skin pattern excision is marked in the standing position (Fig. 13.3). Key landmarks include the midline, the breast meridians, the inframammary fold, and plan for the new nipple position. The breast meridians are marked as a vertical meridian, starting at a point that is half the distance from the sternal notch to the end of the clavicle; this point is carried down to the nipple to create the breast meridian and onto the chest wall below the inframammary crease. Any asymmetries between the breast meridians should then be adjusted to be equidistant from the midline, which may necessitate setting the new nipple position more medial or lateral, in addition to being elevated, depending on the degree of asymmetry. This new nipple position should be marked slightly higher than Pitanguy's point [21], as the autoaugmentation flap can elevate the nipple position similarly to breast implants [22]. A good standard is to mark the new nipple position at the

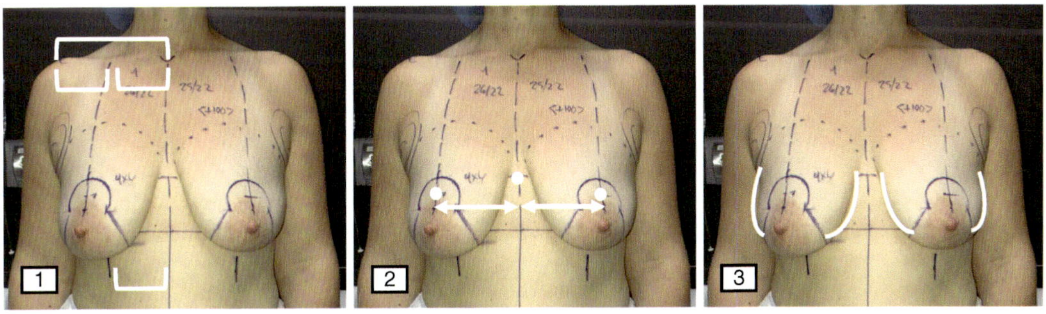

Fig. 13.3 Preoperative markings (1). The midline and breast meridians are marked. The breast meridians are marked at a point that is half the distance from the sternal notch to the end of the clavicle; this point is carried down to the nipple and to the chest wall below the inframammary crease. It is important that the distance of the breast meridian from the midline at the clavicle matches the distance of the breast meridian from the midline and the chest below the breast (2). The new nipple position is marked higher than Pitanguy's point [21], at the point where the inframammary fold crosses the midline. This new nipple position is a guide for positioning the matrix belt to secure the autoaugmentation segment. It is important that the distance of the new breast meridian and new nipple position are both equidistant from the midline (3). The vertical pattern is then completed and marked for skin excision using Lejour's maneuver [23]. The length of skin that is left behind should be equal medially and laterally on each breast

point where the inframammary fold crosses the midline while simulating lower pole skin excision; a 4 × 5 cm areolar window is marked around this new nipple position (4 cm vertical and 5 cm horizontal). This new nipple position is marked at the midline to serve as a guide for later positioning of the matrix belt when securing the auto-augmentation segment. The vertical pattern is then completed and marked for skin excision using Lejour's maneuver [23] by displacing the breast medially and laterally and marking vertical lines that correspond to the breast meridians superior and inferior to the lower pole of the breast. The vertical skin excision pattern should end at least 2 cm from the inframammary fold and can be modified intraoperatively to include a horizontal skin excision to prevent dog ear formation. The skin left behind should be equidistant from the midline and from the anterior axillary line which may mean that the vertical pattern excisions are slightly different in size/width from one breast to another if there is significant breast asymmetry.

Surgical Technique for Auto-augmentation Breast Lift with Matrix Belt

Creating the Auto-augmentation Segment

The vertical skin pattern is de-epithelialized, maintaining a new areolar diameter of 40–42 mm. The nipple is maintained on a superior pedicle. A horizonal incision is made into the breast gland within this pattern, about 1 cm below the new areolar margin to define the top portion of the inferiorly based dermaglandular flap, the auto-augmentation segment (Figs. 13.4 and 13.5).

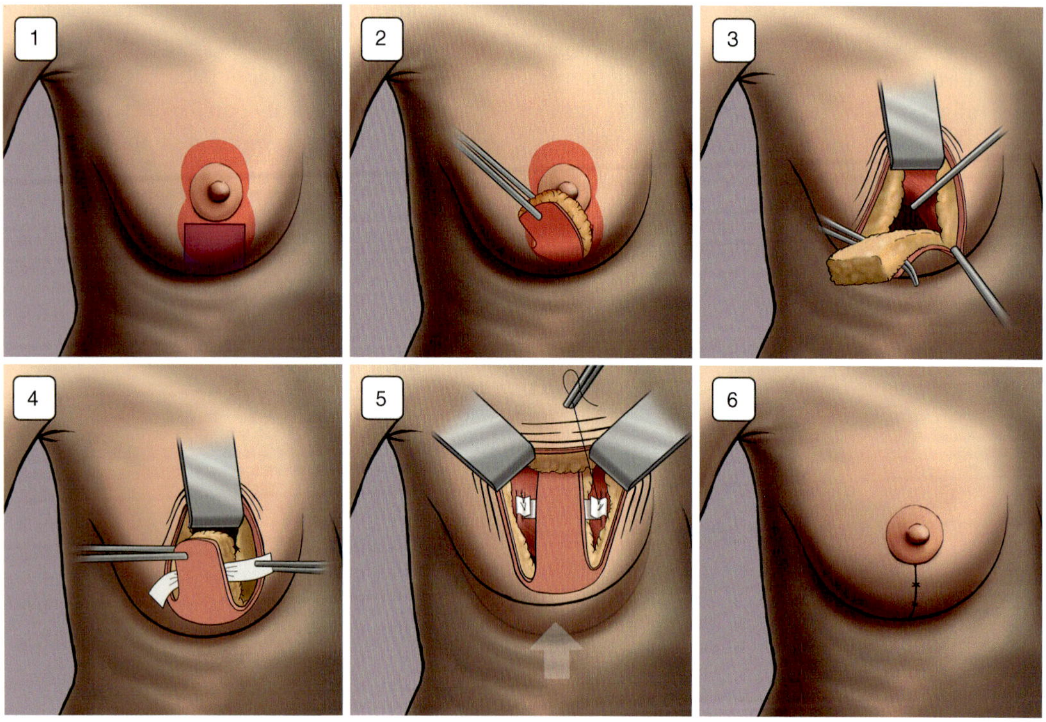

Fig. 13.4 Auto-augmentation astopexy with support matrix. Steps 1 through 3 are the same as the Graf pectoralis muscle sling technique detailed in Fig. 13.1, but differs for steps 4 thru 6 (1). A vertical skin pattern is de-epithelialized (2). An inferiorly based chest wall dermaglandular flap is fashioned and separated from the surrounding medial and lateral breast pillars (3). The flap is folded caudally (4). A horizontal tunnel is made beneath the dermis in the lower portion of the autoaugmentation segment and the matrix is passed through this tunnel (5). The autoaugmentation segment is held in place with the matrix sling which is secured to the underlying pectoralis muscle both medially and laterally by weaving it through and then securing it around a small slip of muscle (6). The medial and lateral breast pillars are sutured together and the vertical incision is closed

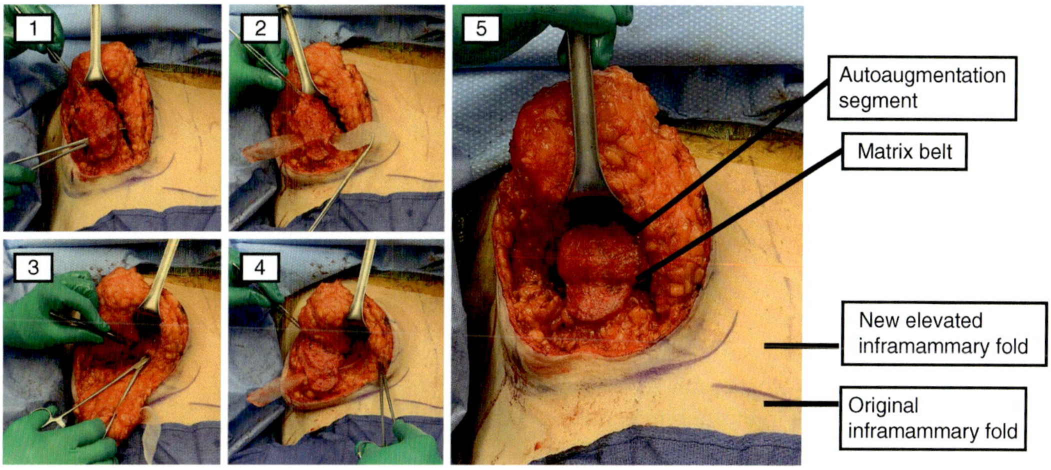

Fig. 13.5 Auto-augmentation mastopexy with a support matrix. This demonstrates the steps illustrated in Fig. 13.4 (1). After preparing the inferiorly based dermaglandular flap as described in Fig. 13.4, a horizontal tunnel is made beneath the dermis in the lower portion of the autoaugmentation segment (2). The matrix is passed through this tunnel. Note that the tunnel is positioned relatively low on the autoaugmentation segment such that it can effectively lift the tissue high into the breast (3). The autoaugmentation segment with matrix attached is reflected caudally and a small tunnel is made in the pectoralis muscle medially at the level of the mid portion of the breast (set at the level of the new nipple position) (4). The matrix is passed through this tunnel, folded back on itself and secured with sutures (5). The autoaugmentation segment is held in place with the matrix sling which is secured to the underlying pectoralis muscle both medially and laterally. Note that the bulk of the tissue sits in the top pole of the breast, which ensures fullness and projection. Also note that this elevation of tissue is significant enough to raise the position of the inframammary fold

Incisions are made medially and laterally at the borders of the vertical skin pattern reduction down to the chest wall to further define the auto-augmentation segment. Care should be taken to preserve symmetric medial and lateral pillars on either side of the segment. This can be achieved by displacing the breast tissue medially and laterally using Lejour's maneuver and ensuring that the breast gland is divided perpendicular to the chest wall, in line with the breast meridian above and below the region of dissection. This auto-augmentation segment is based mainly on the fourth, fifth, and sixth intercostal perforators, (as it is the same pedicle used for an inferior pedicle technique mastopexy or breast reduction, but in this technique the pedicle feeds only the auto-augmentation segment and not the nipple areola complex). The dissection of this auto-augmentation segment should be carried out in such a way that the base of the flap becomes wider as it approaches the chest wall. This auto-augmentation segment can be quite large in patients with large breasts, with a base of up to 8–10 cm and a length of 10–15 cm. The flap should be checked for vascularity and trimmed as needed to prevent future necrosis.

Securing the Auto-augmentation Segment with Prosthetic Matrix

After the inferiorly based auto-augmentation segment has been defined, the remainder of the breast is elevated off the chest wall superiorly in the subglandular plane to make space for the auto-augmentation segment. This dissection should match that of a subglandular dissection for breast augmentation with breast implants. The auto-augmentation segment should be transposed into this space to ensure that the top of the flap has room to sit above the level of the new nipple position. This ensures that there will be adequate fullness in the top of the breast and that it adds to the projection of the breast.

A belt of either synthetic or biologic support matrix is used to hold the breast tissue in place to prevent downward migration and bottoming out over time. This belt should be fashioned out of acellular dermal matrix or long-acting resorbable synthetic matrix and be about 2 cm wide and 20 cm long. For large breasts and large auto-augmentation segments, wider and longer belts may be required. Two matrix materials commonly used for this purpose include Strattice and Galaflex. Strattice is a decellularized, non-crosslinked, porcine-derived biologic material that has been widely used in breast surgery. Since the introduction of Galaflex, a biologically derived scaffold constructed from poly-4-hydroxybutyrate, this synthetic soft tissue support matrix is now the preferred material to provide long lasting support for the auto-augmentation segment. This belt will be positioned horizontally to secure the auto-augmentation segment to the pectoralis major muscle at the level of or slightly higher than the new nipple position (Figs. 13.4 and 13.5). A small horizontal tunnel is made within the autoaugmentation segment using a clamp with gentle spreading to avoid injury to the vascular supply. The belt of matrix is then passed through the tunnel, and the auto-augmentation segment is moved superiorly and woven in place to the underlying muscle. This is accomplished by using a clamp to make a small tunnel within the pectoralis muscle medially and laterally, and the medial and lateral ends of the matrix are respectively passed through these tunnels in the muscle, such that the matrix can be passed through and then folded back onto itself and then secured with a long-acting resorbable suture, such as polydioxanone.

After the auto-augmentation segment has been secured, vascularity should be confirmed, and if there are any concerns, the matrix belt can be adjusted to avoid vascular strangulation and the auto-augmentation segment can be trimmed to prevent future necrosis. While this technique can be done more simply by overlaying the matrix and suturing it to the auto-augmentation segment and the pectoralis muscle, the added steps to weave the matrix in place both within the auto-augmentation segment and into the pectoralis muscle provide a much more durable lift (Fig. 13.6).

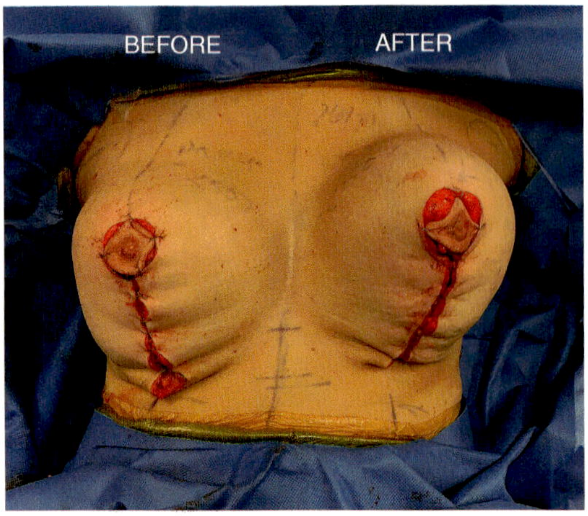

Fig. 13.6 Before and after placement of a matrix belt. This demonstrates the difference in upper pole fullness and inframammary fold position before and after placement of the soft tissue support matrix. The left shows tailor tacking of the breast *before* any soft tissue matrix has been added. The right shows tailor tacking of the breast *after* matrix has been used to secure the autoaugmentation segment superiorly. Note the difference in the fullness of the upper pole of the breast as well as the elevation of the inframammary fold after matrix has been placed

Shaping the Breast

After the auto-augmentation segment has been secured to the chest wall using matrix support, the top portion of the flap is fixed to pectoralis fascia superiorly with short-acting resorbable sutures. The breast tissue inferiorly is coned to create added projection by approximating the medial and lateral pillars with several interrupted sutures. The auto-augmentation segment will not be in the way of this closure, as it will have been transposed superiorly. At this point, the breasts can be tailor tacked with staples, and the nipple lifted into the new elevated position, which sometimes requires some release of the dermis at the edges medially and laterally, being mindful of the blood supply. The patient should be brought into the sitting position to ensure symmetry of the breasts and the auto-augmentation segments (Figs. 13.6 and 13.7). Adjustments can be made to the inframammary region with a horizontal excision of skin and dermis to prevent dog ear formation, but care should be taken to avoid excis-

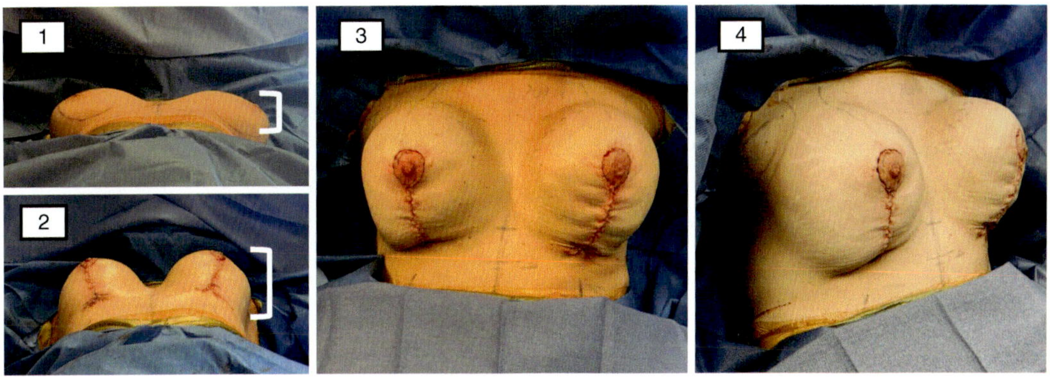

Fig. 13.7 Immediate results after auto-augmentation mastopexy with matrix belt (1). Preoperative view of breasts while patient is supine demonstrating poor projection and lateral breast displacement (2). Immediate postoperative results while patient is supine demonstrating increased projection and centralization of breast tissue volume (3). Immediate postoperative results with frontal view of breasts in sitting position. A small horizontal T incision at the inframammary fold prevents dog ear formation. Wrinkling on the bottom of the breast is expected with a vertical technique (4). Immediate postoperative results with side view of breasts in sitting position. Note that the upper pole of the breast has significant volume and projection. Also note that the breast should have an initial appearance of an "upside down" breast with fullness on the top and flatness on the bottom

ing any of the auto-augmentation segment as this could compromise the inferior vascular supply. Liposuction and contouring of the lateral chest and axillary regions are performed at this time to further shape the breast and its transition to the chest wall. Because the tissues are so well opposed, surgical drains are not required. Closure of the superficial layers is carried out with subcutaneous sutures in the vertical incision to relieve tension. The skin is then closed with a single bidirectional barbed suture (Quill™; Surgical Specialties Corp., Westwood, MA), which can be started where the vertical closure meets the peri-areolar closure and run around the areola in subcuticular fashion. The other limb of the suture can be run down the vertical incision in the deep dermis and back up in the subcuticular plane.

The results of this auto-augmentation technique have been excellent and durable. Figure 13.8 shows an illustrative patient a year and a half after auto-augmentation with a Galaflex matrix belt to correct post-partum breast ptosis. The patient had bilateral lipofilling at the time of the mastopexy to maximize breast volume and upper pole fullness.

Pectoralis Major Muscle Sling Versus Matrix Belt for Auto-augmentation Breast Lift

The pectoralis muscle sling technique as originally described by Graf et al. [3] is a similar technique to the matrix belt technique described above. Instead of matrix, a bipedicle muscle flap in the upper portion of the pectoralis muscle is fashioned in line with the muscle fibers, and the auto-augmentation segment is passed through the muscle and secured in place with sutures. The muscle is snug and robust enough to hold the breast tissue in place for long-lasting results [24]. This muscle sling technique is appropriate for patients who do not want any foreign material placed in their body and for small breasts with auto-augmentation segments that are relatively limited. For patients with moderate to large breasts, and those with dense breast tissue, there is often not enough space to tuck the auto-augmentation segment under the muscle sling, and therefore a matrix belt is necessary in these cases.

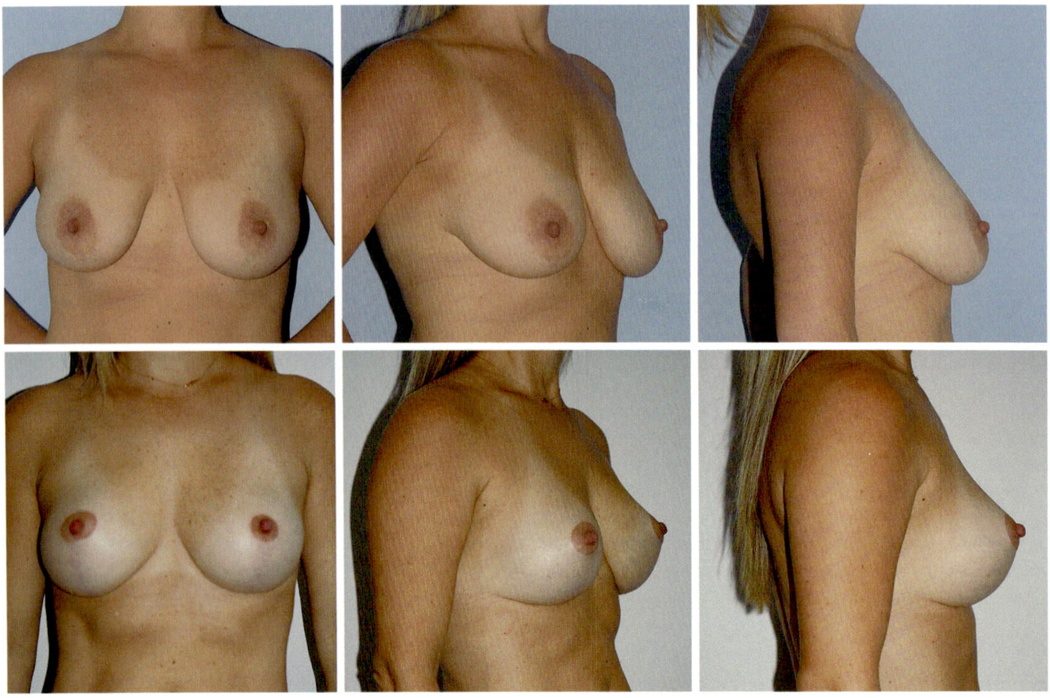

Fig. 13.8 Long term results with matrix belt and lipofilling. This demonstrates preoperative (above) and postoperative (below) results at 18 months following autoaugmentation with matrix belt and lipofilling. Note the round appearance of the breasts in postoperative frontal view, and the lift and projection in the postoperative side views

Auto-augmentation Breast Lift Combined with Breast Reduction

This auto-augmentation technique is an effective tool for creating upper pole fullness in patients who want an overall decrease in breast size, but still want fullness in the breast. The technique is carried out in a similar fashion, with a vertical pattern skin reduction and creation of an inferiorly based dermaglandular auto-augmentation segment, but tissue is then also removed from the upper lateral breast (Fig. 13.9). In general, a breast lift without removal of tissue can make the breast size feel and look smaller by up to one cup size [25]. A small reduction of lateral breast tissue can accomplish further modest breast reduction (volumes 100–200 cc) and can provide a further cup-size reduction. These patients are more likely to have large auto-augmentation segments and often have dense breast tissue, making a belt of matrix necessary to hold the tissue in place. They often also have larger amounts of skin to manage and are, therefore, more likely to need a small horizontal skin excision in the inframammary fold to prevent dog ear formation.

Auto-augmentation Breast Lift: A Valuable Option After Removal of Breast Implants

There is an increasing trend towards breast implant removal, given some of the current controversies in breast augmentation, as well as a changing breast aesthetic to a slightly smaller and more natural appearance [1]. Many patients will develop significant ptosis and loss of fullness in the upper breast after implants have been removed. The auto-augmentation technique can be used to fill the space left behind after an implant is removed and can produce a smaller breast with excellent youthful contours. Ideal

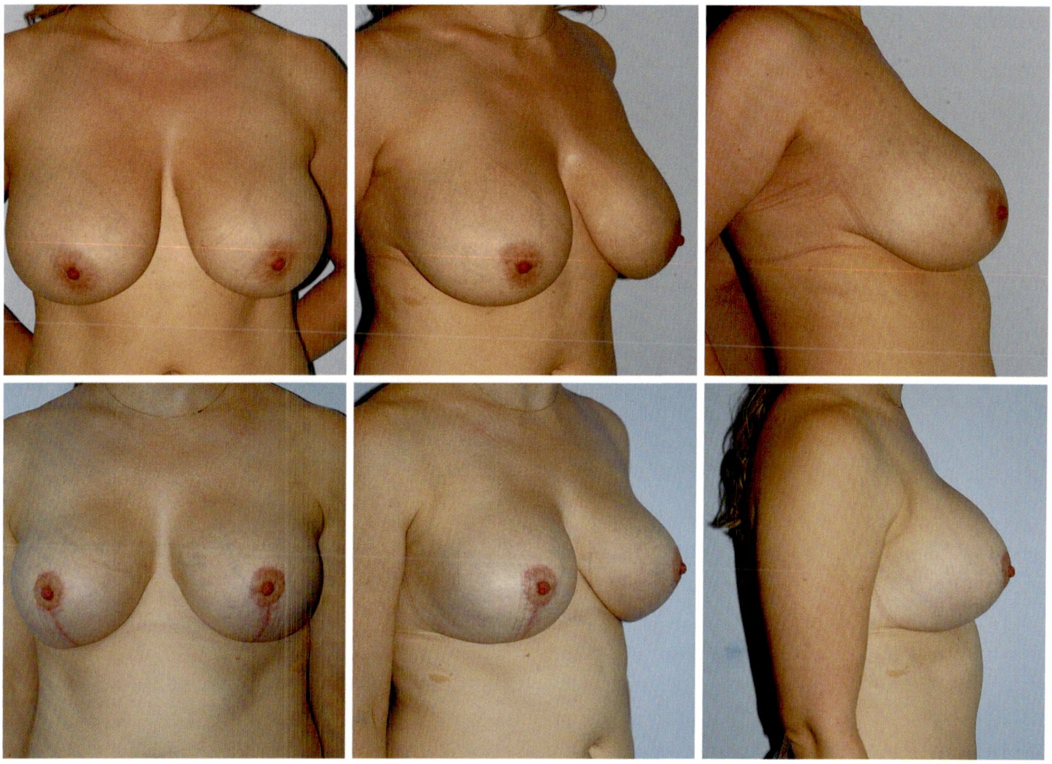

Fig. 13.9 Long term results with matrix belt and breast reduction. This demonstrates preoperative (above) and postoperative (below) results at 12 months following auto-augmentation with matrix belt and small reduction. Note, in the postoperative views, the round appearance of the breasts in frontal view, and the lift and projection in the side views

candidates have an even distribution of breast volume over their implants. Patients with very thin tissue and those with disproportionately thin lower poles are not good candidates.

Prior incisions must be carefully assessed in these patients. Patients with prior breast implant placement through axillary and periareolar incisions are ideal candidates, as there has been no disruption of the vascular supply of the inferiorly based dermaglandular auto-augmentation segment. For patients with implants placed through an inframammary incision, this vascular supply has been interrupted, and therefore, a laterally based auto-augmentation segment can be fashioned (Fig. 13.10). This segment can be moved medially and superiorly and fixated to the chest wall with a pectoralis sling or a belt of matrix. The muscle sling or belt of matrix must be vertically oriented to adequately hold the tissue in place. This laterally based auto-augmentation segment is often thinner and has higher risk of necrosis, so caution should be taken to avoid tension, and the segment should be trimmed to ensure good vascular supply.

When implants are being removed from the submuscular position, the technique can be more challenging and requires a few extra steps to ensure an adequate aesthetic and stable result, compared to removal of implants from the subglandular position. The reason the technique is a challenge in this setting is that submuscular implants often stretch and thin the pectoralis major muscle. When implants are removed from this submuscular position, with or without capsulectomy, the muscle must be stitched to the chest wall with an appropriate amount of tension and with multiple quilting sutures. The overlying breast tissue is often pulled and can be tethered and puckered by its natural adherence to the underlying muscle when the muscle is

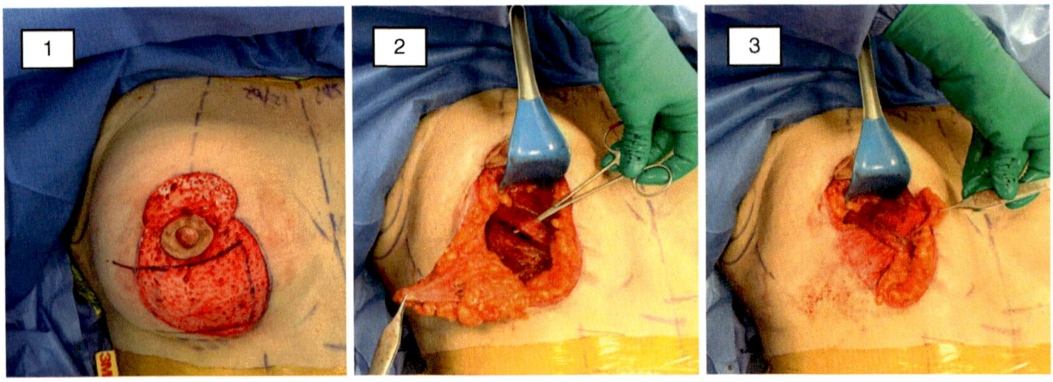

Fig. 13.10 Laterally based auto-augmentation segment (1). A laterally based dermaglandular flap is designed (2). The flap is reflected laterally and a pectoralis sling in defined (3). The autoaugmentation segment is pulled underneath a muscle sling and into superior and medial position to provide upper medial breast fullness

repaired. Therefore, the breast tissue must be dissected off the anterior surface of the underlying pectoralis major muscle in the subglandular plane for full release. This maneuver will make space for the auto-augmentation segment and allow the rest of the breast to appropriately re-drape over the segment. It is important to keep the pectoralis muscle fascia intact on top of the muscle to help hold the thinned-out fibers together. If the breast implant capsule can be left in place after implant removal, its position on the posterior surface of the muscle acts as an additional stabilizing force to hold these thinned muscle fibers together.

When implants are removed with a capsulectomy, and the capsule is removed from the posterior surface of the muscle, the muscle can be friable. In this setting, a pectoralis major muscle sling can be impossible to perform, as it may tear and lacks stability because the bipedicle muscle flap is not stable at the medial/inferior side. In the setting of removal of submuscular implants, a matrix belt is a more robust and reliable way to secure the auto-augmentation segment. This procedure must be performed carefully to ensure the matrix belt is adequately secured to the muscle. Figure 13.11 demonstrates long term results after breast implant removal and reshaping with a laterally based auto-augmentation segment, secured with a belt of Galaflex matrix.

Combining Auto-augmentation Breast Lift with Lipofilling

Lipofilling is a great addition to the auto-augmentation technique for patients who want a modest increase in breast size and a natural fullness of the upper pole of the breast. Patients who want a high degree of fullness in the upper pole and a convex curvature of their cleavage are not good candidates for lipofilling and require breast implants to achieve a more satisfying result. As previously mentioned, the auto-augmentation technique with matrix belt is an excellent method to restore a youthful and perky, albeit smaller breast, after removal of breast implants. In this setting of volume loss and lack of adequate shape when implants are removed, thinned out breast tissue can be addressed with lipofilling. Lipofilling, or autologous fat transfer to the breast, can give added volume and be placed strategically to fill irregularities. Many patients who want implant removal are pleased by the idea of using their own natural tissue to achieve volume.

When lipofilling is performed at the same time as the auto-augmentation breast lift technique, it is important that the fat that is injected is highly purified. When doing a lift, the tissues are often tight, and there is limited space to place fat before interstitial fluid pressure increases to impair capillary blood flow, potentially leading to poor graft-to-recipient interface, decreased oxygen

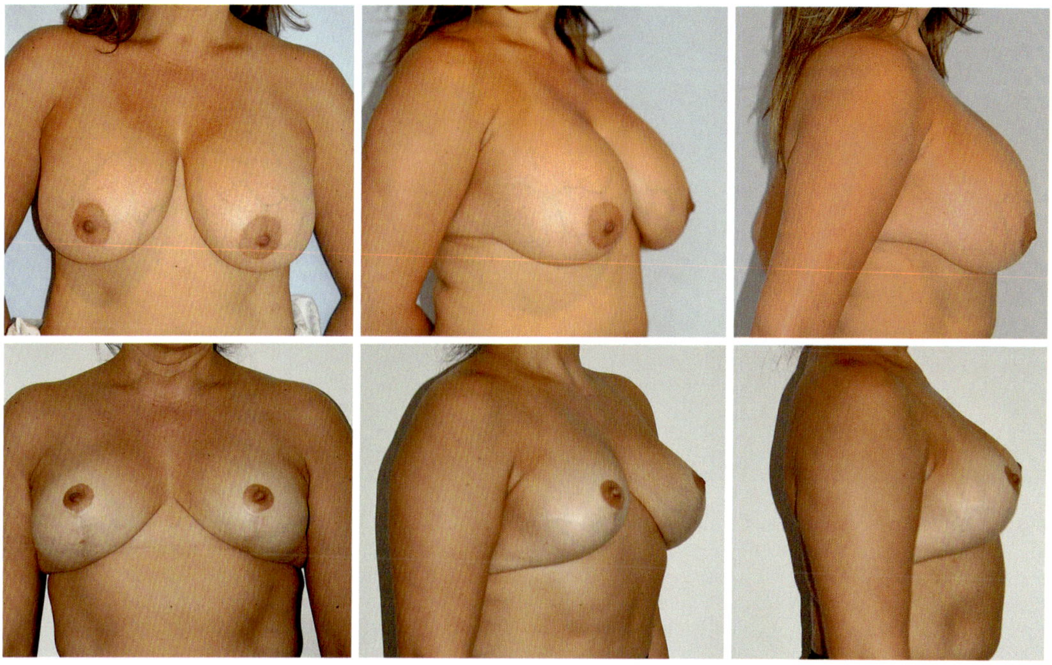

Fig. 13.11 Long term results with matrix belt and removal of breast implants. This demonstrates preoperative (above) and postoperative (below) results at 24 months following autoaugmentation with a matrix belt after the removal of submuscular implants. A laterally based autoaugmentation segment was used because the prior breast augmentation was performed through an inframammary incision making an inferiorly based dermaglandular flap not possible. The matrix belt was oriented vertically to hold the laterally based dermaglandular in place. Note, in the postoperative views, the fullness created in the medial cleavage from the autoaugmentation segment

delivery to the grafted adipocytes, and central graft necrosis [26]. Because there is limited capacity in the recipient site, every attempt should be made to use highly purified, viable adipose tissue, with minimal contaminants (e.g., blood cells, free lipids), to promote predictable long-term graft take and survival.

Achieving Predictable Results with Lipofilling

There are many techniques available for processing and purifying fat grafts, including strainers, centrifugation, and closed systems such as Revolve™ (Allergan, Inc., Dublin, Ireland) and Puregraft® (Puregraft LLC, Solana Beach, CA). In vivo studies have shown that the Puregraft system produces the highest concentration of viable fat cells and the lowest levels of contaminants [27–29]. This single-use, low-cost, consumable filtration system dialyzes harvested fat, removing blood, free lipids, fluid, and fragmented cells in a simple and sterile, closed system (Fig. 13.12). To use the system, harvested lipoaspirate is either suctioned directly into or transferred by injecting into the device and then filtered through a built-in membrane, which removes free lipids and other contaminants. The concentrated graft is then washed with lactated Ringer's or saline solution and then removed from the device with a syringe for use. Long-term MRI studies have demonstrated the durable stability of these fat grafts with an overall significantly better long-term retention rate than other methods. A decade of personal experience corroborates these findings.

A few steps should be considered when lipofilling a breast at the time of initial aesthetic breast surgery in conjunction with the autoaugmentation technique. Depending on the vol-

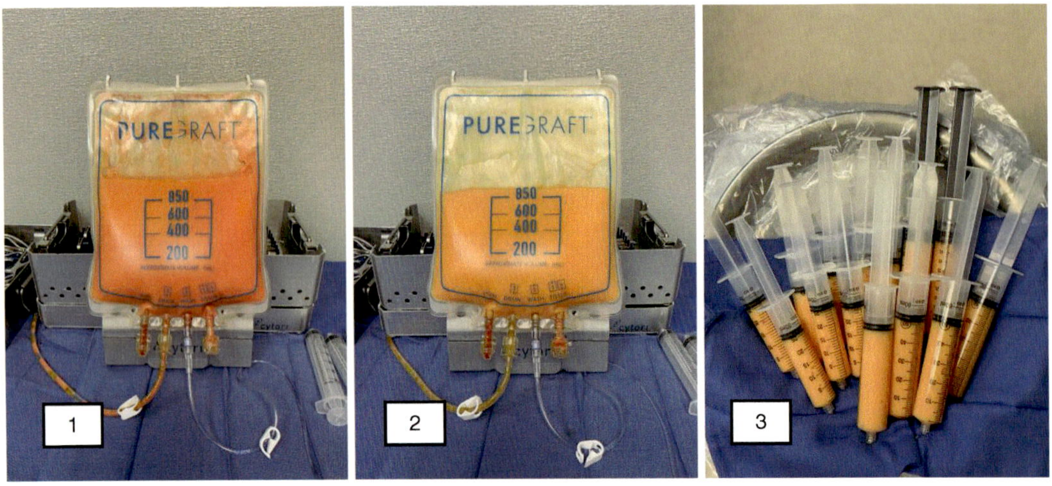

Fig. 13.12 Use of Puregraft for fat transfer and lipofilling. This shows intraoperative filtration of lipoaspirate with the Puregraft system (1). Lipoaspirate is collected directly into a large puregraft device. While the lipoaspirate overall looks relatively clean, it is first drained of excess free fluid and then washed with LR containing gentamycin and again drained to remove contaminants (2). The lipoaspirate has been cleaned and concentrated as demonstrated by a cleaner yellow color and a decrease in volume (3). Fat is drawn up into 25 cc syringes

ume of fat to be transferred (i.e., small [100–200 cc] vs. large [200–450 cc] volumes), the mastopexy markings should be slightly looser when Lejour's maneuver is performed to mark the vertical skin excision. This ensures that the recipient site will have adequate capacity to receive the volume of fat grafted. Making the skin very snug limits the capacity of the recipient bed; therefore, it is important to maintain a little extra skin to leave room for lipofilling.

The surgical technique should proceed first with defining and securing the auto-augmentation segment up to the point of tacking the skin temporarily with staples and the completion of lipocontouring. Puncture holes should be made at points remote from the incisions to avoid fat from interfering with incisional healing. Puncture holes can be made in the periareolar region, and from this area, fat can be grafted into the subcutaneous plane and into the breast tissue. Care should be taken to inject fat predominantly into the upper pole of the breast and to fill the upper lateral breast as much as the upper medial breast. This ensures that patients will not develop a lateral dip, which is a significant contributor to a "droopy" appearing breast after mastopexy. The auto-augmentation segment itself should not be filled with fat, as this could lead to vascular compromise. For patients with additional fat available to graft, and a limited capacity in the actual breast tissue, the pectoralis muscle can be filled, but should be filled in the central and lower regions to avoid a masculine appearance with excessive fullness in the top of the muscle. Prior to closure, the wound should be irrigated copiously to ensure that fat is not free floating within any of the open spaces between the tissues, and there should be a low threshold to place a surgical drain to minimize the risk of seroma.

For significant breast asymmetry in patients undergoing auto-augmentation mastopexy, patients should be advised that two rounds of fat transfer will often be required to achieve symmetric results. The competitive forces of tightening and lifting with volume expansion often limit the volume increase achievable with one round of fat transfer. Patients should be advised that a follow-up procedure can be done to provide additional volume to the smaller breast (Fig. 13.13).

For patients undergoing breast implant removal with immediate auto-augmentation breast lift, caution must be taken with lipofilling in patients with thin tissues, as there is limited capacity in the recipient bed. When the breast implant capsule can be kept in place, it helps to hold the fat in position. Often times, however, patients want the implant capsule removed, which can make it difficult to keep the fat in

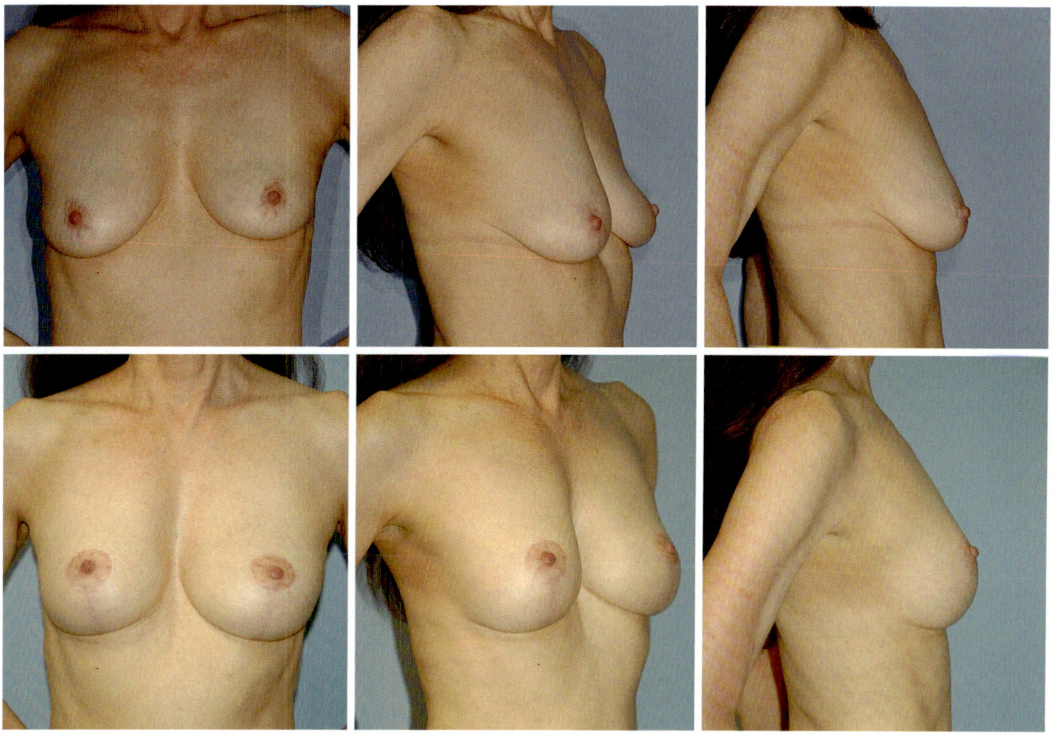

Fig. 13.13 Long term results with matrix belt and serial lipofilling. This demonstrates preoperative (above) and postoperative (below) results at 24 months following autoaugmentation with matrix belt and two rounds of lipofilling. This patient had significant preoperative asymmetry and wanted as much fullness as possible. She underwent autoaugmentation with a Strattice matrix belt and lipofilling with more fat placed on her smaller side, followed by a second round of lipofilling on her smaller side a few months later. Note that her postoperative breast size is much larger

place, particularly in the lower pole, which often needs it most. Sometimes fat can be grafted into the pectoralis major muscle if it is not too friable, but caution must be taken to keep the fat central and low in the muscle to ensure that the results are not masculinizing. These patients should be advised to expect a secondary and possibly a tertiary lipofilling procedure to add further volume and achieve a pleasing contour, particularly in the lower pole of the breast.

Auto-augmentation Technique for Breast Reconstruction after Lumpectomy in Irradiated Patients

This technique can be used to achieve symmetry in patients who have undergone lumpectomy with adjuvant radiation for breast cancer as an oncoplastic type of reconstruction. Extreme caution should be taken on the radiated side due to the risk of fat necrosis and unpredictable results as the tissue heals [30–32]. Furthermore, the auto-augmentation segment is at high risk for fat necrosis given the fibrosis and overall compromised vasculature of the radiated tissue. When doing a bilateral breast lift with or without reduction in the setting of breast asymmetry due to prior lumpectomy and radiation, the radiated side should be treated with a skin-only excision lift and central mound technique without any dermaglandular rearrangement and without the placement of any matrix. The fibrosis of the skin is usually adequate to hold the tissue for a long-lasting result. The nonradiated side can be treated as has been described with an auto-augmentation technique, with matrix belt, with or without lipofilling (Fig. 13.14). Patients undergoing this procedure should be advised that residual asymmetry will likely persist and that additional lipofilling may be required.

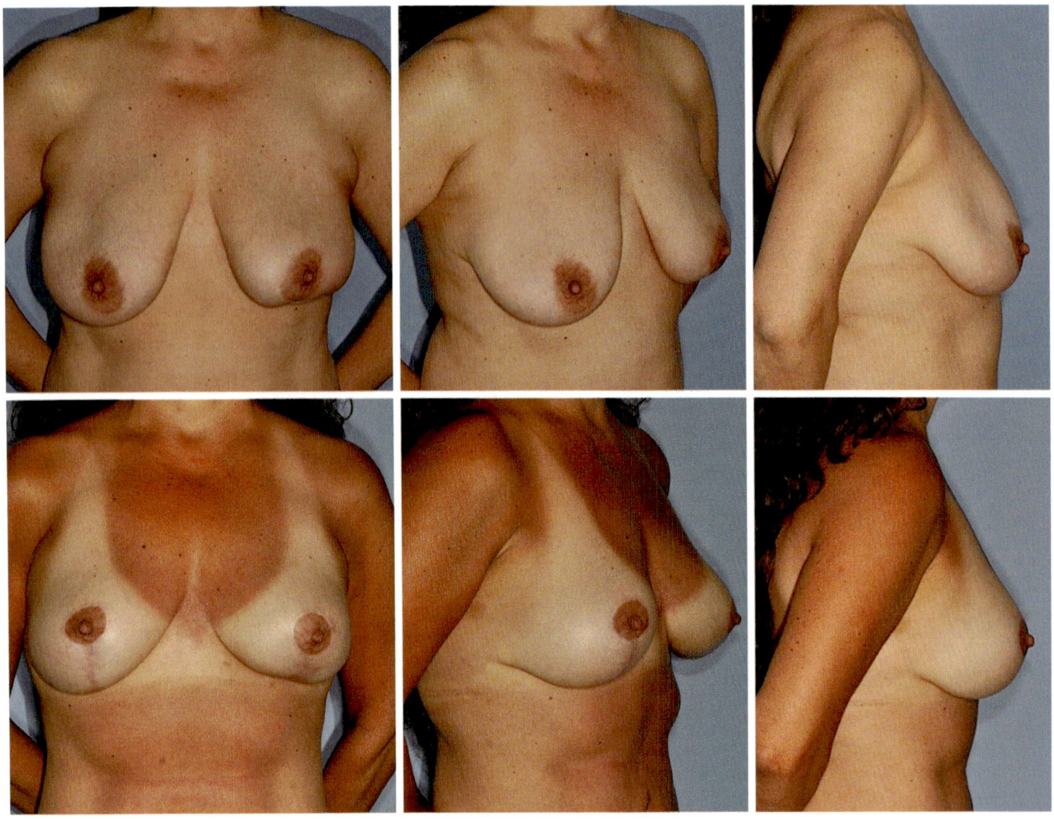

Fig. 13.14 Long term results with matrix belt and lipofilling after lumpectomy for breast cancer. This demonstrates preoperative (above) and postoperative (below) results at 24 months following differential autoaugmentation. This patient had previously undergone a left sided lumpectomy with adjuvant radiation. A traditional autoaugmentation technique was done on her right non-radiated side, and a skin only mastopexy was done on her left radiated side. Both sides were differentially lipofilled, with preferential filling in the top pole on her right non-radiated side and an overall larger volume and more central distribution on her left radiated side. Note, in the postoperative views, the improvement in symmetry, shape and projection

Summary

Established mastopexy techniques allow for implant-free breast augmentation and volume reduction, but remain susceptible to insufficient upper pole fullness and bottoming out over time. The auto-augmentation technique described by the author improves on established mastopexy techniques by utilizing a belt of biologic or synthetic soft tissue support matrix to increase the durability of upper pole fullness and prevent bottoming out. The addition of lipofilling using highly purified fat grafts contributes to upper pole stability and fullness and allows the surgeon to achieve an aesthetically pleasing and natural-looking, symmetric result. This implant-free technique may be appropriate for many patients without prior surgery or to correct deficits following implant removal. Although caution should be exercised following radiation treatment, the auto-augmentation technique may also be applied following lumpectomy for breast cancer. To date, long-term results have been excellent.

References

1. American Society of Plastic Surgeons. 2019 Plastic surgery statistics report. 2019; Available at: https://www.plasticsurgery.org/documents/News/Statistics/2019/plastic-surgery-statistics-full-report-2019.pdf. Accessed 7 Nov 2019.

2. Ribeiro L. A new technique for reduction mammaplasty. Plast Reconstr Surg. 1975;55(3):330–4.
3. Graf R, Biggs TM, Steely RL. Breast shape: a technique for better upper pole fullness. Aesthet Plast Surg. 2000;24(5):348–52.
4. de la Plaza R, de la Cruz L, Moreno C. Mastopexy utilizing a dermoglandular hammock flap. Aesthet Surg J. 2005;25(1):31–6.
5. Ritz M, Silfen R, Southwick G. Fascial suspension mastopexy. Plast Reconstr Surg. 2006;117(1):86–94.
6. Lejour M. Vertical mammaplasty and liposuction of the breast. Plast Reconstr Surg. 1994;94(1):100–14.
7. Kim P, Kim KK, Casas LA. Superior pedicle autoaugmentation mastopexy: a review of 34 consecutive patients. Aesthet Surg J. 2010;30(2):201–10.
8. Hall-Findlay EJ. Pedicles in vertical breast reduction and mastopexy. Clin Plast Surg. 2002;29(3):379–91.
9. Foustanos A, Zavrides H. A double-flap technique: an alternative mastopexy approach. Plast Reconstr Surg. 2007;120(1):55–60.
10. Hammond DC, Alfonso D, Khuthaila DK. Mastopexy using the short scar periareolar inferior pedicle reduction technique. Plast Reconstr Surg. 2008;121(5):1533–9.
11. Bonomi S, Salval A, Settembrini F, Gregorelli C, Musumarra G, Rapisarda V. Inferiorly based parenchymal flap mammaplasty: a safe, reliable, and versatile technique for breast reduction and mastopexy. Plast Reconstr Surg. 2012;130(1):116e–25e.
12. Abboud L, Watfa W, di Summa PG, Raffoul W. An original and simple autoaugmentation mastopexy in mild to moderate breast ptosis: superior pedicle frontal division to achieve upper pole fullness. Gland Surg. 2017;6(6):751–2.
13. Honig JF, Frey HP, Hasse FM, Hasselberg J. Inferior pedicle autoaugmentation mastopexy after breast implant removal. Aesthet Plast Surg. Aug 2010;34(4):447–54.
14. Hall-Findlay EJ. Vertical breast reduction. Semin Plast Surg. 2004;18(3):211–24.
15. Goes JC. Periareolar mammaplasty: double skin technique with application of polyglactine or mixed mesh. Plast Reconstr Surg. 1996;97(5):959–68.
16. de Bruijn HP, Johannes S. Mastopexy with 3D preshaped mesh for long-term results: development of the internal bra system. Aesthet Plast Surg. 2008;32(5):757–65.
17. van Deventer PV, Graewe FR, Wuringer E. Improving the longevity and results of mastopexy and breast reduction procedures: reconstructing an internal breast support system with biocompatible mesh to replace the supporting function of the ligamentous suspension. Aesthet Plast Surg. 2012;36(3):578–89.
18. Adams WP Jr, Moses AC. Use of Poly-4-Hydroxybutyrate mesh to optimize soft-tissue support in mastopexy: a single-site study. Plast Reconstr Surg. 2017;139(1):67–75.
19. Goes JC, Landecker A, Lyra EC, Henriquez LJ, Goes RS, Godoy PM. The application of mesh support in periareolar breast surgery: clinical and mammographic evaluation. Aesthet Plast Surg. 2004;28(5):268–74.
20. Swanson E. A retrospective photometric study of 82 published reports of mastopexy and breast reduction. Plast Reconstr Surg. 2011;128(6):1282–301.
21. Pitanguy I. Surgical treatment of breast hypertrophy. Br J Plast Surg. 1967;20(1):78–85.
22. Swanson E. Prospective photographic measurement study of 196 cases of breast augmentation, mastopexy, augmentation/mastopexy, and breast reduction. Plast Reconstr Surg. 2013;131(5):802e–19e.
23. Lejour M, Abboud M, Declety A, Kertesz P. Reduction of mammaplasty scars: from a short inframammary scar to a vertical scar. Ann Chir Plast Esthet. 1990;35(5):369–79.
24. Graf R, Ricardo Dal Oglio Tolazzi A, Balbinot P, Pazio A, Miguel Valente P, da Silva Freitas R. Influence of the pectoralis major muscle sling in chest wall-based flap suspension after vertical mammaplasty: ten-year follow-up. Aesthet Surg J. 2016;36(10):1113–21.
25. Weichman K, Doft M, Matarasso A. The impact of mastopexy on brassiere cup size. Plast Reconstr Surg. 2014;134(1):34e–40e.
26. Khouri RK, Rigotti G, Cardoso E, Khouri RK Jr, Biggs TM. Megavolume autologous fat transfer: part I. Theory and principles. Plast Reconstr Surg. 2014;133(3):550–7.
27. Zhu M, Cohen SR, Hicok KC, et al. Comparison of three different fat graft preparation methods: gravity separation, centrifugation, and simultaneous washing with filtration in a closed system. Plast Reconstr Surg. 2013;131(4):873–80.
28. Schafer ME, Hicok KC, Mills DC, Cohen SR, Chao JJ. Acute adipocyte viability after third-generation ultrasound-assisted liposuction. Aesthet Surg J. 2013;33(5):698–704.
29. Gerth DJ, King B, Rabach L, Glasgold RA, Glasgold MJ. Long-term volumetric retention of autologous fat grafting processed with closed-membrane filtration. Aesthet Surg J. 2014;34(7):985–94.
30. Voineskos SH, Frank SG, Cordeiro PG. Breast reconstruction following conservative mastectomies: predictors of complications and outcomes. Gland Surg. 2015;4(6):484–96.
31. Terao Y, Taniguchi K, Fujii M, Moriyama S. Postmastectomy radiation therapy and breast reconstruction with autologous tissue. Breast Cancer. 2017;24(4):505–10.
32. Rochlin DH, Jeong AR, Goldberg L, et al. Postmastectomy radiation therapy and immediate autologous breast reconstruction: integrating perspectives from surgical oncology, radiation oncology, and plastic and reconstructive surgery. J Surg Oncol. 2015;111(3):251–7.

14 An Algorithm for the Management of Explantation Surgery

M. Bradley Calobrace, Neil Tanna, and Chet Mays

Introduction

Whereas breast implants had very little regulation during the 1960s, the following decade was characterized by growing public concerns of the risks associated with breast implants such as rupture and removal resulting in increased FDA regulation [1]. During the 1980s, there were several reports of patient-reported autoimmune conditions that were allegedly caused by silicone breast implants. This led to a large-scale inquiry and eventually to a 14-year moratorium on the use of silicone gel implants [2]. In the USA, saline implants became the only option for the majority of plastic surgeons with silicone gel implants being used in the industry supported core studies that were designed to assess safety and efficacy. Based on numerous studies demonstrating safety and efficacy of silicone gel breast implants, the FDA approved these devices for both cosmetic and reconstructive purposes in 2006 [1, 2].

Whether for breast reconstruction or cosmetic breast augmentation, it is well known that breast implants are not lifetime devices. Common reasons for explantation include rupture and capsular contracture; however, recent discussions pertaining to the safety of silicone breast implants are fueling increasing demand for explantation. Rates of explantation have increased from 19,857 procedures in 2009 to 30,000 in 2018, making explantation one of the top ten most commonly performed plastic surgery procedure performed in the US [3, 4]. Given that these procedures are becoming increasingly popular, this review serves as a comprehensive look at the indications for explantation, capsulectomies and the correction of the breast aesthetics without the use of implants. The ability to utilize techniques such as mastopexies, fat grafting and auto-augmentations is critical to achieving beautiful aesthetics after the removal of breast implants.

Indications for Explantation with or without Capsulectomy

The indications for implant removal are numerous, and have included not only complications associated with breast implants such as implant

M. B. Calobrace (✉)
Private Practice, CaloAesthetics Plastic Surgery Center, Louisville, KY, USA

Clinical Faculty, University of Louisville, Division of Plastic Surgery, Louisville, KY, USA

Clinical Faculty, University of Kentucky, Division of Plastic Surgery, Lexington, KY, USA
e-mail: drbrad@calobrace.com

N. Tanna
Faculty, Northwell Health, Zucker School of Medicine, Division of Plastic Surgery, Great Neck, NY, USA

C. Mays
Private Practice, CaloAesthetics Plastic Surgery Center, Louisville, KY, USA

Clinical Faculty, University of Louisville, Division of Plastic Surgery, Louisville, KY, USA

M. B. Calobrace et al. (eds.), *Augmentation Mastopexy*,
https://doi.org/10.1007/978-3-030-48226-8_14

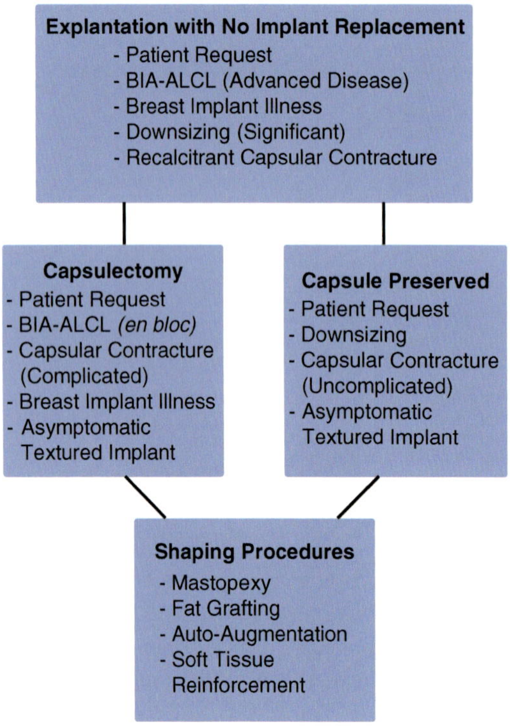

Fig. 14.1 Algorithm for the Management in Explantation Surgery

rupture, capsular contracture and patient's desire for an aesthetic change, but more recently due to issue such as concerns of breast implant illness, treatment of BIA-ALCL (breast implant associated- anaplastic large cell lymphoma), and risk reduction by explantation of textured devices. When performing an explantation, a decision must then be made as the necessity or appropriateness of capsule removal, whether it be total, partial or en *bloc*. This ultimately requires a significant amount of discernment by the plastic surgeon as the ultimate surgical approach is dependent on a myriad of factors designed to ensure the surgery addresses not only the aspects related to the disease process, but also addresses adequately the issues related to the patient's concerns. An algorithm for the management with an understanding of the indications and contraindications facilitates the navigation in surgical decision-making and execution (Fig. 14.1).

Indications for Explantation Surgery and Capsulectomy

Capsular Contracture For implant patients presenting with breast pain and deformity constituting Baker grade III or IV capsular contracture, treatment is indicated. Studies report rates of capsular contracture ranging from 2.8% to 18.9% for augmentation patients, and recent large-scale and long-term analyses have provided new insights [5–8]. It has long been accepted that total capsulectomy is the most effective treatment for capsular contracture demonstrating superiority over partial capsulectomy and capsulotomy. However, a recent systematic review concluded that site change, implant exchange, and addition of acellular dermal matrix were the only aspects of surgery associated with lower capsular contracture recurrence rates and that is was unclear whether a total capsulectomy was superior to a partial capsulectomy. [9] Thus, in face of a capsular contracture, explantation or implant exchange is warranted. In fact, when capsular contractures are recalcitrant and have failed previous attempts at correction, an explantation may be the most prudent approach. In patients with subpectoral implants, a complete capsulectomy is associated with an increased risk of chest wall injury and pneumothorax as the capsule is dissected off the chest wall. In some cases, the capsule is excised anteriorly but retained posteriorly to minimize soft tissue trauma with the new implant placed anterior to the dissected capsule [10] (Fig. 14.2). There has also been good evidence the use of a neosubpectoral pocket with placement of ADM significantly reduced the risk of capsular contracture recurrence, but this would require maintaining the capsule [11]. Finally, a retrospective review by Swanson concluded that capsulotomy alone for capsular contracture demonstrated good results with low rates of recurrence [12]. If a capsulotomy only is done to treat the capsular contracture, the logic for implant exchange is less clear.

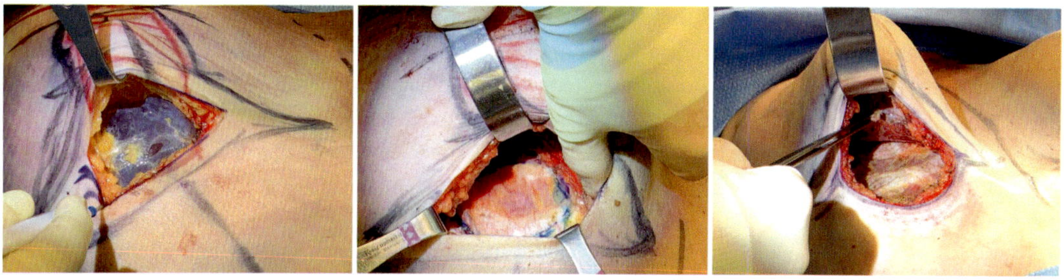

Fig. 14.2 Breast Implant Illness Case. (Left) Near Total (Partial) Capsulectomy performed for submuscular capsule that is extremely thin making a total capsulectomy technically challenging and inappropriate for this patient. (Center) Small portion of extremely thin capsule retained on the chest wall. (Right) The retained capsule after destruction with cauterization. Notice the capsule is obliterated with the chest wall nearly devoid of any remaining capsule

A capsular contracture itself is not necessarily an indication for a capsulectomy if no implant is to be replaced, and sometimes can be used advantageously, as in the SIEF (simultaneous implant exchange with fat grafting) procedure [13]. The capsule can provide support for the soft tissue envelope, provide enhanced circulation to the overlying breast, and create an inner lamellae for fat grafting.

Implant Rupture Rupture of a silicone implant is an indication for implant removal. In many cases, rupture of the device can occur with no other outward sign that the integrity of the shell has been lost. Such "silent ruptures" of silicone gel devices often remain intracapsular and are often asymptomatic and only incidentally detected on mammogram or MRI. Implant rupture rates can vary based on surgeon and manufacturer, but average around 10–25% at 10 years. Different implant models vary in their propensity to rupture, with one model having a 3000-day risk of 33% [14]. Diagnosis of silicone gel implant rupture is usually made using MRI or ultrasound. Due to its lesser expense, high-definition ultrasound is preferred over MRI for the initial evaluation of a possible rupture, although MRI results may be more accurate [15]. Importantly, a high concordance has been demonstrated between ultrasound and MRI for the detection of implant rupture, potentially obviating the need for MRI evaluation for implants if ultrasound demonstrates a rupture [16]. In fact, the new FDA guidelines include a high-definition ultrasound at 5–6 years and an MRI if results are inconclusive.

Although recommendations concerning the appropriate usage of ultrasound, MRI, and mammography for rupture detection is at present still not fully agreed upon, there is agreement that a ruptured implant is an indication for removal, with or without exchange to a new device. Whereas the capsule does not generally need to be removed for a rupture, a significant rupture with silicone imbedded in the capsule preventing complete removal with washings mandates removal of the capsule as well.

Silicone Implant Illness or Breast Implant Illness (BII) An emerging issue facing plastic surgery is concerns by patients that their implants are the cause of a myriad of symptoms referred to in the news and social media by the term "Breast Implant Illness." Silicone implant illness is characterized by a non-specific and generalized constellation of symptoms that include malaise, fatigue, fibromyalgia, headache as well as other patients reported complaints" In 1997, Peters et al. reported on 100 patients presenting for explantation during the silicone moratorium [17].

These patients were divided into three groups. Group 1 did not meet diagnostic criteria for rheumatic or autoimmune disease and demonstrated a > 80% improvement in physical symptoms and 93% improvement in psychological well-being following explantation. Group 2 had rheumatic but not autoimmune disease and would have an initial improvement (placebo effect) but with recurrence in symptoms at 6–12 months. Group 3 had a diagnosed autoimmune disease and showed no improvement of symptoms or autoantibody levels and went on to suffer from the autoimmune disease. A review of 240 explantation patients by Melmed in 1998 found that patients reported a decrease in flu-like symptoms, depression, and fatigue after implant removal [18]. Rohrich in 2000, demonstrated that in patients who underwent explantation, improvements were documented for musculoskeletal symptoms, general pain, and mental health [19]. . De Boer et al. conducted a review of 23 case reports and cohort studies dating from 1994 to 2014, in which 75% of a combined 622-patient sample noted improvements in their overall health and systemic illnesses after the removal of their breast implants. However, explantation alone helped to alleviate symptoms in only 16% of patients who were definitively diagnosed with an autoimmune disorder [20].

However, improvement in symptoms following explantation is variable and breast implants alone may not be the cause of any specific autoimmune or systemic illness [21]. To date, there are no studies demonstrating a cause-effect relationship between silicone implants to what is now termed breast implant illness [21–23]. No test for BII currently exists and it may be that BII is a manifestation of the hyper-stimulation of the immune system that represents an allergic-type response to breast implants, but this remains a conjecture. It is also important to note that BII can occur in the setting of silicone gel or saline-filled breast implants and that it may be the result of the implant shell that is made of silicone. Nevertheless, patient complaints about BII should be taken seriously, and symptomatic patients should be given the option of implant removal with or without capsulectomy (Fig. 14.3). In BII concerned patients, whereas a near total or total capsulectomy may be a reasonable option based on the clinical scenario, there is no indication for an *en bloc* capsulectomy and the use of this term and this type of treatment should be discouraged and reserved only for confirmed malignancy.

Breast Implant-Associated Anaplastic Large Cell Lymphoma Breast implant-associated anaplastic large cell lymphoma (BIA-ALCL) is

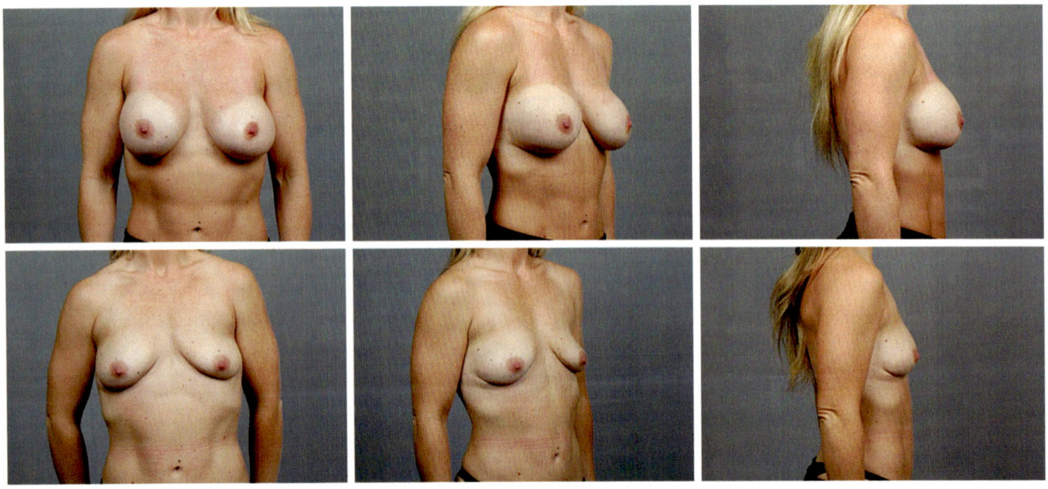

Fig. 14.3 Patient concerned with Breast Implant Illness. Patient who underwent near-total (partial) capsulectomy only with no reconstruction. (Upper) Preoperative views (Lower) 6 months Postoperative views

associated with textured breast implants and has been the focus of research and discussion in the plastic surgery community [24]. The most common presentations include seroma, pain and/or swelling in the breast, capsular contracture, and a mass or lump around the implant [25]. The current incidence of BIA-ALCL varies based on the type of implant. Patients should be counseled that BIA-ALCL is not breast cancer, often follows an indolent course, and that removing the implants and surrounding capsules is often sufficient to achieve complete remission [26]. The capsule, periprosthetic effusion, and any associated masses should be completely removed with the implants through an *en bloc* resection which results in better overall survival and event-free survival outcomes compared to partial or no capsulectomy [27, 28]. Whereas leaving a part of the capsule when performing a capsulectomy may be appropriate for other indications such as capsular contracture or BII, when treating BIA-ALCL, a complete and total capsulectomy surrounded by a contiguous rim of healthy margin (*en bloc* capsulectomy) is warranted. Incomplete removal and persistent margins are associated with recurrence and disease progression.

Asymptomatic Textured Implant Patients When treating patients with textured implants who desire removal for risk reduction from BIA-ALCL in the future, there is no evidenced-based data to support a capsulectomy in an asymptomatic textured implant patient with a normal appearing capsule at surgery. When it can be removed easily, such as in a subglandular augmentation, removal of the capsule adds very little to the morbidity and may prove beneficial. Likewise, if performing an explantation and a worrisome capsule is encountered with a mass, fluid or abnormal thickening, the surgeon may deem it appropriate to remove the capsule with appropriate pathological evaluation. Currently, without supporting data for a prophylactic capsulectomy in an asymptomatic textured implant patient, each surgeon will ultimately need to counsel patients on the best course of treatment with the understanding that a prophylactic capsulectomy may or may not reduce the patients risk of future BIA-ALCL, is associated with increased operative complexity and morbidity, can often impair the final aesthetic result and is associated with a greater financial burden. In asymptomatic patients, explantation alone or exchange to a smooth implant may be appropriate treatment, is less costly and has a much lower risk profile.

Patient Preference Unsatisfactory breast aesthetics due to age-related changes, pregnancy, weight gain or loss, or changes in public opinion concerning breast implants, may result in a non-medically related desire for explantation. As the body acceptance movement gains popularity on social media platforms and concern regarding the safety of silicone implants persists, an increase in the number of patients who seek breast implant removal is anticipated [2, 29].

Surgical Management of the Capsule

The surgical approach appropriate for each patient requires a significant amount of discernment by the plastic surgeon as a myriad of factors must be considered to ensure the surgery addresses not only the issues related to the disease process, but also considers issues related to the patient's concerns, whether evidence-based or solely based on personal perception.

The management of the capsule requires a thorough understanding of the indications for the explantation. The capsule may be considered "friend or foe." The appropriateness as to whether capsule removal is indicated is not always clear and can be quite controversial based on the various indications. This has significant implications as a total capsulectomy can be challenging and can significantly impact the surgical morbidity, financial burden and ultimate aesthetic outcome.

If the capsule is calcified, has a mass present, or is embedded with silicone product, removal of the capsule is warranted. Additionally, patients concerned with breast implant illness will desire any retained silicone left behind by rupture, particle shedding, or gel bleed be removed as completely as possible and will therefore be best served with removal of the entire capsule to ease concerns with inadequate treatment. A confirmed diagnosis of BIA-ALCL requires an *en bloc* resection.

Capsulotomy

Capsulotomy is the simplest, and safest, of the procedures used to manage the capsule in explant patients. Despite this, it has traditionally been considered inferior to capsulectomy as a treatment for capsular contracture. Capsulotomies are performed by scoring the capsule radially and sometimes in a checkered board pattern to achieve expansion of the breast pocket. The dissection is sometimes carried into the breast tissue as well to allow for greater expansion (Fig. 14.4). The advantages of a capsulotomy include preservation of support for the overlying skin envelope when soft tissue coverage is thin, improved circulation for the overlying breast skin soft tissue envelope especially when a mastopexy is planned, and improved pocket control and support for the implant if an implant replacement is planned. Capsulotomies are not adequate in cases of BIA-ALCL, patients concerned with illness from breast implants, complicated capsular contractures such as calcified capsules, when silicone is embedded in the capsule, or an associated capsular mass is identified (Fig. 14.5).

Partial Capsulectomy

In a recent study, partial capsulectomy (anterior capsulectomy) was reported as the most common modality for the treatment of capsular contracture with 46.1% of surgeons opting for partial capsulectomy and 35.1% opting for total capsulectomy [30]. The decision between a partial and total capsulectomy is sometimes best made in the operating room based on the location of the implant.

Whereas subglandular capsules can be more easily removed due to the pectoralis muscle on the floor of the pocket, attempting to remove the posterior section of the capsule in a submuscular augmentation is more prone to injure of the chest wall and the potential for a pneumothorax [10]. In these cases, the posterior capsule is often retained and destroyed through cauterization in attempt to destroy the remaining capsule that may laden with biofilm. Additionally, scoring the posterior portion of the capsule has been suggested to facilitate the closure of the implant pocket if implant exchange is not being performed. In subpectoral partial capsulectomies, dissection is carried between the capsule and the

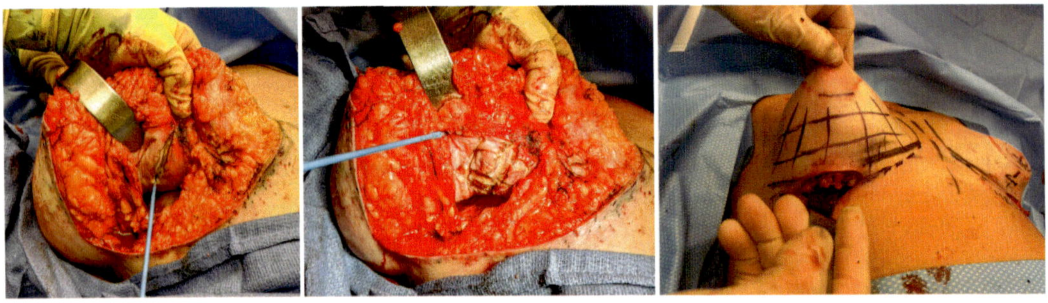

Fig. 14.4 Capsulotmy Technique (Left) Capsulotomies are performed by scoring the capsule radially through the capsule for expansion of the breast pocket. (center, right) Multiple capsulotomies including creating a checkered board pattern is sometimes employed to achieve greater expansion of the breast pocket

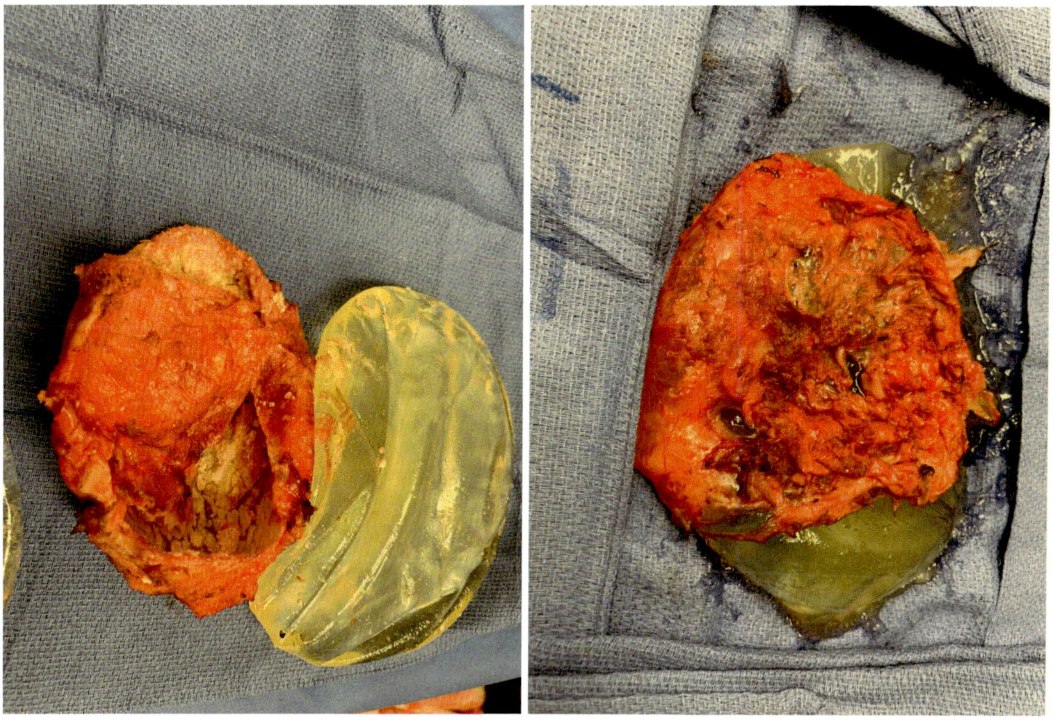

Fig. 14.5 Capsulectomies and not capsulotomies are indicated when the capsule has pathology, including a mass, (Left) calcifications or (Right) silicone embedded in the capsule

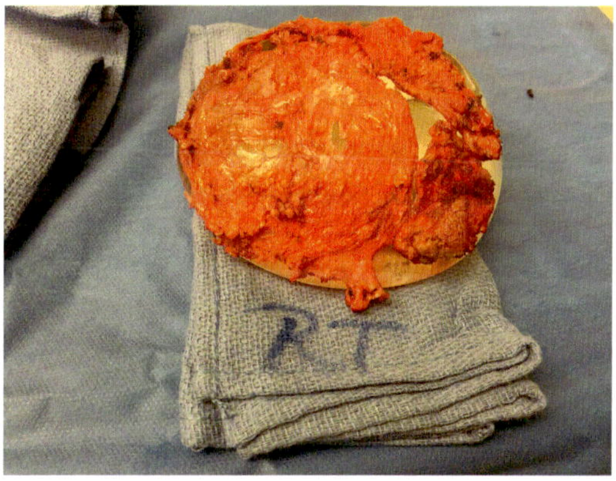

Fig. 14.6 Partial capsulectomy removes the majority of the capsule including the anterior capsule and leaves a portion of capsule on the chest wall

overlying breast tissue. Ultimately, when visualization is impaired, the implant is removed and the remainder of the anterior capsule removed (Fig. 14.6). Laterally, the capsule can be removed off of the floor due to the underlying serratus anterior and pectoralis minor muscles. The most adherent central piece of posterior capsule is retained and destroyed with electrodessication.

Total Capsulectomy

Total capsulectomy is defined as the removal of the anterior and posterior capsule. Although some in the lay press and on social media have referred to an *en bloc* resection as removal of the capsule and implant as a single unit, this is an inaccurate use of this oncologic term (Fig. 14.7). An *en bloc* resection includes removal of the entire capsule and implant including obtaining healthy margins of tissue, removal of any associated masses and/or lymph nodes. This type of resection is appropriate only for a diagnosed case of BIA-ALCL and not for the treatment of suspicious, non-malignancy diseases or prophylactic surgeries [27, 28]. Total capsulectomy with incomplete resection of a mass has led to hyper

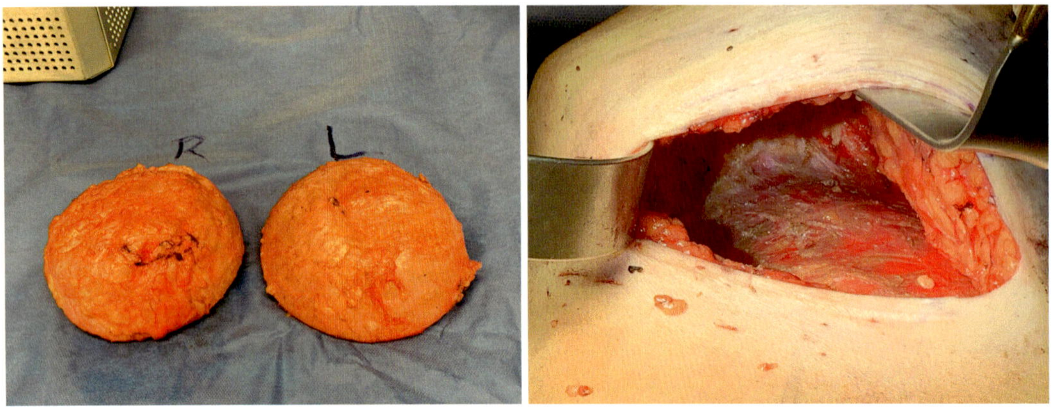

Fig. 14.7 (Left) Bilateral implants and capsules removed in-situ from a patient with subglandular implants and concerns of BII. (Right) the subglandular pocket devoid of implant and capsule. This type of total capsulectomy with implants remaining in-situ for the explantation should not be inaccurately described as an *en bloc* resection, which is a much more extensive resection and reserved for the treatment of cancer

progression of BIA-ALCL with bone marrow metastasis and death [36, 37]. Therefore, a simple prophylactic capsulectomy in an textured implant patient that has active but undiagnosed disease could result in disease progression and dire consequences.

Total capsulectomy is a more invasive procedure that carries a higher risk of bleeding and other perioperative complications compared to partial capsulectomy or capsulotomy [9, 31, 32]. Most patients with subglandular implants will have a total capsulectomy with removal of the implant. The dissection is easily accomplished with minimal risk to the chest wall. Achieving intact removal of the capsule may be more difficult for implants placed in a submuscular plane. In addition, total capsulectomy is exceedingly challenging when the capsule is very thin and fragile (Fig. 14.2a). In these cases, complete excision and removal in situ may not be possible and strip capsulectomy may be performed instead. Alternatively, it is strategically appropriate to remove the capsule in sections as needed as long as the entire capsule is eventually successfully removed. One helpful technique is to hydrodissect the capsule off of the chest wall with infiltration of fluid between the posterior capsule and chest wall. The decision to proceed with a total capsulectomy should be considered carefully, taking into account the specific indications for performing a capsulectomy, the risk tolerance of the patient and the specifics of the procedure.

En Bloc Capsulectomy

En Bloc capsulectomy is defined as an oncologic procedure in which a margin of normal-appearing tissue around the capsule is removed as part of the specimen which also contains the implant, an intact implant capsule, and associated masses. Currently available evidence indicates the use of *en bloc* capsulectomy only in patients with BIA-ALCL. For patients without concern for breast implant associated malignancy, there is no evidence supporting the excision of healthy tissue around the capsule and doing so increases the risk of surgery as well as the difficulty in achieving an aesthetic outcome after explantation.

While patient preference is important to consider when determining how to care for a patient, it is not as critical as performing the correct procedure for the patient with an acceptable risk profile. Therefore, these risks and benefits must be carefully and accurately discussed with the patient to insure the most appropriate procedure is performed on each patient based on the surgeon's evaluation and clinical judgment, the patient's clinical scenario and concerns, and the currently available evidence-based data to guide the ultimate recommendation and treatment course.

Aesthetic Breast Procedures After Explantation

Implant removal will change the appearance of the breast dramatically, especially at larger implant volumes. Procedures such as mastopexy and/or fat grafting are often necessary to maintain satisfactory aesthetics after explantation. Patients who undergo explantation alone often experience disappointment and sometimes even mutilated [17]. Additionally, Netscher et al. conducted a study of 85 consecutive breast implant removal patients using external raters and found that patients received lower aesthetic scores if they did not undergo mastopexy or reconstruction after explantation [33]. Currently, for patients who choose not to undergo implant exchange, or for whom implant exchange is not indicated, a variety of options exist to improve the postoperative appearance of the breast.

Mastopexy Some patients may choose to have no treatment except the explantation with or without the capsulectomy (Fig. 14.3). However, mastopexy is often the best choice to remove excess breast skin in patients requiring additional aesthetic management after implant removal. Some patients may actually choose to stage the procedure in order to take "wait and see" how things look with only removal and then undergo a mastopexy at a later date if deemed necessary (Fig. 14.8).

Preoperative markings are developed for the mastopexy based on the estimated skin excess and nipple position after explantation (Fig. 14.9). The explantation is performed with or without a capsulectomy. The incision location is determined based on the type of mastopexy performed, usually in the IMF or vertically from the NAC to the IMF (Fig. 14.10). After explantation, the mastopexy design is confirmed. This is often done with tailor-tacking but this can be challenging with larger breasts. The design involves locating the position of the NAC and the vertical medial and lateral pillars (Fig. 14.11). The mastopexy is generally performed using as a superiomedial or

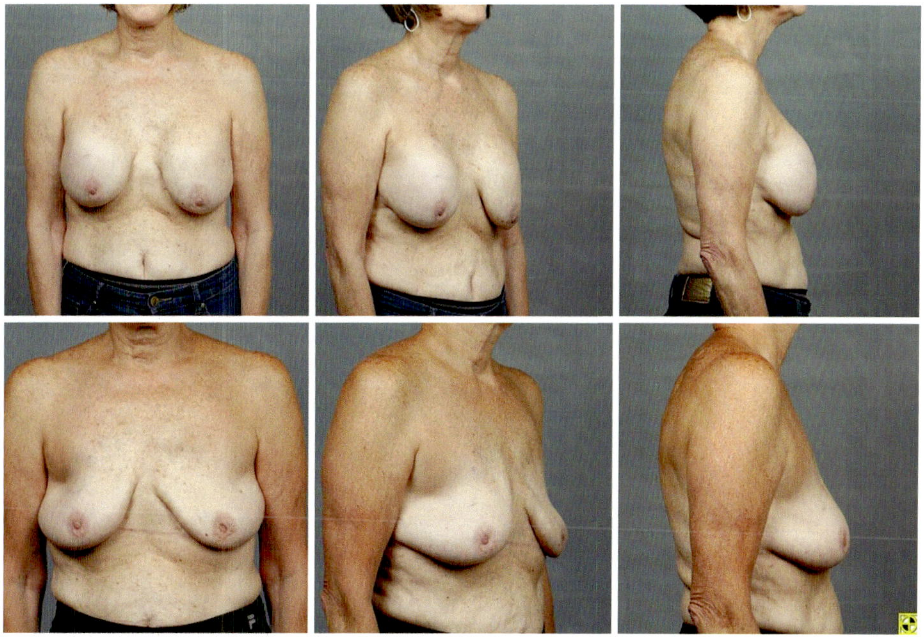

Fig. 14.8 70 year old with bilateral grade 4 capsular contracture underwent bilateral total capsulectomies with explantation of her subglandular implants and no reconstruction. Note the loss of central projection with flat, ptotic breasts

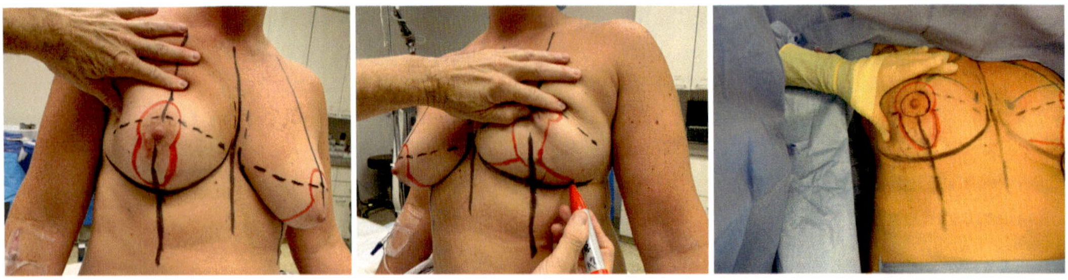

Fig. 14.9 Preoperative markings are developed for the mastopexy based on the estimated skin excess and nipple position after explantation. (Left) Vertical design (center) vertical with inverted-T design (right) Final assessment in the operating room prior to making an incision

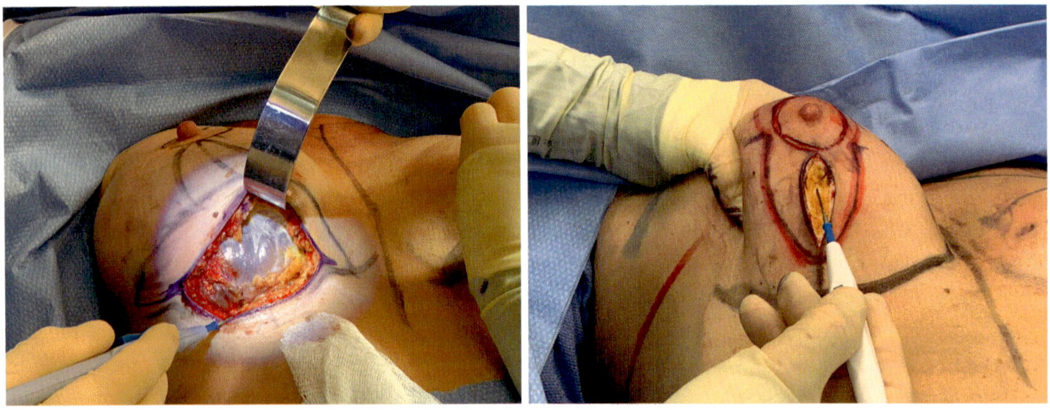

Fig. 14.10 The incision location is determined based on the type of mastopexy performed, usually in the (left) IMF or (right)vertically from the NAC to the IMF

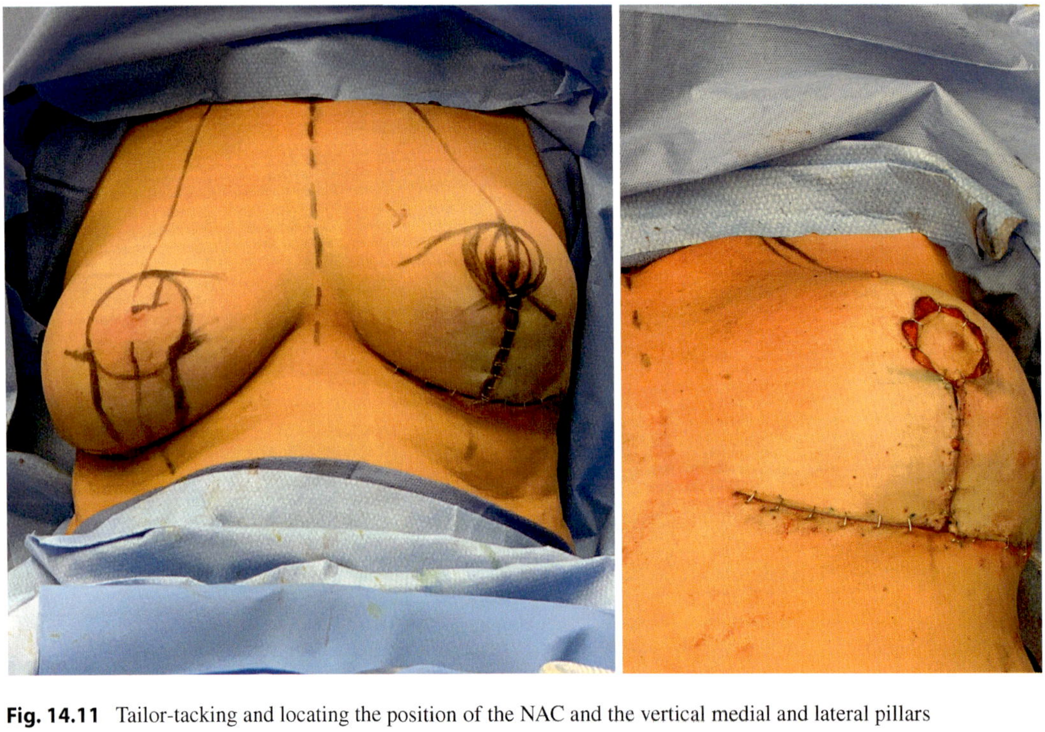

Fig. 14.11 Tailor-tacking and locating the position of the NAC and the vertical medial and lateral pillars

superior pedicle as the central pedicle supplying the inferior or central pedicle has been sacrificed with the original implant placement (Fig. 14.12). Once the pillars are developed, the skin excision pattern is confirmed, either vertically, vertically with a small horizontal wedge or as an inverted-T. The vertical limbs usually are 6–8 centimeters long based on the ultimate size of the breast. The mastopexy provides reduction in the skin envelope and reshaping and lifting of the breast (Fig. 14.13). The limitations in the final aesthetic results are based on the quality and amount of breast tissue available. It can be challenging to achieve any significant upper pole volume in the explantation patient with a mastopexy only (Fig. 14.14). Additional maneuvers may be incorporated, including auto-augmentation of fat grafting.

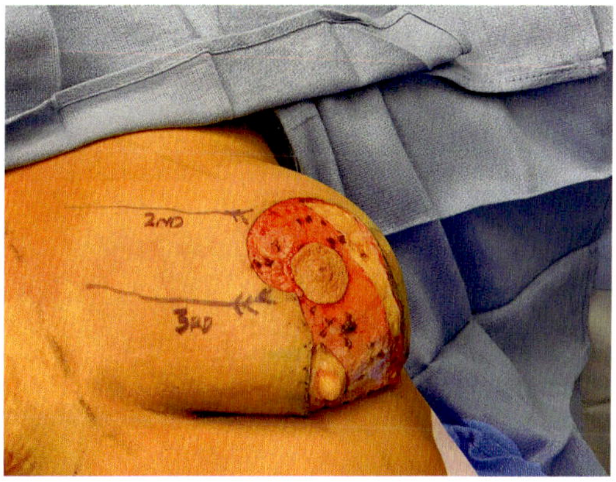

Fig. 14.12 The mastopexy is typical performed with a superior or superiomedial pedicle based off superficial branches of the internal mammary artery, either the 2nd (superior) or the 2nd and 3rd (superiomedial) as the central pedicle was sacrificed with the original breast augmentation

Auto-augmentation Flaps Options for auto-augmentation of the breast after implant removal are relatively limited. The auto-augmentation in an explantation patient includes a superiorly based mastopexy with a de-epithelialized inferior dermoglandular flap to re-orient existing breast volume [34, 35]. This flap is generally based off of the areola superiorly and can be flipped under the breast to create core projection with central breast volume (Fig. 14.15). Fat grafting with

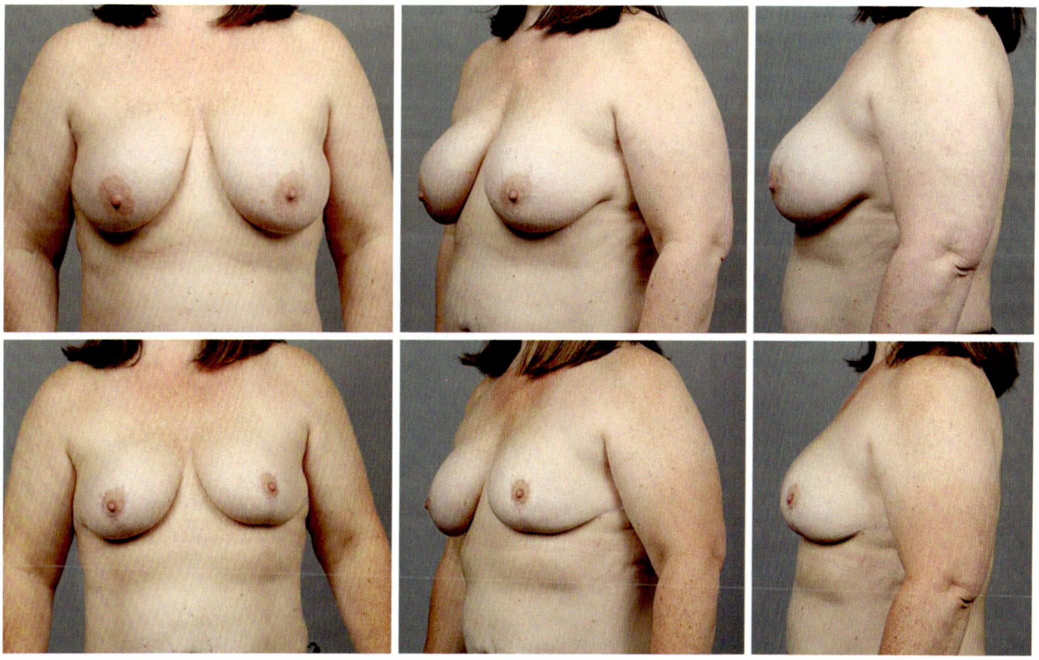

Fig. 14.13 47 year old desiring removal of implants and smaller breasts underwent bilateral explantation with total capsulectomies, mastopexy and fat grafting, 350 cc to the right breast and 290 cc to the left breast. (Upper) Pre-operative views and (Lower) Post-operative views 7 months after surgery

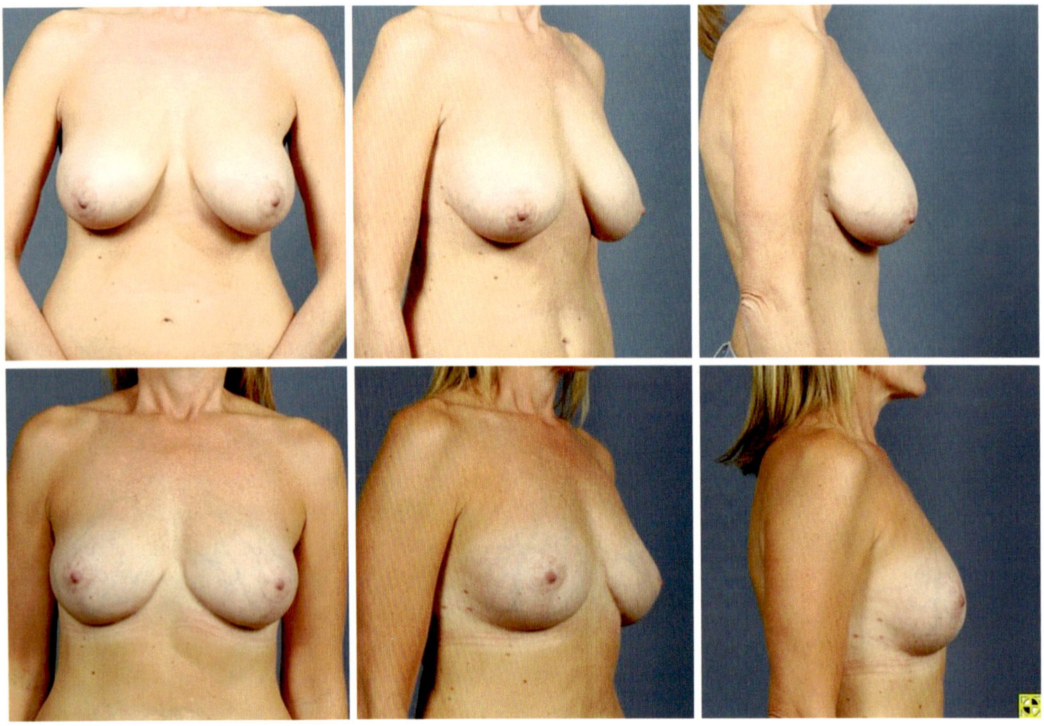

Fig. 14.14 39 year old had undergone a mastopexy augmentation in the past and presented due to recurrent ptosis and desired smaller breasts. She underwent explantation, preservation of the capsule, and an inverted-T mastopexy only. The mastopexy corrected the ptosis, but she lacked upper pole volume due to the limitations in volume of the breasts after the implants were removed. (Upper) Pre-operative views and (Lower) post-operative 9 month views

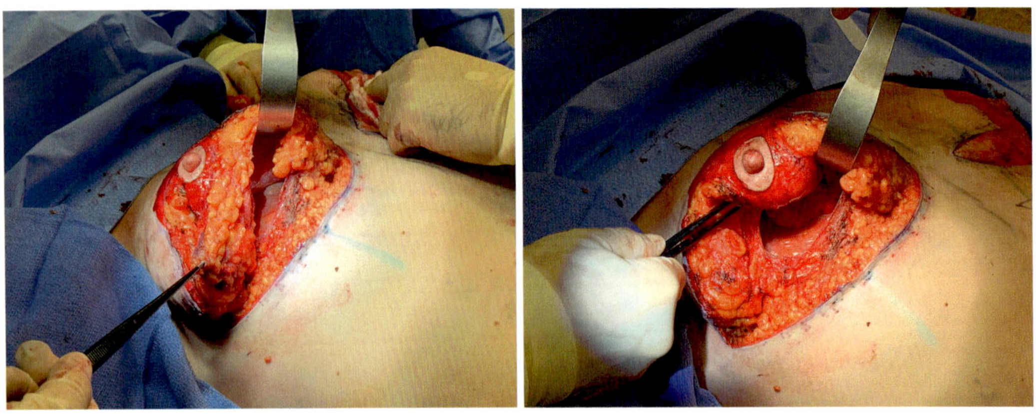

Fig. 14.15 The auto-augmentation in an explantation patient includes a superiorly-based mastopexy with a de-epithelialized inferior dermoglandular flap to re-orient existing breast volume.[3] (Left) The auto-augmentation flap based off of the areola superiorly and (right) shown being flipped under the areola

auto-augmentation can be very effective with the auto-augmentation creating core projection and the fat grafting added to the peripheral breast to enhance the overall size, upper pole volume and cleavage.

During the superiorly-based mastopexy, the inferior central segment of breast tissue between the medial and later pillars can be developed to auto-augment the central breast core. This lower island of tissue is de-epithelialized and released from the pillars, its vascular supply from the areola above. This flap is then flipped under the areola and sutured to the overlying breast tissue with 2-0 vicryl sutures. It is important to release the dermis just below the areola to allow for a smooth transition. Prior to inset, it is important to check the blood supply to the distal portion of the flap and resect any tissue with precarious circulation (Fig. 14.16). This flap preserves the volume to the breast, but places the tissue in a more beneficial location to provide much needed central core volume. The flap is sutured with 2-0 vicryl from the distal end to the pectoralis fascia in the upper chest (Fig. 14.17). The pillars are then re-approximated and final skin excision determined (Fig. 14.18). A mastopexy with auto-augmentation can provide an excellent aesthetic results in the appropriately selected patient (Figs. 14.19, 14.20, and 14.21).

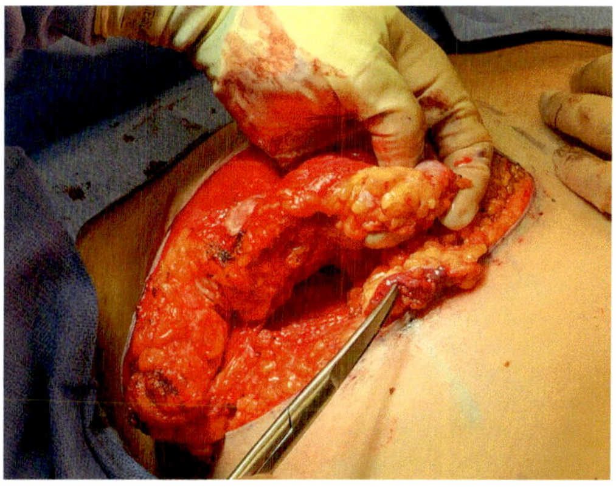

Fig. 14.16 The flap in cut to evaluate the adequacy of blood supply to the distal portion of the flap. If blood supply is inadequate, the flap is resected proximal until good blood flow is observed

Fat Grafting For those patients who require post-explantation augmentation with autologous tissue, fat grafting may be an option. This is best accomplished when the capsule is still present as it prevents the fat from slipping into the old implant pocket. One method for capsular contracture treatment is the simultaneous implant exchange with fat (SIEF), which utilized pre-expansion in the subcutaneous space of the breast and a two-phase fat transfer technique after explantation (but with retention of the capsule) [13]. Patients should be counseled that fat grafting cannot provide the same guarantee of volume as an implant, due to individual differences in the absorption and loss of fat. Additionally, fat graft-

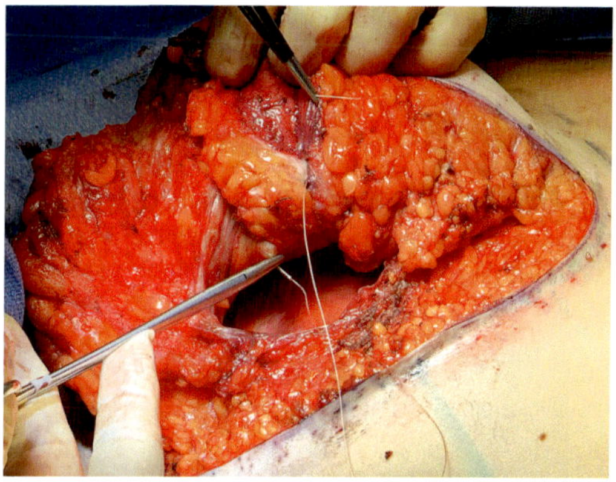

Fig. 14.17 The distal end of the auto-augmentation flap is flipped under the areola and then sutured with 2-0 vicryl to the overlying breast tissue to enhance the projection of the central breast

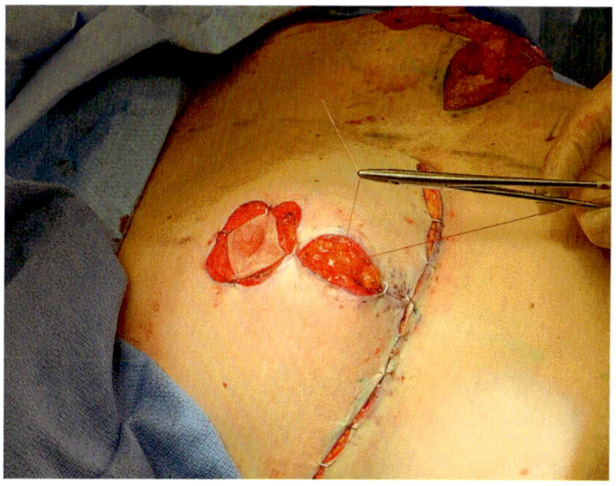

Fig. 14.18 The pillars are then re-approximated with 2-0 vicryl sutures and final skin excision is accomplished

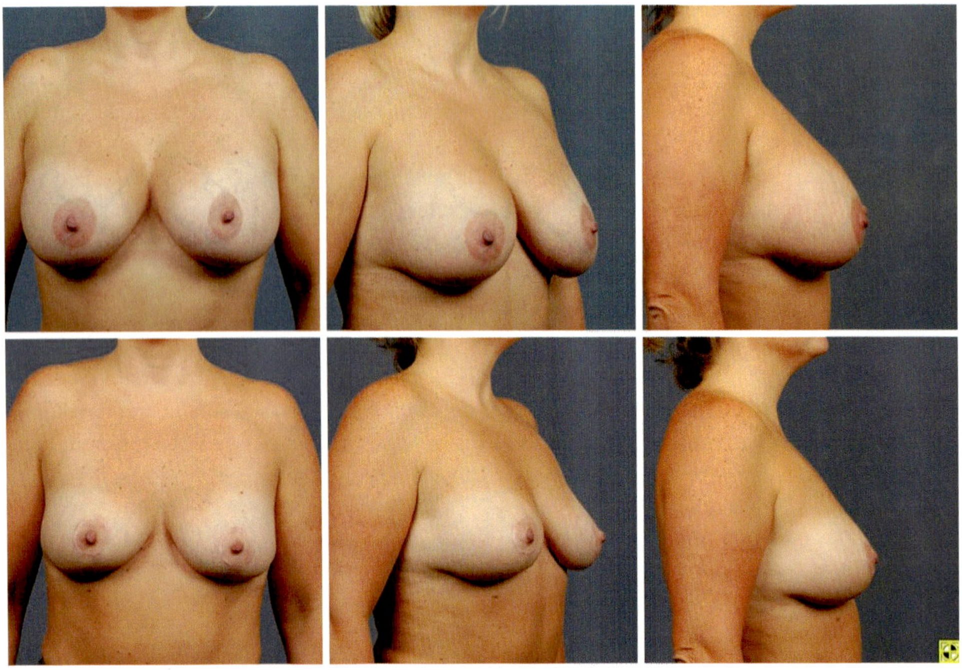

Fig. 14.19 39 year old G4P4 desired smaller, more uplifted breasts. She underwent bilateral explantation, popcorn capsulorraphy of the residual capsule to improve central projection, and a vertical masopexy with auto-augmentation. (Upper) Preoperative photographs and (Lower) 3-year postoperative views

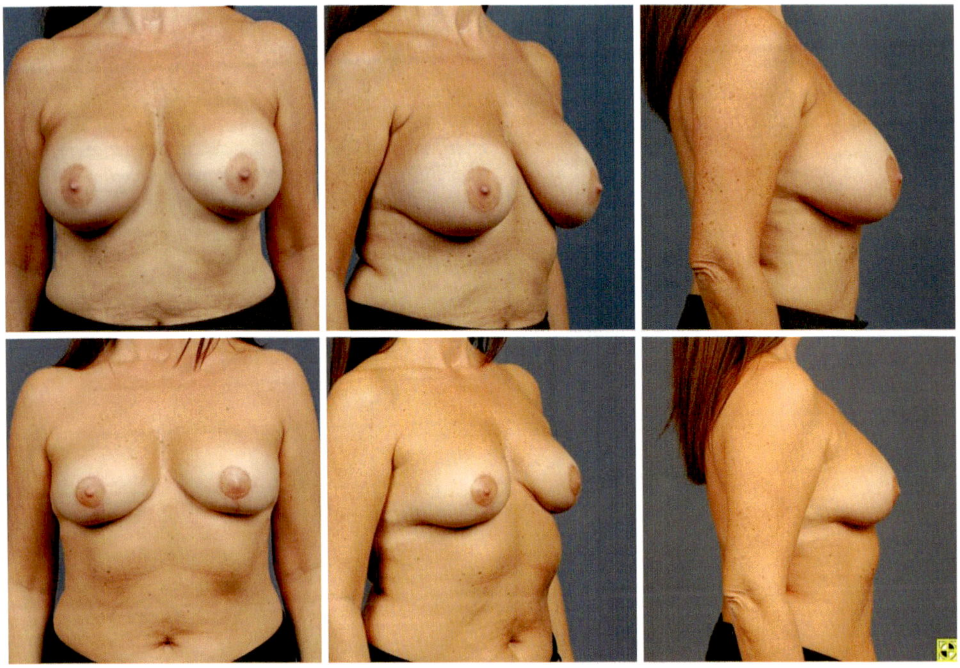

Fig. 14.20 52 year old G2P2 with 15 year history of saline implants with heavy, ptotic breasts desiring asmaller more uplifted apppearance. She underwent explantation, mastopexy and auto-augmentation. (Upper) Preoperative views and (lower) Postoperative views 6 months after surgery

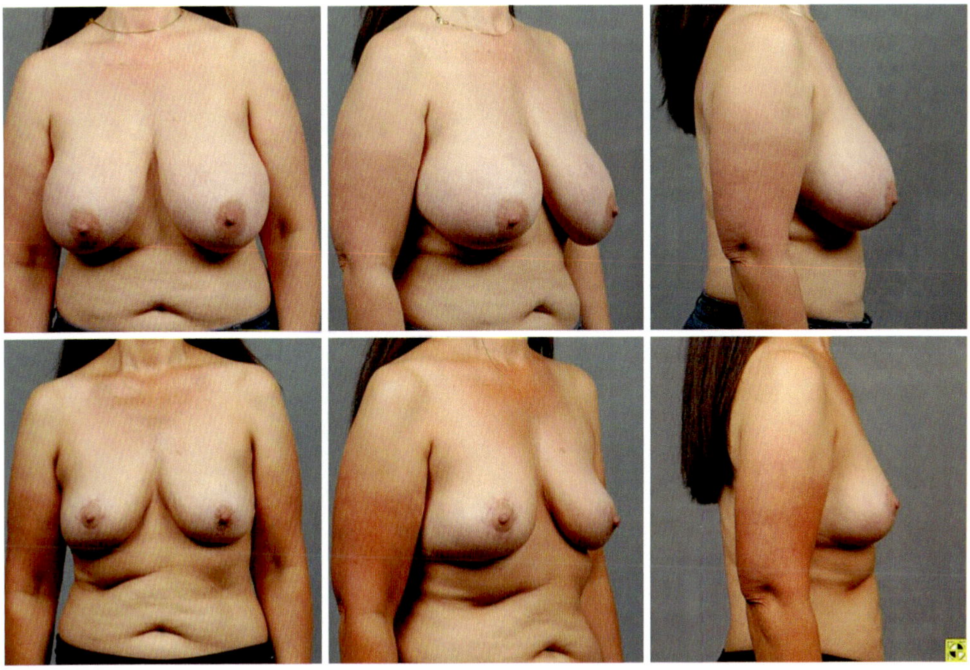

Fig. 14.21 47 year old G2P2 with saline implants and wearing a DDD bra desired more uplifted breasts and a downsize to a full C cup. She underwent saline explantation with popcorn capsulorraphy, an inverted-T mastopexy with auto-augmentation. (Upper) pre-operative views and (Lower) post-operative views 7 months after surgery

ing can provide improvement in global volume including upper volume and cleavage, but is poor at creating core projection and can be less effective as a stand alone procedure if core breast projection is lacking (Fig. 14.22).

For patients without core projection, combining procedures is commonly performed, including mastopexies with or without auto-augmentation and fat grafting (Figs. 14.13 and 14.23).

In fat grafting, the fat is prepared and placed into the subcutaneous tissue of the breast with no significant attempt to place the fat into the breast parenchyma, although undoubtedly some fat most likely is injected into the breast tissue itself. Fat is placed most significantly along the upper poles of the breast and along the medial cleavage. If a mastopexy and/or auto-augmentation arc per formed, the fat is placed in the areas of the breast requiring additional volume. If the anterior capsule has been removed, fat grafting can be more challenging. In thin patients or patients with thin breast flaps, fat grafting may have to be delayed until after the breast and skin flaps have healed and become adherent. When placing the fat, it can be helpful to leave the incisions open until after fat grafting to insure fat has not inadvertently placed deep to the breast flaps into the central breast. The amount of fat that can be injected is variable, but in general, the capacity for fat is thought to be about 1:1. So, if a remaining breast after implant removal is deemed to be around 200 grams, then 200 cc of fat can be placed as a maximal capacity. Retension varies, but is thought to be about 50% based on many variables including flap vascularity and the quality of fat infiltrated. Additional fat grafting session can be performed, offered usually after 6 months from time of initial fat injections.

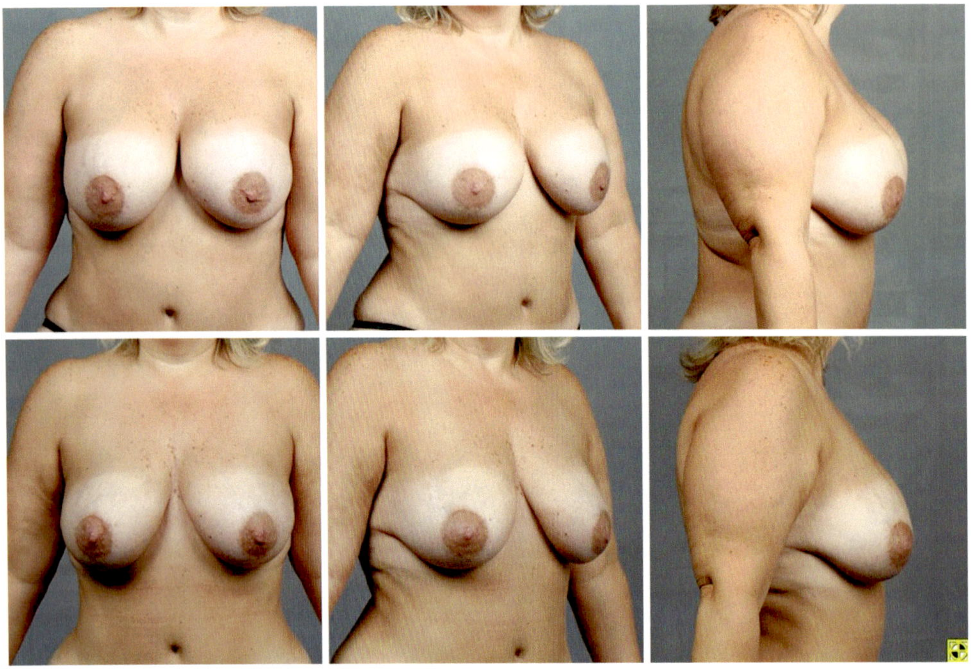

Fig. 14.22 46 year old desired implant removal and no mastopexy. She underwent explantation with placement of 600 cc of fat per breast. This can provide volume but does little to correct the breast ptosis. (Upper) Preoperative views and (Lower) postoperative views 9 months post surgery

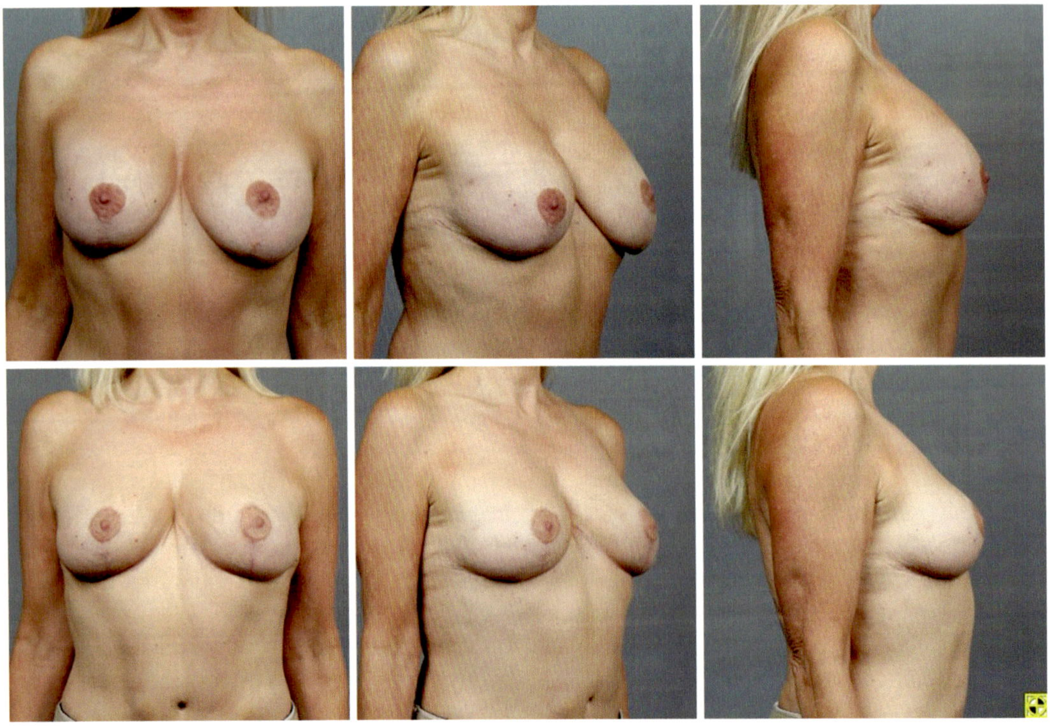

Fig. 14.23 64 year old whom has had a breast reduction 40 years prior and an augmentation mastopexy 4 years ago presented for implant removal and a breast lift. She underwent an explantation inverted-T mastopexy, auto-augmentation and fat grafting, 120 cc to the right breast and 60 cc to the left breast. (Upper) Preoperative views and (Lower) postoperative results 6 months post surgery

Conclusion

Topics in breast implant removal are closely intertwined with issues in the study of capsular contracture, implant rupture, breast implant illness, and BIA-ALCL. Significant advancements have been made in the management of breast aesthetics following breast implant removal. However, decisions concerning breast implant removal are complex and further study is needed to ensure optimal outcomes for explantation patients. While evidence-based research strongly supports implant rupture, capsular contracture, and ALCL as indications for explantation, it is ambiguous for breast implant illness or connective tissue disease. Furthermore, data is lacking on the appropriateness of a more complex and costly prophylactic total capsulectomy procedure in the management of asymptomatic patients with textured implants. The lack of data and ongoing uncertainty in decisions related to explantation and/or capsulectomies requires an even greater need for appropriate discussion with each patient concerning the risk and benefits of potential treatment options. The final recommendations and management can then be determined uniquely for each patient, taking into consideration all evidence-based data as it becomes available, the minimization of unnecessary risks, an appreciation and understanding of all the patient concerns as it relates to her breast, and ultimately sound surgical judgment.

References

1. Spear SL, Parikh PM, Goldstein JA. History of breast implants and the food and drug administration. Clin Plast Surg. 2009;36(1):15–21.
2. Cole NM. Consequences of the U.S. food and drug administration-directed moratorium on silicone gel breast implants: 1992 to 2006. Plast Reconstr Surg. 2018;141(5):1137–41.
3. American Society of Plastic Surgeons. 2010 report of the 2009 statistics. Accessed at https://www.plasticsurgery.org/documents/News/Statistics/2009/plastic-surgery-statistics-full-report-2009.pdf; July 2019.
4. American Society of Plastic Surgeons. 2018 plastic surgery statistics report. Accessed at https://www.plasticsurgery.org/documents/News/Statistics/2018/plastic-surgery-statistics-report-2018.pdf; July 2019.
5. Headon H, Kasem A, Mokbel K. Capsular contracture after breast augmentation: an update for clinical practice. Arch Plast Surg. 2015;42(5):532–43.
6. Spear SL, Murphy DK. Natrelle round silicone breast implants: core study results at 10 years. Plast Reconstr Surg. 2014;133(6):1354–61.
7. Blount AL, Martin MD, Lineberry KD, Kettaneh N, Alfonso DR. Capsular contracture rate in a low-risk population after primary augmentation mammaplasty. Aesthet Surg J. 2013;33(4):516–21.
8. Calobrace MB, Stevens WG, Capizzi PJ, Cohen R, Godinez T, Beckstrand M. Risk factor analysis for capsular contracture: a 10-year Sientra study using round, smooth, and textured implants for breast augmentation. Plast Reconstr Surg. 2018;141(4S Sientra Shaped and Round Cohesive Gel Implants):20S–8S.
9. Wan D, Rohrich RJ. Revisiting the management of capsular contracture in breast augmentation: a systematic review. Plast Reconstr Surg. 2016;137(3):826–41.
10. Seigle-murandi F, Lefebvre F, Bruant-rodier C, Bodin F. Incidence of breast implant rupture in a 12-year retrospective cohort: evidence of quality discrepancy depending on the range. J Plast Reconstr Aesthet Surg. 2017;70(1):42–6.
11. Maxwell GP, Gabriel A. Acellular dermal matrix in aesthetic revisionary breast surgery. Aesth Surg J. 2011;31:65S–76S.
12. Swanson E. Open capsulotomy: an effective but overlooked treatment for capsular contracture after breast augmentation. Plast Reconstr Surg Glob Open. 2016;4(10):e1096.
13. Del Vecchio DA. "SIEF" – simultaneous implant exchange with fat: a new option in revision breast implant surgery. Plast Reconstr Surg. 2012;130(6):1187–96.
14. Maisel Lotan A, Retchkiman M, Tuchman I, Binenboym R, Gronovich Y. Analysis of 109 consecutive explanted breast implants: correlation between suspected implant rupture and surgical findings. Aesthet Plast Surg. 2016;40(5):739–44.
15. Ikeda DM, Borofsky HB, Herfkens RJ, Sawyer-glover AM, Birdwell RL, Glover GH. Silicone breast implant rupture: pitfalls of magnetic resonance imaging and relative efficacies of magnetic resonance, mammography, and ultrasound. Plast Reconstr Surg. 1999;104(7):2054–62.
16. Hold PM, Alam S, Pilbrow WJ, et al. How should we investigate breast implant rupture? Breast J. 2012;18(3):253–6.
17. Peters W, Smith D, Fornasier V, Lugowski S, Ibanez D. An outcome analysis of 100 women after explantation of silicone gel breast implants. Ann Plast Surg 1997;39(1):9–19.
18. Melmed EP. A review of explantation in 240 symptomatic women: a description of explantation and capsulectomy with reconstruction using a periareolar technique. Plast Reconstr Surg. 1998;101(5):1364–73.

19. Rohrich RJ, Kenkel JM, Adams WP, Beran S, Conner WC. A prospective analysis of patients undergoing silicone breast implant explantation. Plast Reconstr Surg. 2000;105(7):2529–37.
20. De Boer M, Colaris M, der Hulst RRWJ V, Cohen Tervaert JW. Is explantation of silicone breast implants useful in patients with complaints? Immunol Res. 2017;65(1):25–36.
21. Rohrich RJ, Kaplan J, Dayan E. Silicone implant illness: science versus myth? Plast Reconstr Surg. 2019;144(1):98–109.
22. Magnusson MR, Cooter RD, Rakhorst H, Mcguire PA, Adams WP, Deva AK. Breast implant illness: a way forward. Plast Reconstr Surg. 2019;143(3S A Review of Breast Implant-Associated Anaplastic Large Cell Lymphoma):74S–81S.
23. American Society of Aesthetic Plastic Surgery. Breast implant illness – frequently asked questions/ talking points. Accessed at https://www.surgery.org/sites/default/files/downloads/BII-Talking-Points-FINAL-1.15.19.pdf; July 2019.
24. Mccarthy CM, Loyo-berríos N, Qureshi AA, et al. Patient registry and outcomes for breast implants and anaplastic large cell lymphoma etiology and epidemiology (PROFILE): initial report of findings, 2012–2018. Plast Reconstr Surg. 2019;143(3S A Review of Breast Implant-Associated Anaplastic Large Cell Lymphoma):65S–73S.
25. Food and Drug Administration. Medical device reports of breast implant-associated anaplastic large cell lymphoma. Accessed at https://www.fda.gov/medical-devices/breast-implants/medical-device-reports-breast-implant-associated-anaplastic-large-cell-lymphoma; July 2019.
26. Leberfinger AN, Behar BJ, Williams NC, et al. Breast implant-associated anaplastic large cell lymphoma: a systematic review. JAMA Surg. 2017;152(12):1161–8.
27. Clemens MW, Medeiros LJ, Butler CE, et al. Complete surgical excision is essential for the management of patients with breast implant-associated anaplastic large-cell lymphoma. J Clin Oncol. 2016;34(2):160–8.
28. Tevis S, Hunt KH, Clemens MW. Stepwise en-bloc resection of breast implant associated ALCL with oncologic considerations. Aesthet Surg J Open Forum. 2019;1(1):1–12.
29. Cohen R, Irwin L, Newton-john T, Slater A. #bodypositivity: a content analysis of body positive accounts on Instagram. Body Image. 2019;29:47–57.
30. Hidalgo DA, Sinno S. Current trends and controversies in breast augmentation. Plast Reconstr Surg. 2016;137(4):1142–50.
31. Dickson JK, Gorman M, Palmer J. The V-Y capsulotomy release for correcting capsular contracture. J Plast Reconstr Aesthet Surg. 2015;68(12):1768–9.
32. Collis N, Sharpe DT. Recurrence of subglandular breast implant capsular contracture: anterior versus total capsulectomy. Plast Reconstr Surg. 2000;106(4):792–7.
33. Netscher DT. Aesthetic outcome of breast implant removal in 85 consecutive patients. Plast Reconstr Surg. 2004;113(3):1057–9.
34. Graf RM, Closs Ono MC, Pace D, Balbinot P, Pazio ALB, De Paula DR. Breast auto-augmentation (mastopexy and lipofilling): an option for quitting breast implants. Aesthetic Plast Surg. 2019;43(5):1133–14.
35. Rohrich RJ, Parker TH. Aesthetic management of the breast after explantation: evaluation and mastopexy options. Plast Reconstr Surg. 2007;120(1):312–5.
36. Loghavi S, Medeiros LJ, Javadi S, Lin P, Khoury JD, Nastoupil L, Hunt KK, Clemens MW, Miranda RN. Breast implant-associated anaplastic large cell lymphoma with bone marrow involvement. Aesthet Surg J. 2018;38(7).
37. Collins MS, Miranda RN, Medeiros LJ, Silva de Meneses MP, Iyer SP, Butler CE, Liu J, Clemens MW. Characteristics and treatment of advanced breast implant-associated anaplastic large cell lymphoma. Plast Reconstr Surg. 2019;143:41S–50S.

Mastopexy with Fat Graft Augmentation

15

James D. Namnoum

Introduction

Mastopexy is the second most common aesthetic breast procedure and has increased in frequency by 99% since the year 2000 [1]. Autologous fat grafting for aesthetic breast surgery has been rising steadily over past decade. A survey of members of the American Society of Plastic Surgeons conducted in 2013 showed that 28% of respondents were using autologous fat grafting for aesthetic breast surgery procedures; this number has almost certainly increased since then [2]. Fat grafting for aesthetic breast surgery has been used to improve the soft tissue environment around breast implants [3], for primary breast augmentation [4–6], as a volume replacement for women undergoing explantation with or without pre-expansion [7], and as a method to reduce intermammary distance and improve symmetry in women undergoing breast reduction, mastopexy, and augmentation [8].

Traditionally, mastopexy alone has been performed far less commonly than augmentation with mastopexy in the US. This reflects preferences of American women for larger, firmer breasts with excessive upper pole convexity and high cleavage. However, a closer evaluation of trend setting fashion standards such as those created by bra manufacturers such as Victoria's Secret, demonstrates that their models have very small breasts which are dramatically altered by pushup bras to appear larger and more voluptuous. While there are no studies documenting changes in women's preferences for breast size, two studies have shown that more financially secure men with greater resources prefer smaller breasted women, and that men with a long-term mating strategy preferred smaller breasts than those seeking a short-term relationship [9, 10]. Concerns about the potential risks of breast implants, breast implant associated-ALCL, and breast implant associated illness may potentially affect women's willingness to undergo augmentation in conjunction with mastopexy. This coupled with changing attitudes regarding the aesthetic value of larger breasts may increase the number of women seeking mastopexy alone.

Mastopexy Techniques

Mastopexy combines nipple elevation, areolar reduction, and skin tailoring to improve the shape of the breast. Often glandular flaps, plication, or a rearrangement of local redundant tissues such as those seen following massive weight loss are used to enhance central projection and upper pole fill; these procedures have the added benefit of relocating ptotic tissues superiorly to prevent

J. D. Namnoum (✉)
Private Practice, Atlanta Plastic Surgery, Assistant Clinical Professor, Emory University, Atlanta, GA, USA
e-mail: jdnamnoum@atlplastic.com

M. B. Calobrace et al. (eds.), *Augmentation Mastopexy*,
https://doi.org/10.1007/978-3-030-48226-8_15

relapse. In some instances, removal of ptotic lower pole tissues may be a good option especially when significant asymmetry exists. This concept of plus minus mastopexy has been shown to be a powerful option to remove ptotic parenchyma while replacing parenchymal volume with implants or autologous fat. Many options exist for glandular reshaping such as superior based flaps, inferior based flaps, chest wall based flaps and laterally based tissues [11–14]. Additional measures such as the use of permanent or absorbable mesh are becoming more commonplace in an effort to maintain the integrity of the reshaped breast [15, 16].

Skin reduction patterns are determined by the degree of skin excess and glandular ptosis. Periareolar mastopexy has traditionally been reserved for patients with minimal ptosis who require nipple elevation of 1–2 cm; Goes has shown it to be a more versatile technique with potentially greater application especially when combined with glandular plication or reduction and reshaping using mesh. Circumvertical mastopexy has more potential to reshape and cone the breast and is valuable for correcting periareolar and horizontal skin excess. The addition of an IMF incision in either a 'T','L', or 'J' permits the tailoring of vertical skin excess potentially decreasing the risk of inferior pole stretch.

Once the gland and skin are reshaped, fat grafting can be used to correct step off deformities of the upper chest, narrow the intramammary distance by filling the décolletage, correct underlying acquired or native shape discrepancies, and equalize volume differences (Fig. 15.1). Grafting can be performed in the subcutaneous plan as well as parenchyma. Preferential fat grafting should begin in the superficial planes and then proceed to deeper delivery in the parenchyma if there is availability of enough lipograft.

The process of proper fat grafting can be broken down to three components: harvest, fat processing, and injection of the fat. In order to harvest correctly, proper tumescent SAFE liposuction techniques need to be performed. Each and every donor site needs to be addressed effectively and respected to prevent contour irregularities while providing an improved shape of the donor site.

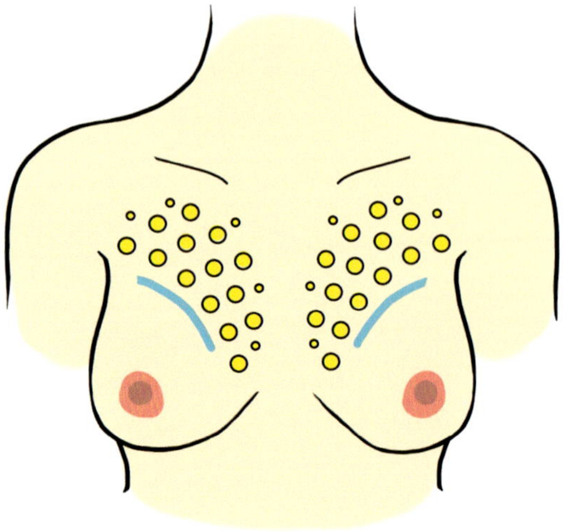

Fig. 15.1 Fat grafting typically is performed to the upper chest to soften the transition from the clavicle and parasternal areas to enhance the cleavage and narrow the intermammary distance. Fat may also be grafted asymmetrically to correct volume and shape asymmetries to other parts of the breast

Multiple techniques exist to perform lipoharvest. Tumescent fluid is instilled into donor sites and allowed to take effect prior to suction. Methods of suction include traditional suction assisted liposuction (SAL), SAFE liposuction techniques, as well as with multi-holed hand harvest methods. Once the fat has been collected it must be processed appropriately. Numerous methods exist for processing fat including decant method, straining, centrifugation, and filtration/washing devices for processing. Critical concepts in processing include washing fat to remove excess oils, drying the fat to remove excess tumescent fluid, and ensuring uniformity of the lipograft to maximize take. Proper processing can reduce the risk potential oil cysts, fat necrosis, and negative sequelae associated with injection of other lipoaspirate components.

After the fat is processed, proper injection methods need to be performed to ensure maximum take. Different methodologies exist to inject but all the procedural tenants remain the same. Fat needs to be injected into healthy tissue in small aliquots to minimize potential necrosis and absorption. In addition, the fat cannot be placed within empty spaces such as an old implant pocket or in large clumps. Injection techniques vary from expansion vibration lipofilling (EVL) techniques to the using fine Coleman cannulas in a linear retrograde fashion. EVL methods utilize a small basket canula and Power Assisted Liposuction (Microaire) device to inject fat in either antegrade and retrograde fashion as long as the canula is in motion. The purpose of the vibration allows for easy passage of the canula and creation of space to allow uniform deposition of fat.

Technical Details: Mastopexy with Chest Wall Based Flap for Auto Augmentation and Fat Grafting

Case 1 (Fig. 15.2)

Presentation: 36-year-old, presents for mastopexy and body contouring. Grade II ptosis (horizontal and vertical skin excess); minimal volume asymmetry. Deficient tissues in upper pole of breast with mild step-off deformity. (see Fig. 15.2 a–c)

Preoperative Markings: Markings are created with the patient in a standing position. A large caliper is used to determine Pitanguy's point (P). The nipple height is set by measuring upwards 3 cm from Pitanguy's point (N); the top of the areola is marked 2 cm above the new height of the nipple (A). Confirmation of the suitability of the designated nipple and areola position is done by grasping the areola and positioning superiorly on the breast mound until a pleasing aesthetic result is confirmed. This is the correlated with the bottom up markings performed earlier and any needed adjustment is made. Further visual confirmation of nipple symmetry is made by having the patient stand in front of a full-length mirror and looking at the reflected placement of the markings. Preliminary marking of the horizontal skin excess is made by a sliding rotation of the breast to the right and left and dropping a vertical line to the breast meridian at the IMF. Definitive marks will be created in the operating room by tailor tacking. Areas of the breast designated for autologous fat grafting is marked over the upper chest and cleavage (dḗcolletage).

Intraoperative markings: the centrally based chest wall flap (measuring 5 × 5 cm). This ptotic tissue from the lower pole will be advanced superiorly to fill the central and upper portion of the breast increasing central projection. Upward relocation of ptotic tissue is used to help prevent relapse of the lower pole (see Fig. 15.2 f).

Intraoperative view: chest wall flap design. Blood supply derived from chest wall perforators entering base of the flap. Flap is advanced superiorly to fill upper pole and increase central projection. The flap is secured into position by suturing to the upper pectoralis fascia superior to the new areolar apex and to the undersurface of the superior gland. Then the pillars are closed. Fat is grafted to the upper pole and cleavage through the open incision around the areola. After completion 100–200 ccs of fat grafted to the decollatage (see Fig. 15.2 g–o).

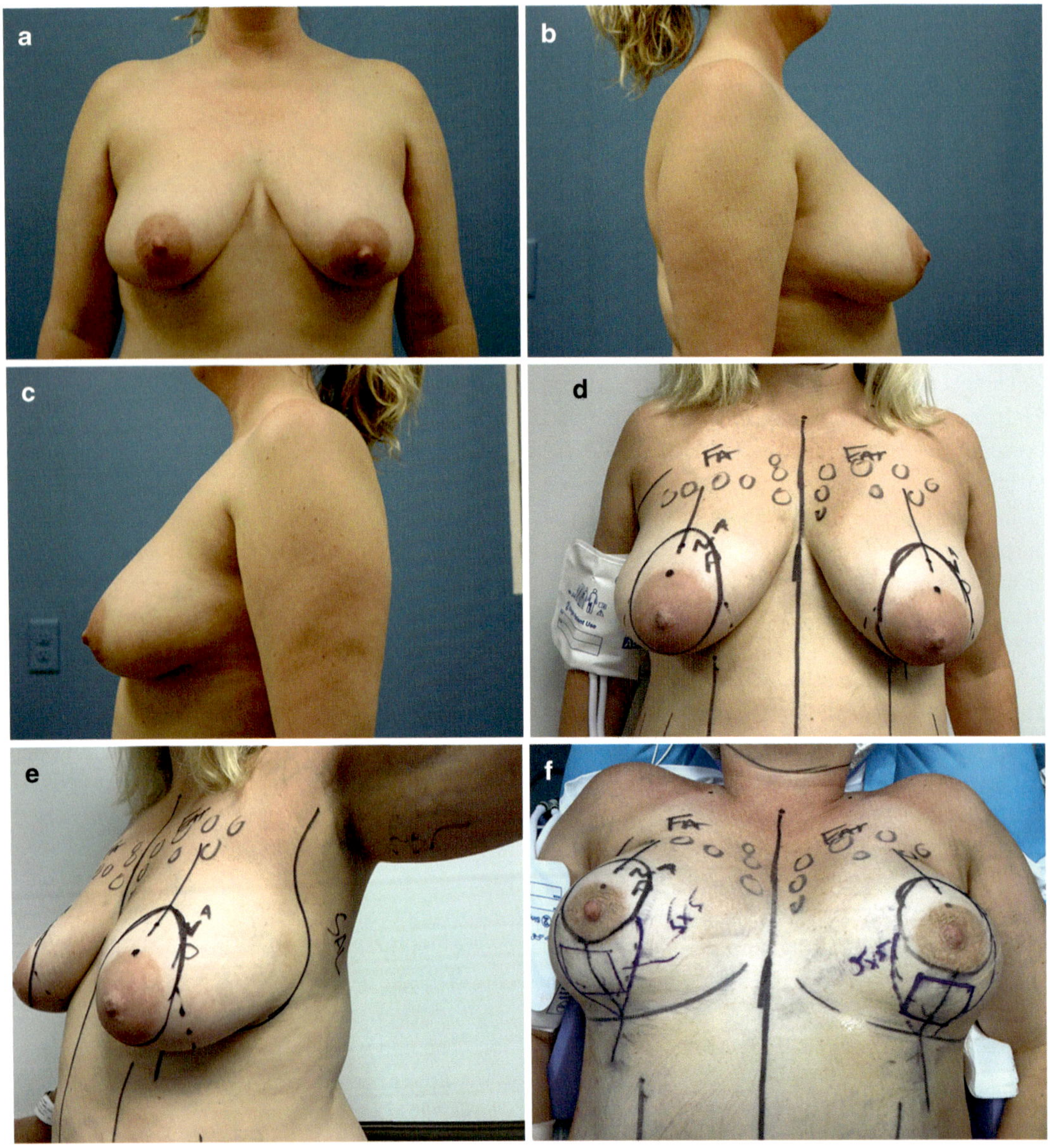

Fig. 15.2 (**Case 1**): 36 year old, presents for mastopexy and body contouring. Grade II ptosis (horizontal and vertical skin excess); minimal volume asymmetry. Deficient tissues in upper pole of breast with mild step-off deformity. **Preoperative views:** (**a**) Frontal (**b**) Right lateral (**c**) Left lateral. Markings (**d–f**). **Intraoperative markings** including the centrally based chest wall flap (measuring 5 × 5 cm). (**g–o**) **Intraoperative view** of chest wall flap design

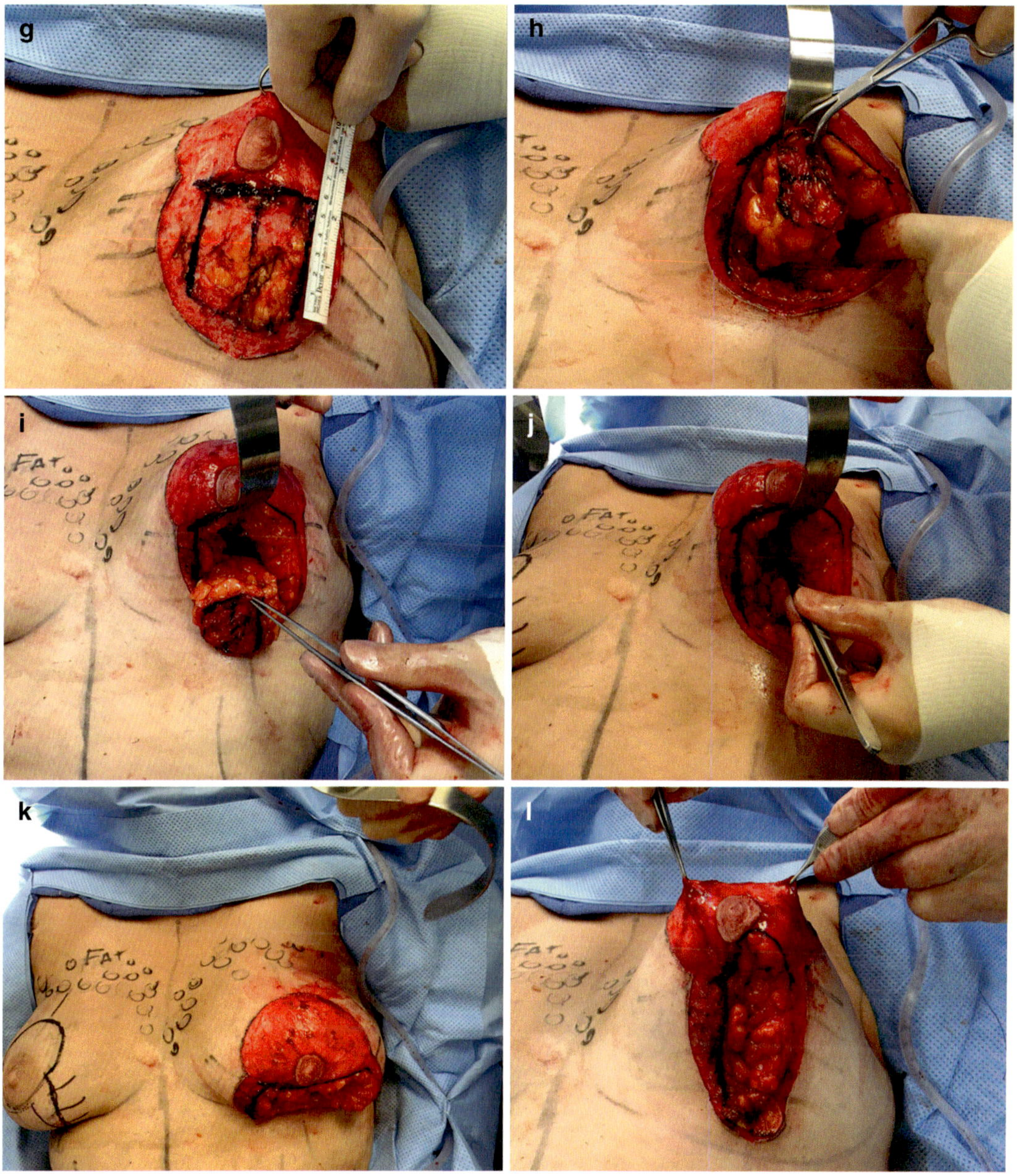

Fig. 15.2 (continued)

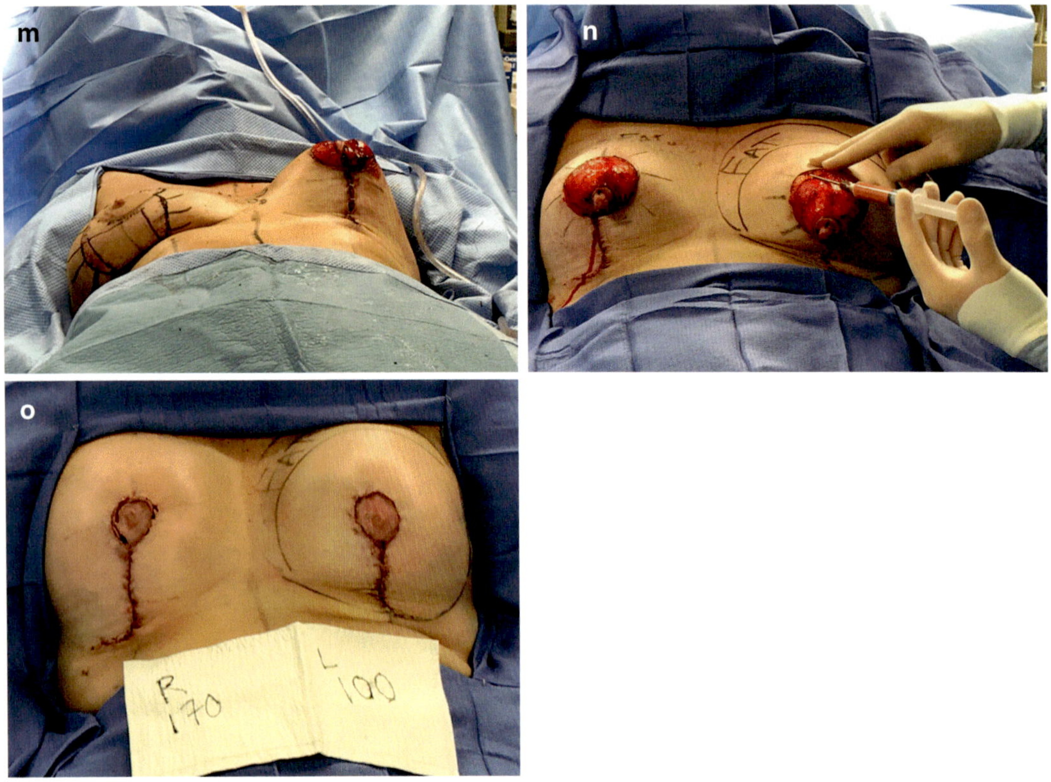

Fig. 15.2 (continued)

Case 2: (Fig. 15.3)

Presentation: 46 year old presents for mastopexy and liposuction. Happy with current size but wants breast lift and liposuction. Fat from hips designated for redistribution to cleavage and upper chest (see Fig. 15.3).

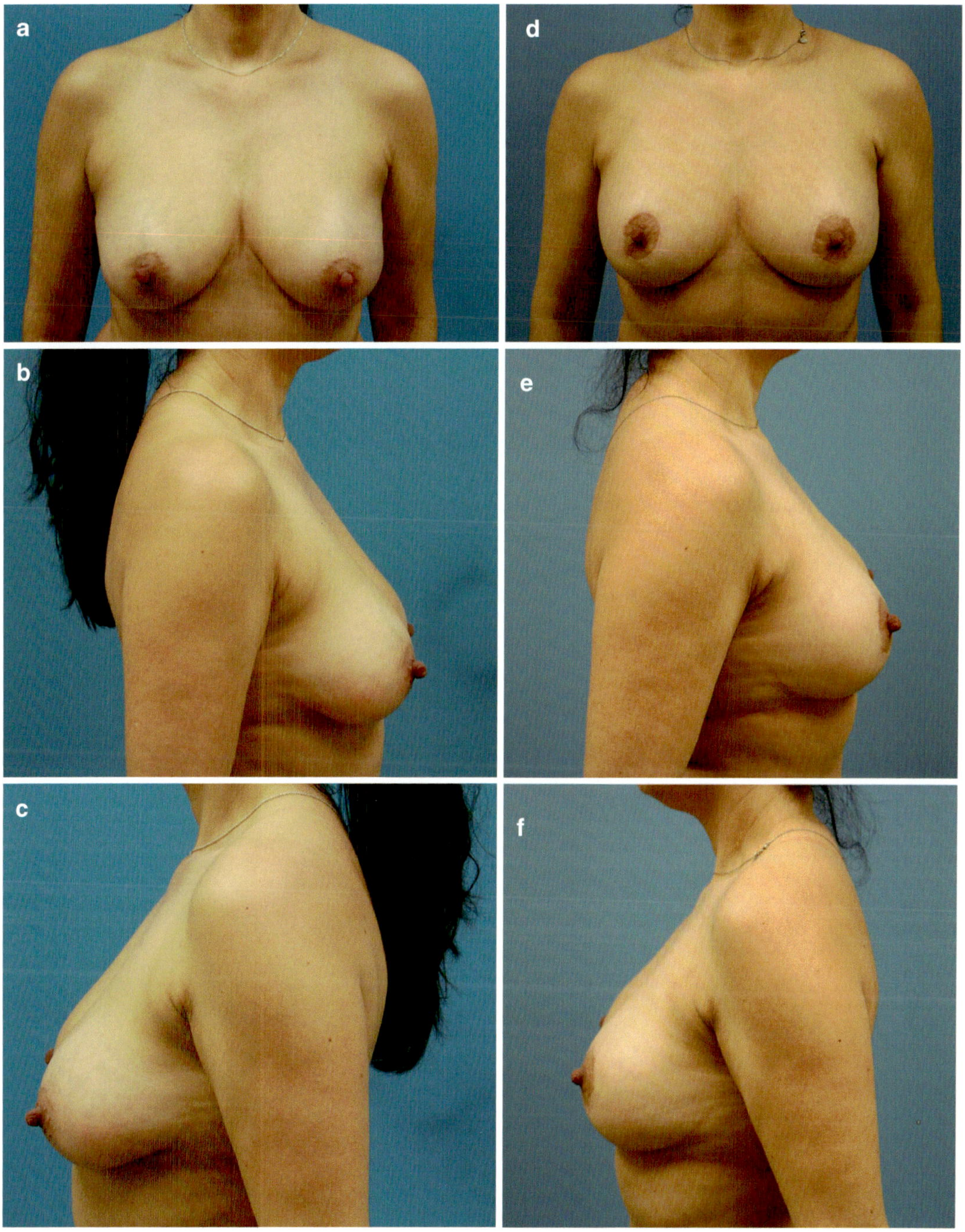

Fig. 15.3 **(Case 2)**: Mastopexy with Fat Grafting. 46 year old presents for mastopexy and liposuction. Happy with current size but wants breast lift and liposuction. Fat from hips designated for redistribution to cleavage and upper chest. **Preoperative views.** (**a**) Frontal. (**b**) Right lateral. (**c**) Left lateral. **Postoperative views** at 2.5 years. Bilateral Mastopexy with chest wall based flaps and fat grafting cleavage and upper chest 120 ccs per side. (**d**) Frontal. (**e**) Right lateral. (**f**) Left lateral

Mastopexy with Auto Augmentation, Glandular Resection and Fat Grafting

In many instances, patients desire and need a small glandular resection in addition to mastopexy. Glandular tissue may be resected from areas of excess fullness centrally, laterally, and inferiorly as needed. Liposuction can be added to refine the lateral breast border and contour axillary fullness. Suctioning of the lower pole may eliminate the need for transverse incision or reduce the size of the skin resection from a 'T' to a 'J' or 'L'. Liposuction of the upper abdomen below the breast contour and down to the costal margin can further improve the transition of the lower breast and upper abdomen. Fat grafting can serve the purpose of adding volume to the parasternal area and soften the transition from the clavicle to the upper breast border. Fat grafting has the added benefit of helping equalize the breast volume and footprint.

Case 3 (Fig. 15.4)

Presentation: 52-year-old woman with macromastia, breast asymmetry and ptosis. Desires mastopexy and a small reduction with contouring of lateral breast and axilla. Hypertrophic upper abdominal scar from previous mole excision (see Fig. 15.4).

Case 4 (Fig. 15.5)

Presentation: 50-year-old woman desires mastopexy and a small reduction. Breast asymmetry and ptosis with right breast larger than left (see Fig. 15.5).

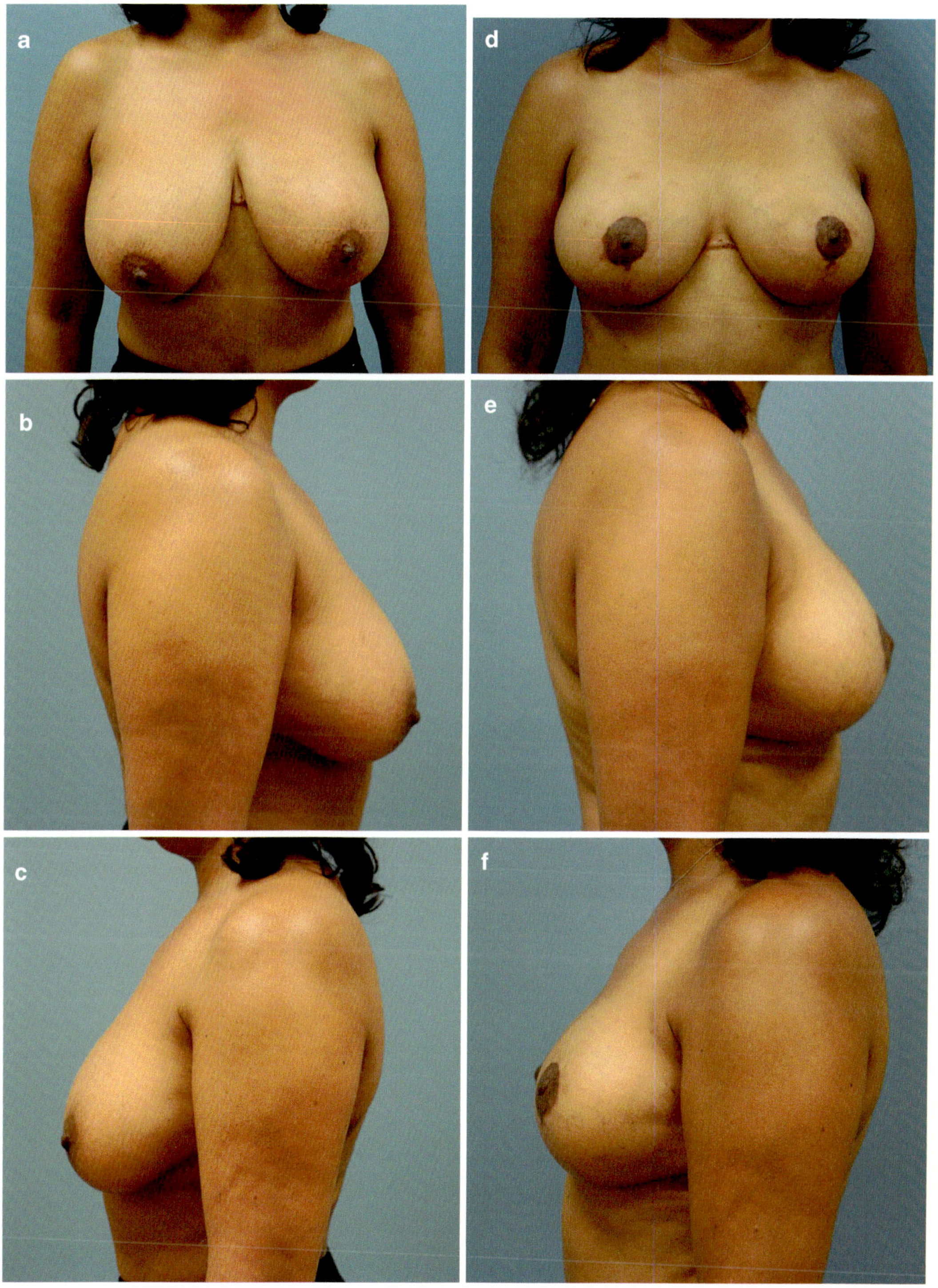

Fig. 15.4 (**Case 3**): 52 year old woman with macromastia, breast asymmetry and ptosis. **Preoperative views**. (**a**) Frontal. (**b**) Right lateral. (**c**) Left lateral. **Postoperative** view at 8 months. Auto augmentation with glandular flap. Tissue resection deep central and lateral breast, right 186 gm; left 108 gm. Fat grafting upper pole and cleavage, right 100 ccs; left 140 ccs. Liposuction upper abdomen 200 ccs; liposuction lateral breasts 150 ccs per side. (**d**) Frontal. (**e**) Right lateral. (**f**) Left lateral

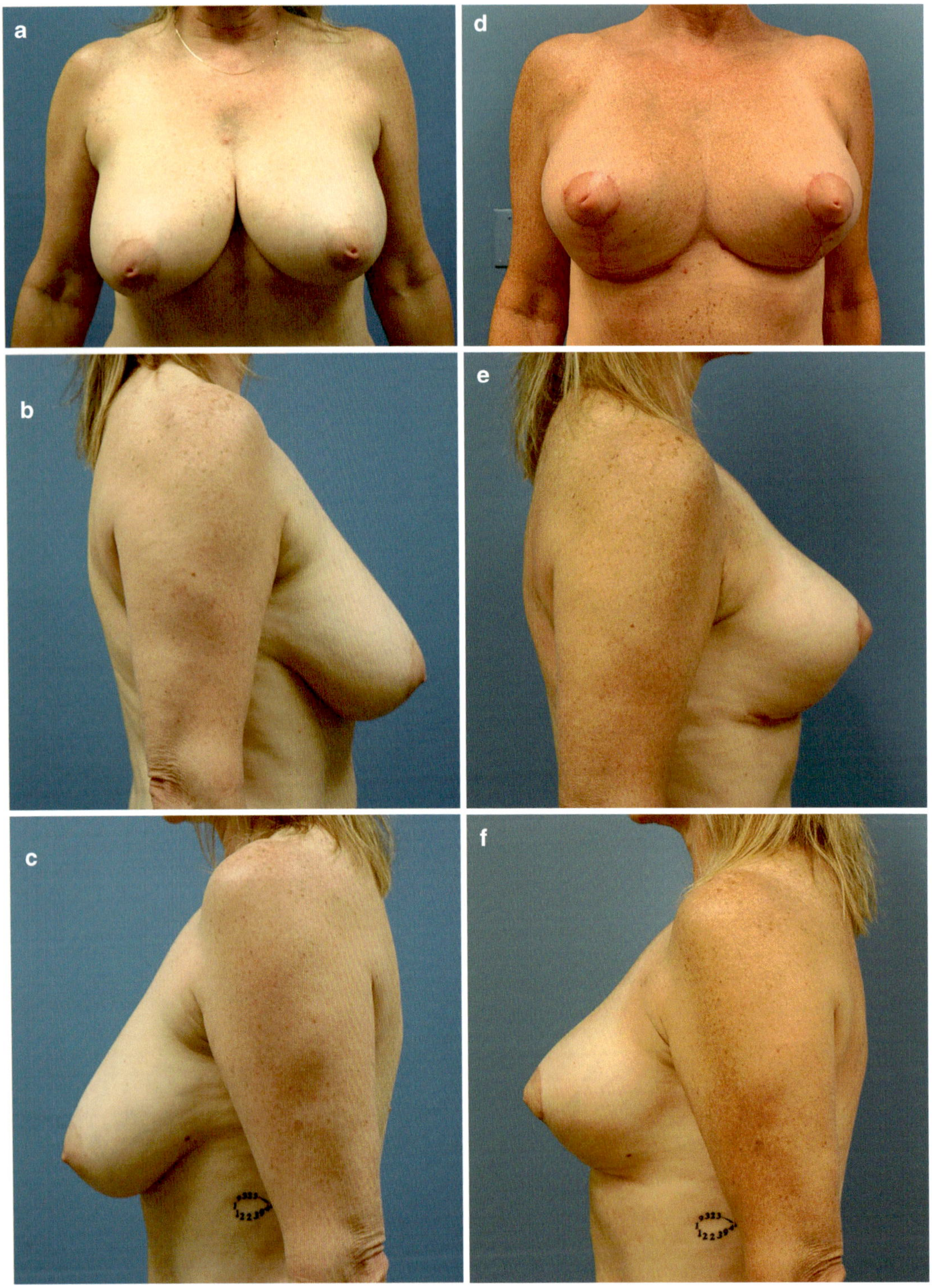

Fig. 15.5 (**Case 4**): 50 year old woman desires mastopexy and small reduction. **Preoperative views**. (**a**) Frontal. (**b**) Right lateral. (**c**) Left lateral. (**d–f**) **Early postoperative** result at 3 months. Auto augmentation with chest wall based flap. Glandular resection from deep central and lateral breast right 166 gm; left 98 gm. Liposuction lateral and axillary breast 100 ccs per side. Fat grafting upper chest and cleavage 300 ccs per side. (**d**) Frontal. (**e**) Right lateral. (**f**) Left lateral

Explantation Mastopexy with Auto Augmentation and Fat Grafting

As patients age and gain weight, they often elect to remove implants placed at an earlier age and undergo mastopexy. These patients are often candidates for explantation combined with mastopexy and fat grafting to avoid a deflated central breast and upper chest. Fat grafting can be a useful tool to restore volume to the entire breast. These patients must have realistic expectations and understand the volume increase will be modest and less than that of what their prior implant volumes were. Donor site liposuction of the lateral breast, axilla, and upper abdomen may be of value. Care must be taken to respect the donor site and practice SAFE liposuction techniques to avoid any deformity.

Case 5 (Fig. 15.6)

Presentation: 34-year-old with a history of breast augmentation with silicone devices, 350 ccs placed subpectorally 12 years previously. Has experienced 25 lb weight gain since. Desires explantation, mastopexy and fat grafting with liposuction of abdomen and hips.

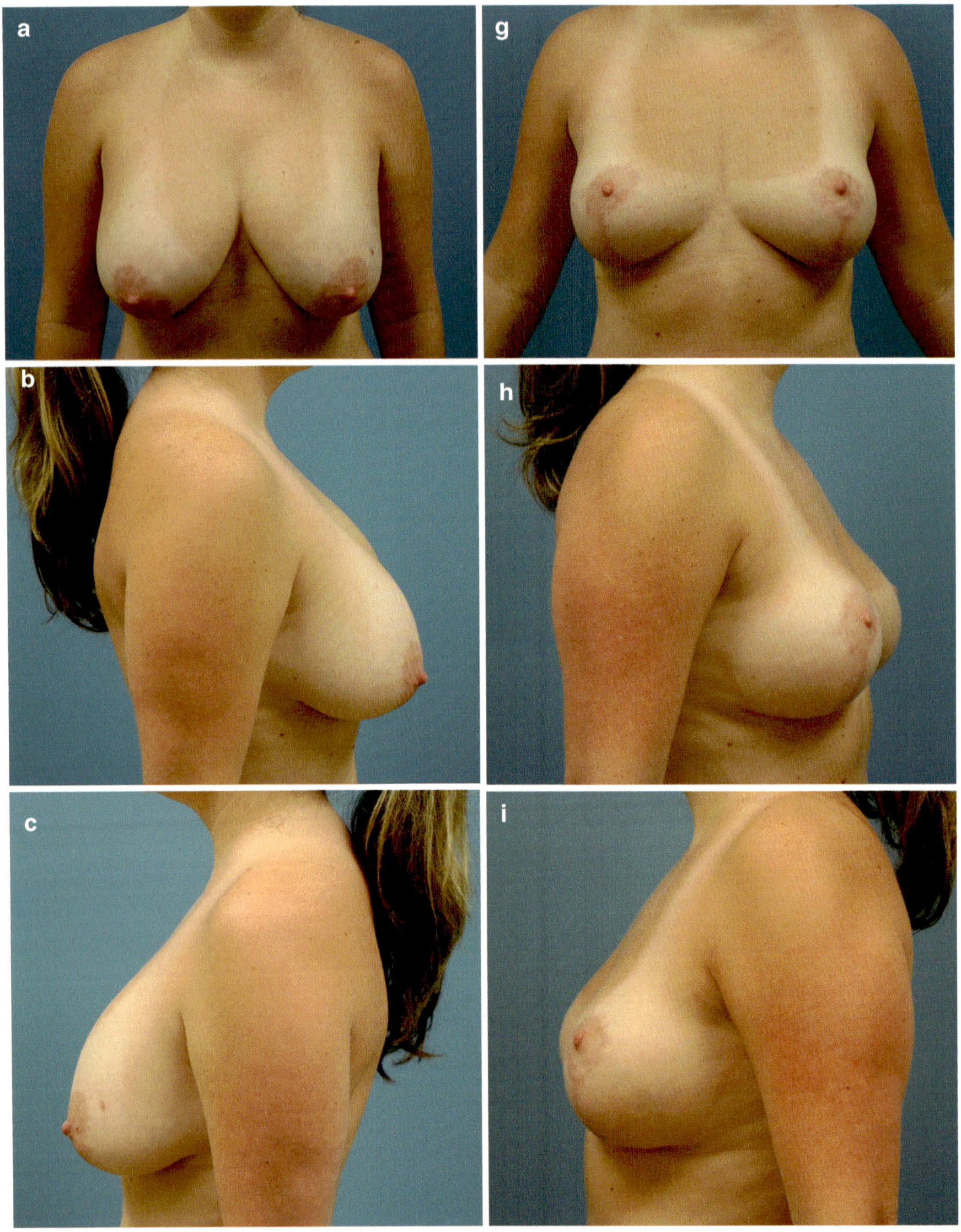

Fig. 15.6 (**Case 5**): 34 year old with a history of breast augmentation with silicone devices, Desires explantation, mastopexy and fat grafting with liposuction of abdomen and hips. **Preoperative Views**. (**a**) Frontal. (**b**) Right lateral. (**c**) Left lateral. **Intraoperative views.** (**d**) Following explantation, auto augmentation with superiorly based flap and fat grafting 130 ccs right breast only. Note soft tissue fill upper chest and para sternal area right as compared with left (unfilled). Liposuction of abdomen, hips, and lateral breast performed. (**e**) Following Fat grafting of both breasts, upper chest and para sternal areas 130 ccs per side. (**f**) Final result after closure. **Postoperative Views** at 10 months. (**g**) Frontal. (**h**) Right lateral. (**i**) Left lateral

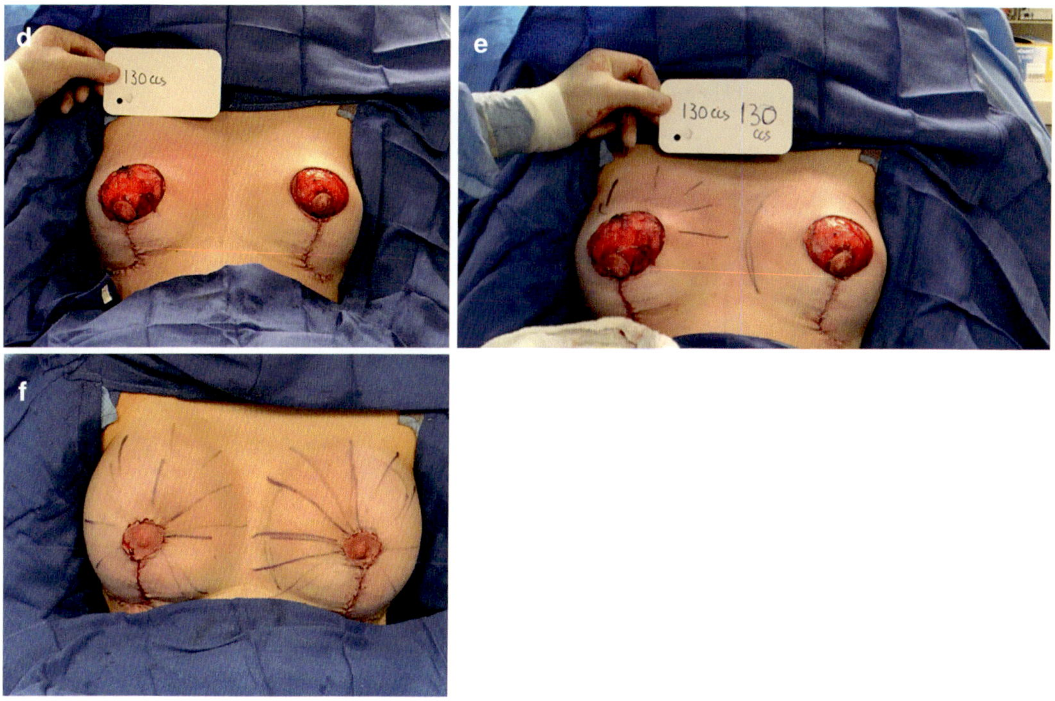

Fig. 15.6 (continued)

Case 6 (Fig. 15.7)

Presentation: 45-year-old woman with previous subpectoral augmentation with saline devices (480 ccs) desires explantation and mastopexy. She has experienced 25 lb. weight gain since initial breast augmentation and complains of breast ptosis and macromastia. 'Sized' by original surgeon to 'fill' breast envelope deflated postpartum.

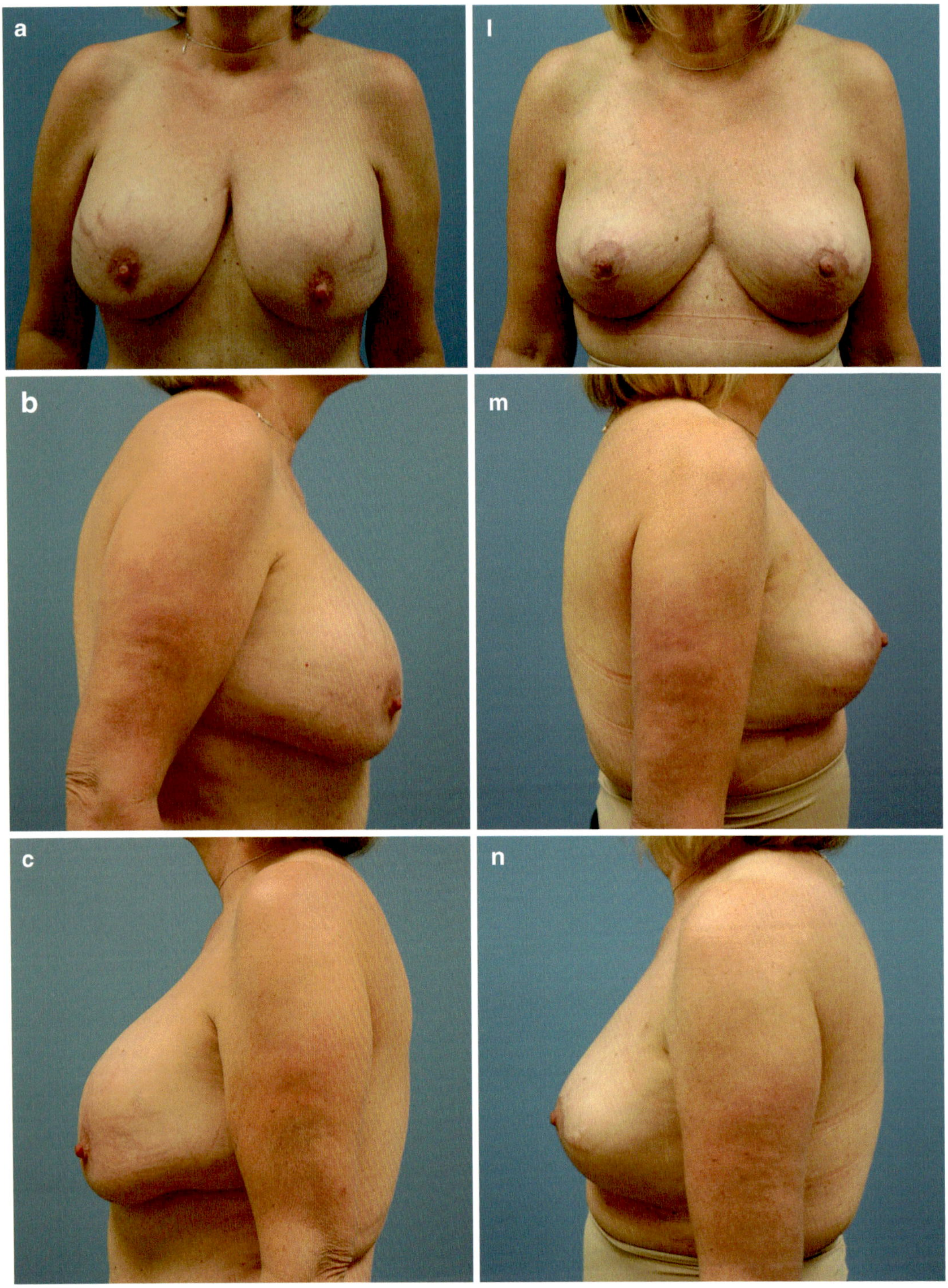

Fig. 15.7 (**Case 6**): 45 year old woman with previous subpectoral augmentation with saline devices. **Preoperative views**. (**a**) Frontal. (**b**) Right lateral. (**c**) Left lateral. (**d**) Immediate Preoperative. (**e–h**) **Intraoperative views**. (**e**) Following explantation. Native breast tissue assessed in preparation for tailor tacking. Arms position down on abdomen to minimize distortion. (**f**) Tailor tacking completed and breast marked for skin excision and fat grafting. (**g**) Skin deepithelialized and superiorly based flap designed. (**h**) Superiorly based flap developed and ready for inset. (**i**) Flap inverted and sewn to the pectoralis muscle filling the upper pole and central portion of the breast. Pillars closed. (**j**) Fat grafting of upper pole and parasternal region performed using a reverse flow pump. (**k**) Filling completed. 200 ccs grafted per side. **Post-operative views** at 3 months. (**l**) frontal. (**m**) right lateral (**n**) left lateral

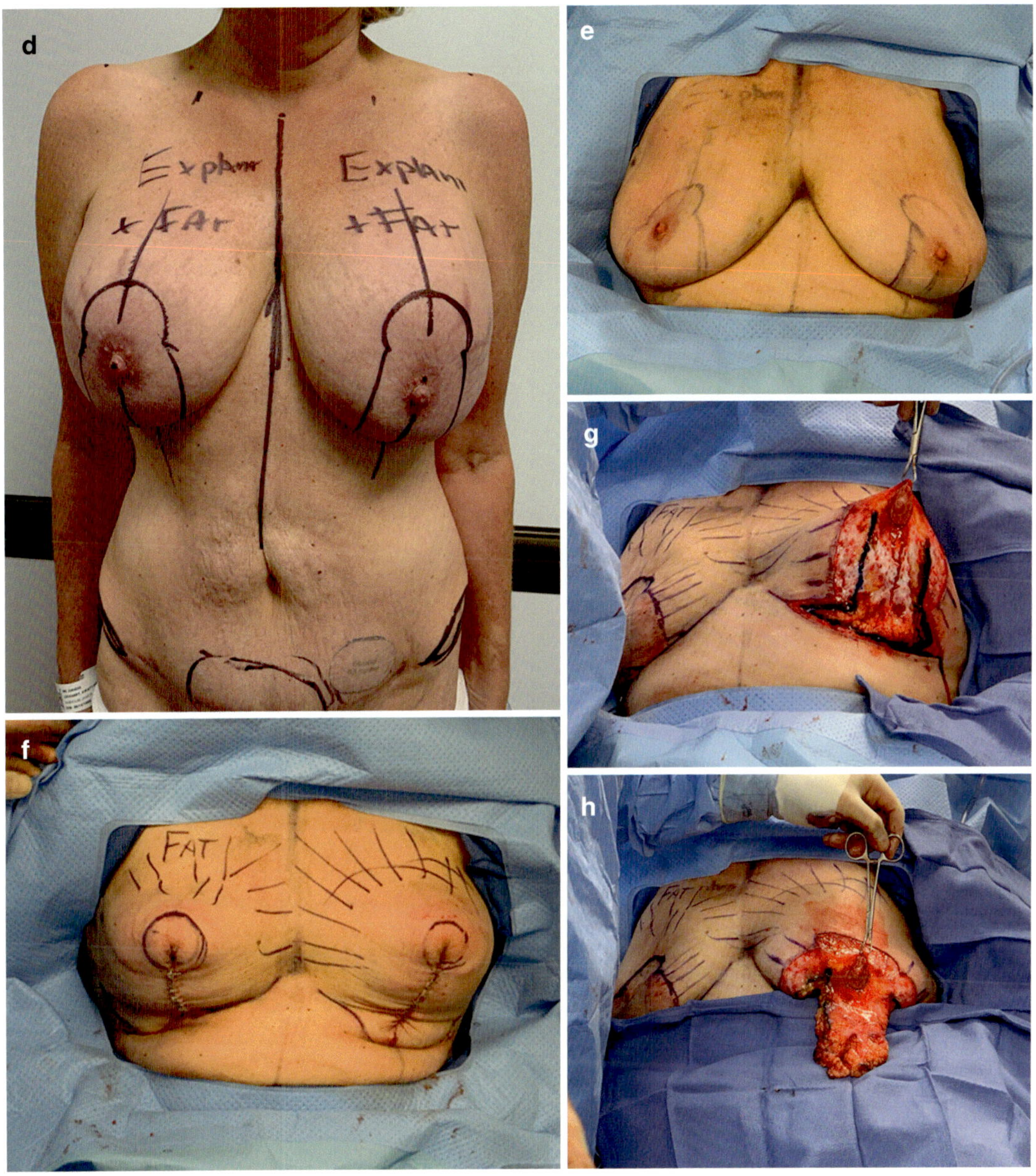

Fig. 15.7 (continued)

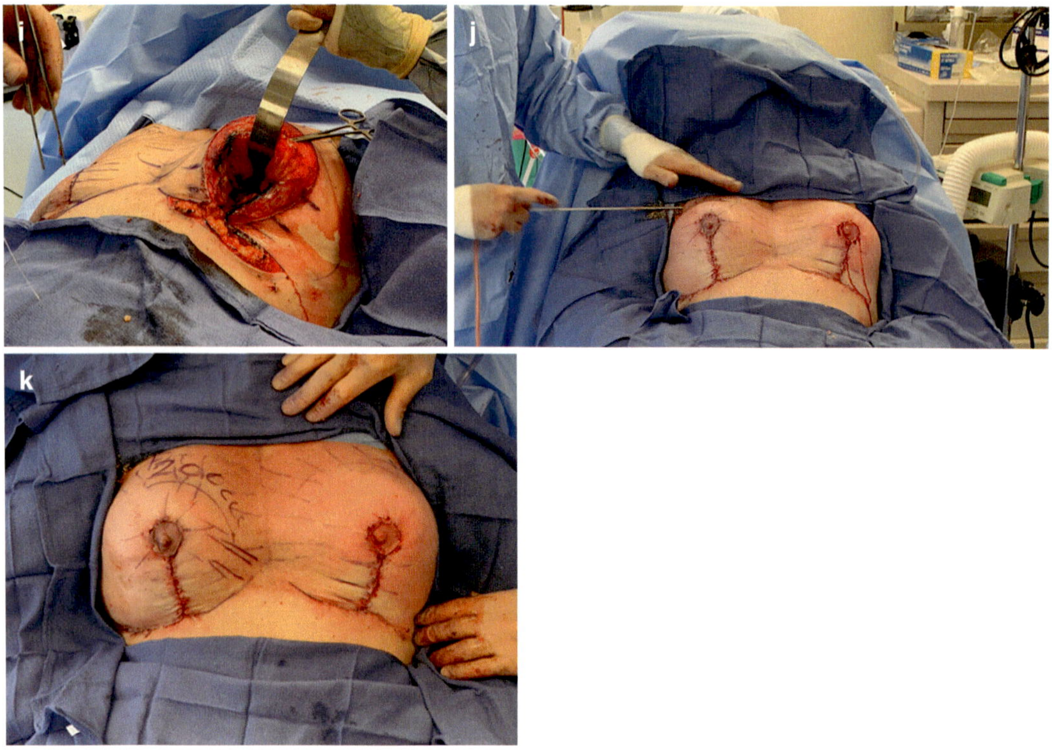

Fig. 15.7 (continued)

Conclusions

Mastopexy has become a more popular procedure as the augmented appearing breast becomes less fashionable for certain groups of women. Technical approaches that combined glandular tissue rearrangement in combination with targeted tissue removal and fat grafting give an unparalleled opportunity to remake the breast shape. This approach has proven useful in the patient seeking mastopexy alone or mastopexy following explantation. The addition of fat grafting permits equalization of breast volume, balancing of footprint asymmetries, filling of parasternal and upper chest breast deficiencies and correction of contour deformities following explantation or prior breast surgery. Fat grafting also provides a useful fallback for correction of underappreciated volume, shape, or chest wall asymmetries that can be best realized near the end of a complicated revision case. In addition, fat grafting offers the plastic surgeon the opportunity to treat the donor site for the patient to improve overall body contour. Although the typical volumes injected are in the range of 100–150 ccs larger volumes for grafting are possible as long as the graft to capacity ratio of the breast is respected.

References

1. 2017 Plastic surgery statistics report, America Society of Plastic Surgeons. ASPS National Clearing House of Plastic Surgery Procedural Statistics. 2017.
2. King RE, Mehara BJ, Pusic AL, et al. Trends in autologous aft grafting to the breast: a national survey of the American society of plastic surgeons. Plast Reconstr Surg. 2013;132(1):35–46.
3. Auclair E, Blondeel P, Alexander D, et al. Composite breast augmentation: soft-tissue planning using implants and fat. Plast Reconstr Surg. 2013;132(3):558–68.
4. Del Vecchio DA, Bucky LP. Breast augmentation using preexpansion and autologous fat transplantation: a clinical radiographic study. Plast Reconstr Surg. 2011;127(6):2441–50.

5. Khouri RK, Eisenmann-Klein M, Cardoso E, et al. Brava and autologous fat transfer is a safe and effective breast augmentation alternative: results of a 6-year, 81-patient, prospective multicenter study. Plast Reconstr Surg. 2012;129(5):1173–87.
6. Khouri RK, Khouri RK Jr, Rigotti G, et al. Aesthetic applications of Brava-assisted megavolume fat grafting to the breasts: a 9-year, 476-patient, multicenter study. Plast Reconstr Surg. 2013;133(4):796–807.
7. Del Vecchio DA. 'SIEF' - simultaneous implant exchange with fat: a new option in revision breast implant surgery. Plast Reconstr Surg. 2012;130(6): 1187–96.
8. Serra-Mestre JM, Fernandez PR, Foti V, et al. Breast cleavage remodeling with fat grafting: a safe way to optimize symmetry and to reduce intermammary distance. Plast Reconstr Surg. 2017;140(5):665e–72e.
9. Swami V, Tovee MJ. Resource security impacts men's female breast size preferences. PLoS One. 2013;8(3):e57623.
10. Zelazniewicz AM, Pawlowski B. Female breast size attractiveness for men as a function of sociosexual orientation (restricted vs. unrestricted). Arch Sex Behav. 2011;40(6):1129–35.
11. Lassus C. A 30-year experience with vertical mammoplasty. Plast Reconstr Surg. 1996;97(2):373–80.
12. Ribeiro L, Accorsi A Jr, Buss A, et al. Creation and evolution of 30 years of the inferior pedicle in reduction mammoplasties. Plast Reconstr Surg. 2002;110(3):960–70.
13. Graf R, Biggs TM. In search of a better shape in mastopexy and reduction mammoplasty. Plast Reconstr Surg. 2002;110(1):309–17.
14. Miotto GC, Eaves FF 3rd. The circumrotational technique for mastopexy. Aesthet Surg J. 2015;35(7):796–809.
15. Goes JC. Periareolar mammoplasty: double skin technique with application= of polygalactine or mixed mesh. Plast Reconstr Surg. 1996;97(5):959–68.
16. Adams WP, Moses AC. Use of poly-4-hydroxybutyrate mesh to optimize soft-tissue support in mastopexy: a single-site study. Plast Reconstr Surg. 2017;139(1):67–75.

Mastopexy with Auto-augmentation

16

M. Bradley Calobrace and Chet Mays

Introduction

When evaluating a patient with ptosis, it is important to initially understand the underlying cause of the ptosis, whether it be developmental or acquired secondary to weight loss, hormonal changes, pregnancy and/or aging. This will give some understanding to the cause of the ptosis, the loss of upper pole volume and the quality of the breast parenchyma and skin. In the initial assessment, it is important to determine the volume status of the breast, the extent of loss of upper pole volume and the patient's goals for the procedure. The treatment of the ptotic breast can be accomplished through a variety of techniques. Techniques that have been employed focus on the elevation of the NAC and the lower pole of the breast through skin tightening and potentially parenchymal resection. These techniques, however, have traditionally failed to maintain volume in the upper pole long-term.

M. B. Calobrace (✉)
Private Practice, CaloAesthetics Plastic Surgery Center, Louisville, KY, USA

Clinical Faculty, University of Louisville, Division of Plastic Surgery, Louisville, KY, USA

Clinical Faculty, University of Kentucky, Division of Plastic Surgery, Lexington, KY, USA
e-mail: drbrad@calobrace.com

C. Mays
Private Practice, CaloAesthetics Plastic Surgery Center, Louisville, KY, USA

Clinical Faculty, University of Louisville, Division of Plastic Surgery, Louisville, KY, USA

M. B. Calobrace et al. (eds.), *Augmentation Mastopexy*,
https://doi.org/10.1007/978-3-030-48226-8_16

Patients seeking mastopexy with volume deficiencies desiring larger breasts and/or those patients desiring upper pole volume often require placement of an implant with the mastopexy to achieve the desired appearance. The addition of an implant to the procedure, an augmentation mastopexy, is by far the most popular and most successful method for achieving and maintaining upper pole volume post mastopexy.

However, there are many patients who do not want a breast implant but are dissatisfied with their breast shape and are seeking a mastopexy for improvement. There are also patients in whom breast volume is adequate and additional volume would be unacceptable to the patient. There have been a variety of mastopexy techniques described to address the ptotic breast. The techniques are often described in reference to the final scar placement, such as the circumareolar technique, circumvertical technique and inverted-T scar technique [1–5]. However, there is much more variation in the techniques, including the vascular pedicle orientation, management of the parenchyma and additional ancillary procedures to enhance the results. Additionally, the challenge in these patients is in achieving a satisfactory improvement in the upper pole of the breast without the use of an implant. To optimize the mastopexy and upper pole volume, various surgical techniques have been employed, including parenchymal suturing techniques, local flap transpositions, and the use of a pectoralis sling for stabilization of the flap transfer [6–12]. In our experience, the utilization of a lower pole parenchymal transposition flap to auto-augment the upper pole has been an excellent alternative. This is often combined with upper pole fat grafting to further enhance the outcome. The upper pole flap transposition not only creates volume higher in the breast, it unloads the volume from the lower pole of the breast, potentially contributing to a more successful outcome as compared to a traditional mastopexy.

The decision on the appropriate mastopexy approach is based on not only the physical findings but also patient expectations. In the preoperative evaluation, breast measurements, breast tissue density, quality of skin, NAC and breast ptosis, chest wall characteristics, and the breast footprint all must be considered in planning for the procedure. The ideal candidate would be a patient with adequate volume, dense breast parenchyma, mild to moderate ptosis, good quality skin and a high breast footprint. Figure 16.1 shows the ideal mastopexy patient.

Perioperative decision making is critical to a successful outcome in an auto-augmentation mastopexy surgery. In this chapter, we will review our approach to decision making with a focus on patient selection, review of mastopexy options, vascular anatomy of the transposition flap, and selection and planning of the mastopexy auto-augmentation procedure. The operative technique and post-operative care will be reviewed in detail in hopes of providing the best chance for successful outcomes, minimal complications, and satisfied patients.

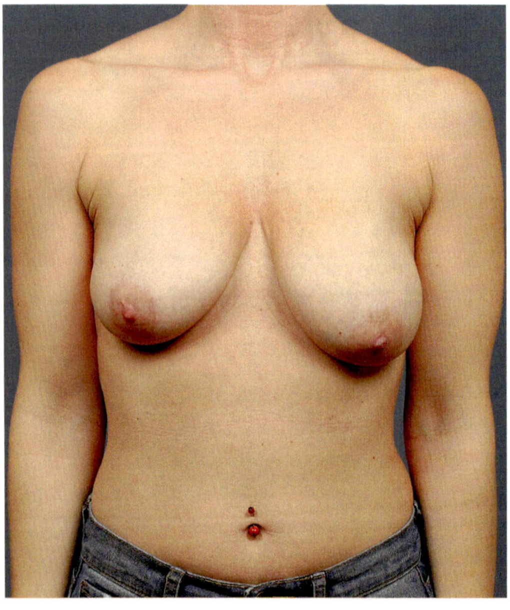

Fig. 16.1 Ideal augmentation mastopexy candidate with adequate volume and dense breast parenchyma

Pre-operative Evaluation

The evaluation should begin with a breast exam with breast measurements including the base width, sternal notch to nipple distance, nipple to fold distance (at rest and under maximal stretch). Figure 16.2 shows Important pre-op measurements.

The amount of ptosis present should also be assessed. Ptosis has classically been described as per Regnault based on the relationship of the NAC to the inframammary fold [13].

Table 16.1 shows Regnault ptosis classification.

Although this provides some information about the degree of breast ptosis, it in of itself is insufficient to describe the true extent of breast ptosis. A more complete assessment of ptosis is summarized in Table 16.2 below.

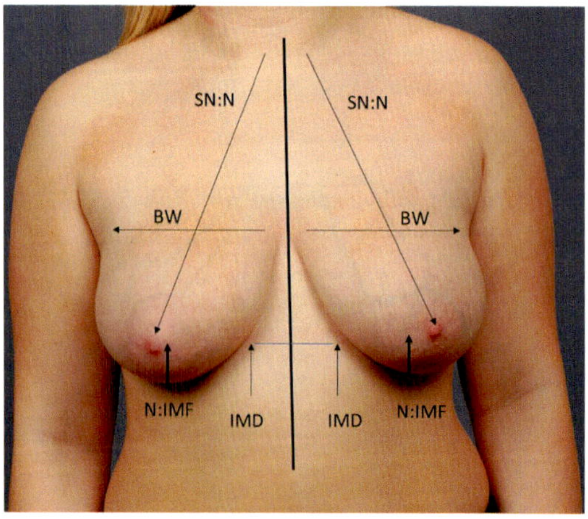

Fig. 16.2 Breast measurements. SN:N Sternal notch to nipple. BW; Breast width. N:IMF Nipple to IMF. IMD; Intermammary distance

Table 16.1 Regnault ptosis classification

Type	Degrees	Description
Grade I	Mild	Nipple position at the level of the inframammary fold
Grade II	Moderate	Nipple position below the inframammary fold but above the lower breast contour
Grade III	Severe	Nipple position below the inframammary fold at the lower contour of the breast
Pseudo-glandular		Nipple position above the fold but the breast is below the fold

Table 16.2 Assessment of breast ptosis

Relationship of the NAC to the IMF (Regnault's degree of ptosis)
(a) *Grade 1*: nipple at the level of the inframammary fold, above the lower contour of the gland (b) *Grade 2:* nipple below the level of the inframammary fold, above the lower contour of the gland (c) *Grade 3:* nipple below the level of the inframammary fold, at the lower contour of the gland
Amount of breast tissue overhanging the fold
Location of the NAC on the breast mound
Amount of vertical excess and horizontal excess
Footprint of the breast on the chest wall – low, medium, high
Quantity and quality of breast parenchyma and skin

Figure 16.3 shows varying degrees of breast ptosis. Ideal candidates for autoaugmentation based on degree of ptosis and breast tissue.

The mastopexy auto-augmentation is a circumvertical or vertical type mastopexy and thus an assessment of the pedicle planned must be evaluated. The most common pedicle for this technique is a superior pedicle, but a superomedial pedicle could also be used. In this procedure, an evaluation must include assessment as to the surgeon's ability to do the mastopexy with a superior or superomedial pedicle. In the senior author's experience, elevation of the NAC beyond 5–6 cm, depending on the quality of the tissue, is less reliable and an inferior based pedicle would be used and a mastopexy auto-augmentation would not be performed. This final judgment as to the viability of this technique is based solely on the surgeon's comfort and experience in utilizing a vertical approach with a superiorly -based or superomedial blood supply. The flap transposition to the upper pole is just a variant of the vertical mastopexy, and individual experience will determine the appropriateness of this approach.

The assessment should also include evaluation of the skin thickness and elasticity, the quantity and distribution of subcutaneous fat, the composition and firmness of the breast parenchyma, the integrity of the Cooper's ligaments, the nature and position of the underlying musculature and the shape and slope of the underlying chest wall. All these aspects of the breast composition influence the shape of the breast and ultimately the outcome after the mastopexy.

One additional aspect in considering the mastopexy with auto-augmentation is the presence of an adequate amount of lower pole tissue to make the transposition possible and worthwhile. In patients with significant nipple descent but with short N-IMF distance, the vertical lower pole segment of tissue would be too short and inadequate to provide any benefit in the upper pole. Also, the footprint should be observed. Whereas this procedure can be performed on any footprint, it is the high breasted patient that benefits the most. In these patients, the short upper thorax requires only a small amount of tissue to produce a significant improvement. In the low-breasted footprint patient, the auto-augmentation does not elevate the upper breast border significantly enough and an implant would be a more appropriate for correcting the upper pole. Most patients are not on either of these extremes, but more in the grey zone and judgment will be necessary. Likewise, assessing the firmness of the parenchyma is important, as patients with more firm, dense breasts do better at holding the shape long-term compared to more lax breast tissue such as a weightloss patient.

Blood Supply

An understanding and thorough assessment of the vascular anatomy is critical to performing the procedure safely. The breast has a rich blood

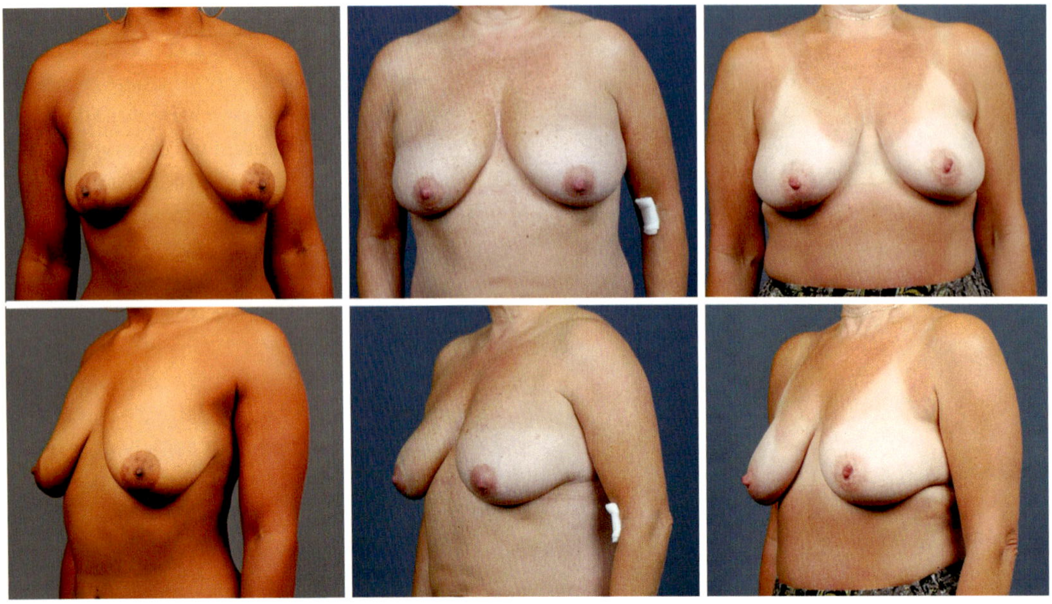

Fig. 16.3 Varying degrees of breast ptosis showing relationships of the Nipple position and breast tissue to the inframammary fold

supply from multiple sources, including the internal mammary artery perforators, the lateral thoracic arteries, the thoracoacromial and the anterolateral and anteromedial intercostal perforators. As mentioned previously, the superior pedicle and occasionally the superomedial pedicles are utilized. The superior pedicle is supplied by the second branch of the internal mammary artery (IMA) that emerges deep from the second interspace and courses superficial across the medial upper breast to enter the NAC slightly medial to the midline and approximately 1 cm deep. The medial pedicle is supplied by the third branch of the IMA that emerges from the third interspace and similarly courses superficially across the breast parenchyma to the medial aspect of the NAC. The superficial position of these vessels in the upper pole allow the entire breast to be elevated off the muscle and chest wall in a subcutaneous plane for the planned flap transposition.

Figure 16.4 is a schematic of the breast blood supply.

The inferior pedicle and central pedicle are supplied by the fourth branch of the IMA that courses deeply across the medial breast to enter through Wuringer's septum approximately 1–2 cm above the IMF and often just medial to the breast meridian.

Figure 16.5 shows the 4th branch of the IMA coming through Wuringer's septum.

The Inferior pedicle also has additional blood supply through contribution from intercostal perforators along the IMF [14].

In the mastopexy auto-augmentation procedure, the lower flap of breast tissue is based solely on the central pedicle. The intercostal perforators are divided when the flap is detached from inframammary fold. An understanding of the location of the 4th branch supplying this lower transposition flap is critical to creating a mobile flap of tissue with a viable pedicle blood supply. Obviously, if a patient has had a breast augmentation in the past or the breast has in any way been elevated off the chest wall previously, the central pedicle would have been divided and the flap transposition would not be possible.

Fat Grafting

In the mastopexy patient, whether an auto-augmentation is utilized or not, fat grafting can be very effective in improving the upper pole

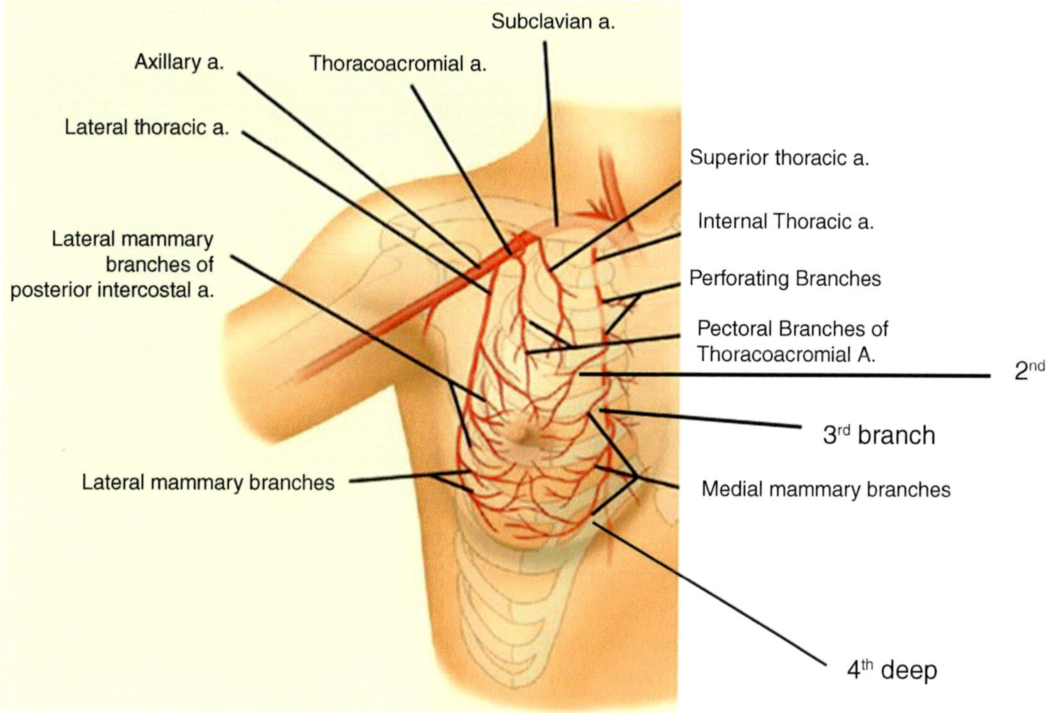

Fig. 16.4 Breast blood supply

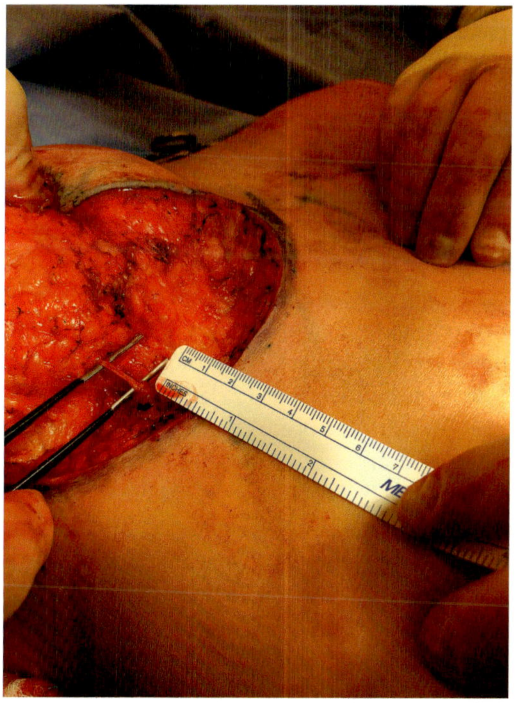

Fig. 16.5 wuringer's septum

volume without the use of an implant. Fat improves fullness, coverage and cleavage, but is not effective at increasing core projection of the breast. Thus, in the mastopexy auto-augmentation patient, it can be very effective to utilize the transposed flap for some added projection and roundness to the upper pole, while using the fat grafting to blend additional volume into the upper pole and cleavage area. The combination appears to have additive benefit in improving upper pole volume without the use of an implant.

Patient Expectations

The most important element of the perioperative planning is patient education and the need to spend some time understanding the patient's desired outcome and expectations with the operation. Patients requiring a mastopexy have more significant changes to the breast than those needing simply a breast augmentation, and often have increased laxity of the tissue, stria, nipple and breast ptosis, and loss of parenchymal volume and/or firmness. Thus, managing expectation in these challenging cases is paramount.

Patients often are unaware of asymmetries, the significant atrophy of the breasts, and differences in the chest wall that affect the final outcome. During the evaluation, it is important to determine what "look" the patient would desire, especially in terms of nipple position and volume in the upper pole. Patients need to understand the limitations in achieving a desired look to the breast as compared to a breast augmentation or even an augmentation mastopexy. Based on the patient's desires, the operative design takes into account the patient's desires in an effort to achieve a satisfactory result for the patient. A patient desiring a more natural look and not requiring extremely full upper poles is an ideal candidate for this procedure. The patient needs to understand that even the auto-augmentation with or without fat grafting will produce a fuller, naturally sloping upper pole at best. The procedure will not create the firm, full roundness that an implant can produce. These patients will also have scars on the breast, which at times can heal unpredictably, and a clear understanding of the location of the scars and anticipated outcome should be discussed. Expert perioperative decision making with an operative approach specifically designed to meet the patient's goals is more likely to provide optimal results for each patient.

Pre-operative Markings

Appropriate preoperative markings provide a roadmap and are essential to planning and performing the vertical mastopexy with auto-augmentation surgery. The markings guide the surgeon in providing symmetrical NAC placement and mastopexy design. The patient is sitting upright during the markings. A line is initially drawn along the midline of the breasts and bilaterally down the meridians. The meridian lines bisect the breast equally and may not intersect though the nipple if there is NAC malposition.

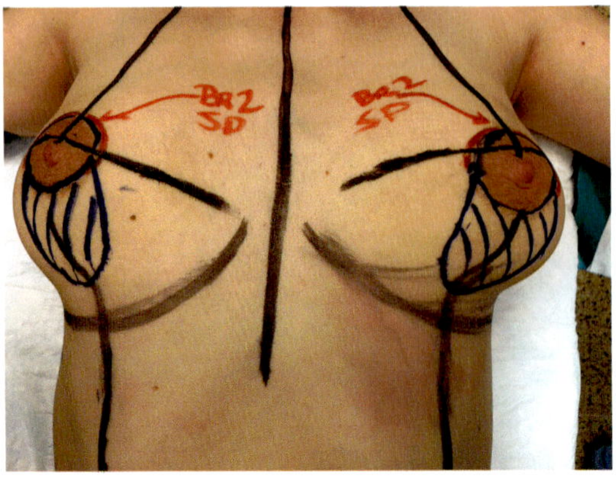

Fig. 16.6 pre-op markings of circumvertical mastopexy with autoaugmentation

The inframammary folds are then drawn, noting any asymmetries to be addressed at surgery. The position of the IMF is then drawn on the anterior breast through the meridian incision. The breasts are then rotated medially and laterally to mark the location of the vertical incisions.

Figure 16.6 shows pre-op markings.

This vertical mastopexy is based on a superior pedicle blood supply and is not dependent on the final skin excision pattern. Decision on nipple placement is performed and is based on the location of the fold and expected location of the new lifted breast's central mound position. This can be approximated by simulating the mastopexy and identifying the probable location of the NAC. The nipple position is usually at or within 2 cm of the reflected inframammary fold, referred to as Pitanguy's point [15]. Placement of the areola is marked, starting approximately 2 cm above the nipple position and extending the curved drawing down to meet the medial and lateral vertical markings. This areolar opening marking should produce an areolar opening of approximately 42 mm. Approximately 7 cm below the bottom of the keyhole opening, a line is drawn marking the inferior extent of the vertical incision. Curved transverse lines are then drawn from these medial and lateral points extending down to the IMF. Approximately 2–3 cm above the fold a u-shaped line connects the medial and lateral vertical markings to define the extent of skin resection.

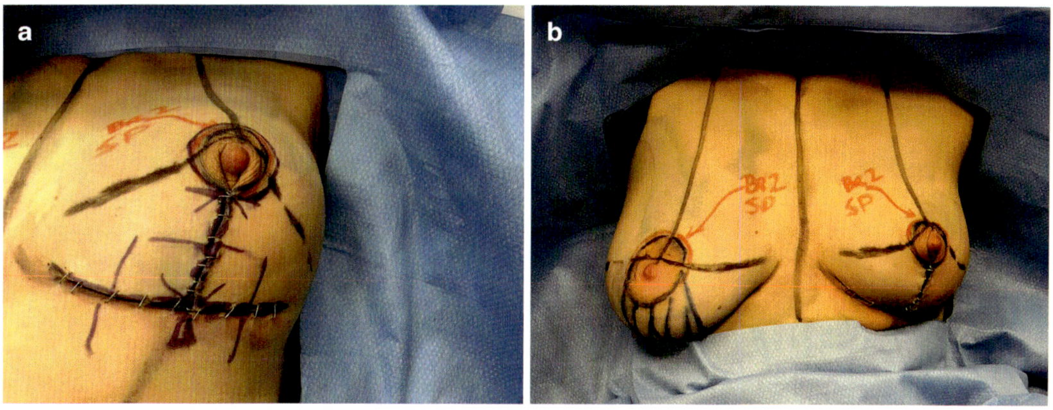

Fig. 16.7 (**a**) Pre-op breast tailor-tacking. (**b**) Tailor tacking on the patient's left side vs. no tailor tacking on the right side

Intra-operative Markings

Once the patient is under anesthesia and has been prepped for the operative procedure, all markings are confirmed and retraced as necessary. The symmetry of the drawings is also confirmed. If any questions exist as to the accuracy of the markings, tailor-tacking can be performed in many cases to reconfirm the markings. Tailor-tacking is performed with a stapler and the patient is placed in the upright position to confirm design, symmetry and NAC positioning.

Figure 16.7a shows Intra-op breast tailor-tacking to confirm design, symmetry and NAC positioning.

Figure 16.7b shows Tailor tacking on the patient's left side vs. no tailor tacking on the right side as the patient is sitting upright.

In the supine position, the staples are removed and the superior pedicle is designed to be positioned in the superior keyhole from the 8 o'clock to 4 o'clock position.

Surgical Technique

The patient is placed on the operating room table with the arms secured to the sides at 45 to 60 degrees. Once the patient is prepped with Chloraprep and draped appropriately, the markings and incision location are confirmed. If feasible, tailor-tacking to confirm location of NAC and markings for the mastopexy can be very helpful. When in doubt about the mastopexy markings, it is advisable to stay conservative and leave a little more skin on the breast flaps. These can be adjusted during the final assessment and contouring prior to the closure. The operative field is then injected with 50 cc per side of local anesthetic solution (Table 16.3) using a spinal needle and a 20 cc syringe.

Figure 16.8 shows a pre-op breast analgesic injection.

Each breast is placed under maximal stretch and the areolas are marked with a 42 mm cookie-cutter (range 38–45 mm depending on desired aesthetics) and incised with a 15 blade scalpel. Utilizing a 10-blade, the entire area within the marks is then de-epithelized and cauterized for hemostasis.

Figure 16.9 shows a de-epithelialized central flap. Areas of blue marking indicated the island of tissue that will be transposed to the upper pole.

The lateral and medial flaps are dissected straight down toward the chest wall. The lateral and medial pillars are then developed keeping them at least 2 cm thick. It is important to maintain good pillar volume to avoid leaving the lower pole to deficient.

Figure 16.10 shows the dissection of medial and lateral breast pillars.

Table 16.3 Concentrations of Breast Analgesic Solution Injected Prior to Prepping the Patient. 25 ml of each of the components listed on the left hand side of the table are combined to make a 100 ml solution. This is split so that 50 ml of the solution is injected into each breast using a 20 cc syringe and spinal needle

Breast local anesthetic formula	Volume
½% Lidocaine Plain	25 ml
½% Lidocaine/1:200,000 epinephrine	25 ml
½% Bupivacaine/1:200,000 epinephrine	25 ml
Injectable Saline	25 ml
	Total
¼% lidocaine, 1/8% bupivacaine, 1:400,000 epinephrine	*100 ml*

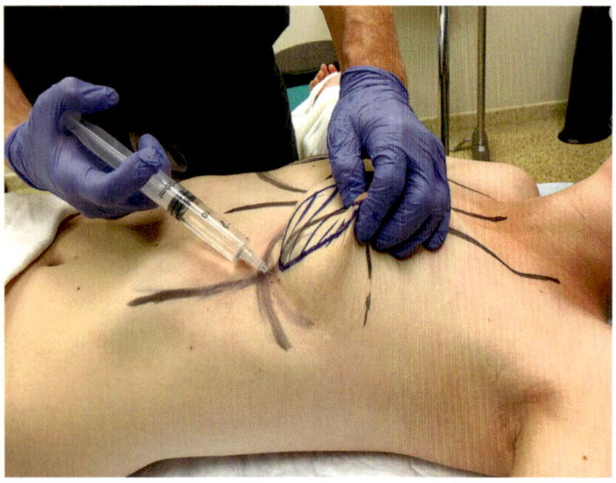

Fig. 16.8 Breast analgesic injection with 20cc syringe and spinal needle

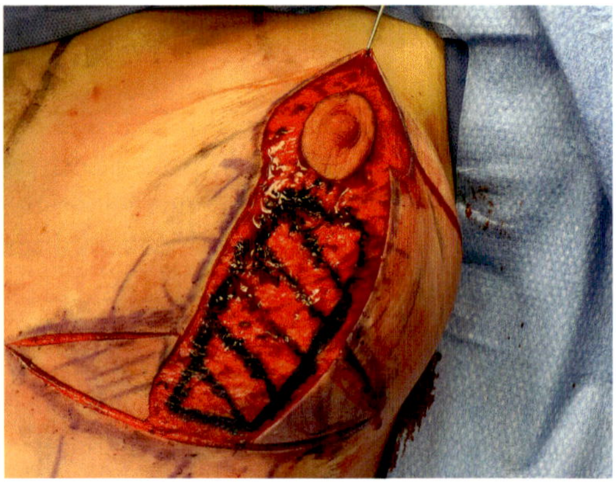

Fig. 16.9 De-epithelialized central flap. Areas of blue marking indicated the island of tissue that will be transposed

The central pedicle in the lower pole is then developed as a flap to transposition into the upper pole. Care must be taken to insure the flap is large enough to be worthwhile and yet leave enough tissue in the lower pole to avoid having a hollow lower pole. Flaps of less than 4 cm's in length are probably not worth transposing. Once the flap is designed, dissection and mobilization of this flap is then performed. The medial and lateral dissections of the flap have already occurred in creating the medial and lateral pillars.

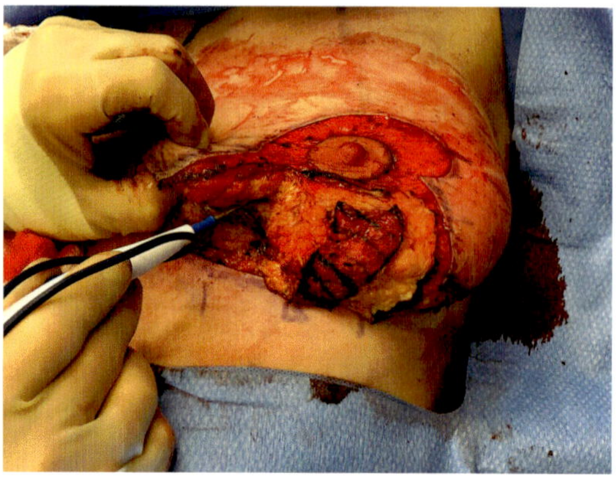

Fig. 16.10 Dissection of medial and lateral breast pillars

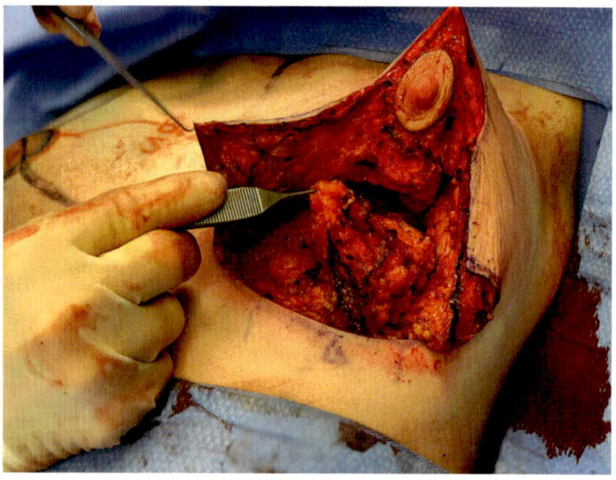

Fig. 16.11 Dissection of the central mound flap

Figure 16.11 shows the dissection of the breast central mound flap .

The flap is then transected at the inframammary fold and the dissection is carried cephalad from the fold staying on the chest wall. This flap is dissected circumferentially, and then incrementally dissected to free its attachment to create a mobile flap still attached to the deep 4th branch of the IMA that courses through Wuringer's sep-

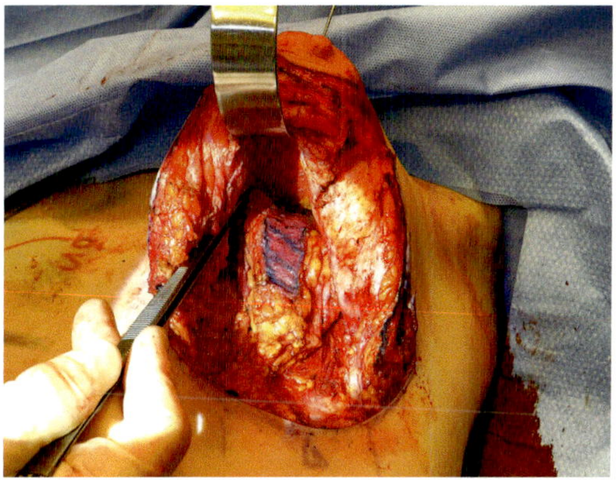

Fig. 16.12 Flap elevation and transposition to the upper pole

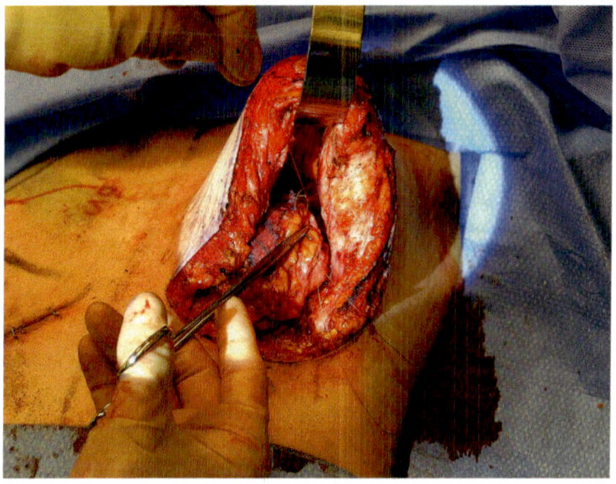

Fig. 16.13 Transposition flap sutured to the pectoralis fascia to maintain upper pole projection

tum. This vessel is identified usually approximately 1–1.5 cm cephalad to the IMF (see Fig. 16.5). Doppler confirmation can also be performed if desired to insure the vessel has not been injured. Once the flap has been dissected and released for mobilization, the remainder of the breast above the flap is elevated off the pectoralis fascia.

Figure 16.12 shows flap elevation and transposition to the upper pole.

The lower island flap is then transposed into the upper pole and sutured into place with approximately four 2–0 Vicryl sutures.

Figure 16.13 shows a transposition flap sutured to the pectoralis fascia to maintain upper pole projection.

Once the flap is positioned and stabilized, tailor-tacking is performed to confirm the shape of the breast. Tailor tacking begins at the inferior areola (6 o'clock position) and proceeds inferiorly towards the IMF. The ideal inferior areola to fold distance varies based on the size of the breast, but is usually 6–7 cm. Adjustments are made with the tailor-tacking to create the desired breast shape.

Figure 16.14a is an anterior view of breast-tailor tacking showing the shape and contour of the breast.

Figure 16.14b is a lateral view of tailor tacked breast.

Once the desired vertical limb length is determined, this location represents the base of the new breast. Any remaining breast tissue or skin below this level must be addressed. As in any vertical mastopexy approach, the skin flaps can be undermined, and the breast tissue resected to allow the skin to re-drape on to the abdomen and the fold of the breast. This can also be accomplished with liposuction under the redundant skin with skin re-draping. This allows the fold to come up and keep the incision vertical only.

Alternatively, a horizontal wedge of skin and breast tissue is excised. The markings for the wedge excisions are extended medially and laterally to create the inverted-T scar and the final tailor-tacking is performed.

Figure 16.15a shows an estimation of horizontal wedge needed along IMF to address the excess tissue after tailor tacking and applying downward force.

Figure 16.15b is a lateral view of the breast after tailor tacking. The downward force aids in determining the amount of tissue resection along the IMF.

Once the breast shape is confirmed, the final excision of tissue is performed in preparation for closure.

The pockets are irrigated with bacitracin saline solution and hemostasis is insured. Deep parenchymal sutures of 2–0 Vicryl are then placed along the vertical incision bringing the medial and lateral pillars together at the midline.

Figure 16.16 shows the medial and lateral breast pillars brought together with 2–0 Vicryl suture.

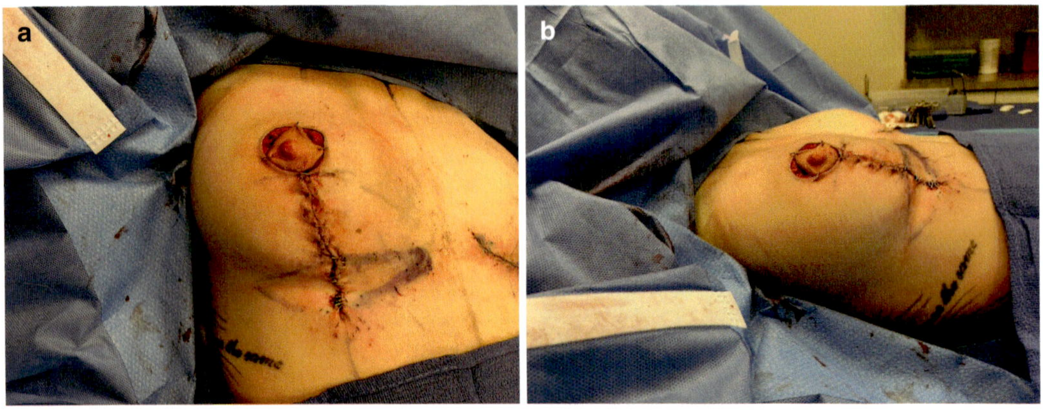

Fig. 16.14 Breast tailor tacking

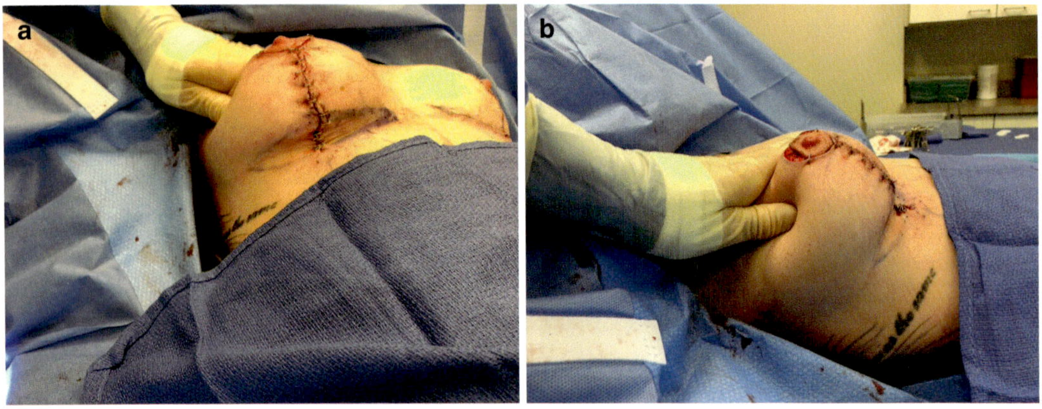

Fig. 16.15 Estimation of horizontal wedge needed based on excess tissue after tailor tacking

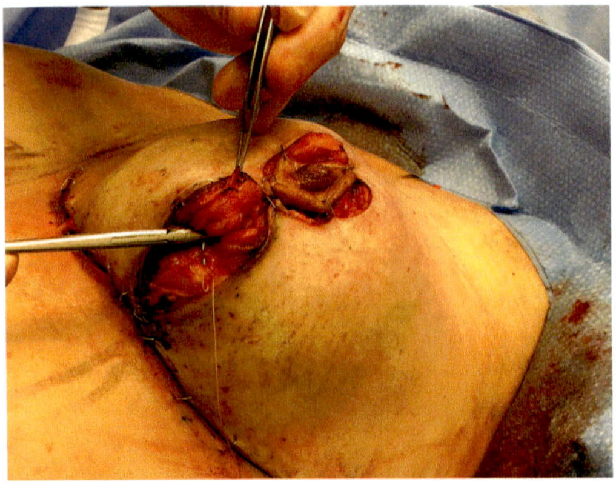

Fig. 16.16 Medial and lateral breast pillars brought together with 2–0 Vicryl suture

All incisions are then closed with interrupted 3–0 PDS dermal sutures. The vertical and horizontal scar are closed with a 4–0 Monocryl running subcuticular suture. The areolas are then closed with a simple running 5–0 nylon suture.

Figure 16.17 shows the final closure of the breast with the patient sitting upright on the OR table.

If fat grafting is to be performed, fat is collected through a variety of techniques for planned injection. The fat is then allowed to settle but no additional processing is performed. The fat is placed into 20 cc syringes and utilizing a 2 mm blunt needle, injected into the upper poles of the breast and medially to create improved cleavage. Approximately 60–100 cc of fat is injected per side. The fat is placed in the subcutaneous fat just under the skin. The area is massaged to allow the fat to spread evenly over the area.

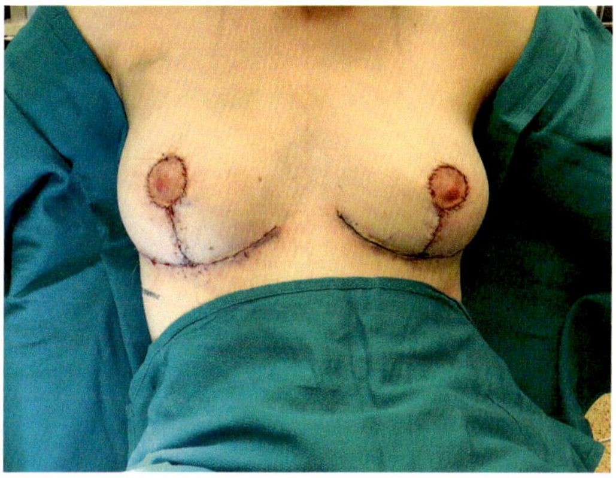

Fig. 16.17 Final closure of the breast with the patient sitting upright on the OR table

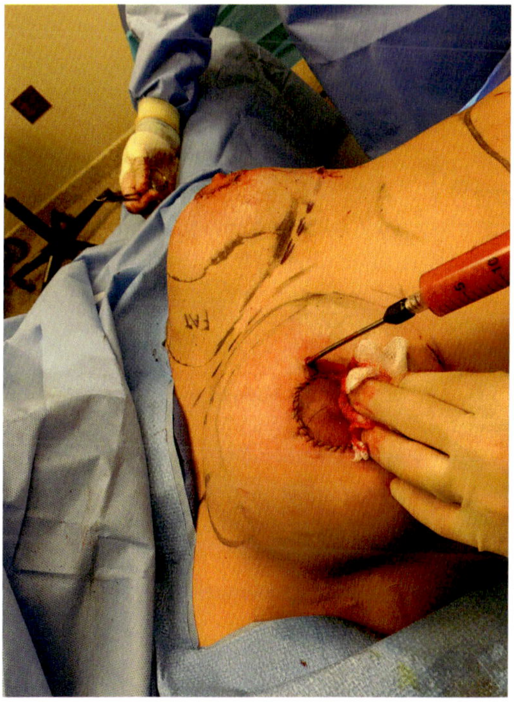

Fig. 16.18 Fat grafting to the breast after final closure into the subcutaneous plane

Figure 16.18 shows fat grafting to the breast after final closure into the subcutaneous plane.

Steristrips are placed over the incision. Contour tape is then placed along the lateral breast border and inframammary fold. The breast are wrapped with a xeroform gauze, Kerlix and ace wrap.

Post-operative Care and Expected Outcomes

The patients are instructed to leave all dressing on for 24 hours. The wraps are then removed and a sports bra is worn for the following 4 weeks. Dressing changes with antibiotic ointment and gauze are used over incisions for 1 week. Patients are allowed to shower after 48 hours. The contour tape is removed at day 4–7. Nylons around the areolas are removed 5–7 days postoperatively. The subcuticular Monocryls are clipped on the ends as they exit the skin at 2 weeks. Scar management with silicone gel or silicone sheeting is initiated on all patients at 2 weeks. Patients are allowed to resume activities of daily living almost immediately. Exercise is usually allowed at 4 weeks with heavy lifting at 6 weeks.

Patients are counseled that they can expect swelling and firmness to develop as her breasts heal. The breasts will continue to soften over time and the breast will relax over the first few months. The results are stable after 6 months, but scars can continue to improve over the first year and some additional relaxation of the breast with loss of upper pole volume can continue for even longer. Whereas inferior pedicle shape looks relatively normal shortly after the procedure, superior pedicle technique may take longer to obtain its natural shape.

Complications

There are very few significant complications in the early postoperative period. The only significant concern early is ischemia to the nipple-areolar complex or skin flaps. Ischemia may be due to the dissection of the pedicle, but often is secondary to excessive tension on the skin closure and underlying volume under the skin flaps. If recognized immediately, all sutures should be removed to evaluate for improved circulation, improved color, good capillary refill and pinprick bleeding. It is important to assure the pedicle is free of tension and not twisted or compromised. Topical nitroglycerin or DMSO (Dimethylsulfoxide) can be used to improved venous outflow. If the closure is too tight due to volume present under the flaps, additional breast volume can be removed in an attempt to reduce the closure tension. If any doubt exists, the wound around the NAC can be left unattached and closed the following day in the clinic. Although conversion to a free nipple graft could be done if inadequate pedicle flow through all of the above mentioned efforts, this is by far more common in a breast reduction and should be extremely rare in a mastopexy procedure.

Hematoma rarely occur within the first 24 hours, but a late hematoma at day 10 to 14 is also occasionally encountered as activity level increases and clots are being resorbed at the end of cauterized vessels. A very small hematoma can be allowed to resolve on its own, but any substantial hematoma should be explored, evacuated of blood and drained. Small amounts of blood within the pocket in a mastopexy without a breast implant is generally less concerning as there is not potential for capsular contracture. Seromas are generally managed conservatively with serial aspiration until resolved.

Secondary Procedures

Late sequalae include poor scarring, recurrent ptosis, bottoming out, asymmetry, contour deformities, fat necrosis and loss of upper pole volume. These may require revisional procedures to improve the final aesthetic outcome. Most procedures are delayed at least 6 months or greater to allow for soft tissue remodeling and stabilization of the results. Scars are often the product of excessive tension on the closure and postoperative swelling and can often be improved with scar revisions when the environment for scar maturation is more optimal. Lower pole stretch deformities and recurrent ptosis are managed with a revision of the mastopexy with or without the addition of some additional support from a mesh or acellular dermal matrix. More commonly, the lower pole can become empty as the flap is transposed to the upper pole, leading to a flattened, empty lower pole contour.

Figure 16.19a shows loss of lower pole volume after autoaugmentation leading to an empty flattened lower pole contour.

Figure 16.19b shows improvement in lower pole volume after revisionary surgery to improve lower pole contour.

This can be avoided by ensuring adequate pillar volume is present to fill the lower pole. The empty lower pole can be treated with revision of the mastopexy with or without fat grafting. Fat necrosis is often simply monitored if it is small and not deforming the shape of the breast. If it involves the transposed flap, it may present as firmness in the upper pole of the breast. If the area of fat necrosis impairs the shape or softness of the breast or is interfering with cancer surveillance, excision of the involved area is appropriate.

Loss of upper pole volume is the most common late finding after mastopexy and has been to

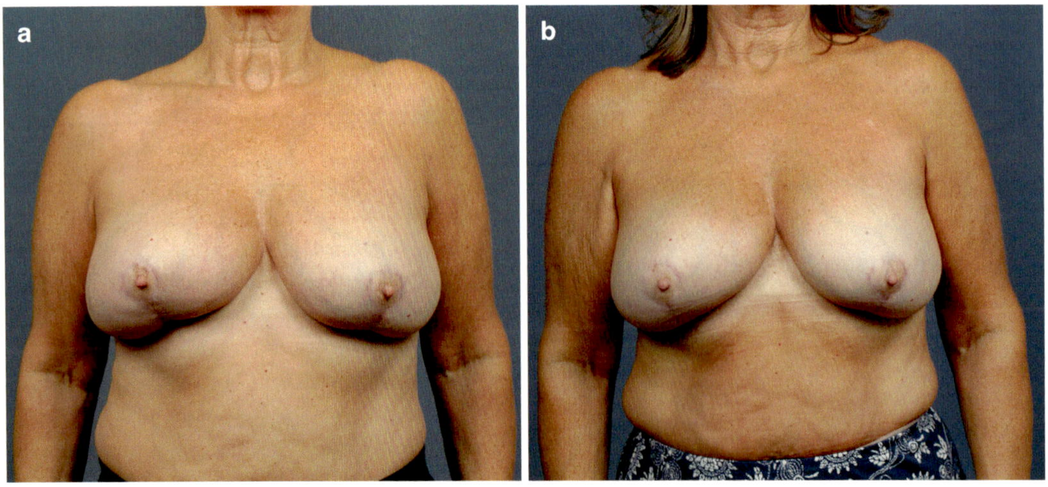

Fig. 16.19 (**a**) Loss of lower pole volume after autoaugmentation leading to an empty flattened lower pole contour. (**b**) Improvement in lower pole volume after revisionary surgery to improve lower pole contour

some degree mitigated by the use of transposition flap into the upper breast. Loss of the upper pole can be secondary to relaxation and loss of lower pole support or simply due to the lack of stable, firm volume in the breast envelope. The most effective management is tightening of the lower pole if needed and the addition of a breast implant.

Conclusion

With proper preoperative evaluation and employing accurate surgical techniques, excellent results can be achieved with mastopexy with auto-augmentation. The significant advantage of the superior pedicle technique in the appropriately selected patient is not the elimination of an inframammary scar, but rather the parenchymal shaping and lower breast pole unloading that provides more stable and predictable results. The added advantage of this technique is the volume unloaded from the lower pole is transposed into the upper pole to provide additional projection and volume. Fat grafting can further enhance the results, adding volume to augment the upper pole and improve postoperative cleavage. This technique is simply a modification of a well-established technique that can be easily mastered and provide optimal results with high patient satisfaction.

Summary Box – Pearls for Success

- Drawings are performed preoperatively as a guide with intraoperative adjustments expected
- Superior pedicle is reserved for modest mastopexies, with NAC elevation limit of 5 to 6 cm's
- Lower pole volume can be resected or auto-augmented to upper pole with a superior pedicle
- Resecting all extra skin through an inverted-T technique provides the most accurate appearance of the breast at the end of the procedure
- Upper pole volumes are less stable with a mastopexy alone, can be improved with auto-augmentation and optimized with a breast implant

Case Examples

Case 1

31 year old female with breast ptosis and asymmetry who underwent bilateral Full wise mastopexy with Ribeiro autoaugmentation transposition flaps to provide breast volume without the use of implants.

Figure 16.20 shows before and after inverted-T mastopexy using Ribeiro autoaugmentation flaps.

Case 2

20 year old female with breast ptosis seeking a lift and volumization of her breast without the use of an implant. An inferior based Ribeiro flap for autoaugmentation was used to transpose lower pole volume into the upper pole.

Figure 16.21 shows before and after photos of an inverted-T mastopexy using Ribeiro flaps for autoaugmentation.

Case 3

19 year old female with breast ptosis and asymmetry. A superior based autoaugmenation flap was used to restore symmetry and provide shape and volume to the breast without the use of implants.

Figure 16.22 shows a 19 year old female before and after inverted-T mastopexy with superior pedicle autoaugmentation.

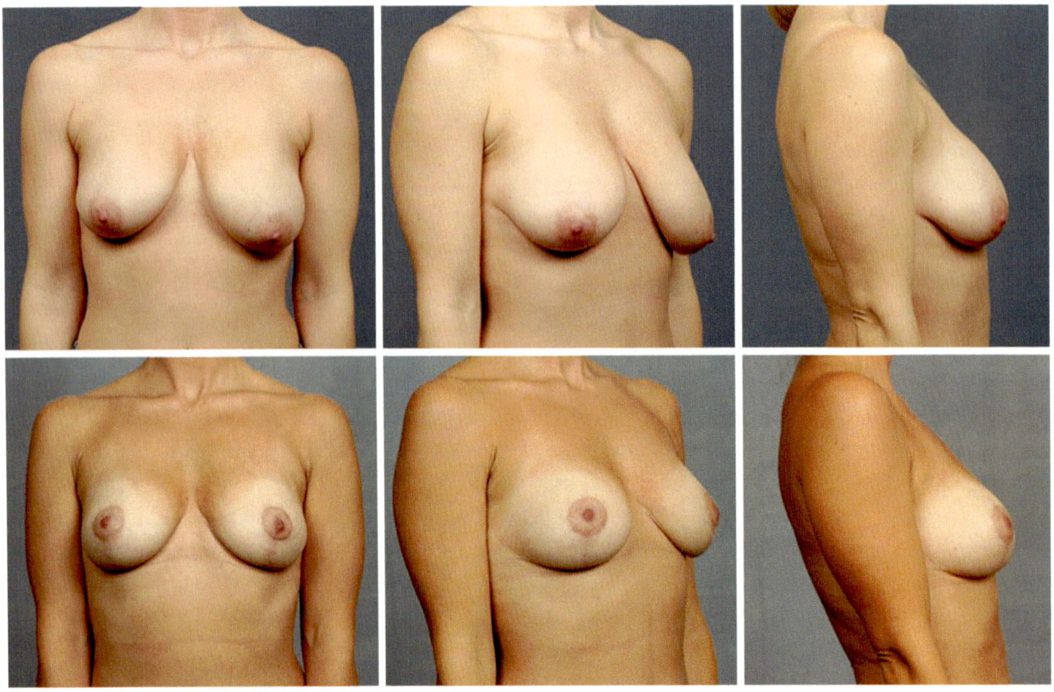

Fig. 16.20 Before and after autoaugmentation with inverted-T mastopexy using Ribeiro flaps

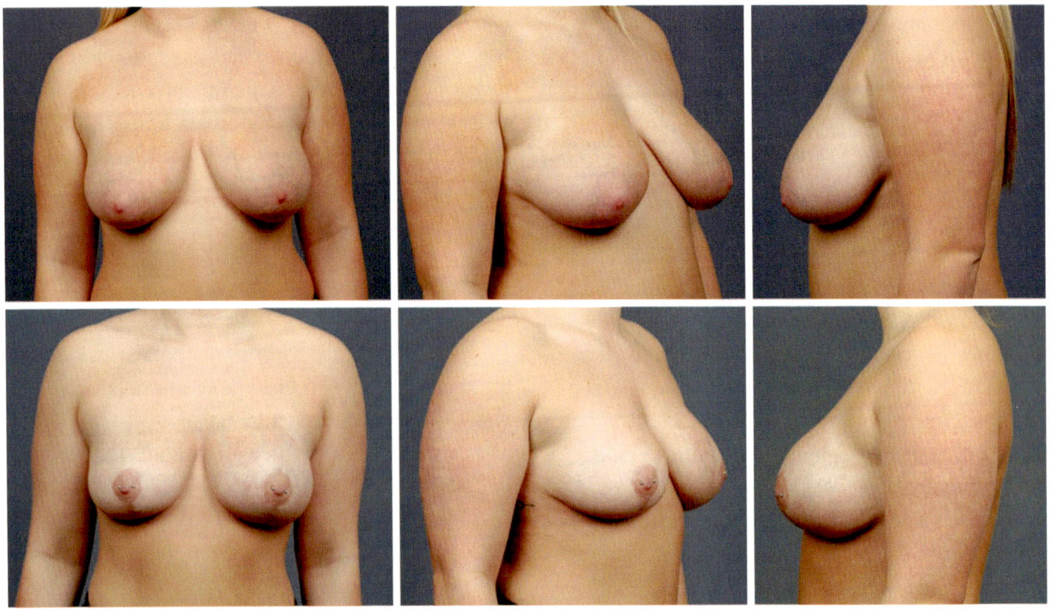

Fig. 16.21 Before and after photos of an inverted-T mastopexy using Ribeiro flaps for autoaugmentation

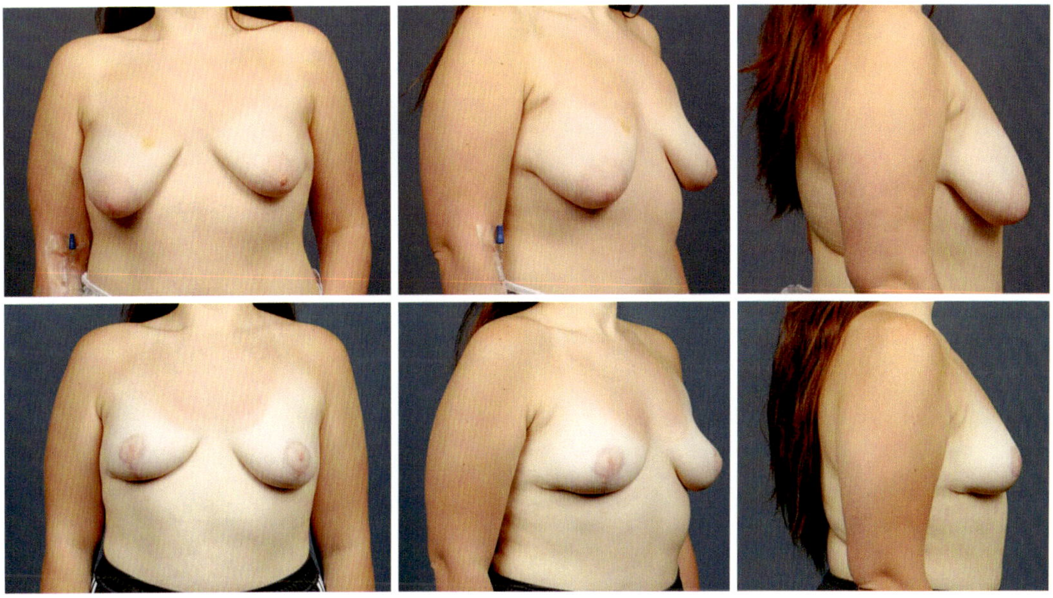

Fig. 16.22 19 year old female before and after inverted-T mastopexy with superior pedicle autoaugmentation

References

1. Binelli L. A new Periareolar mammoplasty: the "round block" technique. Aesth Plast Surg. 1990;14:93–100.
2. Lejour M. Vertical mammoplasty for breast reduction and mastopexy. In: Spear SL, editor. Surgery of the Breast: Principles and Art. Philadelphia: Lippincott-Raven; 1998. p. 73.
3. Hall-Findlay EJ. Pedicles in vertical breast reduction and mastopexy. Clin Plast Surg. 2002;29:379–91.
4. Wise RJ. Treatment of breast hypertrophy. Clin Plast Surg. 1976;3:289–300.
5. Marchac D, Olarte G. Reduction mammoplasty and correction of ptosis with a short inframammary scar. Plast Reconstr Surg. 1982;69:45–55.
6. Graf R, Biggs TIM. In search of better shape in mastopexy and reduction mammoplasty. Plast Reconstr Surg. 2002;110:309–17.
7. Lassus C. A 30-year experience with vertical mammoplasty. Plast Reconstr Surg. 1996;97:373–80.
8. Hall-Findlay EJ. Vertical breast reduction with a medial based pedicle. Aesth Surg J. 2002;22:185–94.
9. Ribeiro L. A new technique for reduction mammoplasty. Plast Reconstr Surg. 1975;55:330–4.
10. Ribeiro L, Accorsi A, Buss A, et al. Creation and evolution of 30 years of the inferior pedicle in reduction mammaplasties. Plast Reconstr Surg. 2002;110:960–70.
11. Rubin JP, Khachi G. Mastopexy after massive weight loss: dermal suspension and selective auto-augmentation. Clin Plast Surg. 2008;35:123–9.
12. Hammond DC, O'Connor EA. The lower island flap transposition (LIFT) technique for control of the upper pole in circumvertical mastopexy. Plast Reconstr Surg. 2014;134(4):655–60.
13. Regnault P. Breast ptosis definition and treatment. Clin Plast Surg. 1976;3:193–203.
14. Hall-Findlay EJ. Applied anatomy: key concepts for modern breast surgery. In: Hall-Findlay, editor. Aesthetic breast surgery: concepts and techniques. Thieme Publishers New York, New York.
15. Pitanguy I. Surgical treatment of breast hypertrophy. Br J Plast Surg. 1967;20(1):78–85.

17 Use of Soft Tissue Support in Augmentation Mastopexy

Bruce Van Natta, Bill G. Kortesis, and Gaurav Bharti

Introduction

Augmentation mastopexy can be a difficult operation for multiple reasons. Either operation alone—augmentation or mastopexy—present multiple variables to control for. Combining these procedures compounds these variables, creating a challenge for even the experienced plastic surgeon. Often, performance of the proper technical aspects of augmentation mastopexy is simply not enough to sustain excellent results. This can be due to a patient's poor tissue quality, inadequate soft tissue envelope and the use of large implants. The combination of simultaneously attempting to tighten and lift the skin envelope while placing an implant to increase size creates forces that are inherently working against each other.

Poor quality elasticity of the soft tissues, in particular the skin itself, can result in lower pole stretch when a round implant is used. With the use of shaped devices, pseudoptosis or waterfall deformity can occur. In other instances the implant may be malpositioned and the repair may call for additional reinforcement. In these cases enhanced structural support of the parenchyma and/or implant pocket may be employed to correct the deformity.

Historically a variety of materials and methods have been used to attempt to maintain mastopexy results achieved initially on the operating table. These have included absorbable Vicryl® mesh and Tigr® mesh, as well as permanent meshes made from polypropylene, nylon, and Marlex® [1]. A breast-shaped formed permanent mesh product has been utilized outside the United States known as Brefit® [2]. An absorbable multifilament woven silk mesh, Seri Scaffold® was recently available for soft tissue support in mastopexy but suffered from a significant number of adverse events and is not currently being used [3].

Although multiple mesh constructs have been utilized to enhance soft tissue support over the years, currently two products are used: (1) Acellular Dermal Matrix (ADM) such as Alloderm®, Strattice®, FlexHD® and others, and (2) Poly-4-hydroxybutyrate (P4HB) sold as GalaFLEX® [4, 5]. GalaFLEX scaffold is manufactured by Galatea Surgical in Lexington MA. It is a monofilament, biologically derived polymer that serves as an initial scaffold while tissue ingrowth occurs. The P4HB polymer is fully resorbed in 18–24 months. Strattice and Alloderm are sold by Allergan. These are forms of animal or human cadaver derived acellular dermal tissues that have been chemically and or

B. Van Natta (✉)
Private Practice, Meridian Plastic Surgery Owner/Partner, Indianapolis, IN, USA
e-mail: bvannatta@indy.rr.com

B. G. Kortesis · G. Bharti
Private Practice, Hunstad/Kortesis/Bharti Cosmetic Surgery, Charlotte, NC, USA

M. B. Calobrace et al. (eds.), *Augmentation Mastopexy*,
https://doi.org/10.1007/978-3-030-48226-8_17

radioactively treated to decellularize the dermis to create a supportive construct. In addition to soft tissue support, they can add some additional thickness in cases of thin tissues.

The focus of this chapter will be the use of poly-4-hydroxy butyrate (P4HB) absorbable monofilament scaffold, GalaFLEX, to provide soft tissue support in mastopexy augmentation.

History and Histology of P4HB

Poly-4-hydroxybutyrate is a naturally occurring polyester—a resorbable polymer with long term strength retention. Derived biologically from bacterial fermentation, it degrades by bulk hydrolysis into 4HB, a naturally occurring substance in multiple human tissues. 4HB is eliminated via the Krebs cycle as CO2 and water. The breakdown products are much less inflammatory than polyglycolic acid (Dexon®) or polylactic acid (PLA). The GalaFLEX scaffold retains approximately 70% of its strength after 12 weeks and is fully resorbed by 18–24 months.

GalaFLEX received 510 K approval by the FDA in 2007 for "reinforcement of soft tissue in plastic and reconstructive surgery and general soft tissue reconstruction." It was first used in humans as a suture (Monomax®) in 2008 and the first mesh configuration was used in humans in 2010. Bard licenses P4HB mesh as Phasix® for abdominal wall and hernia repair. Phasix mesh preclinical trials were completed in 2012 and the product was launched in 2013. In a porcine preclinical test the collagen repair was shown to have a burst strength 3.5 times greater than the native porcine abdominal fascia at 52 weeks [6, 7]. This study in a porcine model demonstrated that the burst strength contribution of the P4HB scaffold declined to near zero by 1 year but the collagen construct that replaced it was significantly stronger than the native porcine fascia [6, 7] (Fig. 17.1).

Based upon the initial success of P4HB mesh in hernia repair and abdominal wall reconstruction, Galatea Surgical was formed to explore other options for use in soft tissue support in the body [8]. The initial product was a flat mesh. Later 3-D shaped versions were offered (GalaSHAPE®) and finally a 3-D shaped product with a supportive rim (GalaFORM®) was introduced (Fig. 17.2a–c). Currently the authors typically prefer the shaped rimmed product for soft tissue support of the breast in mastopexy augmentation. A clinical trial using P4HB mesh in mastopexy was published in 2018 [9]. This study concluded that:" GalaFLEX scaffold safely and successfully supports and elevates breast tissue in mastopexy and reduction mammaplasty, with maintained support at 1 year. Surgeon and patient

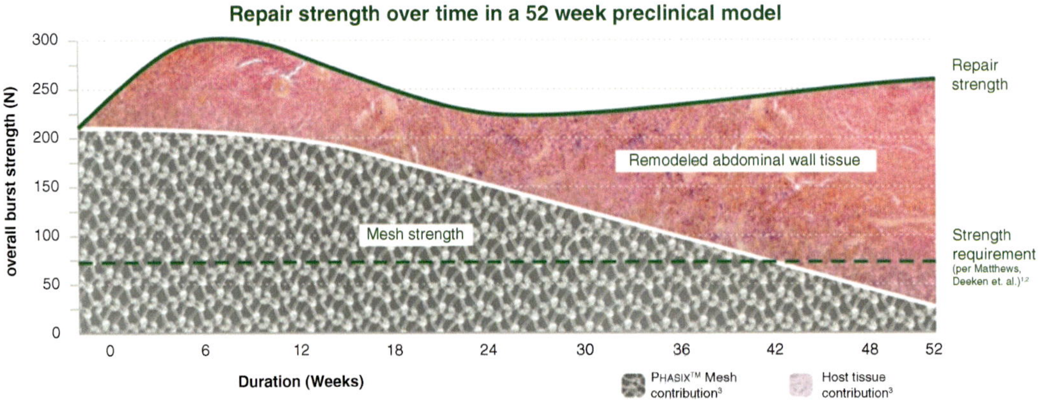

Fig. 17.1 This image of a study in a porcine model demonstrated that the burst strength contribution of the P4HB scaffold declined to near zero by 1 year but the collagen construct that replaced it was significantly stronger than the native porcine fascia

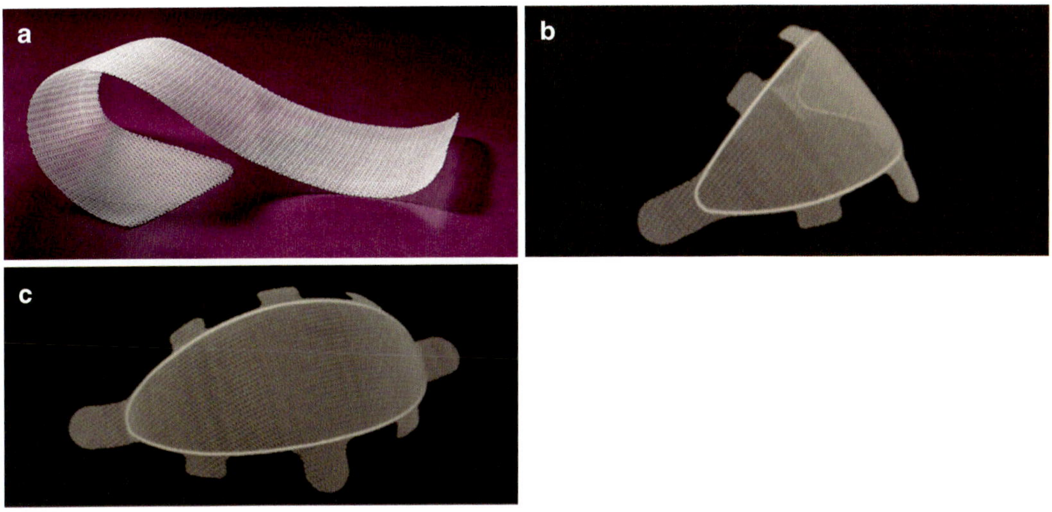

Fig. 17.2 (**a**–**c**) The initial Galatea product was a flat mesh show in (**a**). Later 3-D shaped versions were offered (GalaSHAPE®) and finally a 3-D shaped product with a supportive rim (GalaFORM®) was introduced shown in (**b**, **c**)

satisfaction were high. No mammogram or ultrasound interference was detected."

Histologically P4HB scaffold is seen to have early vascularization and complete coverage of the mesh by tissue ingrowth at 6 weeks with a thickness of 1 mm of the combined tissue/scaffold construct. The original mesh is 0.6 mm thick. By 7 months the combined tissue/mesh construct is over 3 mm in thickness with rich vascularization and abundant Types 1 and 3 collagen being demonstrated (Fig. 17.3a–d).

Indications

Currently both ADMs and GalaFLEX mesh do not have a specific indication for use in the breast by the FDA. They do however each have 510 K approval for soft tissue support generally in the body. Cost is a significant issue for the use of adjunctive support products. Generally speaking the cost for P4HB scaffold is roughly half of that for ADMs. In light of this cost factor and because of excellent clinical success with low adverse events, we see GalaFLEX scaffold as the preferred option for use in mastopexy augmentation.

Typical Indications for Use of P4HB Scaffold Include

1. Massive weight loss patients whose poor tissue quality generally cannot support the parenchyma with the added weight of an implant.
2. Patients requiring implants larger than 375 cc.
3. A previous smoker or someone with genetically poor quality soft tissue.
4. Post-partum female with significant striae, a lax soft tissue envelope and mobile inframammary fold (IMF).
5. Revision augmentation mastopexy patient with recurrent ptosis or implant malposition.
6. Peri-areolar mastopexy patient such as when performed for tubular breast deformity to prevent areolar restretch and recurrent herniation.

Placement Options

Implant Pocket Reinforcement

The scaffold can be placed internally along the breast fold in the pocket, but only in cases with minimal soft tissue cover. In most cases of

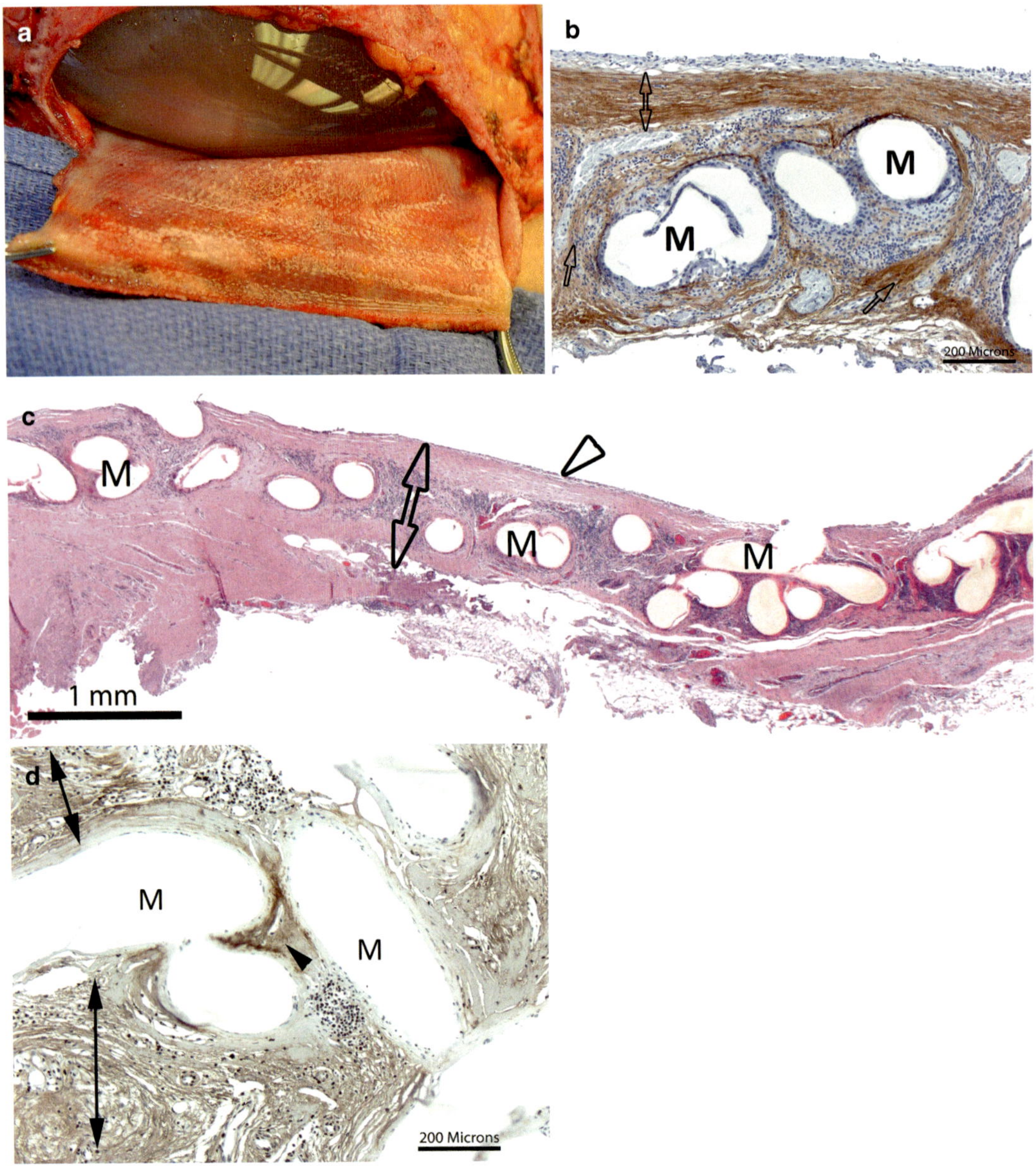

Fig. 17.3 (**a**) Appearance of GalaFLEX scaffold against implant at 6 weeks. (**b**) Histology demonstrating mature fibrous collagen forming along the implant (double arrow). (**c**) Newly formed connective tissue developing on either side of the scaffold (double arrow). (**d**) 7 month specimen showing intervening collagen between the scaffold loops staining positive for Collagen I (double arrows)

augmentation mastopexy the P4HB scaffold should be placed under the flaps. These flaps should be no thicker than 1–2 cm or glandular ptosis can result leading to a waterfall deformity. When the scaffold is placed within the pocket this serves the purpose of strengthening both the pocket and the IMF. It is recommended that in the first 15–20 cases the surgeon sit the patient up to confirm the position of the implant. It is best to leave it on the table as you want to see it long term—the scaffold support will not stretch to fill out the lower pole as commonly occurs without scaffold support. Either a flat mesh sheet or a 3D GalaSHAPE or GalaFORM may be used (Fig. 17.4a, b. Massive weight loss large volume simultaneous augmentation mastopexy 770 cc

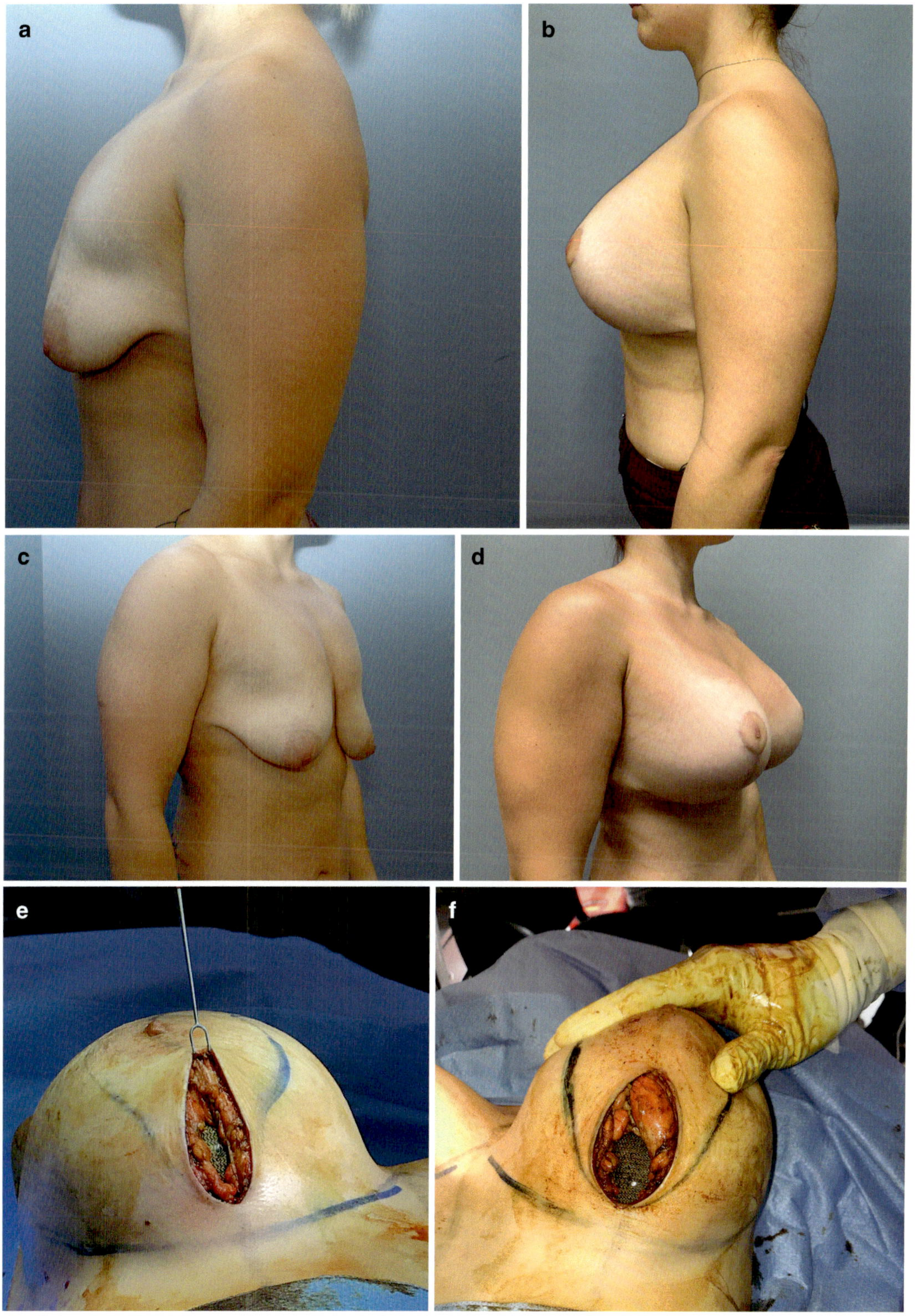

Fig. 17.4 (**a–d**) Preoperative and postoperative lateral and obliques views of a Massive weight loss patient that underwent large volume simultaneous augmentation mastopexy using 770 cc Allergan Natrelle Inspira Cohesive smooth implants in dual plane submuscular space with Galaform mesh pocket reinforcement. (**e**, **f**) Intraoperative views showing placement of the Galaform mesh adjacent to the breast implant

Allergan Natrelle Inspira Cohesive smooth implants in dual plane submuscular space with Galaform mesh pocket reinforcement).

Vertical Pillar Reinforcement

A small triangular piece can be used in the parenchyma to reinforce pillar sutures . With vertical mastopexy, pillar creation and apposition in the midline is crucial. Addition of P4HB scaffold allows for a stronger closure and better central support leading to reduction of glandular ptosis. Some surgeons choose to undermine flaps medially and laterally for mesh placement as well (Fig. 17.5).

Inferior Pole Parenchyma Reinforcement

Generally a shaped option (GalaSHAPE or GalaFORM) is preferred in this application. The scaffold can be anchored to the chest wall to delineate the exact location of the IMF. The tabs are suture securely to the deep chest tissues to avoid distorting the lower edge of the 3D mesh (Fig. 17.6a, b).

Combination Mesh Placement

P4HB scaffold can be used inside of the pocket and in the soft tissue for cases that require both forms of added support.

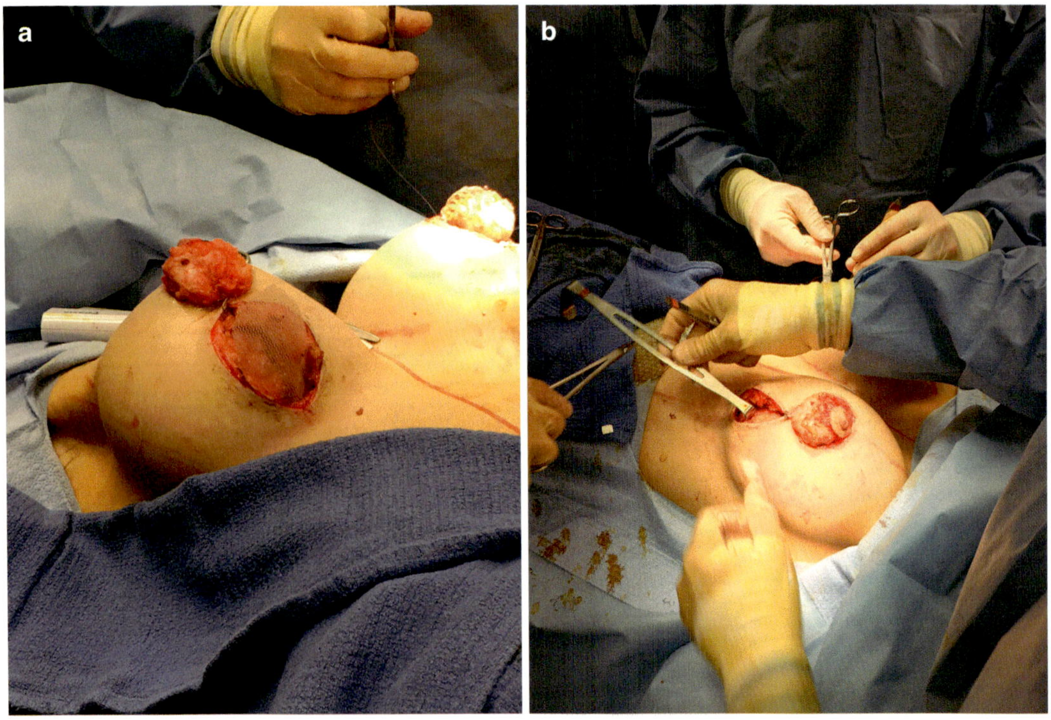

Fig. 17.5 (**a**, **b**) Intraoperative view of P4HB mesh in a vertical augmentation mastopexy draped around the lower pole parenchyma following lateral and medial skin flap elevation. The mesh is secured to the chest wall and laterally and medially. (Courtesy of Bill Kortesis and Gaurav Bharti)

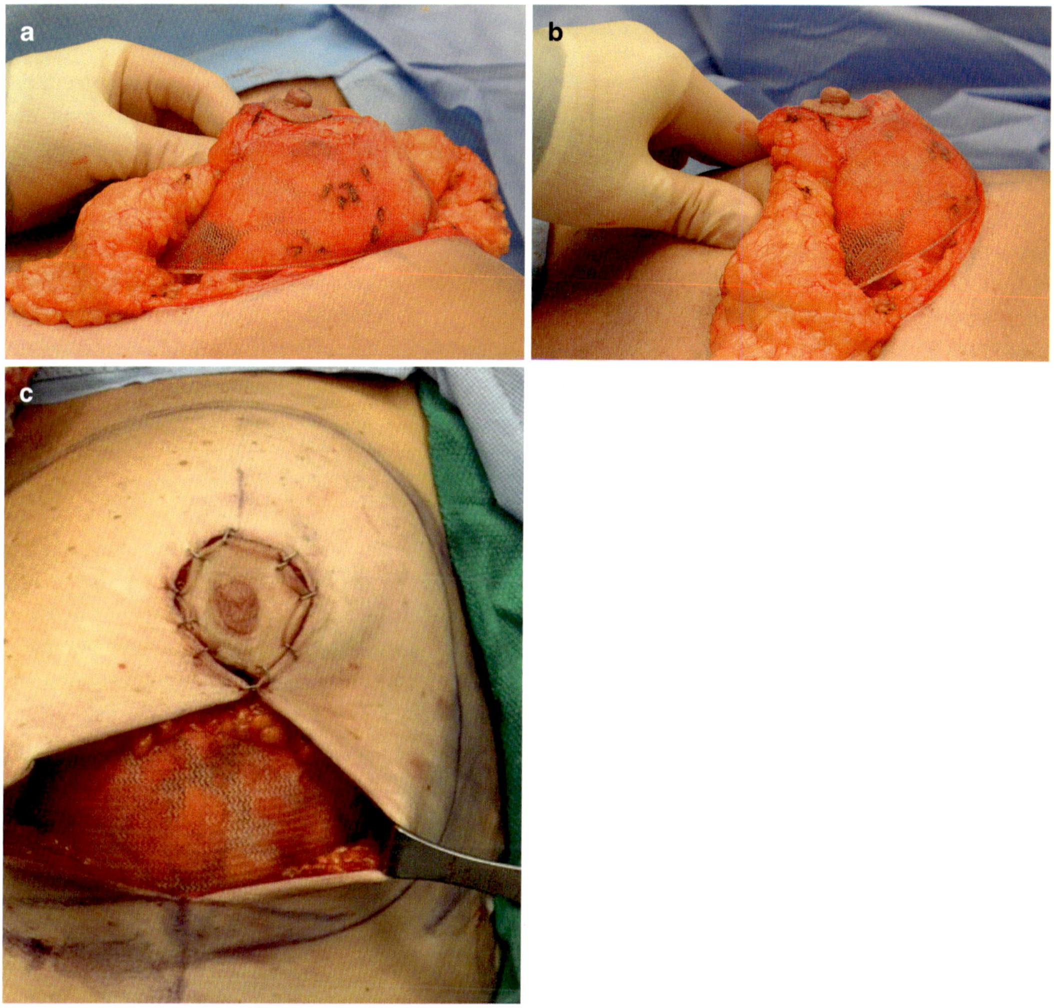

Fig. 17.6 (**a**–**c**) Intraoperative views of GalaFORM 3D scaffold with top rim removed. Lower tabs are sutured to the deep chest tissues to anchor and define the inframammary fold. C, courtesy of Braun Graham

Technical Aspects

P4HB scaffold should be treated similarly to a breast prosthesis. Contact with the skin should be avoided and the scaffold should be rinsed with the same antiseptic/antibiotic used for implants.

Scaffold should ideally lay smoothly against the parenchyma or implant without folds. Folding of mesh will generally heal well but does increase palpability.

When using P4HB scaffold under mastopexy flaps it is best to not over tension it. Doing so will result in an abnormal creasing in the breast that may not resolve without surgical correction. It is best to sit the patient up before finishing the case to confirm the shape and effectiveness of scaffold support. The rule of thumb is to: "leave it on the table as you want to see it long term". The mesh does not stretch over time.

As noted previously, it is best to leave the mastopexy flaps no thicker than 1–2 cm to avoid glandular ptosis of the soft tissue away from the remainder of the breast tissue-implant. Placing the scaffold within the implant pocket should only be done if the flaps are quite thin—otherwise it is best to place the mesh just under the flaps. If the rimmed version GalaFORM is being used we typically trim off the top rim, using the lower rim as an underwire type of support and to assist with shaping. This avoids buckling of the top rim when closing the flaps vertically.

Consider marking the nipple position approximately 0.5–1.0 cm higher than usual. Typically in mastopexies, with or without augmentation, there is stretching of the lower pole which results in a slight upward rotation of the nipple areolar complex (NAC). Since there is so little lower pole stretch when the P4HB scaffold support is used, this rotation won't occur and can result in a less than optimal aesthetic appearance. Additionally, we find that there when P4HB scaffold is used the flaps can be cut more generously since we are not using the skin to lift and support the mound. Much like the evolution if face lifting, we now only need to remove the excess skin. The skin is not providing support when GalaFLEX is used.

Generally it is best to avoid suturing the upper edge of the scaffold to the lower edge of pectoralis muscle. Suturing to muscle eliminates the dual plane effect and may lead to glandular ptosis of the parenchyma away from the implant.

Complications When Using Mesh

Overall it is the authors' experience that device related complications have been very rare. To date, with over a combined total of 800 cases of use of P4HB scaffold we have never had to remove the P4HB scaffold in its entirety due to infection or patient reaction. A few cases of exposure at the inverted T incision have occurred which have been managed with wet to dry dressings with resultant granulation. Alternatively, excision of the small exposed piece of scaffold and delayed primary closure of the flaps may be performed with uneventful healing. A few cases have required revision as a result of incorrect technique of placement such as over tensioning at the time of initial placement.

Most all patients will be able to palpate their scaffold for up to a year depending upon the thickness of the tissue cover. Patients should be told to expect to be able to palpate the material for the first few months.

Seromas are extremely rare when using P4HB open weave scaffold. They are much more common in using ADMs. The authors rarely use drains when using P4HB scaffold but always do in cases using ADM.

Patient Acceptance

Many surgeons and some patients question if the additional cost of P4HB scaffold is justified in self pay cosmetic cases. In situations where some form of soft tissue support is absolutely indicated, such as the massive weight loss patient, P4HB mesh is much less expensive than ADM and does not carry the issues of source of origin, seromas or "red breast" syndrome. We often recommend that the patient view the use of GalaFLEX® somewhat as an insurance policy. The cost of the scaffold is much less than the cost of a revision surgery. We typically show patients photos of cases done with and without GalaFLEX to demonstrate the advantages.

The question of "how long will it last?" occasionally comes up. There are currently cases out 7–8 years with no loss of support, indicating that the collagen sheet that remains after scaffold resorption is capable of maintaining the clinical result over time.

The overall concept of the use of P4HB scaffold is generally appealing to patients. They readily understand the need for support and the concept of an "internal bra". The additional fact that the GalaFLEX is absorbable is attractive to most patients as well.

Conclusions

The use of P4HB in mastopexy augmentation offers an answer to the vexing problem of dealing with tissues that have already failed. We ask those same failed tissues to support not only the weight of the breast tissue, but the added weight of the implant as well. The long term results that can be achieved using P4HB scaffold are superior to those obtained without the additional soft tissue support (Figs. 17.7a–d and 17.8a–f). Although there is a learning curve with any new device or technique, the concept is fairly straight forward and the advantages are significant. The paucity of adverse events is an added bonus. Reoperations are reduced and outcomes are maximized. Use of this support device can significantly enhance results and provide for increased surgeon and patient satisfaction.

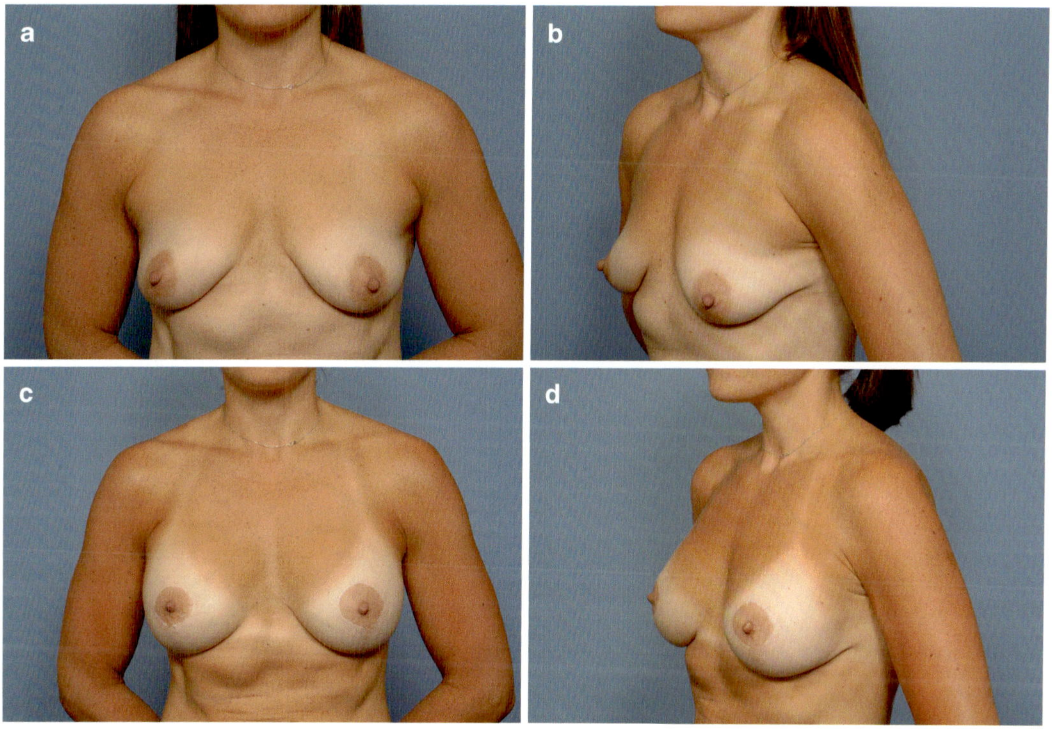

Fig. 17.7 (**a–d**) Case Example: 1 year post op views of Wise pattern mastopexy augmentation combined with P4HB mesh soft tissue support and 235 cc smooth gel implants

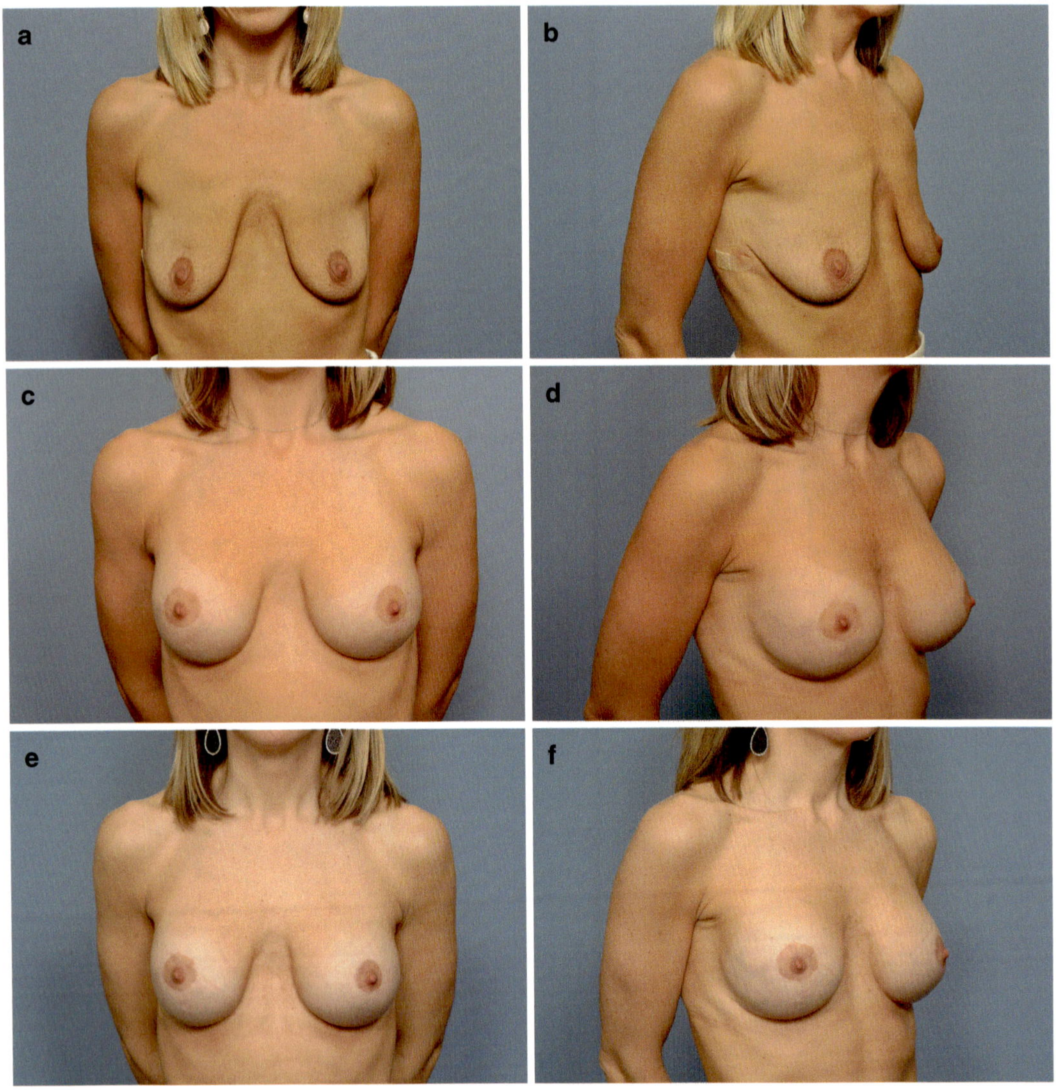

Fig. 17.8 (**a**–**f**) Case Example: 2 year (**c** and **d**) and 5 year (**e** and **f**) post op views of a mastopexy augmentation patient with GalaFLEX mesh and 339 cc implants. Note virtually no change in the appearance of the result between 2 and 5 years. The absorbable scaffold would be nearly completely gone at 2 years and certainly at 5 years indicating long term support from the remaining collagen tissue

References

1. Becker H. The use of synthetic mesh in reconstructive, revision, and cosmetic breast surgery. Aesthet Plast Surg. 2013;37:914–21.
2. De Bruijn HP. Mastopexy With 3D Preshaped Mesh for Long-Term Results: Development of the Internal Bra System. Aesthet Plast Surg. 2008;32:757–65.
3. MAUDE Database: accessdata.fda.gov. Accessed 6/23/19.
4. Bengtson BP. Emerging applications for acellular dermal matrices in mastopexy. Clin Plast Surg. 2012;39:159–66.
5. Adams WP. Aesthet Surg J. 2016;36(Suppl_2):S23–S326.
6. Williams SF, Martin DP, Moses AC. Aesthet Surg J. 2016;36(Suppl_2):S33–S42.
7. Adams WP, Toriumi DM, Van Natta BW. Aesthet Surg J. 2016;36(Suppl_2):S23–S32.
8. Adams WP, et al. Aesthet Surg J. 2018;38(5):502–18.
9. Deeken CR, Abdo MS, Frisella MM, Matthews BD. Physicomechanical evaluation of absorbable and non absorbable barrier composite meshes for laparoscopic ventral hernia repair. Surg Endosc. 2010;25(5):1541–52.

Augmentation Mastopexy in the Massive Weight Loss Patient

18

Bill G. Kortesis, Gaurav Bharti, and Charalambos "Babis" Rammos

Introduction

There has been a dramatic rise in obesity over the past several years. Accordingly, weight loss surgical procedures as well as diet and exercise programs have gained popularity. The soft tissue network and overall anatomy of a massive weight loss patient is very different from a traditional case undergoing an augmentation mastopexy (Fig. 18.1). The possibility of complications is much higher in the weight loss patient population frequently needing revision procedures. Careful planning must be performed when approaching breast volume enhancement and reshaping with a mastopexy. These procedures can typically be performed simultaneously, but in certain instances may need to be staged. Goals and expectations of the patient are discussed in detail during consultation, and a thorough personal and family history is performed. Patients need to be counseled regarding the high rate of revision surgery that can be necessary to achieve the ideal aesthetic outcome [1].

B. G. Kortesis · G. Bharti
Hunstad/Kortesis/Bharti Plastic Surgery Center, Charlotte, NC, USA
e-mail: DR.K@hkbsurgery.com; DR.B@hkbsurgery.com

C. "B." Rammos (✉)
PSG Plastic Surgery, Peoria, IL, USA

Department of Surgery, Division of Plastic Surgery, University of Illinois, College of Medicine, Peoria, IL, USA

Pre-operative Evaluation

- A thorough history and physical examination is performed focusing on:
  - History of any breast disease and breast cancer.
  - History of pregnancy.
  - Desire for future pregnancy.
  - Mammogram: Screening mammogram is obtained for any patient over 35 years old.
  - Current Body Mass Index (BMI), goal weight, time elapsed since goal weight was achieved
  - The main exclusion criteria for augmentation mastopexy in the massive weight loss patient is active nicotine use. Use of nicotine in the general population leads to 5 times increase of overall complication rates. With large transpositions of the NAC, the risks in a massive weight loss smoker are exponentially higher than a non-smoker.
  - Patients with a positive history of smoking are screened with a cotinine urine test. They are instructed to refrain 4 weeks before and after surgery.

M. B. Calobrace et al. (eds.), *Augmentation Mastopexy*,
https://doi.org/10.1007/978-3-030-48226-8_18

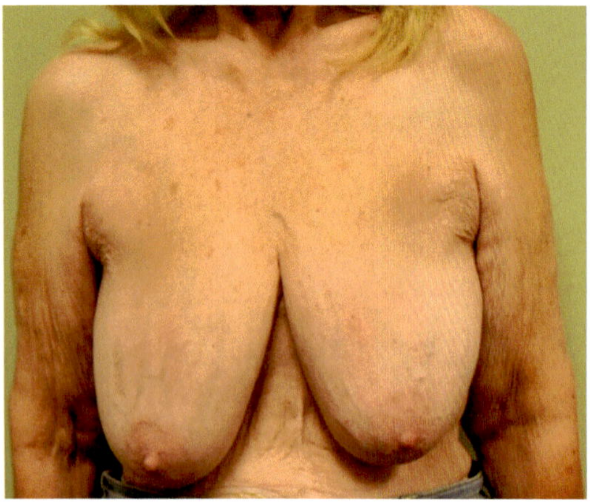

Fig. 18.1 Patients with massive weight loss present with deflated breasts, ptosis and loss of projection

- Current height and weight.
- Current breast size and desired breast size.
- Palpation for any breast masses, lymph nodes, or nipple discharge.
- Observation of breast ptosis and degree of ptosis
- Observation of chest wall and breast asymmetries, such as differences in inframammary fold height, nipple areola complex (NAC) height, breast volume, and breast shape. Often, in the massive weight loss patients the IMF is freely mobile and lacks true integrity. In situations of the very mobile and non-adherent IMF, internal support measures need to be considered such as internal sutures or synthetic mesh placement.
- Observation of the location of the breasts on the chest wall. It is imperative to note that massive weight loss patients have inherently low lying breasts on the chest wall. The footprint of these breasts are such that they cannot be elevated to a more apical position without direct volume addition to the upper pole. Volume addition is more reproducibly provided with the use of prosthetic implants.
- Cardinal Breast Measurements
- Breast width at its widest point.
- Nipple to Inframammary fold (N-IMF) distance.
- Sternal notch to Nipple distance.
- Breast height.
- Assessment of breast parenchyma and skin
- Elasticity: This is performed with deflection of the skin, and observation for resistance.
- Pinch test: This is performed at the superior and medial portion of the breast, between the examiner's thumb and index finger.
- Choice of implant volume. Sizers are placed in a bra and compared to any images obtained by three-dimensional imaging.

Pertinent Anatomy

- The breast extends from the second or third rib down to the sixth or seventh rib (cephalad to caudad) and from the lateral sternum to the anterior axillary line (medial to lateral)
- The major blood supply to the breast is from the internal mammary artery
- Lateral and anterior branches of the second through sixth intercostal nerves provide innervation to the skin overlying the breast

Perioperative Decision Making

Specific techniques that need to be discussed as it pertains to the massive weight loss patient is the amount of excess skin, amount of soft tissue support/loss, relative nipple position to new proposed position, and amount of volume required to address upper pole deficiency. Upper pole deficiency can be corrected with use of implants, fat, autologous flaps, and a potential combination of the prior. Pedicle preference depends on surgeon capabilities as well anatomy of the current breast. Authors prefer a superior or superior medial pedicle depending on the length of transposition, with small elevations just requiring a superior, and with anything greater than 4–5 cm requiring a superior medial one. This pedicle has a robust blood supply and is reliable.

A detailed discussion of patient preference for replacement of upper pole fullness is required. Those requiring minor fullness with a preference for autologous reconstruction, fat grafting serves as a viable option. Our process for fat grafting is as follows: We use proper tumescent as well as SAFE liposuction techniques for harvesting. This is usually done using a 4 mm microaire Mercedes tip cannula. We prefer to process the fat using the Revolve System by Allergan Medical for fat processing. The fat is injected in an antegrade and retrograde manner using a Microaire 3 mm basket cannula using external vibrational lipofilling. Care is taken to only inject small aliquots at a time and to avoid over deposition. It is imperative to not overfill and create a high pressure environment. The upper pole is preferentially filled first followed by the remainder of the breast. Fat grafting is halted once firmness is noted of the soft tissue to avoid any risks of pressure related necrosis or ischemia.

For those that want non implant-based augmentation, a number of autologous flaps have been described to help. Core concepts revolve around de-epithelializing skin redundancies and coning the breast. These parenchymal flaps are often based off of central chest wall perforators.

Most patients actually desire a stable upper pole and thus require an implant to do so. And with the advent of newer form stable cohesive gel implants, upper pole stability can be gained with lower profile projection options. Therefore, a surgeon can accommodate a patient's ideal breast width measurements with even a low profile cohesive implant and still maintain that stable upper pole without any potential collapse.

A choice needs to be made with the patient in regards to subpectoral dual plane versus prepectoral. Patients still require an adequate 2 cm pinch test to place implants in the pre-pectoral space. For those who do not have such a pinch test we suggest a subpectoral dual plane approach. With the potential disassociation of the breast parenchyma with the sub-pectoral space, adequate dual planning needs to be performed to place all tissues in congruity.

In addition, stabilization of the lower pole from potential stretching and implant malposition needs to addressed properly. This is with removal of excess lower pole tissue and potential support with mesh like products. A full detailed explanation of potential mesh options and positions will be addressed within the soft tissue support chapter.

Correction of the dramatic skin laxity and NAC ptosis is of paramount important in augmentation mastopexy with a massive weight loss patient. Almost all of these patients will require maximal incision line length of a wise pattern resection to eliminate vertical and horizontal excess and to properly cone and shape the breast mound. There can be significant variability in the amount and distribution of the breast parenchyma in these patients. There can be instances where there is only a skin envelope that is devoid of parenchyma and others where there is still parenchymal excess. Instances where there is parenchymal excess of the lower pole will require aggressive debulking as this tissue will tend to lead to recurrent glandular ptosis. Instances of lack of parenchyma will need to consider using the most cohesive implant to avoid rippling and wrinkling.

In certain instances an augmentation mastopexy sequence may need to be staged for a massive weightloss patient. Instances where staging would be prudent include: extreme cases of ptosis with highly exaggerated N:IMF or SN:N distances, medical comorbities, or any situation where the surgeon is not comfortable with the numerous variables at play when combining these procedure in a massive weight loss patient. These patients will often require revisions of their augmentation mastopexy when performed in combination or in a staged approach. This should be discussed upfront with the patient during consultation. The need for revisions is well tolerated by massive weight loss patients as they are frequently addressing another concurrent body contouring concern at that time.

Patient Expectations

Severe grade II or grade III ptosis with synchronous flattening of the upper pole is an indication for wise pattern augmentation mastopexy. However, the two techniques work against each other. Mastopexy is designed to reposition the nipple areola complex, and reduce the vertical and horizontal skin excess, all without tension at the wound closure. Augmentation on the other hand, increases the size of the breast, and exerts more tension at the wound closure. Careful selection of implants and modest skin resection are of paramount importance to prevent complications. With a massive weight loss patient these issues become more prominent and occur more often. Often there can be recurrent ptosis even though the surgeon may have felt that they had resected enough skin and parenchyma. Having to perform revision surgery on the weight loss patient can frequently occur. Most often the revision procedure will be a revision mastopexy requiring further skin and parenchymal resection and or implant/pocket repositioning. Pitfalls are discussed in detail:

- **Scars:** Patient should make an informed decision based on the knowledge that the scars will be located centrally and will be visible to an extent. In the massive weight loss patient, to achieve an improved shape and position, longer scars are produced. Patients with massive weight loss must understand the necessity for longer scars to eliminate skin excess.
- **Breast Size:** Tightening of the lower pole only is not sufficient to restore upper pole fullness. Patient expectations and the need for an implant to restore volume are discussed in detail during consultation. In addition, details discussions must be had regarding the need to understand limitations of implant volume to prevent complications such as lower pole stretch and implant malposition.
- **Implants:** Capsular contracture, malposition, rupture and need for reoperation should be discussed with the patient when implants are used. Implant malposition is a common complication in massive weight loss patients
- **Recurrent Ptosis:** There is a detailed discussion with the patient that the conditions that caused the initial ptosis will still progress after surgery likely making necessary a revisionary operation after a period of time. Early postoperative ptosis is common in the massive weight loss patient population, as early as 3 months. Adequate intraoperative correction of excess and ptotic skin is of paramount importance to achieve longer lasting results.
  - Waterfall deformity can occur when an adequate dual plane is not performed or if the muscle prevents implant from adequately settling. Therefore, the muscle must be released adequately to prevent such issues.
  - Also, inadequate resection of the lower pole can create a bottoming out affect. Therefore, adequate resection of the lower pole tissue needs to be performed. In cases where tissues are too thin to resect soft tissue support with mesh is encouraged.
- **Symmetry:** Nipple position, and differences between the two breasts in terms of volume and shape should be taken into consideration in the massive weight loss patient. Asymmetric breast resection, different implant use and lateralization of the nipple are planned accordingly

Operative Approach

Superior Pedicle Wise Pattern Augmentation Mastopexy with a Smooth Round Silicone Implant

Markings

Preoperative markings are similar to those for reduction mammoplasty. Because an implant will be used, less skin is marked for excision. Additional skin is excised after the implant has been placed. The patient is marked in the upright standing position, and the following markings are made: midline, from sternal notch to xiphoid, inframammary fold and breast meridian (Fig. 18.2). The new nipple location is marked by transposition of the inframammary fold to the front of the breast, at the level of the meridian. Massive weight loss patients present with nipple medialization. Placement of the nipple more lateral at the true breast meridian is of paramount

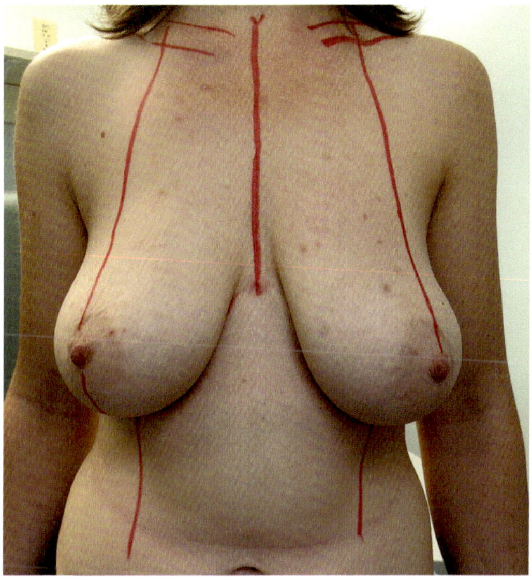

Fig. 18.2 The patient is marked in the upright standing position, and the following initial markings are made: Midline, from sternal notch to xiphoid, Inframammary Fold, Breast meridian

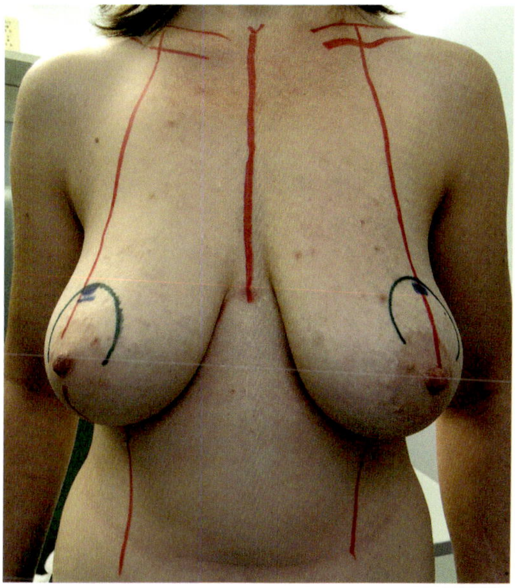

Fig. 18.3 The new areola opening is transferred on the superior breast parenchyma. The top of the areola is about 1–2 cm above the inframammary fold

importance. The top of the areolar opening is marked 1–2 cm above the new nipple position. With the use of a keyhole breast reduction marker (42 mm), the areola opening is marked (Fig. 18.3). The breast is displaced, first laterally and then medially. Vertical lines are drawn from the lower portion of the new areola to a point 1 cm above the inframammary fold (Fig. 18.4). Measurements are made bilaterally, from sternal notch to nipple, and from midline to ensure symmetry. Finalized markings are shown (Fig. 18.5).

Operating Room

The patient is brought to the operating room and placed in the supine position on the operating table with the arms extended up to 90 degrees and well secured to the arm boards. Both shoulders should be at the same height. The patient is sat up to evaluate the preoperative status (Fig. 18.6a, b). Local anesthesia containing a mix of lidocaine and Marcaine with epinephrine is injected into the marked pattern, and as a breast block. A vertical incision is made sharply within the mastopexy resection pattern, dividing the breast tissue, and carried down with cautery

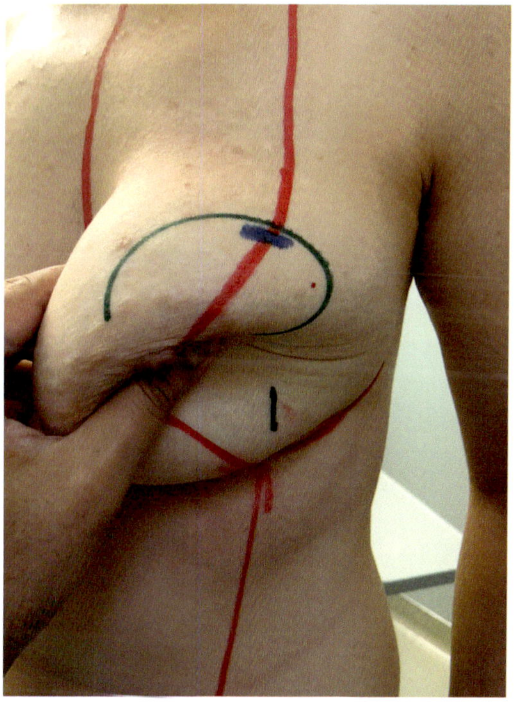

Fig. 18.4 The breast is displaced, first laterally and then medially. Vertical lines are drawn from the lower portion of the new areola to a point 1 cm above the inframammary fold

to the pectoralis fascia. The pectoralis muscle is grasped and divided till the areolar space under the muscle is identified. A lighted retractor is then placed below the pectoralis major muscle and strong upward traction is placed so as to separate the pectoralis major from the pectoralis minor muscle (Fig. 18.7). Pocket dissection is performed with the monopolar electrocautery and there is no use of blunt dissection. Prevention of bleeding is paramount to avoid capsular con-

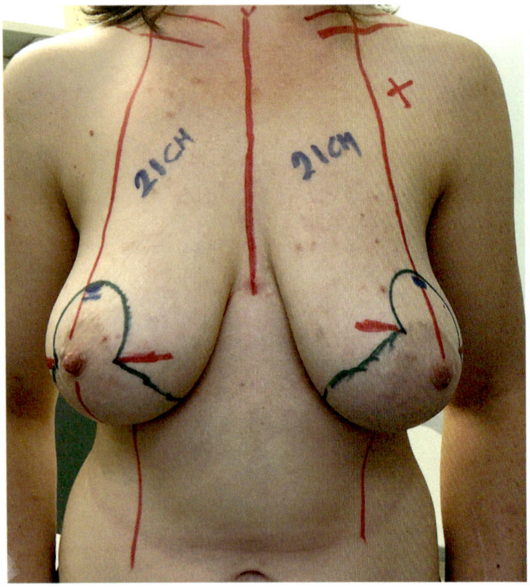

Fig. 18.5 Preoperative frontal view markings of a 40-year-old female with grade II ptosis

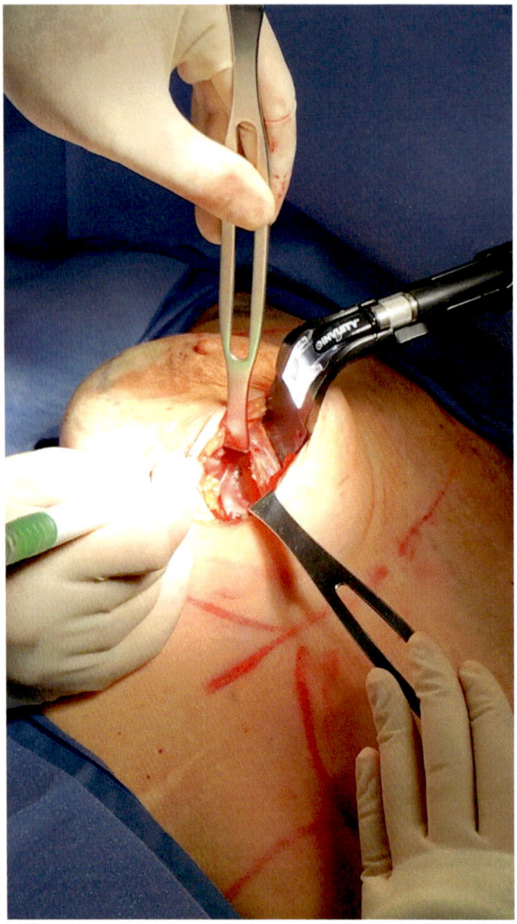

Fig. 18.7 After breast tissue division, the pectoralis major muscle is encountered. The pectoralis major muscle edge is divided and dissection proceeds in an areolar plane

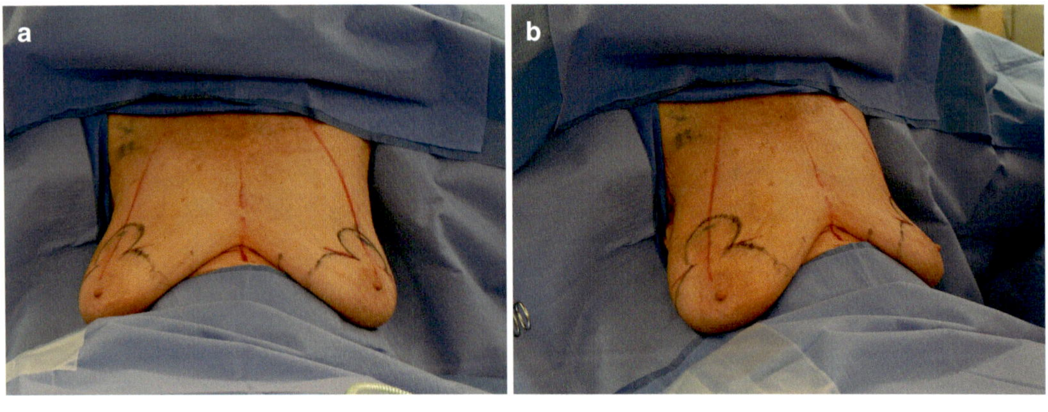

Fig. 18.6 (**a**) Intraoperative frontal view of the patient positioned on the operating table. The patient is placed in an upright seated position for initial appreciation. (**b**) Intraoperative oblique view of the patient positioned on the operating table. The patient is placed in an upright seated position for initial appreciation

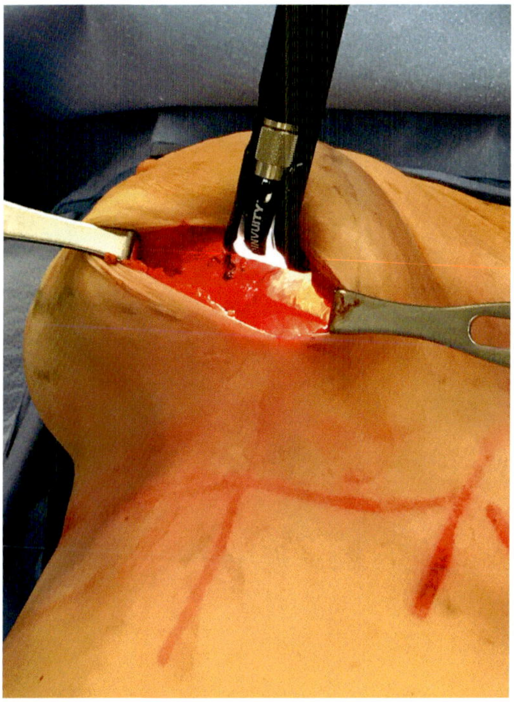

Fig. 18.8 A submuscular pocket is created under direct visualization to accommodate the implant. Dissection is performed with cautery, and excellent hemostasis is achieved. Pectoralis minor muscle fibers are left intact

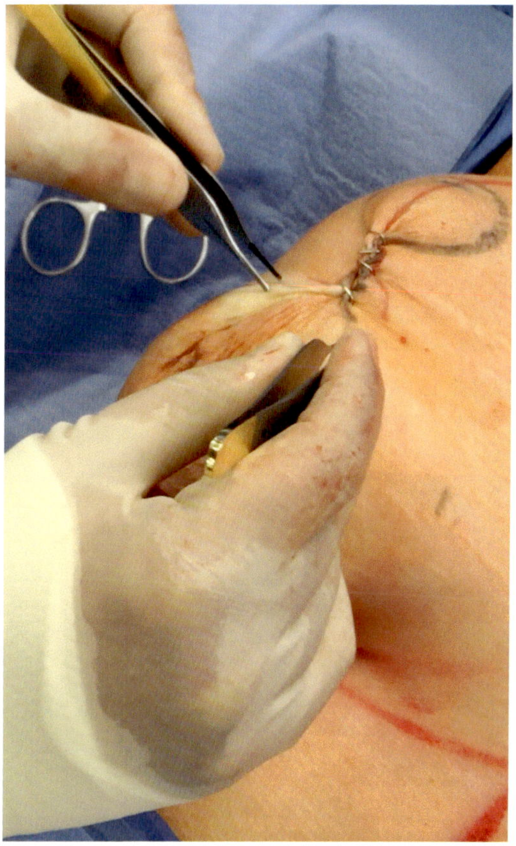

Fig. 18.9 After placement of the tester gel implants, the breasts are temporarily stapled closed

tracture. Submuscular dissection proceeds from medial to lateral in a clockwise fashion for the left breast and in an anticlockwise fashion for the right breast, until the pocket is of appropriate size (Fig. 18.8). Care is taken to avoid any contact with the ribs so as to decrease postoperative pain. The medial origin of the pectoralis major muscle is disinserted, so as to achieve adequate expansion of the lower pole and avoid a constriction deformity. Meticulous hemostasis is achieved. It is imperative to avoid over dissection laterally. In cases of asymmetries sizer implants are placed and the breasts are temporarily stapled closed (Fig. 18.9). A 6–8 cm inframammary fold-areola distance is used, and an appropriate elliptical mastopexy pattern is designed (Fig. 18.10). The patient is placed in the upright seated position and symmetry is confirmed. If there are areas for additional dissection, these are marked. The pockets are irrigated with triple antibiotic solution. The formal implants are then placed in a sterile manner using the no-touch technique. The implant is transferred to the Keller funnel avoiding any contact with the operating table or the surgeon's gloves (Figs. 18.11 and 18.12). A Deaver retractor is used by the assistant to facilitate placement of the implant (Fig. 18.13). The pockets are closed with 3-0 Vicryl (Fig. 18.14). The skin is then tailor tacked, and the patient is placed in the upright position again to verify the mastopexy marks. The nipples are traced with a 42 mm cookie cutter. The areola is left in situ (Fig. 18.15). The marks are incised sharply and the intervening skin de-epithelialized. An incision is made with the cautery around the periphery of the vertical limbs. The inferior portion of the areola pedicle is released with cautery, thus

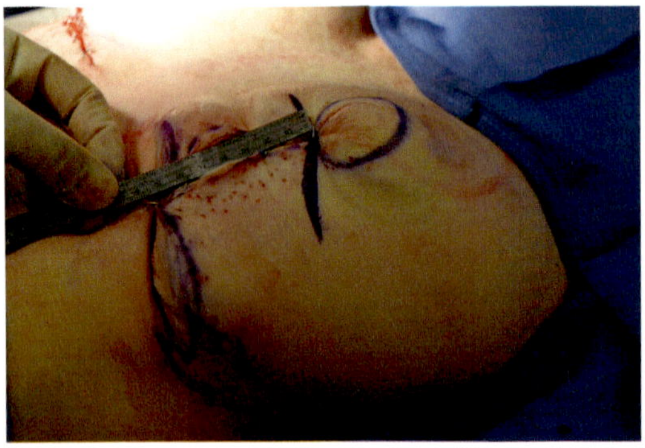

Fig. 18.10 A vertical limb of approximately 7 cm is created

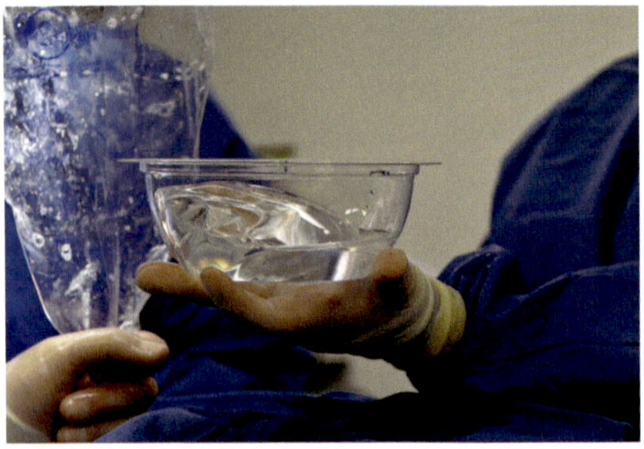

Fig. 18.11 The formal implant package is opened, and will be transferred to the Keller funnel

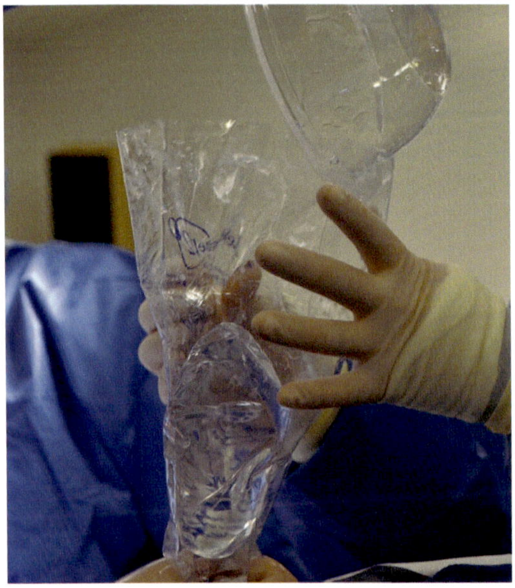

Fig. 18.12 The no touch technique is used. The implant is transferred to the Keller funnel without being touched

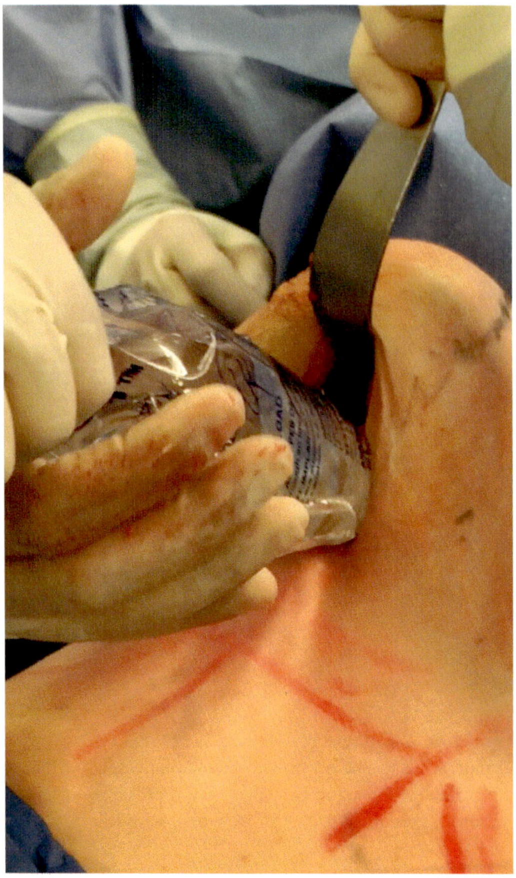

Fig. 18.13 A Deaver is used for retraction and exposure of the pocket, and the implant is transferred with the Keller funnel

creating a superior pedicle, to allow for superior motion and inset without tension. A small wedge of tissue is removed from the vertical limb to improve the contour. The elliptical mastopexy pattern is removed full-thickness with great care not to enter the implant pocket, and the resected amounts are recorded. With the shape and size confirmed with the patient sitting up, vertical pillar breast sutures are placed, on average a total of 3 interrupted sutures (2-0 Vicryl). The skin is closed in layers with interrupted 3-0 Monocryl for the deep dermis and a running subcuticular 3-0 Monocryl more superficially. The patient is placed again in an upright seated position for final assessment (Fig. 18.16). The before (Fig. 18.17) and after on table result (Fig. 18.18) are shown for comparison.

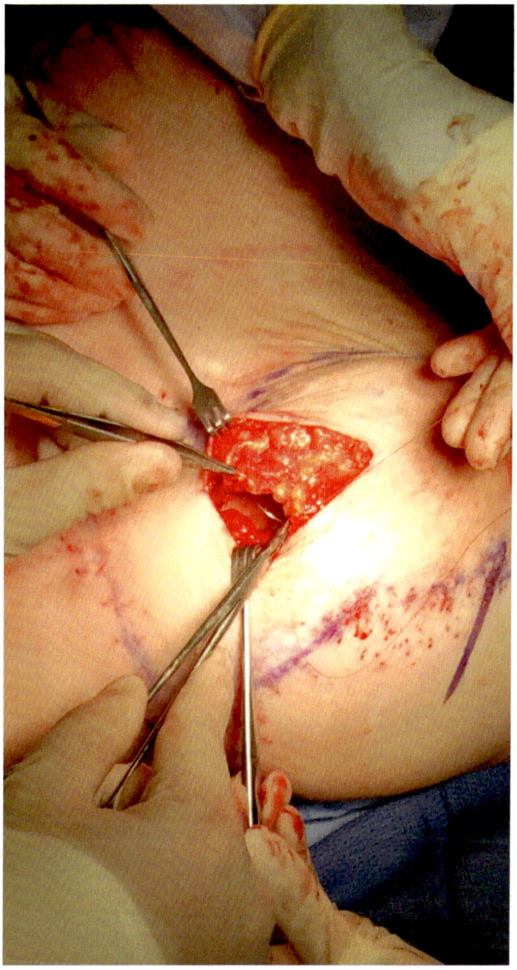

Fig. 18.14 Closure of the deeper breast tissue and pocket is performed

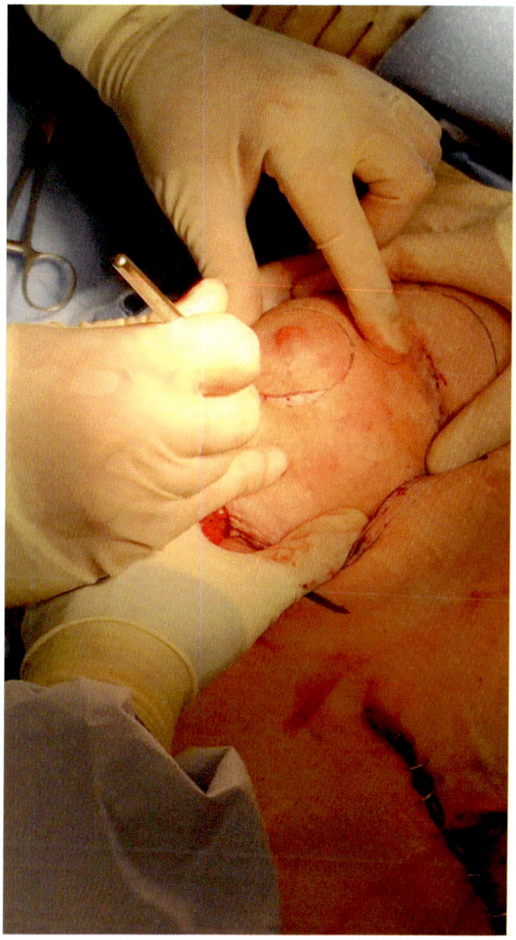

Fig. 18.15 The areola is incised first

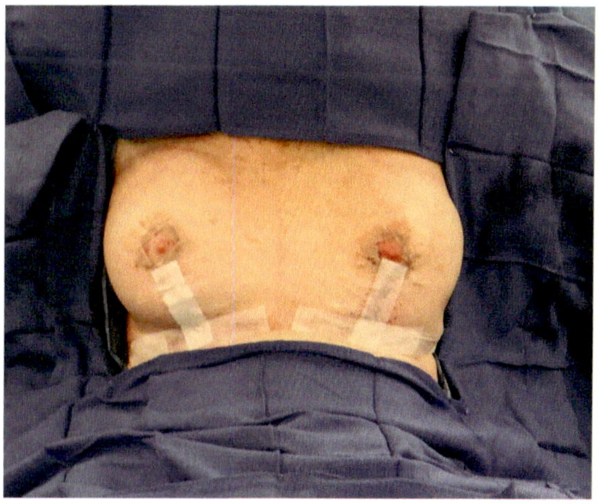

Fig. 18.16 Patient at the seated upright position with the formal implants in place, and skin wounds closed

Auto Augmentation with Creation of Parenchymal Flaps and Dermal Suspension

This technique is used when patients have enough volume of native breast tissue and lateral chest wall excess. This technique is widely used and is thought to contribute to a more natural appearance and a lower rate of ptosis over time [2, 3].

The wise pattern is marked as follows: The apex of the inverted T is chosen by transposing the inframammary fold anteriorly onto the breast. An angled inverted V pattern is then drawn from

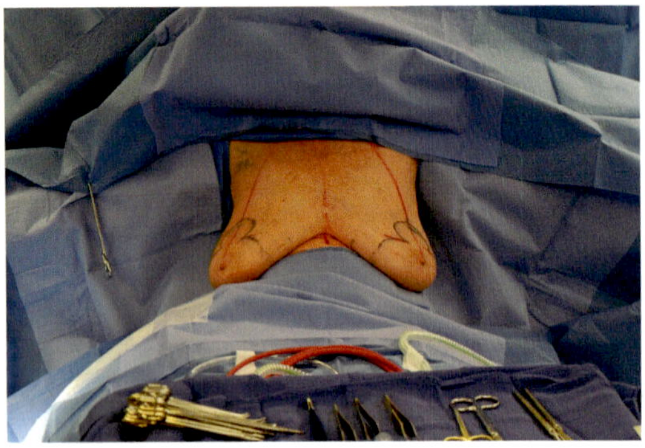

Fig. 18.17 Intraoperative frontal view of the patient positioned on the operating table. The patient is placed in an upright seated position for initial appreciation

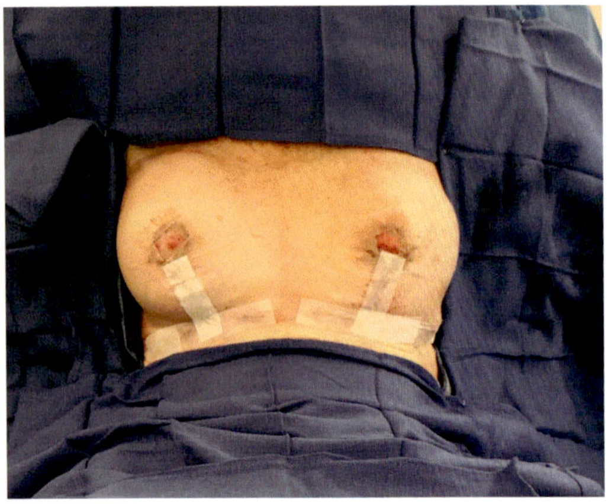

Fig. 18.18 Intraoperative frontal view of the patient positioned on the operating table. The patient is placed in an upright seated position for final appreciation. A bilateral Wise pattern augmentation mastopexy was performed

this point downward. Care is taken to include in this pattern the entirety of the areola. Average length of the vertical limbs is 8 cm. A medial and lateral extension is then drawn, meeting the inframammary fold marking. The entire dermis lying within the Wise pattern is then deepithelialized. A pedicle of approximately 10 cm is then marked. Medial and lateral flaps are then raised and rotated, and dermal suspension is performed. Finally, plication of the flaps with the pedicle is performed.

Augmentation Mastopexy with Soft Tissue Reinforcement

Massive weight loss patients present with lack of structural soft tissue support and often a need for reinforcement of the inframammary fold. Multiple mesh constructs are available to provide support. Currently, two products are used most often to provide this structural support: Galaflex and Strattice. Galaflex is manufactured by Galatea and is a synthetic mesh construct made of P4HB that serves as a scaffold for soft tissue ingrowth to help provide a stronger soft tissue construct long term. Strattice is a porcine acellular dermal matrix that has been treated to decellularize the dermis to serve as supportive construct that can also serve to add additional thickness with soft tissue coverage.

Post-operative Management

Patients are discharged at the same day of surgery after they recover in the postoperative anesthesia care unit (PACU). Postoperative medications include limitation of oral analgesics. The authors prefer oral anti-inflammatories such as Advil or Tylenol. Prior to awakening in the surgical suite the patient is often given a one-time dose of Toradol, 30 mg. In addition to anti-inflammatories, the patient is given a 7-day course of oral antibiotics. All patients are placed in a soft bra without an underwire. Patients are instructed to avoid heavy lifting, no more than10 lbs. for a period of 10 days. Minimal exercise programs (walking, light cardio, light leg activities) can be initiated after a few days. Patients may shower in postoperative day 1 (POD #1). Follow up appointment is scheduled for day1, 1 week, 3 weeks, 3 months, 6 months, and 1 year.

Complications include and are not limited to:

- Hematoma formation is usually less than 5% in most reported series. Patients are screened for any use of anticoagulation, and medication is temporarily held preoperatively.
- Infection is rare and occurs in less than 1% of the patients. There is no clear evidence for better outcomes with the use of postoperative antibiotics.
- Wound healing issues are more frequent in the wise pattern technique, especially in the smoking population. Patients need to quit smoking at least 4 weeks before the operation
- Implant malposition can occur in massive weight loss patients. This can occur as the inframammary fold is not fixed or hypermobile. It is imperative in these cases to perform maneuvers to reinforce and secure the IMF to the chest wall when possible.
- Asymmetry is not uncommon. Large differences between the 2 breasts require revisional surgery
- Nipple-Areola Necrosis may be prevented with monitoring options that include clinical examination.
- Recurrent ptosis over time will occur due to gravity and aging. Parenchymal support with the use of vertical pillar sutures is thought to decrease the likelihood of recurrent ptosis.
- Capsular contracture is due to inflammation, which in turn may be due to tissue trauma, bacteria, and blood. The use of the Keller funnel has been shown to lead to a statistically significant reduction in the incidence of reoperations performed due to capsular contracture within 12 months of primary breast augmentation

Conclusion

Augmentation mastopexy in the massive weight loss patient requires careful preoperative planning and recognition of changes that occur with weight fluctuations. These procedures have a large impact on quality of life of massive weight loss patients [4, 5].

Case Examples

Case 1

This 69-year-old female developed severe Grade III ptosis after massive weight loss (Figs. 18.19a, b). A dual plane augmentation with a Wise pattern skin resection and reshaping of the breast gland was performed. A 295 ml smooth round moderate profile silicone implant was used. The vertical and horizontal scar technique, previously described, was used, with a breast resection of 42 gr from the right side and 21 gr from the left side. She is shown 2 weeks postoperative (Figs. 18.20a, b).

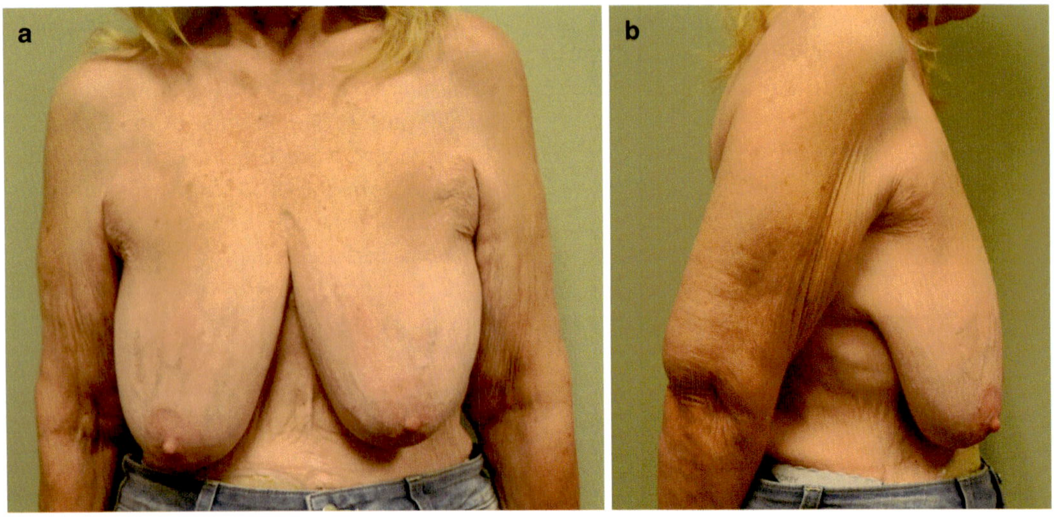

Fig. 18.19 (**a**) Preoperative frontal view of a 69-year-old female with grade III ptosis. (**b**) Preoperative right lateral view of a 69-year-old female with grade III ptosis

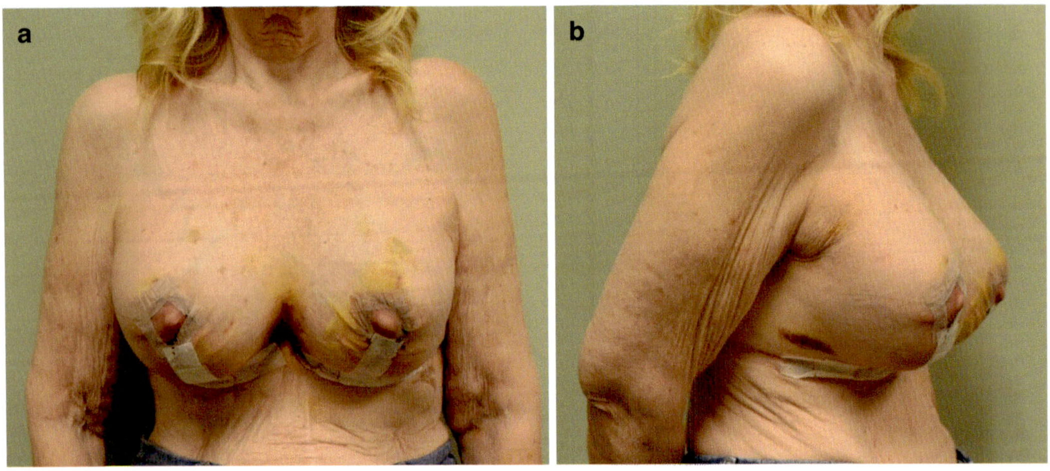

Fig. 18.20 (**a**) Postoperative frontal image obtained at 2 weeks follow up after wise pattern mastopexy augmentation with a 295 ml smooth round implant with moderate projection. (**b**) Postoperative right lateral image obtained at 2 weeks follow up after wise pattern mastopexy augmentation with a 295 ml smooth round implant with moderate projection

Case 2

This 32-year-old female developed Grade III ptosis after massive weight loss (Fig. 18.21 a–c). She requested a mastopexy and expressed the desire for superior pole fullness. The Wise pattern technique, described previously, was used. A 485 ml smooth round moderate cohesive silicone implant (Allergan Inspira 485 cc SCM) was placed in the dual plane subpectoral space, and a superior pedicle was used. The patient is shown 8 months after the procedure (Fig. 18.22 a–c).

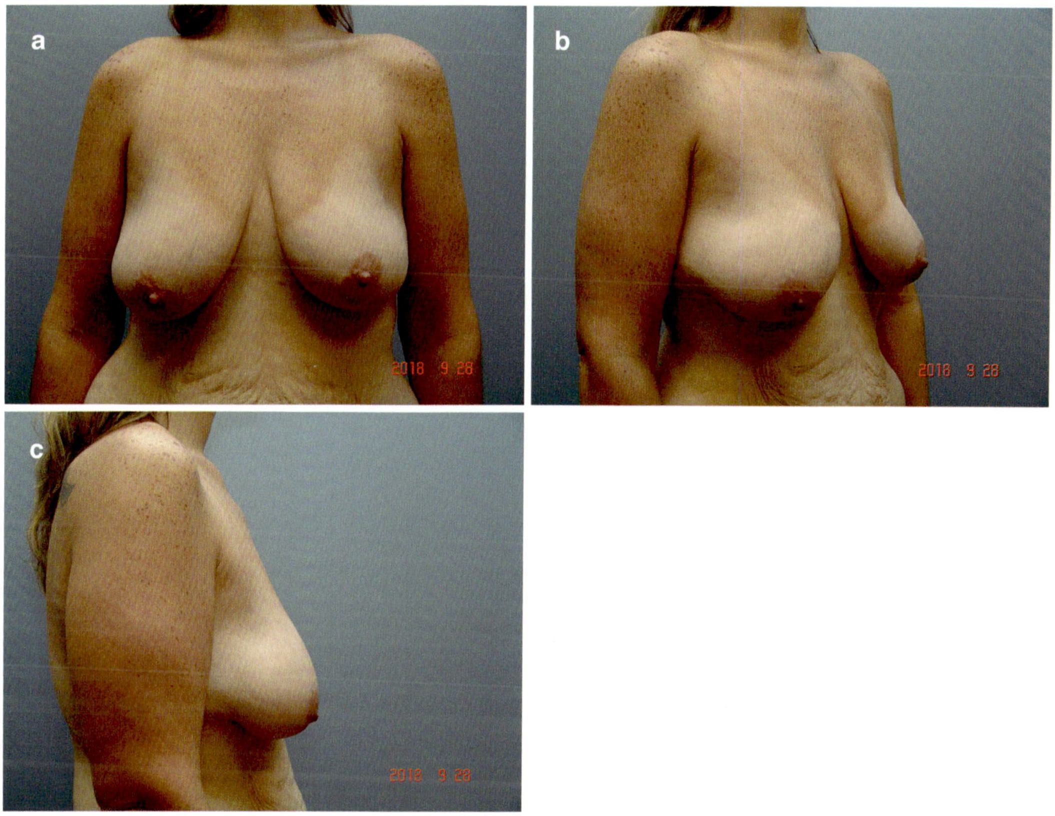

Fig. 18.21 Preoperative frontal, oblique, and lateral views of a 34-year-old female with grade III ptosis

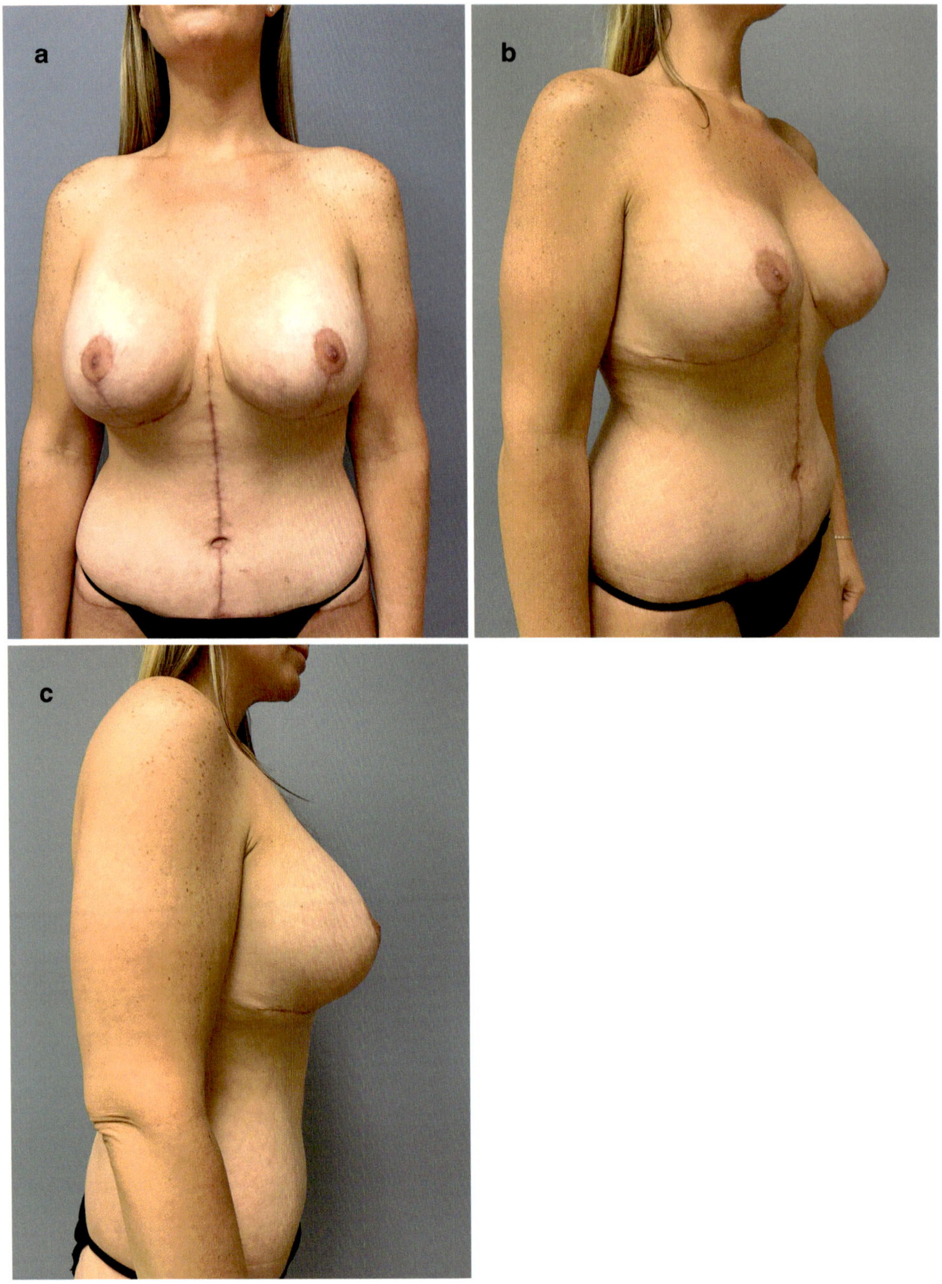

Fig. 18.22 Postoperative frontal, oblique, and lateral images obtained at 8 months follow up after wise pattern mastopexy augmentation with a 485 ml smooth round implant with moderate projection, Allergan Inspira SCM

References

1. Coombs DM, Srivastava U, Amar D, Rubin JP, Gusenoff JA. The challenges of augmentation mastopexy in the massive weight loss patient: technical considerations. Plast Reconstr Surg. 2017;139(5):1090–9.
2. Rubin JP. Mastopexy in the massive weight loss patient: dermal suspension and total parenchymal reshaping. Aesthet Surg J. 2006;26:214–22.
3. Rubin JP, Khachi G. Mastopexy after massive weight loss: dermal suspension and selective auto-augmentation. Clin Plast Surg. 2008;35:123–9.
4. Sarosiek K, Maxwell GP, Unger JG. Getting the most out of augmentation-mastopexy. Plast Reconstr Surg. 2018;142(5):742e–59e.
5. Hidalgo DA, Spector JA. Mastopexy. Plast Reconstr Surg. 2013;132(4):642e–56e.

19 Pitfalls in Augmentation Mastopexy

Gaurav Bharti, Bill G. Kortesis, and Jeffrey R. Claiborne

Introduction

Augmentation mastopexy is a challenging combination of procedures that requires careful preoperative planning and intraoperative decision-making. When executed appropriately results are fantastic, but when performed without proper planning and execution, complications can happen. Multiple pitfalls exist which lead to complications requiring re-operative augmentation mastopexy. The key to success is proper preoperative assessment and planning to recognize what maneuvers need to occur for a predictable outcome. In addition, surgeons must develop true understanding of the dynamics of aging breast tissue and how implants can affect these dynamics. The pitfalls of augmentation mastopexy can be related to improper technique in dealing with the breast tissue or the implant itself. In this chapter, we will examine some of the common pitfalls and complications associated with this procedure and ways to avoid them.

G. Bharti · B. G. Kortesis
Private Practice Hunstad/Kortesis/Bharti Cosmetic Surgery, Charlotte, NC, USA
e-mail: Dr.b@hkbsurgery.com; Dr.k@hkbsurgery.com

J. R. Claiborne (✉)
Private Practice, Northshore Plastic Surgery, Mandeville, LA, USA

Common Pitfalls

Waterfall Deformity (High Riding Implant and/or Tissue Ptosis)

The waterfall deformity can occur for several reasons. In all situations the cause for the distorted appearance is that the implant is sitting in a higher position than the bulk majority of the breast (Figs. 19.1 and 19.2). This may be because the implant is superiorly malpositioned and the tissue, although in normal position, appears to be falling off the implant. It also can occur from an implant being in normal position, but appears high riding as the breast tissue is ptotic and inferiorly malpositioned. Often it can be a combination of both. Correction of the deformity requires proper identification of the cause. This occurrence is common with a massive weight loss patient who undergoes simultaneous augmentation mastopexy.

High Riding Implant

A high riding implant is where the implant stays too high on the chest wall relative to the breast footprint (the inferior edge of the implant lies several centimeters above the IMF) (Fig. 19.3). This can be due to malposition (poor planning and execution) or capsular contracture (excessive and abnormal pocket scarring).

M. B. Calobrace et al. (eds.), *Augmentation Mastopexy*,
https://doi.org/10.1007/978-3-030-48226-8_19

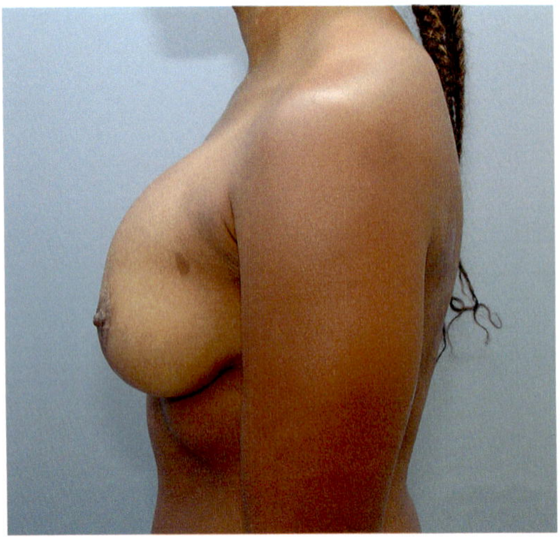

Fig. 19.1 Waterfall deformity, lateral view showing high riding implant and ptotic breast tissue inferioly hanging off the implant

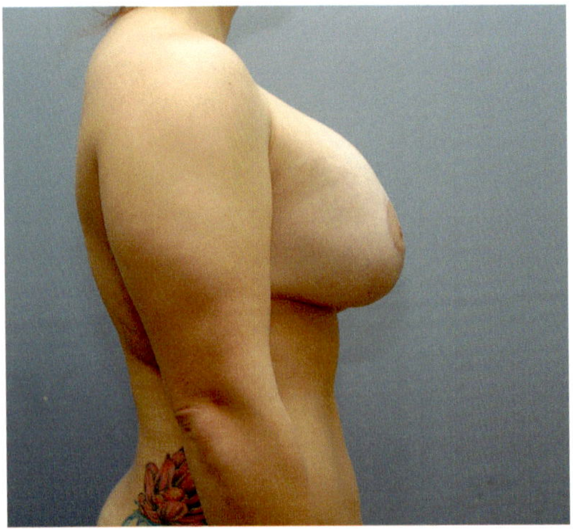

Fig. 19.2 Waterfall deformity, lateral view showing high riding implant and ptotic breast tissue inferioly hanging off the implant

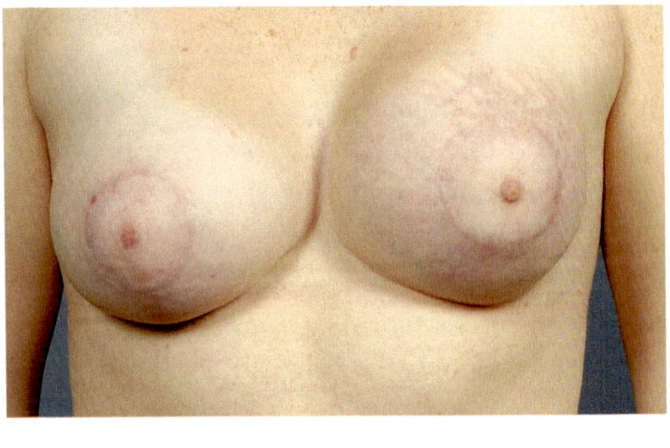

Fig. 19.3 Unilateral high riding implant with a periareolar mastopexy

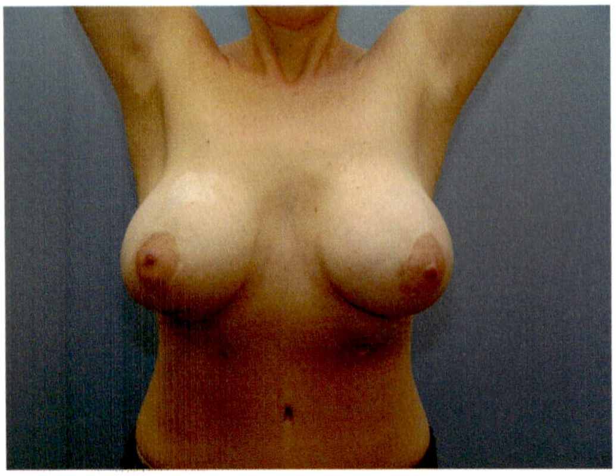

Fig. 19.4 Inferior implant malposition/double-bubble on the right breast AP view

Precise pocket planning is critical to avoid superior malposition. Implants will settle and drop inferiorly in their pockets until they reach a site of firm fascial or muscular attachment. Pectoralis-rib muscle attachments can prevent adequate implant descent and is one etiology of superior malposition. If the pectoralis origin is 2–3 cm above the inframammary fold (IMF), the implant will be unable to settle to the desired IMF level. The advantage of the dual plane technique is that the pectoralis-rib attachments are released, and therefore the implant will drop to the IMF ligament complex. With a dual-plane technique, the surgeon depends on the IMF ligament complex to determine the implant's inferior final position, therefore the surgeon must be careful to preserve this complex during pocket dissection or the surgeon must recreate the IMF complex with polydioxanone suture (PDS). If the surgeon purposefully performs a dual-plane pectoralis release but inadvertently damages the IMF complex, the implant will descend below the IMF and lead to inferior malposition (Figs. 19.4 and 19.5). For pocket dissection, a total submuscular approach is an option but must be performed cautiously; the surgeon must release some of the pectoralis attachments from the muscle's posterior surface down to the level of the IMF to allow adequate implant descent. The inferior extent of the submuscular pocket must correspond to the IMF. To help ensure that smooth implants drop fully to the desired level and to keep pockets soft, a proper postop-regimen of displacement

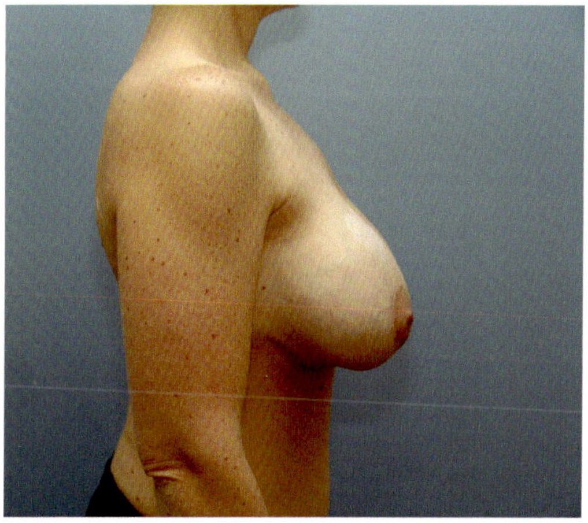

Fig. 19.5 Inferior implant malposition/double-bubble on the right, lateral view

exercises can help (1) the muscle to relax and stretch, (2) the implant to settle completely, and (3) the pocket capsules to remain supple [1].

Textured implants for breast augmentation provide a reliable option for breast augmentation, but care must be taken when performing this procedure as textured implants perform differently than smooth. Textured devices have a dramatically increased overall surface area when compared to smooth implants which allows for more contact with adjacent soft tissue creating a stability by either a frictional effect or more adherent Velcro-like effect. Textured implants typically do not undergo the drop and settling like a smooth device; they stay in the position placed at the time of surgery. Since textured devices will remain in a stable position, it is imperative to place the devices with the inferior edge at the IMF and seat them low in the breast pocket to avoid a malposition that would require reoperation.

Use of synthetic or biosynthetic mesh for implant pocket support also alters implant descent. Similar to the textured devices, use of synthetic mesh for pocket support such as Galaflex (Galatea Surgical) limits implant movement postoperatively. These synthetic mesh constructs do not stretch. The on-table result needs to be exactly what the surgeon wants long term. This requires sitting the patient in the upright position and looking at the position of the implant with the mesh in place. This will ensure appropriate placement and prevent this avoidable malposition.

Postoperative Pseudoptosis

Ptotic breast tissue (excessive lower pole fullness) within the first year after mastopexy is usually driven by poor markings and technical failure of inadequate (1) tissue debulking and resection, (2) tissue support and stability, or (3) both.

Plus-minus (or addition-subtraction) augmentation mastopexy refers to the concept of debulking the lower pole of the breast to alleviate the glandular ptosis and replenishing lost volume (especially in the upper pole) with an augmentation using an implant or autologous fat grafting. Inadequate lower pole resection and repair will lead to persistent or recurrent glandular ptosis.

This pitfall frequently occurs with surgeons trying to preserve parenchyma (1) to keep breast volume, (2) out of fear of vascular compromise, or (3) concern for removing all the tissue covering and protecting the implant. The surgeon cannot be afraid to remove lower pole breast tissue. With a proper understanding of anatomy and technique, aggressive resection can be performed safely and effectively. If a surgeon is uncomfortable with mobilization and debulking of the excess breast tissue then a staged procedure may be warranted.

With a superior and superior-medial pedicle technique, tissue resection is performed between the vertical pillars, the edges of which were marked preoperatively by medial and lateral breast displacement. All of the breast parenchyma between the pillars is excised. The depth of resection stops when the surgeon reaches the breast fascia which is a very distinct plane providing secure implant coverage and support [6]. After parenchymal resection between the pillars, the surgeon should only see the deep breast fascia – the implant is not exposed/visible and no parenchyma persists. One of the problems with the inferior pedicle techniques is that all of this lower pole tissue which is normally resected during a superior pedicle technique must be preserved for NAC viability. The inferior pedicle technique is setup and predisposed to early recurrence of breast ptosis. The central pedicle through Wuringer's septum is the dominant blood supply to the inferior pedicle which is sacrificed with the augmentation may lead to vascular compromise.

Even with a technically sound resection of breast parenchyma, early recurrence of breast ptosis can occur due to inadequate repair. The breast parenchyma pillars should be re-approximated so that the lower pole tension is on the parenchymal sutures rather than skin. When placed correctly, the lower pole has a flattened appearance intraoperatively and the skin edges are in close proximity before the final superficial layer of sutures. Not only does this prevent early recurrence of ptosis, but it also reduces skin tension and dehiscence.

It is imperative not to have the pillar sutures be too superficial within the subcutaneous fat to decrease the risk of fat necrosis. In addition, the pillar sutures should approximate the tissue and not strangulate. When placing the pillar sutures the authors typically start with the most inferior pillar suture first to help adequately cone the breast.

It is worth noting that massive weight loss patients have a greater propensity for recurrence of breast ptosis due to tissue dynamics. As seen with any body contouring procedure in this patient population, their tissues have little elasticity and tend to lose the intraoperative "tightness" quite quickly. Lower pole pillar repair needs extra attention to ensure adequate support and stability.

Overly Elevated Nipple Areolar Complex

A critical step in any mastopexy is setting the position of the NAC. The position is carefully determined with preoperative markings but can be assessed and adjusted intraoperatively through sitting-up and tailor-tacking if needed. We believe it is critical for the position to be largely determined preoperatively; there is significant change of landmarks and orientation of the breast soft tissue structure on the operating room table both supine and in an elevated sitting up position. It also can be difficult to assess for torso twisting and shoulder height discrepancies intraoperatively.

The authors' preferred method for determining the location of the NAC with augmentation mastopexy is multistep. The breast meridian IMF height is marked on the sternal midline and IMF height discrepancies between the breasts are noted. Pitanguy's point is then transposed onto the anterior surface of the breast, and this point should line up with the sternal IMF marking. Breast coning is simulated to show where the proposed NAC would appear to be on the maximum projecting point of the breast. Use of ideal breast measurements of sternal-notch:nipple (SN:N) distances of 21 cm can be utilized as a guide, but due to significant variation in breast footprint position, using the SN:N as a guide is unreliable. Height symmetry between breasts can be checked with SN:N measurements or a leveling ruler. It is important to note the new NAC position marking for an augmentation mastopexy often needs to be 0.5–2 cm higher than a for breast reduction. When the upper pole of the breast is volumized in an augmentation mastopexy, the most projecting part of the breast will be elevated and can alter the ideal NAC position.

Excessively Long Nipple Areolar Complex to Fold Distance

One of the most common and rather underreported complications from augmentation mastopexy is the long nipple areolar complex to fold distance. There is no absolute consensus on the exact distance that this measurement needs to be set. However, there are multiple authors who describe a relative standard. A measurement of approximately 6–8 cm should be obtained with the breast not on stretch. A distance of greater than 8 cm can create a breast that is not ideal by displacing the nipple to a higher positon than at the most projected portion and leading to a bottomed out appearance. This stargazing phenomenon can cause the nipple to peak thru bathing suits and common bras. It is important for surgeons to set the ideal distance and to debulk the excess in the lower pole of the breast to prevent recurrent and pseudoptosis.

Poor Implant Selection

It is extremely important to abide by appropriate tissue based planning in choosing an implant during an augmentation mastopexy procedure. Wrong choices can either create too much tension during closure or an empty breast appearance. The ideal choice of implant width needs to be within 1 cm of the ideal breast width. The ideal breast width is the distance from the anterior axillary line to 0.5 cm from the sternum. This avoids having a gap in the midline (cleavage area) or laterally from a highly projected smaller implant. Ideally in patients with larger breasts seeking enhancement this can be achieved with a lower profile cohesive device. It is important not to oversize or stuff larger implants even if it is what the patient desires.

Widened Mastopexy Scars

Poor scar formation following any aesthetic procedure is always a deleterious outcome. Multiple factors can contribute to this occurrence. The most common cause of this relates to excess skin tension upon closure of the mastopexy following an augmentation. Opposing forces are introduced with a volume addition of an implant and tightening of the breast soft tissue envelope. The pitfall is to try to make the skin closure very tight in hopes of providing the highest and tightest look. This is a mistake. Overly tightened skin envelopes will always stretch long term and will likely scar poorly.

The surgeon must be mindful about the size of implant being placed, the amount of breast soft tissue, and the degree soft tissue laxity. When marking the mastopexy, the tension exerted with medial and lateral distraction when marking the vertical pillar resection needs to be uniform. Compared with a breast reduction, the augmentation mastopexy medial and lateral distraction tension during marking should be less – volumizing the breast takes up some of the vertical wedge skin excess. Assessment of the pillar width intraoperatively after augmentation (with intraoperative tailor tacking or distraction) adds a level of security. Intraoperatively reconstruction of the central support of the breast with pillar sutures is critical for success. This removes the tension on the skin and relies on the breast parenchyma to be the soft tissue support and brassier rather than the skin (Figs. 19.6, 19.7, 19.8, 19.9, 19.10, and 19.11).

NAC Necrosis and Pedicle Selection

NAC necrosis is a dreaded complication of any nipple repositioning aesthetic intervention such as mastopexy or reduction mammoplasty (Fig. 19.12). Causes of this deformity all relate to ischemic injury secondary to either poor arterial inflow or venous insufficiency.

We prefer superior or superior-medial pedicles as they tend to have the most robust and reliable blood supply [7, 8]. Inferior pedicle techniques and central mound techniques are not as robust and often require the surgeon to leave redundant lower pole tissue. The inferior parenchyma must be preserved with an inferior pedicle technique, predisposing these patients to early recurrence of tissue ptosis. Superior and superior-medial techniques not only preserve the desired upper pole volume and resect the superfluous lower pole ptotic tissue, these techniques also are faster and easier.

When performing an augmentation mastopexy, the placement of the implant divides the 4th – 5th deep intercostal perforators which supplies the central pedicle and a significant amount of the inferior pedicle (IMF perforators also supply inferior pedicle). If incisions are made at the fold for the mastopexy, these perforators are also sacrificed. Thus, with inferior pedicle and central pedicle techniques, a pedicle blood supply is not possible and only random blood supply provides circulation to the NAC. For this reason, we believe an inferior or central pedicle should never be used in an augmentation mastopexy.

Venous insufficiency is related to venous obstruction from pressure or an inadequate venous network (Figs. 19.13, 19.14, and 19.15). Considering the rich venous network throughout the superior-medial breast, venous insufficiency is most commonly related to closure under too much tension. During pedicle inset, careful attention should be made to tension and a low threshold should exist to aggressively debulk the deep surface of the pedicle. Surgeons often are too timid to resect volume from the deep surface of the pedicle which has no role in vascular preservation. For arterial preservation, le Roux showed that at the NAC boundary, the mean arterial depth was 10.3 mm (standard deviation (SD): 2.5) and

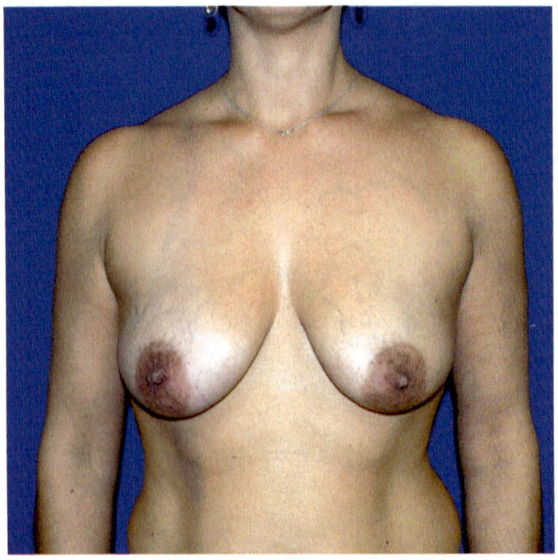

Fig. 19.6 Before and after photos illustrating how high implants settle postoperatively. Preop ap

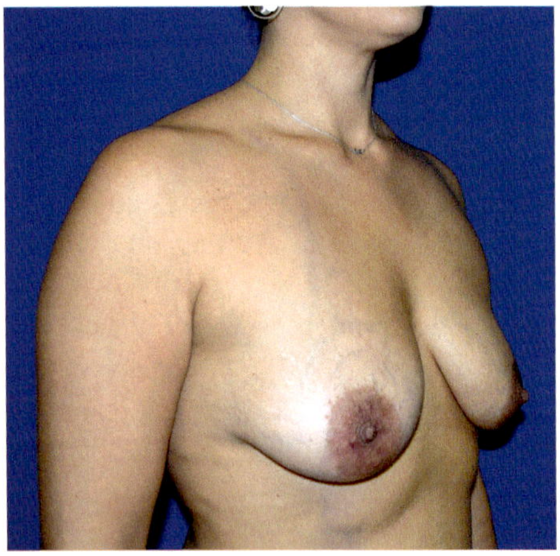

Fig. 19.7 Before and after photos illustrating how high implants settle postoperatively. Preop oblique

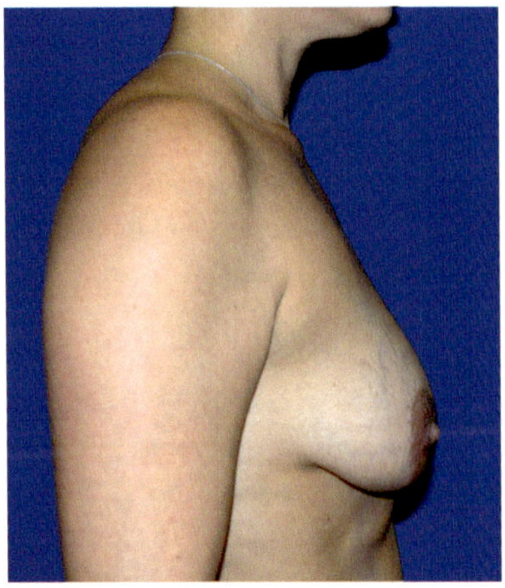

Fig. 19.8 Before and after photos illustrating how high implants settle postoperatively. Preop lateral

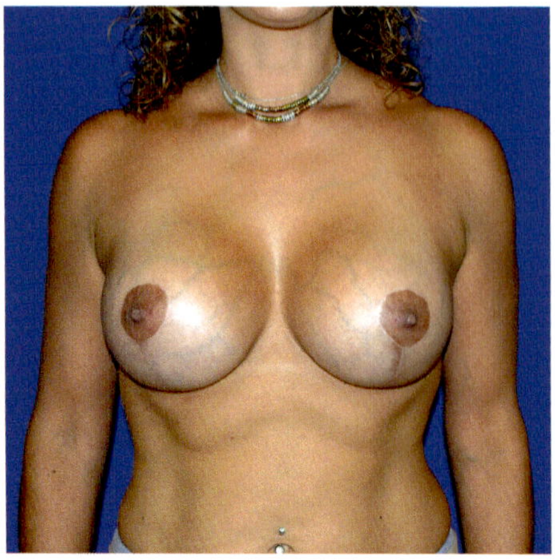

Fig. 19.9 Before and after photos illustrating how high implants settle postoperatively. Postop ap

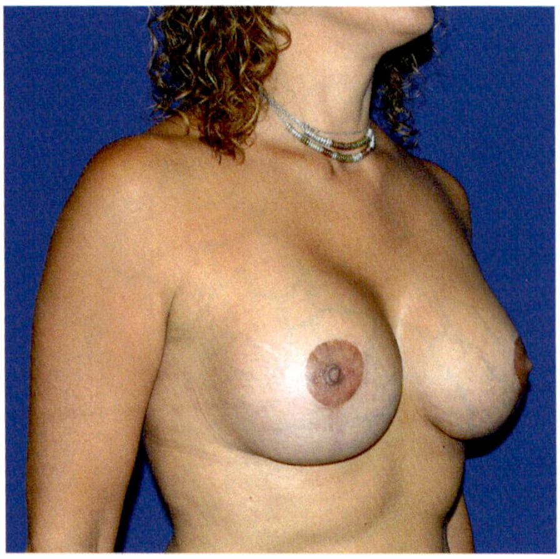

Fig. 19.10 Before and after photos illustrating how high implants settle postoperatively. Postop oblique 2

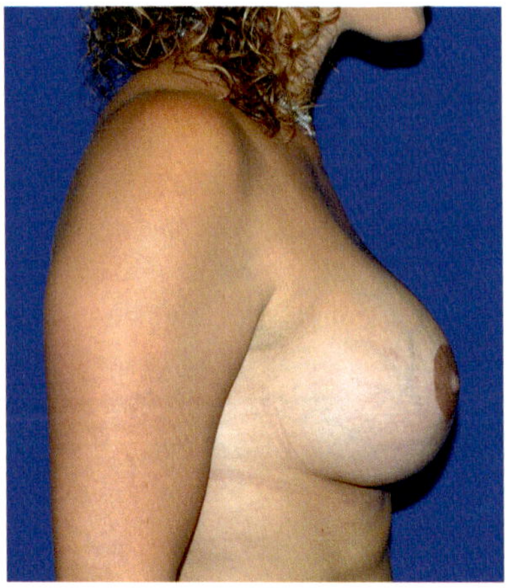

Fig. 19.11 Before and after photos illustrating how high implants settle postoperatively. Postop lateral

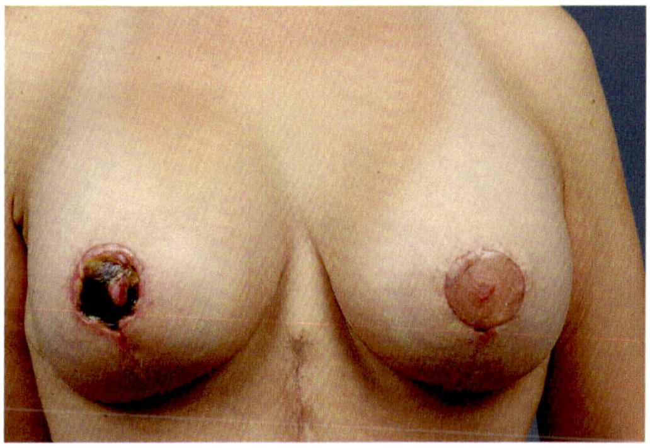

Fig. 19.12 Example of unilateral nipple necrosis following augmentation mastopexy

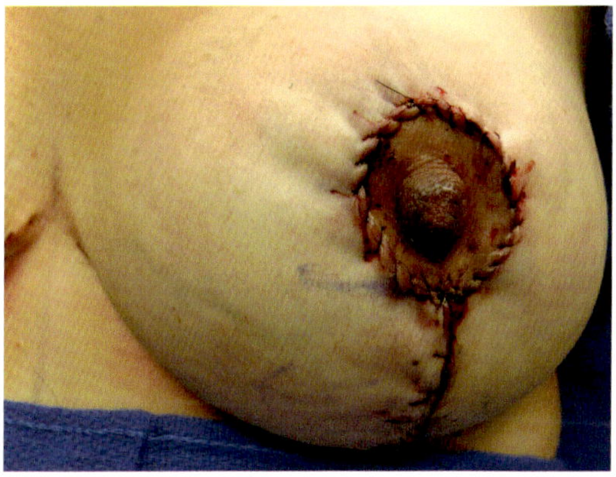

Fig. 19.13 Example of venous insufficeny of nipple areolar complex

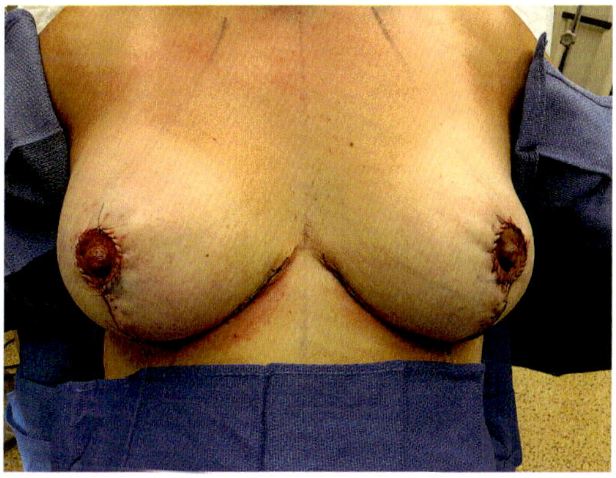

Fig. 19.14 Example of venous insufficeny of nipple areolar complex

at 3 cm from NAC the mean depth was 14.2 mm (SD 4.6) [7]. Critical veins run in the superficial 5 mm [7]. Therefore, superomedial pedicles can be safely trimmed to 3 cm thickness if needed.

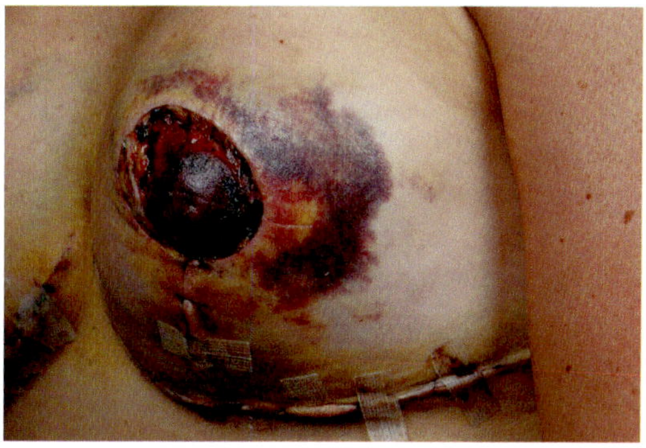

Fig. 19.15 Example of venous insufficeny of nipple areolar complex. Following periareolar release of sutures and progressing to necrosis

In all situations, vascular related issues must be addressed immediately. If there is any concern on the operating room table then they need to be addressed prior to leaving the operating room. The first step should be removing the NAC inset sutures and assessing if vascularity improves. If perfusion improves, then tension needs to be reduced by adjusting inset sutures, resecting more parenchyma or reducing implant volume. Placement of DMSO or nitroglycerin can be used to improve venous outflow as well. Communication with anesthesia is also critical; vasoactive medications and patient temperature also have a very significant impact on skin perfusion.

Smokers should not undergo major elective surgery as their risks of vascular related complications are elevated 2–5 fold [9]. They should quit smoking for a minimum of 4 weeks prior to surgery and avoid smoking after surgery for at least 4 weeks. This needs to be clearly explained to the patient. This means no nicotine-related product. Given the high rates of deception and non-compliance among smokers, the nicotine status of patients should be tested [10]. Systemic vascular disorders can also increase the risk of NAC loss and should be considered preoperatively.

Periareolar Mastopexy for Wrong Patient

The periareolar mastopexy is a procedure that can be fraught with problems. It is often utilized improperly and for the wrong patients (Figs. 19.16 and 19.17). A periareolar mastopexy does not correct tissue ptosis – it only elevates the NAC. Any patient with a significant degree of tissue ptosis or a NAC position that requires more than 1–2 cm of elevation is not a good candidate for a periareolar mastopexy. This technique may elevate the NAC up 2 centimeters, but this technique does not lift the breast itself. The periareolar technique also flattens the breast, which may be totally appropriate and helpful in a tuberous breast deformity, but creates a horrible shape typical ptotic breast. When combined with an augmentation, this technique has historically led to large amounts of areolar spreading. To combat this, wagon-wheel procedures utilizing a permanent Gortex suture have been advocated by some, but care must be taken as these techniques can be problematic and can lead to permanent suture related issues such as infection, extrusion, and poor aesthetic outcomes [11]. In the vertical technique, combining a coning pattern with resection of skin and parenchyma of the lower pole very reproducibly shapes the breast and helps regulate areolar diameter.

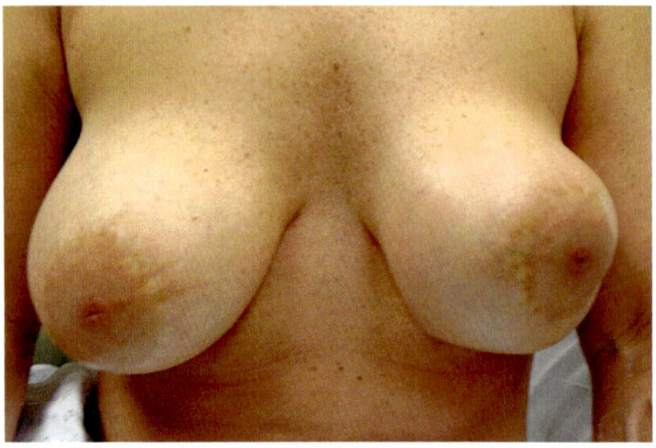

Fig. 19.16 Example of poorly selected case for periareolar augmentation mastopexy

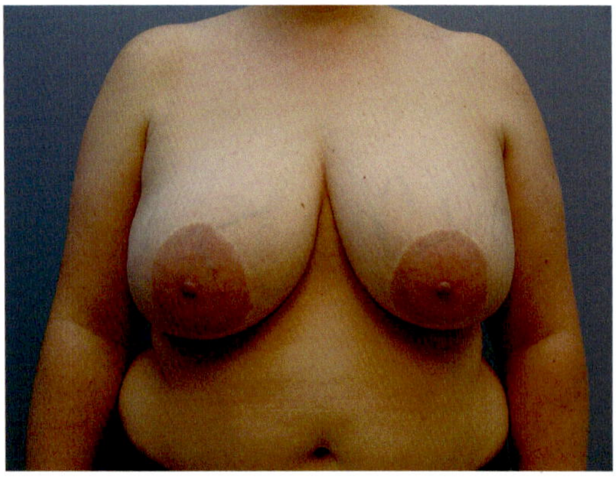

Fig. 19.17 Example of poorly selected case for periareolar augmentation mastopexy

Management and Operative Approach

High Riding Implant

Superiorly malpositioned implants (unilateral or bilateral) in the first few weeks postop should be initially managed with massage and inferior displacement exercises. It is normal for smooth round submuscular implants to start high and then slowly drop into position postoperatively (Figs. 19.18, 19.19, and 19.20). For implants that do not appear to be dropping, firm pressure applied to the upper pole of the implant helps the implant stretch lower pole tissue fibers that were not completely released that are holding the implant too high. If implant position does not improve or resolve by 2–3 months, then the implant position is not likely to correct itself with conservative management. If failed conservative management with displacement exercises, treatment of superiorly malpositioned implants involves pocket revision (lowering capsulotomy) or formal implant pocket conversion (creation of a new pocket).

Capsular contracture is another cause of high riding implants, and although it can appear similar to superior malposition, it's management is different. With capsular contracture, the implant capsule stiffens and shrinks. While superior malposition can usually be managed with inferior capsulotomy (a relatively quick and simply procedure), often capsular contracture has created marked fibrosis and the capsule requires partial or total removal to restore the normal pliability of the breast. A variety of options exist to manage capsular contracture without a clear consensus on the best management technique [2, 3]. For primary capsular contracture where the capsule is

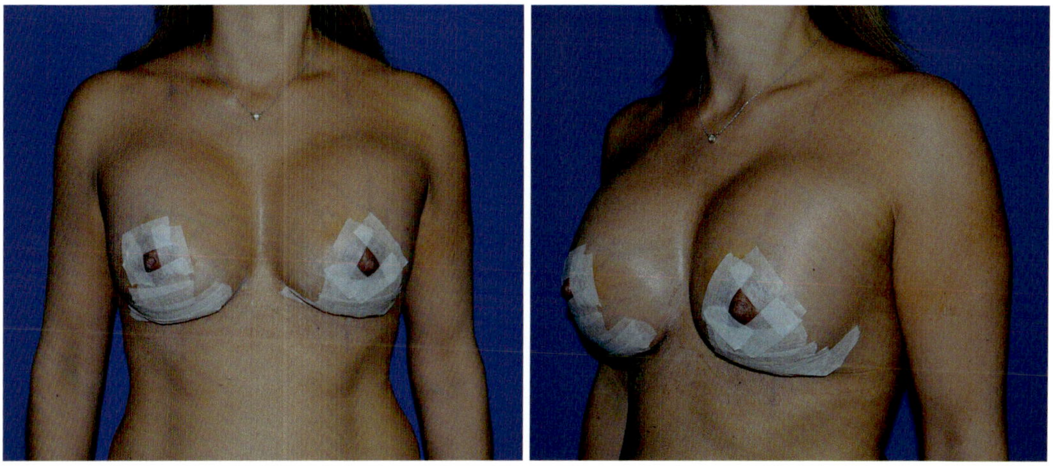

Figs. 19.18 and 19.19 High implants at 1 week postop (see Figs. 19.6, 19.7, 19.8, 19.9, 19.10, and 19.11 for her before and after photos illustrating how implants settle postoperatively). AP, Oblique

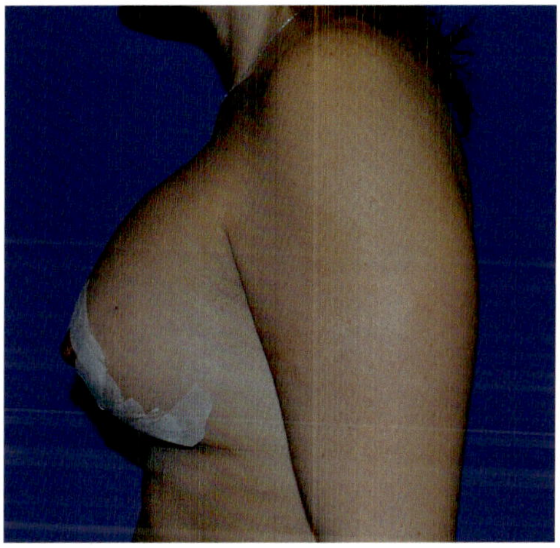

Fig. 19.20 High implants at 1 week postop. Lateral

not overly rigid, multiple options are reasonable [capsulotomy, capsulectomy (partial/total), neo-subpectoral pocket creation]. Recurrent capsular contracture cases or very stiff capsules cannot be managed with a capsulotomy and should be treated with creation of a new implant pocket: neo-supectoral pocket or capsulectomy ± acelluar dermal mesh. It is worth noting that leukotriene antagonists have shown success in the prevention and treatment of capsular contracture and should be considered as an adjunct or alternative to surgery [4, 5].

Postoperative Tissue Ptosis

All patients are at risk for recurrence of breast ptosis with aging and time, but if breast ptosis recurs within the first few years after surgery without patient lifestyle changes, the surgeon should take a critical look at his technique. Treatment of recurrent glandular ptosis requires a revision mastopexy with resection and repair of the lower pole. As previously discussed, during the repair the tissue support needs to rely on the breast parenchymal pillars rather than the skin (Figs. 19.21, 19.22, 19.23, 19.24, 19.25, 19.26, 19.27, 19.28, and 19.29).

Overly Elevated Nipple Areolar Complex

It cannot be over-emphasized that the NAC position should not be placed too high. It is a fairly simple procedure to elevate a NAC that is too low, but a very difficult situation to try to lower the NAC. A star-gazing NAC is not positioned on the point of highest breast projection, but rather is on the upper pole of the breast. Most strategies to lower the NAC involve trying to raise the point of highest breast projection by tightening the lower pole of the breast, often using a lower pole wedge resection to try to decrease the NAC:IMF dis-

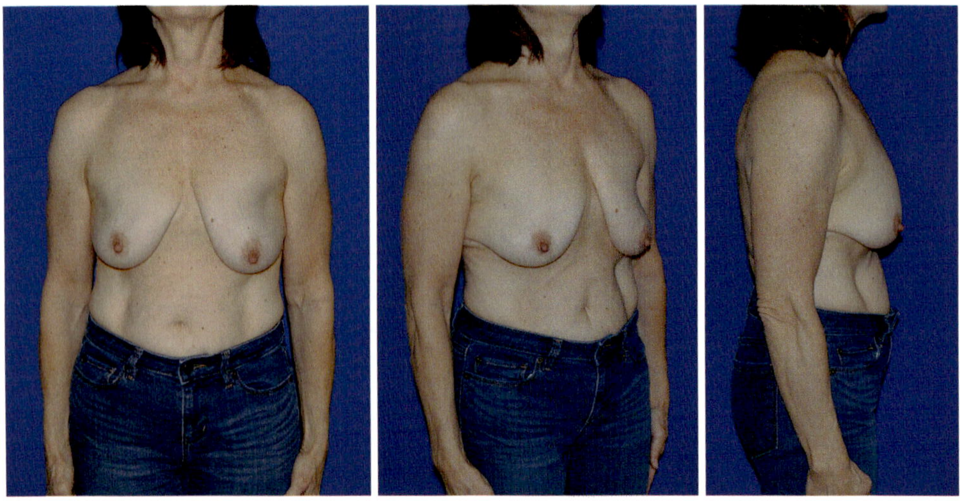

Figs. 19.21, 19.22 and 19.23 Patient treated with an augmentation-mastopexy but developed a waterfall deformity postoperatively due to a high riding implant and tissue ptosis. She was treated with a correction mastopexy and a pocket revision. Her after photos shown are at 1 year postop. Preop AP, Case preop oblique, Case preop lateral

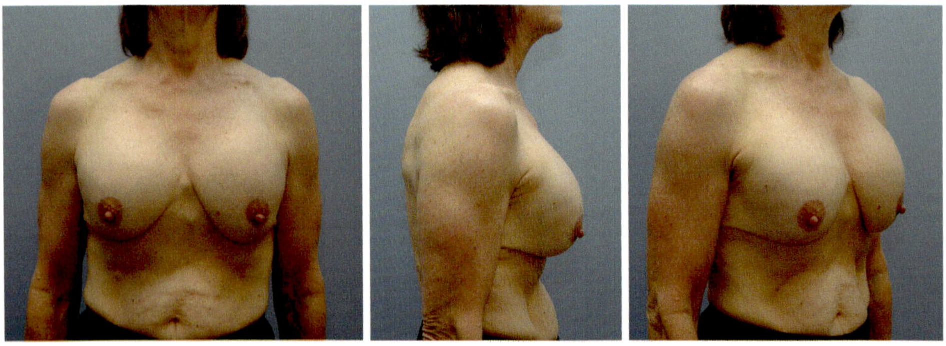

Figs. 19.24, 19.25 and 19.26 Patient treated with an augmentation-mastopexy who developed a waterfall deformity postoperatively due to a high riding implant and tissue ptosis and was treated with a correction mastopexy and a pocket revision. Postop AP, Postop Lateral, Postop Oblique

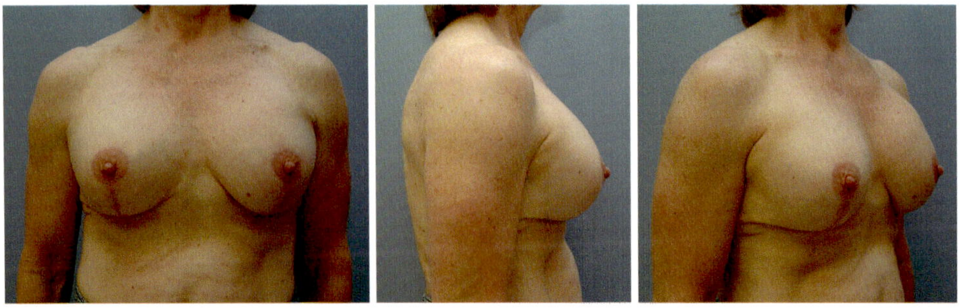

Figs. 19.27, 19.28 and 19.29 Patient treated with an augmentation-mastopexy who developed a waterfall deformity postoperatively due to a high riding implant and tissue ptosis and was treated with a correction mastopexy and a pocket revision. Postop after revision, AP, Postop after revision, lateral, Postop after revision, oblique

tance. Successful correction of an overly elevated nipple is very difficult and usually compromises must be made.

Conclusion

There is steep learning curve with augmentation mastopexy, which is why some surgeons prefer to tackle this operation in two stages. However, this procedure can be accomplished predictably and successfully in one stage with an understanding of anatomy and tissue dynamics. Complications and flawed results are unavoidable, but hopefully this chapter will serve as a resource to minimizing their frequency and impact.

References

1. Sood A, Xue EY, Sangiovanni C, Therattil PJ, Lee ES. Breast massage, implant displacement, and prevention of capsular contracture after breast augmentation with implants: a review of the literature. Eplasty. 2017;17:e41.
2. Rehnke RD, Groening RM, Van Buskirk ER, Clarke JM. Anatomy of the superficial fascia system of the breast: a comprehensive theory of breast fascial anatomy. Plast Reconstr Surg. 2018;142(5):1135–44.
3. Michelle le Roux C, Kiil BJ, Pan WR, Rozen WM, Ashton MW. Preserving the neurovascular supply in the hall-Findlay superomedial pedicle breast reduction: an anatomical study. J Plast Reconstr Aesthet Surg. 2010;63(4):655–62.
4. van Deventer PV, Graewe FR. The blood supply of the breast revisited. Plast Reconstr Surg. 2016;137(5):1388–97.
5. Nolan MB, Martin DP, Thompson R, Schroeder DR, Hanson AC, Warner DO. Association between smoking status, preoperative exhaled carbon monoxide levels, and postoperative surgical site infection in patients undergoing elective surgery. JAMA Surg. 2017;152(5):476–83.
6. Coon D, Tuffaha S, Christensen J, Bonawitz SC. Plastic surgery and smoking: a prospective analysis of incidence, compliance, and complications. Plast Reconstr Surg. 2013;131(2):385–91.
7. Hammond DC, Khuthaila DK, Kim J. The interlocking Gore-Tex suture for control of areolar diameter and shape. Plast Reconstr Surg. 2007;119(3): 804–9.
8. Headon H, Kasem A, Mokbel K. Capsular contracture after breast augmentation: an update for clinical practice. Arch Plast Surg. 2015;42(5):532–43.
9. Wan D, Rohrich RJ. Revisiting the management of capsular contracture in breast augmentation: a systematic review. Plast Reconstr Surg. 2016;137(3):826–41.
10. Graf R, Ascenço AS, Freitas Rda S, Balbinot P, Peressutti C, Costa DF, Dos Santos FH, Ratti MA, Kulchetscki RM. Prevention of capsular contracture using leukotriene antagonists. Plast Reconstr Surg. 2015;136(5):592e–6e.
11. Huang CK, Handel N. Effects of Singulair (montelukast) treatment for capsular contracture. Aesthet Surg J. 2010;30(3):404–8.

Managing Complications in Augmentation Mastopexy

20

Dennis C. Hammond and Ashley R. Chandler

Introduction

Augmentation mastopexy can be one of the most satisfying aesthetic breast procedures performed by a plastic surgeon. In these patients, the shape and size of the breast has been dramatically altered over time as a result of weight gain and/or loss, pregnancy, or simply aging. As a result, what at one time presented as a youthful, full, attractive breast becomes variably deflated, ptotic, and misshapen secondary to tissue atrophy with damage to the skin envelope (Fig. 20.1). This deterioration in the overall aesthetic appearance of the breast over time can be a powerful motivating factor leading patients to seek improvement. By restoring the desired volume and tightening the ptotic skin envelope with lifting of the position of the nipple areola complex (NAC), dramatic improvement in the appearance of the breast can be achieved. However, meshing together these two sometimes competing surgical goals of adding volume while at the same time tightening the skin envelope can require exacting surgical planning and expertise over and above that required for more basic aesthetic surgical procedures such as augmentation or mastopexy alone. In point of fact, for many patients, augmentation mastopexy can be considered more of a reconstructive procedure and it is not surprising that reoperation rates as high as 20–50% have been reported [1, 2].

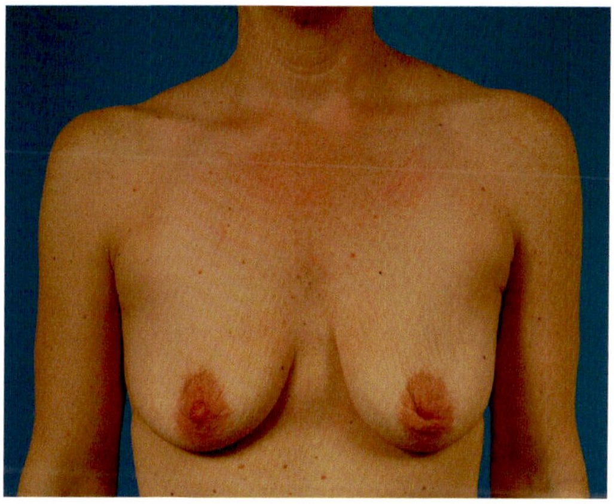

Fig. 20.1 Typical appearance of a patient seeking augmentation mastopexy. Very often these are patients who are multiparous and, after breast feeding, present with loss of skin tone, ptosis to the skin envelope and the nipple/areola complex, and a deflated appearance with loss of volume

D. C. Hammond (✉)
Plastic Surgery, Spectrum Health Medical Education Partners, Grand Rapids, MI, USA

Partners in Plastic Surgery, Grand Rapids, MI, USA
e-mail: drhammond@pipsmd.com

A. R. Chandler
Florida State University College of Medicine, Pensacola, FL, USA

M. B. Calobrace et al. (eds.), *Augmentation Mastopexy*,
https://doi.org/10.1007/978-3-030-48226-8_20

Operative Goals

To understand the goals of managing complications after augmentation mastopexy, it is helpful to review the basic elements of a successful uncomplicated primary augmentation mastopexy procedure.

Addition of Volume

For the augmentation mastopexy patient, adding volume is a very straightforward procedure and almost any implant can be successfully used to accomplish this goal. Identifying the volume of the desired breast can readily accomplished using any of several strategies including looking at results from previous patients to the use of external sizers to the use of three dimensional imaging. Generally as a result of the excessive skin envelope, much more freedom in implant volume selection exists for the augmentation mastopexy patient as opposed to the simple breast augmentation patient. However as a result of the proportionately greater pre-existing breast volume, augmentation mastopexy patients typically need less volume than in breast augmentation, and care must be taken to avoid over-augmentation. As well, smaller implants will typically perform better than larger volume devices as less long term stress is placed on the soft tissue envelope.

Management of the Ptotic Skin Envelope

There is great variability in the degree of ptosis any given patient will present with, and typically every patient will demonstrate some degree of excess skin with sagging of the skin envelope, a low positioned and often widened NAC, and variable descent of the existing breast parenchyma creating a hollowed out upper pole. To manage these combined features, all of the described mastopexy patterns can be effectively utilized including periareolar, circumvertical, and inverted T pattern approaches. All of these patterns will lift the position of the NAC and tighten the skin envelope. However, no matter what approach is used, a common theme associated with them all is gradual loss of shape with stretching of the skin envelope. This so called "bottoming out" phenomenon is one of the most common complications associated with augmentation mastopexy and operative correction accounts for many of the secondary procedures performed in these patients.

Timing of Operative Management of Complications

After augmentation mastopexy, there is a variable degree of edema that accumulates in the soft tissue that can distort the appearance of the breast. In cases where a complication has developed, the over-riding goal is to successfully correct the situation with one operation. Therefore, intervening before the edema and soft tissue settling that normally occurs after surgery can lead to inaccurate intraoperative decision making with regard to a host of variables including breast volume, shape, NAC position, and overall symmetry. In order to accurately plan and correct each of these variables, the breast must be fully healed. Therefore, it is recommended that any operative correction be delayed until at least 6 months have passed to allow full and accurate demonstration of the final result. At that point then, accurate and successful planning and operative correction can be performed.

Complications and Management Strategies

Each of the following represent commonly seen complications associated with augmentation mastopexy. In many instances, some of these complications occur together. By identifying the root cause of each complication, an organized operative strategy can be devised to maximize the quality of the final aesthetic result.

Bottoming out

Postoperative change in the shape of the breast is one of the most common complications that can occur after augmentation mastopexy. This shape change is usually secondary to one of two factors, either excessive stretch of the skin envelope with inferior descent of the NAC or loss of the position of the inframammary fold inferiorly. As well, these two complications can occur together creating a phenomenon referred to as a "double bubble" deformity with the result being a significant deleterious effect on the quality of the result (Fig. 20.2) [3]. Patients who are particularly prone to this complication are those with excessive elasticity to the skin, patients who have experienced significant deflation after pregnancy and breast feeding, and in particular, those patients who have undergone significant weight loss. Successful operative correction requires accurate diagnosis of the problem coupled with an effective plan of management for each contributing factor responsible for the bottomed out appearance of the breast.

Correction of Skin Stretch: Technique

Once the breast has been operated on, any incisions that disrupt the breast parenchyma will inevitably release the Cooper's ligaments which play a major role in maintenance of breast shape.

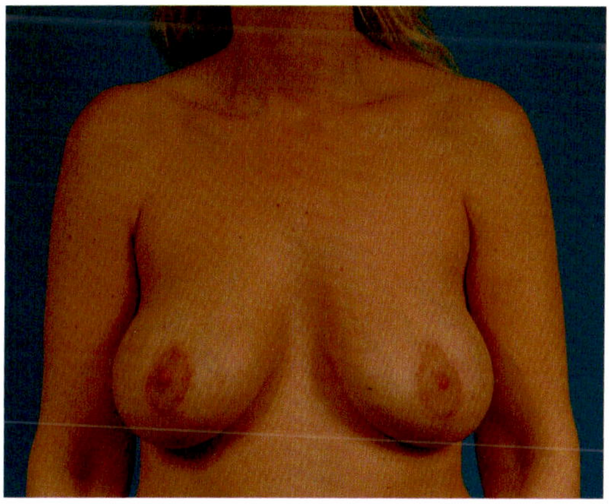

Fig. 20.2 After augmentation mastopexy, it is not uncommon for the skin envelop to stretch under the weight of the implant and breast tissue resulting in a ptotic, deflated appearance

As a result, postoperative stretch of the skin secondary to the weight of the breast coupled with the added stress applied by the weight of the implant can occur as the skin envelope cannot support this stress alone. The result is expansion of the skin envelope, loss of breast shape, and inferior descent of the NAC often with widening of the areola diameter. Fortunately, there is a finite ability of the skin to stretch, and once the complication has declared itself, management with re-tightening of the skin envelope can be quite effective in restoring an aesthetic breast shape.

To correct bottoming out secondary to skin stretch, the new position of the NAC must be set. Typically an effective landmark to determine this point is to set the top of the areola at a point 6 to 7 cm above the inframammary fold. Where this mark intersects the breast meridian then determines the top of the areola position on each side. The pattern is then drawn as a smooth oval around the existing areola such that the old scar and any widened pigmented areolar skin is removed. The new areolar diameter is set at anywhere from 40 to 44 mm. At this point the need for a vertical segment is assessed. A good rule of thumb is to adopt a strategy that adds the vertical segment whenever doing so will improve the shape of the breast. In this manner, issues regarding shape are prioritized over the creation of scar. In cases where already pre-existing circumvertical or inverted T scars are already present, the new skin pattern is simply diagrammed over the top of these scars taking out the required amount of skin needed to reshape the breast (Fig. 20.3).

The procedure itself can be performed under either local anesthesia with or without IV sedation, or general anesthesia. When concomitant implant pocket manipulation is required, general anesthesia is a better choice to allow worry free correction of the problem. The initial new areolar incision is made after first infiltrating all the proposed skin incision areas with a dilute solution of lidocaine with epinephrine to limit dermal oozing. The new skin pattern is then tacked up into position with temporary skin staples. The shape of the breast is assessed with the patient in the

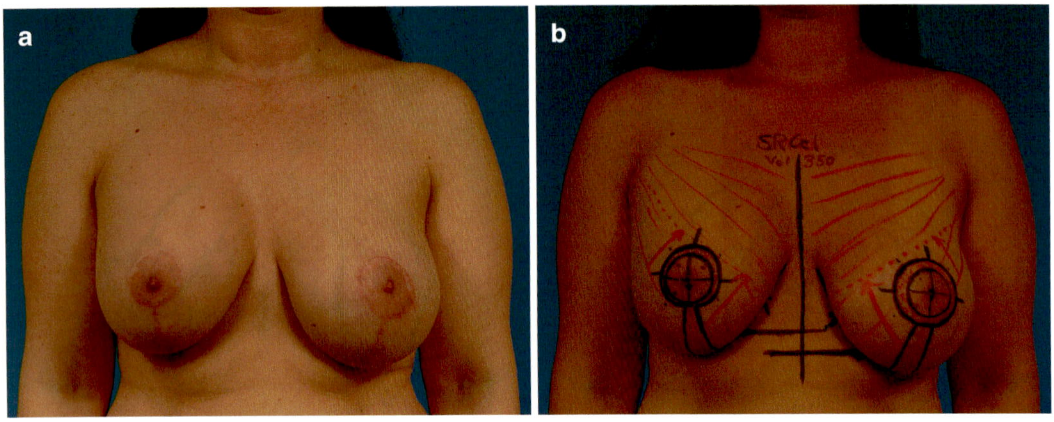

Fig. 20.3 Markings for Correction of Bottoming Out (**a**) Preoperative appearance of a 40 year old woman who has previously undergone an inverted T pattern augmentation mastopexy. She present with ptosis of the skin envelope, asymmetry, and a widened areola. (**b**) Preoperative marks in preparation for bilateral inverted T pattern mastopexy, periareolar revision using the interlocking suture technique, partial capsulectomy, dual plane release of the pectoralis major muscle, and implant re-insertion

upright position and modifications in the degree of lift of the NAC or tightening of the skin envelope are made as needed. Once the desired shape has been created, the margins of the skin pattern are marked with a surgical marker and the staples are removed. The involved segments of skin are de-epithelialized and the pattern is closed over the top of the implant. The periareolar defect is managed using the interlocking suture technique (see below). A strategy of mild overtightening of the vertical segment can be strategically employed to allow for a small degree of postoperative settling to occur. Using this strategy, an aesthetic and long term correction of the problem can be achieved (Fig. 20.4).

Repair of the Inframammary Fold: Technique

In cases where the location of the inframammary fold is malpositioned, it is almost always secondary to unplanned inferior descent of the fold. In these cases, a variable amount of abdominal skin inferior to the breast is inadvertently incorporated into the skin envelope of the lower pole of the breast. As a result, the distance from the actual inframammary fold to the nipple becomes excessively long and the NAC position appears high. Operative correction therefore involves replacing the abdominal skin back down onto the abdominal wall by fixating the bottomed out fold into the correct position. This restores a proportionate distance from the new inframammary fold to the nipple thus creating an aesthetic relationship between the position of the breast footprint and the NAC.

Fold correction is often performed in conjunction with skin envelope tightening as the two complications very often occur together. Typically, one of the incisions used to perform the original mastopexy can be used to access the implant pocket. By gently applying pressure to the lower pole of the breast, the amount of fold elevation required to restore a properly positioned footprint can be estimated and the portion of the pocket capsule that requires excision and repair can be visualized through the incision. Although simple plication of the capsule can be performed, it is advisable to actually excise the redundant bottomed out portion of the capsule so that, once the cut edges are repaired, fresh tissue edges are approximated that can heal together more effectively, thus ensuring a stable long lasting result. Once the position of the fold is chosen, it is recommended to stabilize the repair using permanent sutures to maximally enhance the success of the repair. The use of absorbable suture materials risk premature postoperative rupture with loss of fold

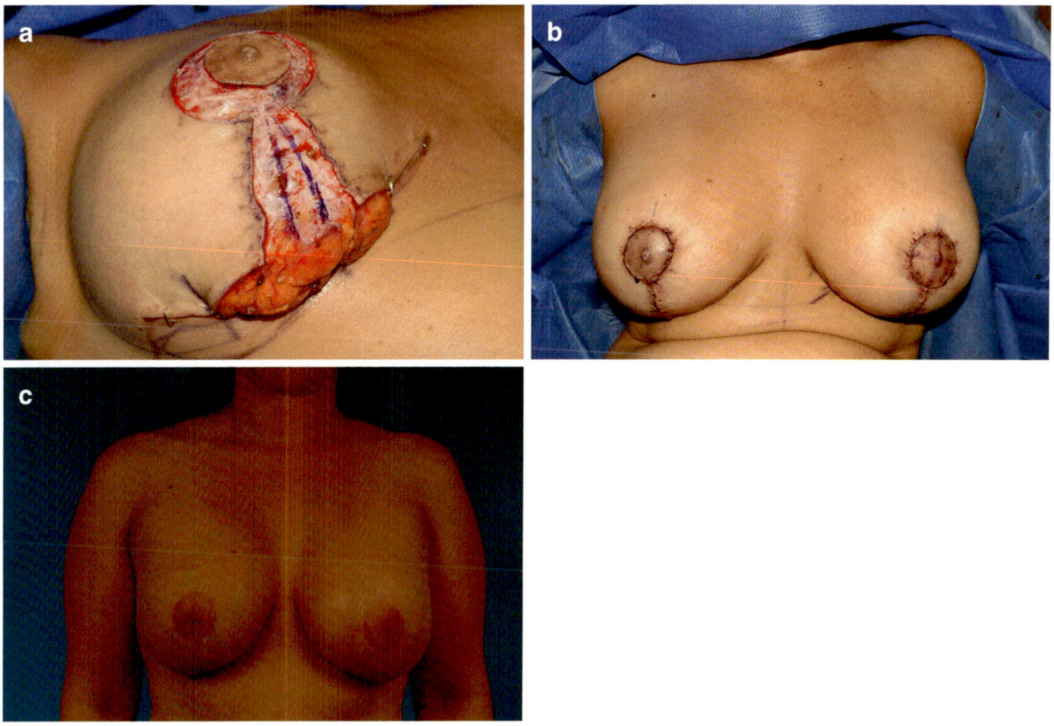

Fig. 20.4 Technique to Correct Bottoming Out (**a**) Intraoperative appearance of the breast after de-epithelialization of the redundant skin envelope, partial capsulectomy, and implant reinsertion. (**b**) Intraoperative appearance after bilateral revision. (**c**) Final appearance demonstrating correction of the soft tissue ptosis, improved symmetry, and an elevated and more aesthetic NAC

position. Care must be taken to create a smooth contour along the inframammary fold by carefully placing each suture in such a way that notching or irregularities are avoided. To assist in this endeavor, it is recommended that the fold repair be performed with the patient in the upright position to ensure that an accurate and smooth repair is accomplished. Although technically demanding, repair of a malpositioned inframammary fold can have a profoundly beneficial effect on the overall shape of the breast after augmentation mastopexy (Fig. 20.5).

Double Bubble Deformity

When stretch of the skin envelope occurs in tandem with loss of fold position in patients where the implant is in the subpectoral or partial subpectoral position, a unique type of deformity can occur called a "double bubble" deformity. In these patients the inframammary fold is malpositioned inferiorly while the old fold is still present as a crease that runs across the lower pole of the breast. The distance from the fold to the nipple is excessively long, and the entire deformity is made dramatically worse with contraction of the pectoralis major muscle. Patients who are particularly prone to this complication include those where the elasticity of the native breast skin is greater than the elasticity of the abdominal skin that has been inadvertently incorporated into the breast mound. In these patients, a natural break point is created that does not completely soften when the fold is lowered, leading to the deformity (Fig. 20.6).

Repair of the Double Bubble Deformity: Technique

To correct a double bubble deformity, the position of the inframammary fold must be relo-

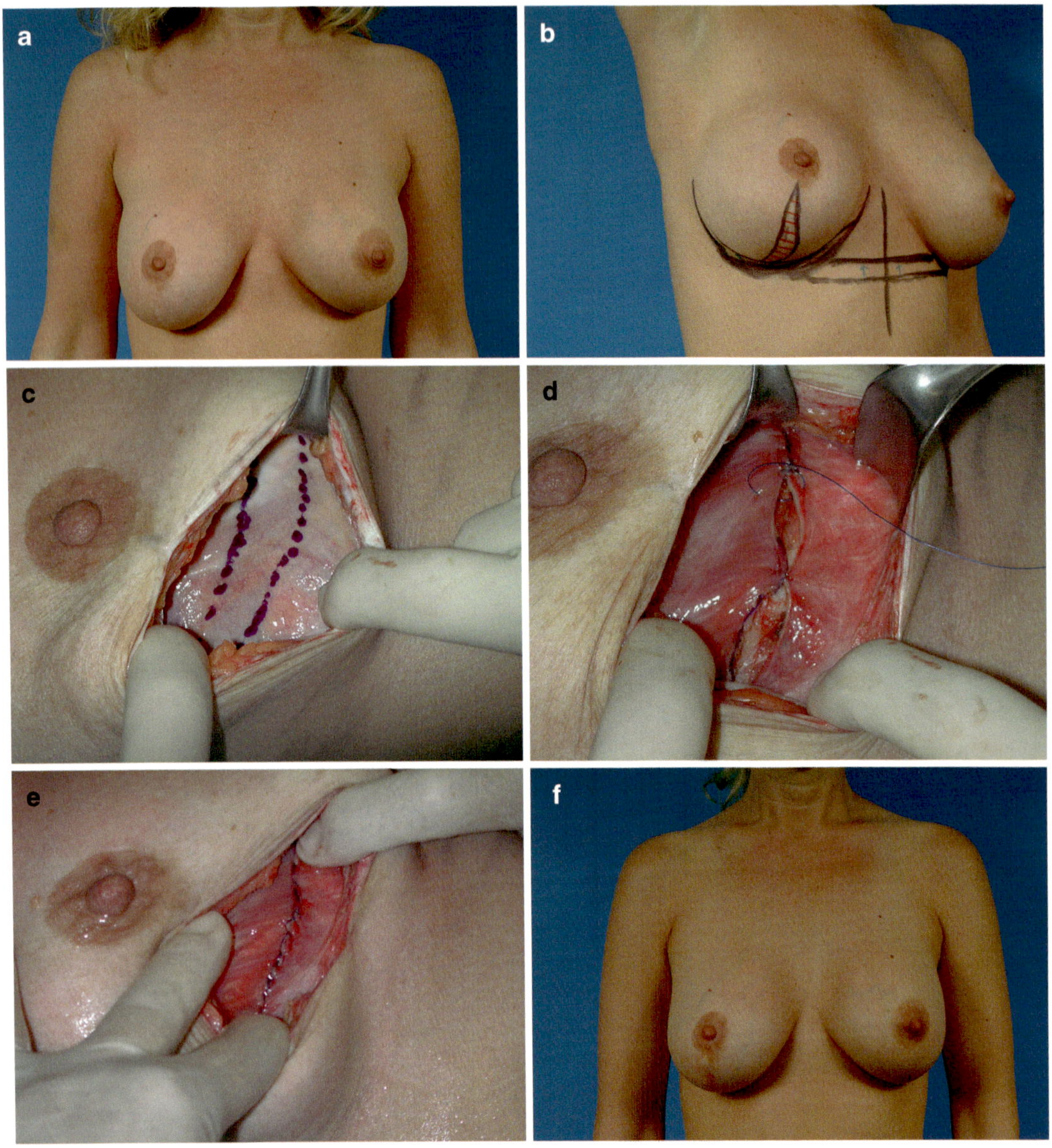

Fig. 20.5 Repair of Fold (**a**) Preoperative appearance of a 39 year old woman 3 years after undergoing a right circumvertical augmentation mastopexy demonstrating descent of the right inframammary fold with inferior implant malposition. (**b**) Preoperative marks in preparation for inframammary fold reconstruction. (**c**) The capsule in the expanded lower pocket along the inframammary fold is marked for excision. (**d**) The redundant capsule is excised and repaired with 3-0 permanent monofilament suture. (**e**) Final appearance of the repaired inframammary fold. (**f**) Final appearance at 9 years demonstrating elevation of the inframammary fold with correction of the inferior implant malposition

cated superiorly using standard fold repair techniques. This will shorten the fold to nipple distance. As well, the crease created by the old fold must be released with internal scoring of the soft tissues along the fold. Finally, the pull of the pectoralis major muscle must be taken out of the equation by either fully releasing the muscle along the lower pole of the breast with an aggressive dual plane maneuver, or simply converting to a subgandular implant position. Combining these operative maneuvers can correct the implant to soft tissue mismatch and

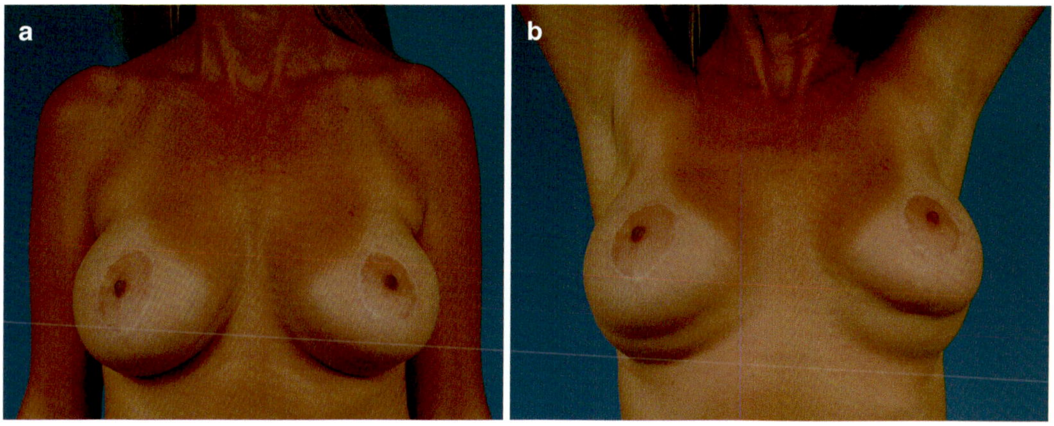

Fig. 20.6 Example of Double Bubble (**a**) Preoperative appearance of a patient who has undergone previous augmentation mammaplasty complicated by loss of the inframammary fold. (**b**) With the hands elevated, the distortion along the inferior pole of the breast becomes more pronounced creating the classic "double bubble" deformity. The inferior descent of the implant below the fold, with inadvertent incorporation of abdominal skin into the lower pole of the breast is readily evident. The persistent crease representing the original inframammary fold position results in a significant deformity in the lower breast contour

restore an aesthetic shape to the augmented and lifted breast (Fig. 20.7).

NAC Malposition

Inherent in any augmentation mastopexy procedure is proper repositioning of the inferiorly located NAC at the apex of the breast mound. Unfortunately, when the NAC is malpositioned, it can dramatically adversely affect the overall result after augmentation mastopexy. In order to successfully manage periareolar problems, two principles are helpful in moving the position of the NAC in relation to the position of the breast. First, any incision made around the areola is most effective if it goes entirely around the areola such that the resulting forces on the areolar closure are evenly distributed. This can minimize distortion in the shape of the areola. Second, the areola/periareolar closure is more secure when it is supported by a permanent purse-string suture type of closure. This can prevent postoperative spreading of the areolar diameter. Both of these principles are incorporated into the design of the interlocking purse-string suture technique for the management of areola diameter and shape [4]. Incorporating this technique into the management of NAC malposition can provide a reliable method to move the position of the NAC on the breast mound in cases where the NAC is malpositioned.

Interlocking Suture: Technique

During the preoperative marking sequence, the desired apex of the top of the areolar pattern is diagrammed onto the breast. This point can be determined directly by lifting the top of the proposed areolar incision superiorly until it is in the middle of the breast and then marking this spot. Alternatively, the position of the inframammary fold can identified and then drawn across the upper abdomen connecting the two breasts. By measuring 6 to 7 cm above this line and carrying this mark over to the breast meridian on each side, the top of the periareolar pattern can be estimated. The pattern is then drawn around the medial, inferior, and lateral margins of the existing areola to create the shape of an oval. This represents the outer incision. A 40 to 44 mm areolar incision is made with the patient upright after applying gentle pressure to the breast to remove the effect of natural skin retraction in the areola. This will optimize the creation of a round shape to the resulting areolar closure. Once the two incisions are diagrammed, each perimeter is evenly divided into eight cardinal points. The goal of the closure will be to join

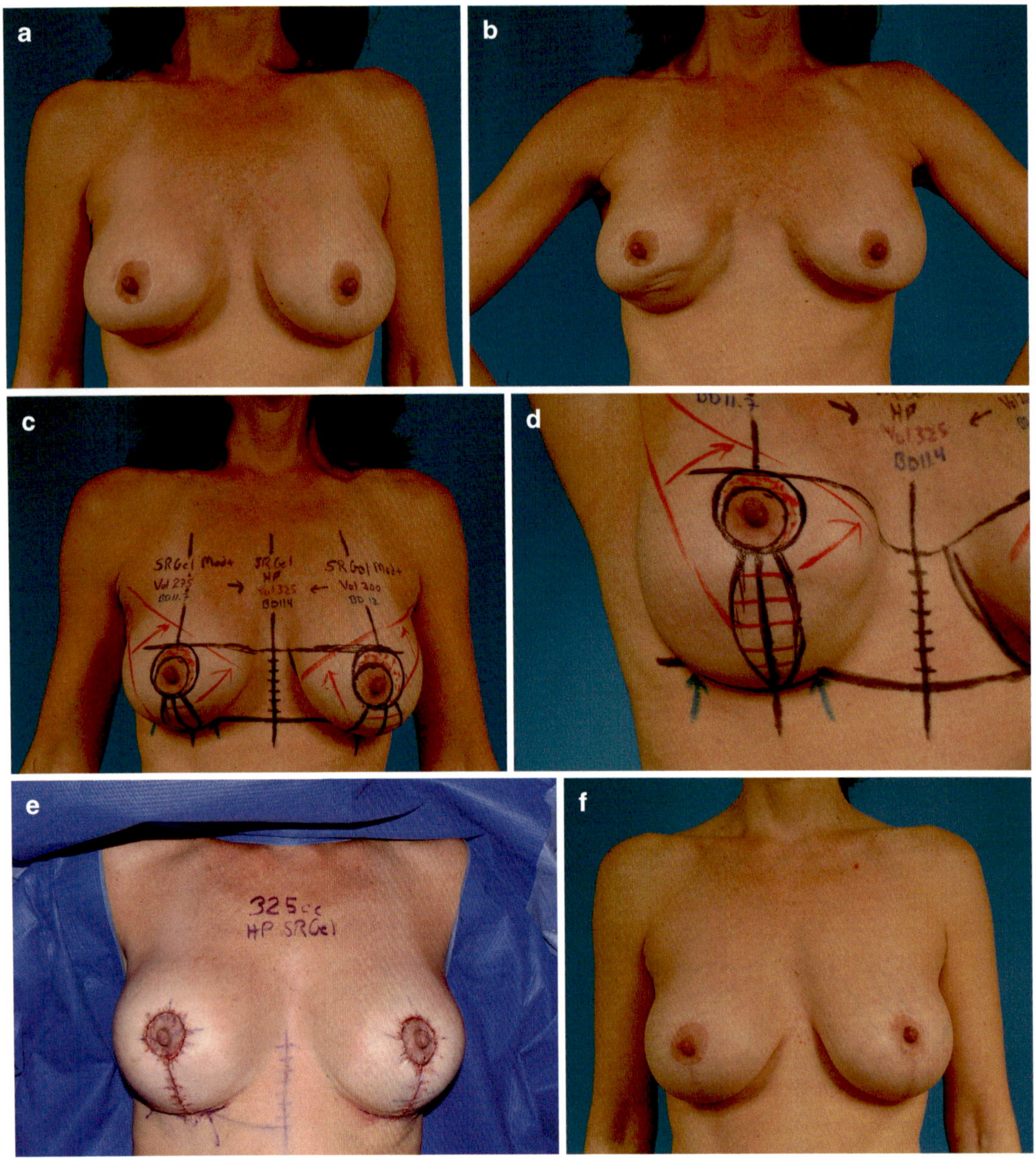

Fig. 20.7 Markings and Technique for Double Bubble Correction (**a**) Preoperative appearance of a 41 year old woman who presents with loss of the right inframammary fold after bilateral periareolar augmentation mastopexy. Several revisionary attempts to correct this deformity have been unsuccessful. (**b**) With contraction of the pectoralis major muscle, the deformity becomes exaggerated and the previous inframammary fold contour becomes more pronounced. (**c**) Preoperative marks in preparation for revision include the use of a short scar pattern to manage the redundant skin envelope, further release of the pectoralis major muscle to allow it to window shade superiorly away from the area of the inframammary fold, a requested slight increase in implant volume, and repair of the right inframammary fold. (**d**) The area of inframammary fold repair is highlighted by the light blue arrows. (**e**) Immediate appearance after soft tissue repair and implant exchange using a 325 cc high profile smooth round gel implant. (**f**) Postoperative appearance at 7 months demonstrates a stable aesthetic revision with complete correction of the "double bubble" deformity. (**g**) With window shading of the pectoralis major muscle superiorly, the pull of the muscle along the inframammary fold is eliminated allowing the creation of a smooth inframammary fold contour

Fig. 20.7 (continued)

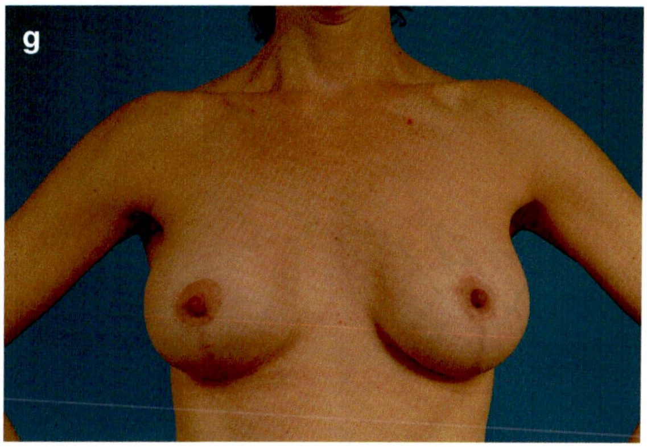

these eight cardinal points together. In essence the inherent dog-ear that results because the outer incision is longer than the inner incision will be taken up evenly over the entire length of the periareolar incision. At surgery, the skin of each incision is scored through the epidermis and the intervening area is de-epithelialized. If it is known that there is reliable blood supply coming to the NAC from below, a dermal shelf is created by incising the dermis along the margin of the outer incision 5 mm from the incision edge. If the blood supply to the NAC is uncertain as it can be in many revision cases, the dermis is left intact and only a small opening is made at either the 3 o'clock position on the right breast or the 9 o'clock position on the left. This is done as it is helpful to always place the knot at the most medial aspect of the pattern so it can be easily identified later should the suture ever have to be removed. Using a permanent suture material, an interlocking pattern between the outer periareolar incision and the areolar incision is made that will "lock" these two wound margins together once the suture is tied down. The best material to use for this purpose is a Teflon suture (Polytetrafluorethylene – PTFE) attached to a straight "Keith" needle as it has a very smooth surface and can slide through the extensive soft tissue framework of the closure easily. The suture pass is started at the most medial aspect of the pattern running from deep to superficial. The strand is run across the defect taking a small bite of the areolar dermis. The stand is then run back to the periareolar incision where the straight needle is passed through the dermal shelf to the next cardinal point. Repeating this process 8 times creates a "wagon wheel" type of appearance to the pattern. The suture strand is finished by passing from superficial to deep directly at the point where the pattern started. By pulling up on the loose suture ends, the defect will close down to the desired diameter. The knot is finished with 6 to 8 throws and then tucked under the dermal edge to prevent postoperative exposure. If the areolar margin is in any way notched or irregular at this point, a small amount of additional de-epithelialization can be carefully performed to create a perfectly round shape. Final closure is performed with a running subcuticular 3-0 barbed absorbable suture (Fig. 20.8). Using this technique can be an extremely helpful tool in managing all types of complications related to malpositioned, irregularly shaped, or asymmetric areolas.

Scarring

Perhaps the most significant disadvantage associated with augmentation mastopexy relates to the amount of cutaneous scar that is variably associated with the procedure. After primary augmentation mastopexy, the new position of the breast and NAC with newly formed relaxed skin tension line relationships along with pressure created by the volume of

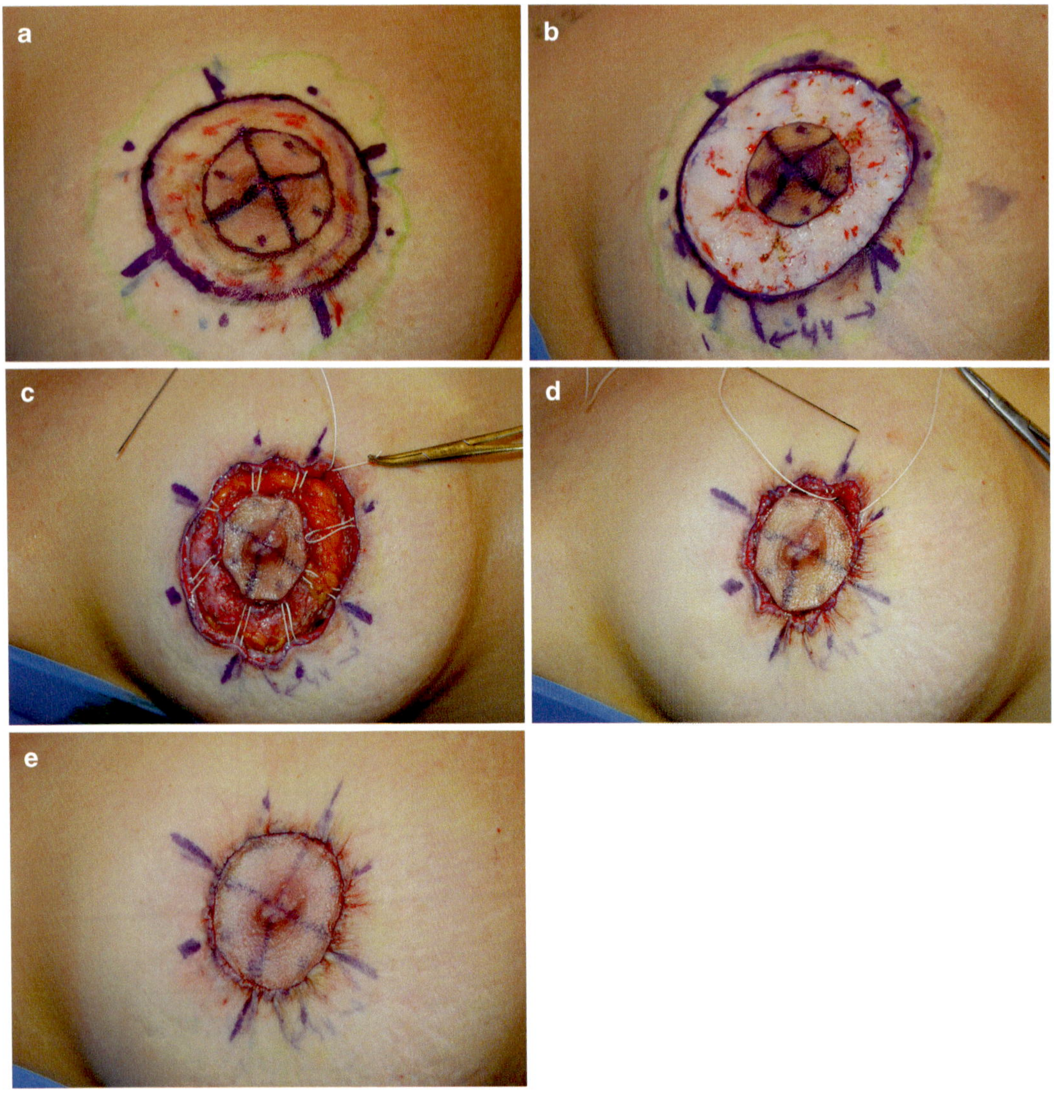

Fig. 20.8 Interlocking Periareolar Mastopexy Suture Technique (**a**) Preoperative marks in preparation for placing the interlocking purse string suture. The inner and outer diameters of the repair are divided into eight evenly spaced points. (**b**) Once the initial incisions are made, the intervening skin is de-epithelialized. (**c**) A 3-0 sized polytetrafluoroethylene (PTFE or Teflon) suture is placed within the defect, joining each of the eight cardinal points together. (**d**) The purse string suture is cinched down to the desired diameter. (**e**) Appearance after final closure with a 3-0 subcuticular barbed absorbable monofilament suture

the implant can lead to suboptimal scarring. However, once full healing has occurred after six months to one year postoperatively, it is very possible to simply revise the cutaneous scars with the expectation that improved healing will occur simply because the new relationships between the various skin flaps and the NAC will have matured.

Scar Revision: Technique

The scars are outlined preoperatively and any adjustments in the skin envelope or NAC are diagramed. The wound margins are excised at a 90 degree angle to the skin surface to help align the skin edges of the incision anatomically without overlap. The edges are undermined slightly to reduce skin tension and a precise dermal approximation using 4-0 absorbable monofilament suture is used to align the skin edges and then, most importantly, a final subcuticular suture using a 3-0 barbed monofilament completes the closure. The use of the barbed suture prevents any micro motion from occurring at the incision line as the body twists and turns, thus preventing micro tears from exacerbating the inflammation associated with healing. By stabilizing the wound edges until full healing can occur, scars of outstanding quality can be result, thus enhancing the overall result after augmentation mastopexy (Fig. 20.9).

Capsular Contracture

As with any breast implant procedure, capsular contracture can be a debilitating complication that can not only adversely affect the shape of the breast, but can also be a source of postoperative discomfort and pain. Treatment in cases of augmentation mastopexy is really no different than in other cases of breast augmentation or reconstruction. Decisions with regard to capsulotomy versus capsulectomy, as well as other considerations such as implant replacement, pocket irrigation, and the use of acellular dermal matrices are all important considerations often made on a

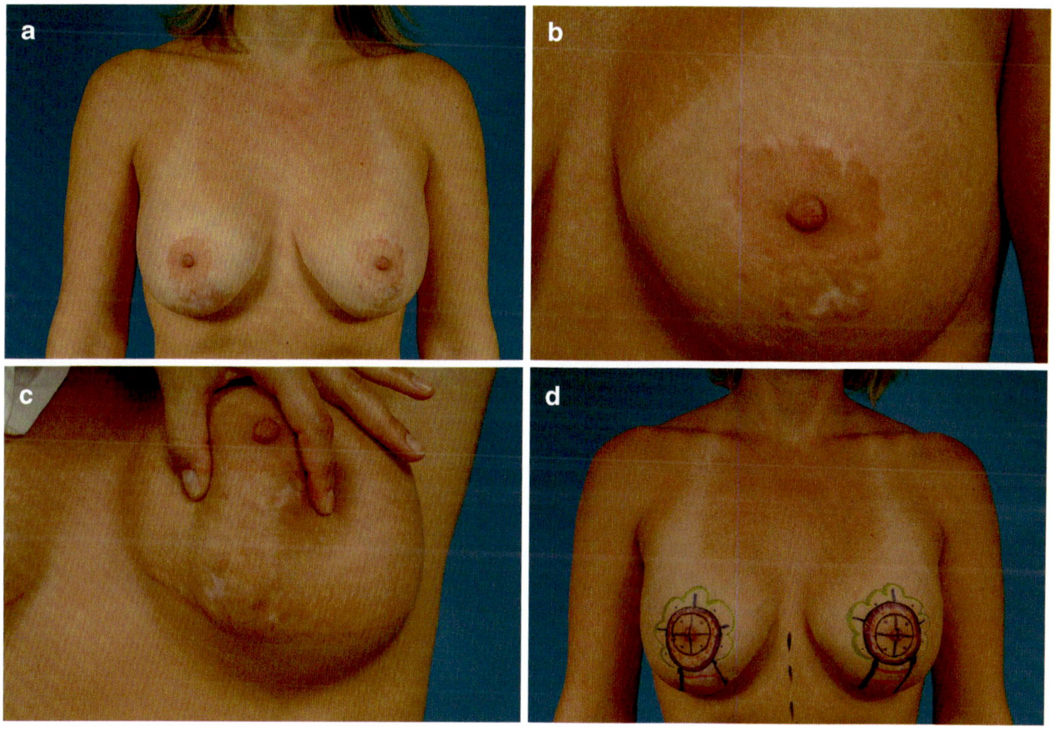

Fig. 20.9 Scar Revision (**a**–**c**) Preoperative appearance of a 43 year old woman with irregular and widened scars after previous augmentation mastopexy. (**d**) Preoperative marks in preparation for circumvertical skin only scar revision including tightening of the lower pole of the breast using a vertical skin takeout along with a periareolar scar revision using the interlocking suture technique. (**e**) Appearance of the lower pole of the left breast after tailor tack plication of the redundant skin envelope. (**f**) When the staples are removed, the extent of skin removal encompassing most of the undesirable scar can be visualized. (**g**) Appearance after removal of the affected skin envelope. (**h**) Final closure. (**i**–**k**) Final appearance 2 years post op demonstrating improved cutaneous scarring in both the vertical as well as the periareolar components, and an overall improvement in the shape of the breast

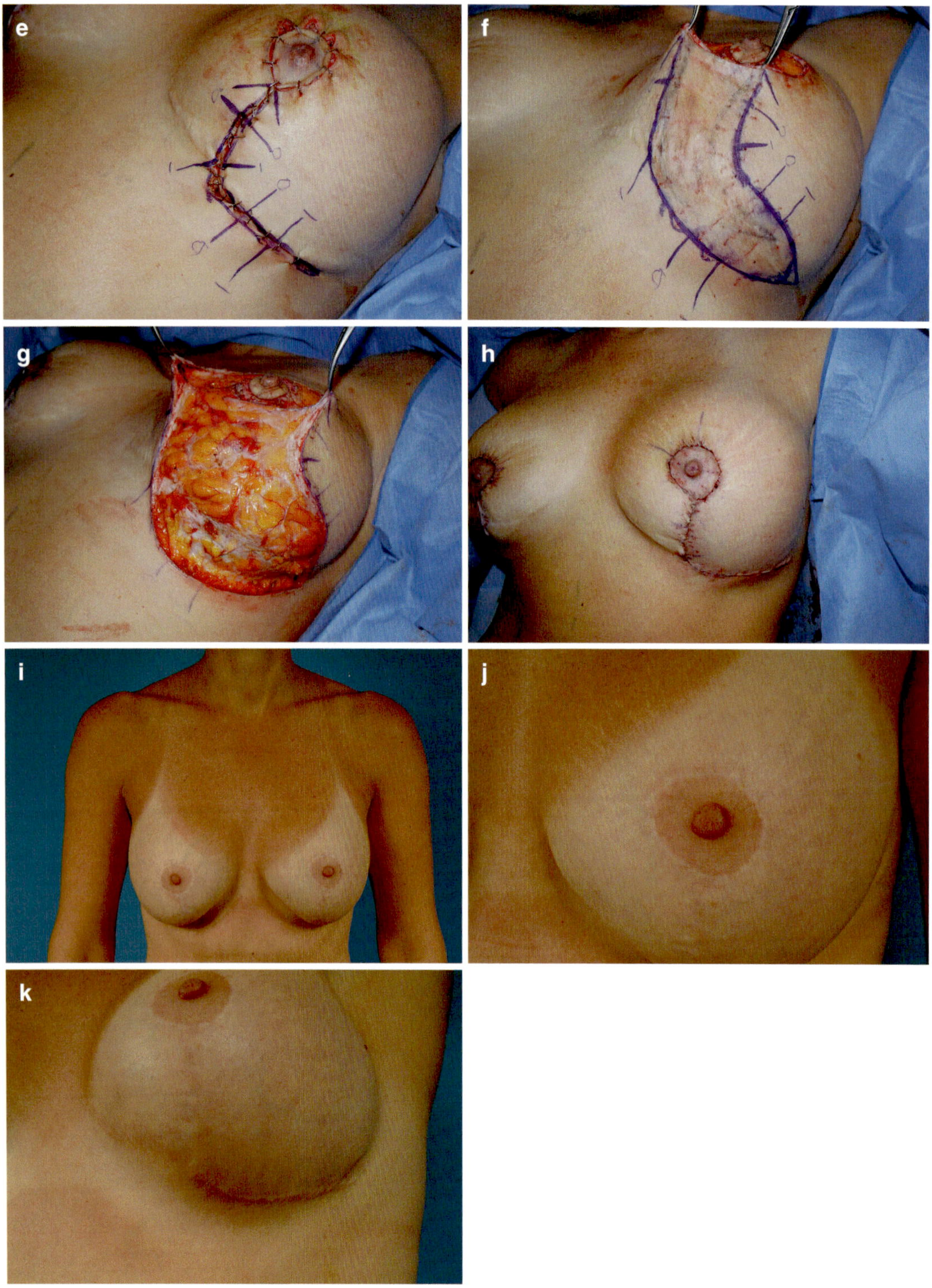

Fig. 20.9 (continued)

case by case basis depending on the experience level of the surgeon. Somewhat unique to augmentation mastopexy however is the observation that, once the tethering effect of the capsule is removed, often a distortion in the shape of the breast secondary to skin stretch can then be unmasked. In these cases, the treating surgeon should be aware of this possibility as a simple redo of the mastopexy pattern may be required to restore an aesthetic appearance to the breast after capsulectomy.

Capsulotomy:Technique

Capsulotomy as a treatment for capsular contracture has the advantage of appropriately treating the problem without creating a significant amount of operative morbidity. By simply releasing the contracted capsule using a multi-axial or checkerboard incision pattern, the surface are of the implant space is expanded to better accommodate the implant, creating a softer, more aesthetic result. In most cases, the creation of raw surface areas is minimal enough that a drain is not needed postoperatively. The procedure is performed best under general anesthesia as the operative field can include the entire anterior capsule of the breast. After accessing the breast pocket, the implant is removed and the capsule is inspected. If it is not overly thick or calcified, a simple scar release can be performed using bovie cautery to divide the capsule along the anterior surface of the pocket. The margins of the pocket can be expanded as need to better accommodate the base diameter and height of the implant. Release of the scar is extended into the surrounding soft tissue of the breast as needed to fully release any scar bands that might have extended into the surrounding fat. Once the implant space has been restored, the pocket is irrigated and the implant re-inserted. Any residual shape distortion is released as needed to create the desired result (Fig. 20.10).

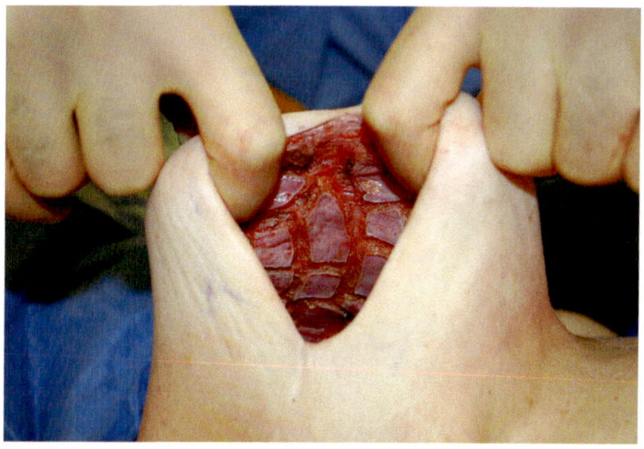

Fig. 20.10 Capsulotomy Technique: Appearance of the capsule after checkerboard capsulotomy

Capsulectomy:Technique

As opposed to simple capsulotomy, a full capsulectomy is required when the surrounding capsule is problematic by either being excessively thick or calcified. In such instances, leaving behind thickened or calcified segments of the capsule can inadequately release the scar contracture leading to an incomplete result. The operation is performed as with a capsulotomy, however, after the capsule has been checker boarded, the individual squares of retained capsule are sequentially removed, leaving behind a soft and compliant soft tissue envelope. Often times a very satisfying snapping type of release can be felt as these scar segments are removed. If the capsule against the chest wall and ribs is overtly thickened, it can be removed as well to avoid any sense of movement restriction to the arm and chest that the patient could potentially experience postoperatively. Otherwise, if it is so thin that it cannot be safely peeled away from the ribs and intercostal spaces, it is left behind. Due to the creation of an entire new implant pocket with raw surfaces, a drain is required to prevent postoperative fluid accumulation. The implant is then re-inserted to complete the procedure (Fig. 20.11).

Breast Animation

Whenever an implant is placed under the pectoralis major muscle, there will be some element of breast animation associated with contraction of the muscle. This animation is almost always manifested as a pull on the implant directed superolaterally as the muscle contracts. As well, the lower inner portion of the pocket can be seen to flatten under the effect of the muscle. When

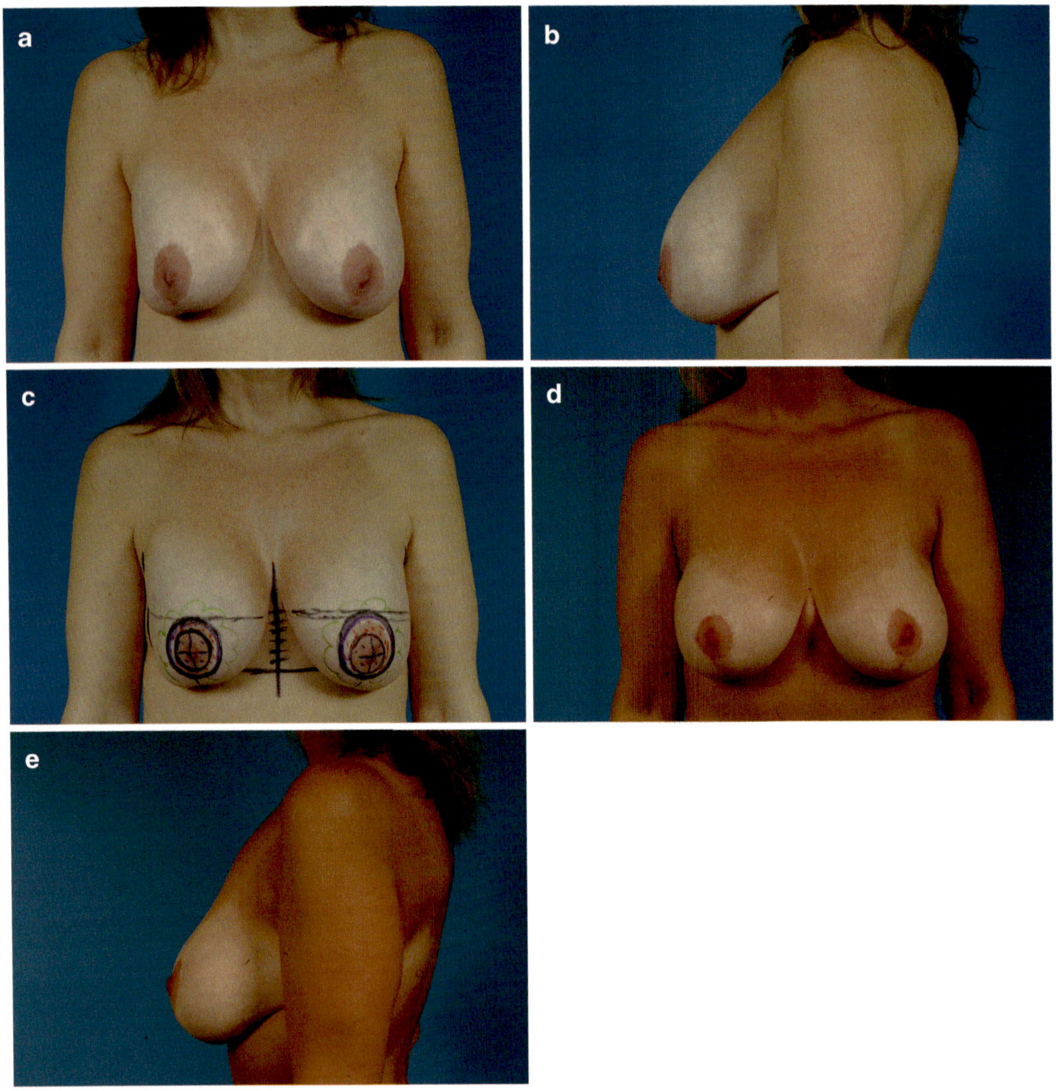

Fig. 20.11 Capsulectomy Case (**a**, **b**) Preoperative appearance of a 39 year old woman with presents with painful Baker Grade 4 capsular contracture after bilateral circumvertical augmentation mastopexy. (**c**) Preoperative marks in preparation for periareolar scar revision along with bilateral capsulectomy. (**d**, **e**) Postoperative appearance at 5 years demonstrates soft breasts without evidence of contracture recurrence and an overall aesthetic result

this distortion in the shape of the breast becomes problematic for the patient, it is reasonable to address it with either a further release of the muscle or a complete pocket change to subgandular or subfascial [5, 6].

Further Release of the Muscle: Technique

In many instances, only a limited release of the pectoralis major muscle is performed for patients undergoing augmentation mastopexy using a partial subpectoral pocket. Therefore to limit the effect of the muscle contraction, and yet still utilize the muscle to cover the upper inner portion of the pocket, the origin of the muscle along the lower and lower inner aspect of the chest wall must be released to approximately the 4 o'clock position on the right breast or the 8 o'clock position on the left breast. As well, the attachments of the muscle to the overlying breast must be released in a dual plane type fashion for a distance of 1–2 cm along the entire lateral border of the muscle all the way up into the axilla to allow the muscle to window shade upwards such that it covers only the upper inner third of the implant. This type of release is called a combination pocket. The breast is entered through an existing incision and the implant is removed. The border of the muscle can be seen through the capsule and the muscle release accomplished as described using bovie cautery. By getting the muscle up "out of the equation", the effect of muscle contraction and subsequent animation of the breast is greatly reduced or eliminated. However the thickness of the muscle can still enhance the cover of the implant in the critical upper inner portion of the breast that is often visible in clothing, the so-called "social" area of the breast. By maintaining the thickness of the soft tissue cover in this area, any chance of implant or wrinkle visibility is eliminated. In this fashion, the beneficial aspect of using the muscle to help soften the breast contour is maintained while at the same time greatly minimizing the disadvantage of excessive breast animation. Once the muscle has retracted superiorly, the implant is replaced and the partially dual-planed leading muscle edge is manually re-draped over the superior aspect of the implant (Fig. 20.12).

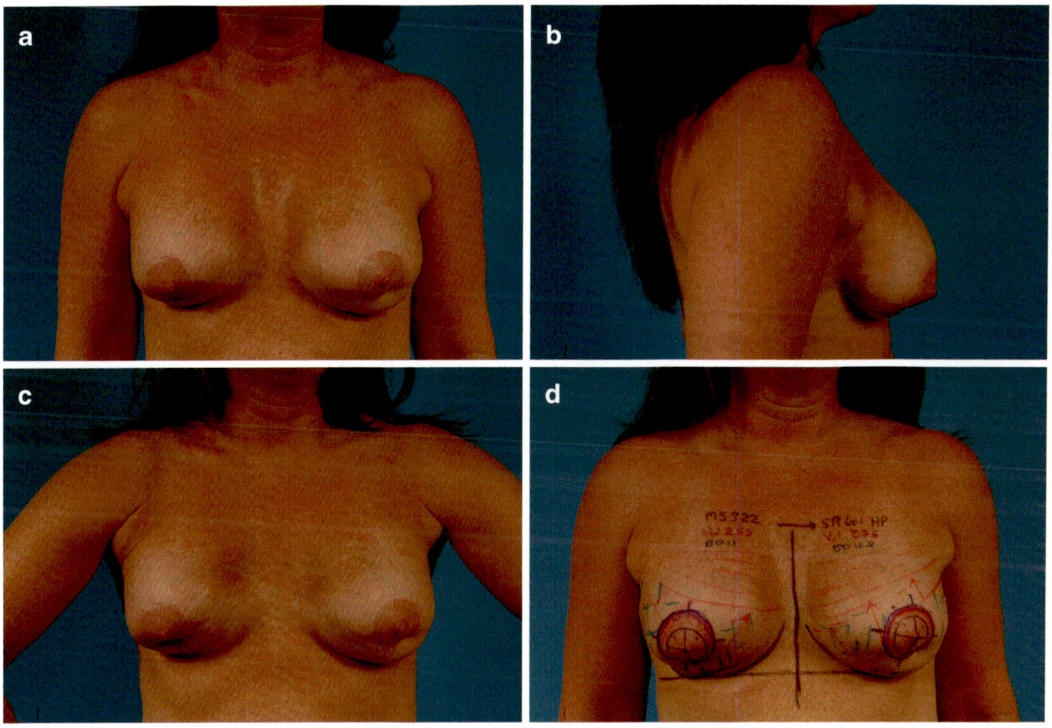

Fig. 20.12 Breast Animation - Combination Pocket (**a**–**c**) Preoperative appearance of a 47 year old woman with significant breast animation and capsular contracture after previous bilateral periareolar augmentation mastopexy. (**d**) Marks in preparation for revision including redo of the periareolar scar, aggressive dual plane release of the pectoralis major muscle to decrease the degree of breast animation, capsulectomy, and implant exchange. (**e**, **f**) Immediate result after first plication of the left breast periareolar pattern and then after bilateral complete revision. (**g**–**i**) Appearance at 6 months demonstrates an improved aesthetic breast appearance with complete correction of the animation deformity

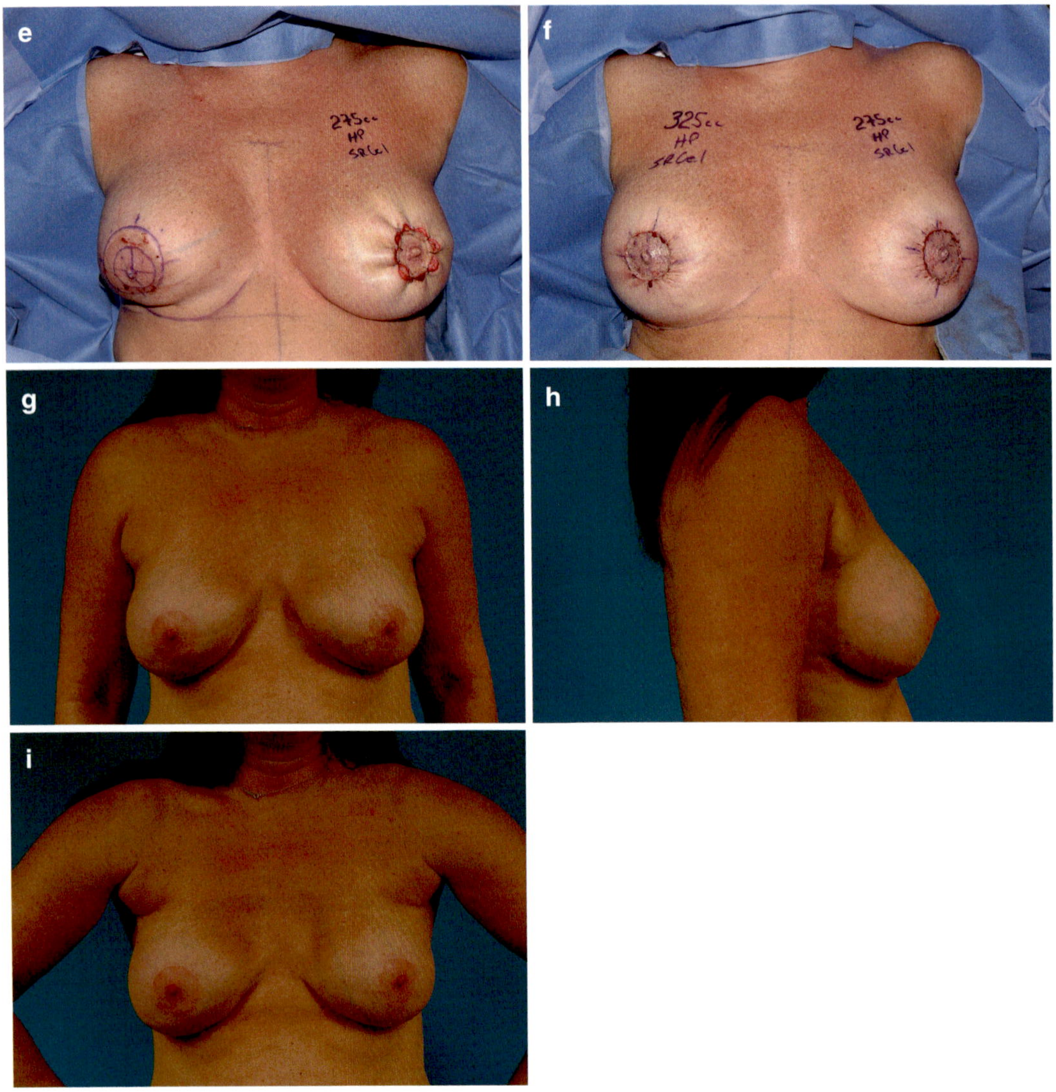

Fig. 20.12 (continued)

Conversion to a Subgandular Pocket: Technique

While partial release of the muscle can be very effective in limiting breast animation, the most certain way to eliminate it is to convert to a subglandular or subfascial pocket. In this case, the implant is removed and the leading edge of the pectoralis major muscle is released from the overlying breast. By applying traction to the inferolateral margin of the muscle, a new subglandular or subfascial pocket can be developed as needed to accommodate the chosen implant. While the capsule on the underside of the muscle and the corresponding area of the chest wall can be removed to create a new raw surface to promote more reliable healing of the muscle against the chest wall, such efforts are generally not required as secure stabilization of the edge of the pectoralis major muscle is sufficient to allow it to stick down into position without performing a partial capsulectomy. By simply applying mild traction on the released pectoralis major muscle to provide a bit of resting tension, the edge of the muscle is sutured down to the chest wall with numerous interrupted figure of eight 2-0 or 3-0 permanent nonabsorbable monofilament sutures. In many instances the muscle cannot be pulled down all the way into an anatomic position along the inframammary fold. In these cases, the muscle is simply attached where it can comfortably lie and secured into position. The implant is then inserted into the new pocket and closed. Generally no drain is placed as this procedure becomes essentially a subgandular or subfascial breast augmentation where drains are only rarely used. In these patients, the shape of the breast is often much improved as the tethering effect of the muscle is removed allowing the implant to more smoothly shape the breast. In cases where significant distortion of the breast is present preoperatively, pocket change can provide for a significant improvement in the overall result (Fig. 20.13).

Size Dissatisfaction

In the augmentation mastopexy patient, there are many variables that are all being addressed at the same time. After the NAC has been lifted, the skin envelope tightened, and the breast parenchyma re-positioned, it can be somewhat difficult to assess the overall volume of the breast. Additionally, in cases where the skin envelope is simply lifted and tightened, the effect at least outwardly is that the breast appears smaller despite the fact that only skin was removed. All these factors make meeting exact demands for a specific cup size or overall breast size hard to meet precisely. With this is mind, when breast size issues do occur postoperatively, it is more common that patients feel they are too big rather than too small. One reason for this relates to the fact that many patients actually have more volume than they realize and it is simply malpositioned inferiorly. Once the breast is lifted, the lack of volume

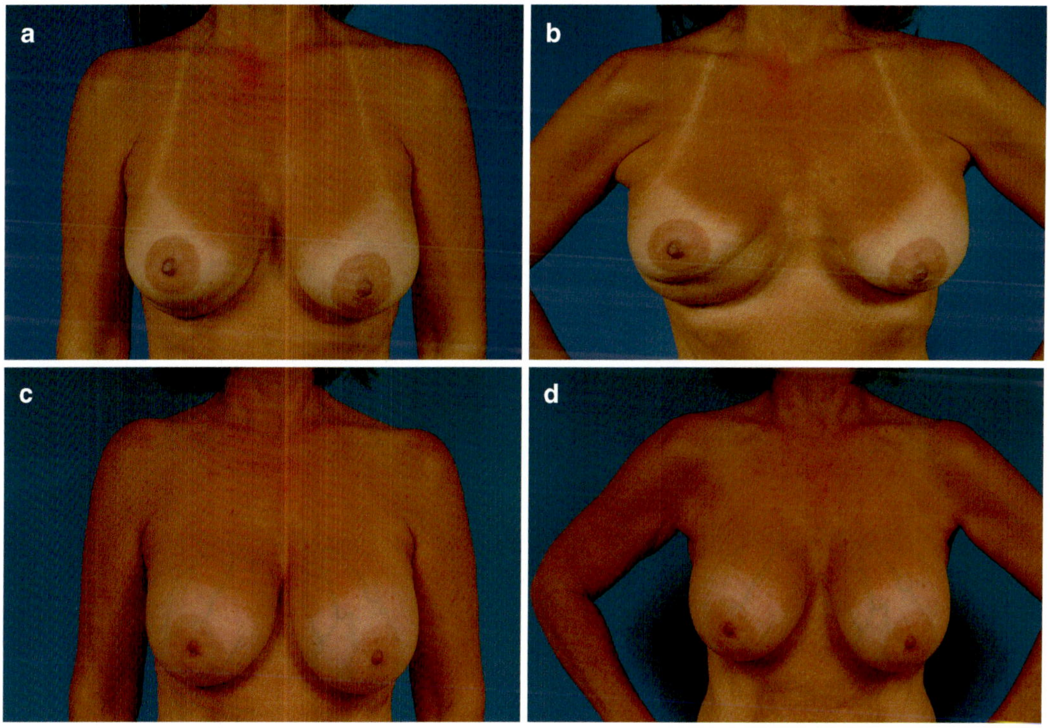

Fig. 20.13 Breast Animation - Pocket Change (**a**, **b**) Preoperative appearance of a 47 year old woman who demonstrates significant animation after subpectoral implant placement. (**c**, **d**) Postoperative appearance at 9 years demonstrates complete correction of the animation deformity after pocket change to the Subglandular plane

becomes less noticeable. Therefore, approaching augmentation mastopexy with the same mindset as augmentation alone can lead to the use of implants that are too big.

Implant Upsizing After Augmentation Mastopexy

When dealing with a patient who feels she is too small, it is fairly easy to use external sizers or three dimensional computer imaging to identify a new implant size that the patient can sign off on. By involving the patient in this decision, further disappointment related to breast size can be avoided. Also, by taking photographs with the sizers in place or saving three dimensional images in the patient record, the decisions made in planning can be documented.

Placing a Larger Implant: Technique

Implant upsizing is a fairly straightforward procedure, once the desired volume implant has been identified. By accessing the breast through an existing incision, the old implant is removed and the capsule inspected. Any thick or firms areas that could affect the shape are removed and the borders of the pocket medially, superiorly, and laterally are opened slightly to accommodate the larger device. Any additional modifications that might be necessary such as repositioning the fold or manipulating the muscle cover can also be performed as needed. However, when the IMF is properly positioned, it is very important to leave it untouched otherwise inadvertent lowering of the fold could result. One very important decision that must be made at this point is how to manage the capsule. In cases of concomitant capsular contracture, capsulotomy or capsulectomy can be performed at this point to good effect. However, when the capsule is not problematic, leaving the anterior capsule untouched is preferable. If the capsule is at all restrictive to providing the desired shape, it can be selectively released with a limited capsulotomy as needed. If the scars associated with the mastopexy are objectionable, or the size, shape, or position of the areola needs to be improved, these adjustments can be made once the new implant volume has been determined. Taken together, these combined techniques can often create very aesthetic and long lasting results (Fig. 20.14).

Implant Downsizing After Augmentation Mastopexy

Reaching a decision regarding implant volume with a patient who feels she is too big is more uncertain. In these cases, external sizers cannot be used and three dimensional imaging is difficult to incorporate into the decision making process. In general, downsizing an implant by 100 cc or less will not make enough of a change to make the operation worthwhile. Depending on the volume of the existing implant, a reduction of 100 to 200 cc is not uncommon. In these cases, a detailed discussion with the patient, often supplemented with photos demonstrating previous results, is required to accurately assess the result the patient is seeking. It is important to document such discussions to ensure that the patient's desires are accurately reflected in her medical record.

Placing a Smaller Implant: Technique

In cases where the patient feels the breast is too big, it is very easy to simply exchange the implant with a smaller device. Often no further capsule modification or pocket manipulation is required. By utilizing an existing incision, the pocket is entered and the old implant removed. The capsule is assessed and any thicker or firm areas that could affect the shape are either released or removed. In particular the lateral margin of the pocket is evaluated and if the pocket is too large, the implant can slide off laterally creating a medial hollow when the patient lies flat. In these situations, the lateral gutter can be closed off by removing the redundant capsule and repairing it with interrupted permanent 2-0 or 3-0 permanent sutures with or without mesh reinforcement. When closing off a lateral gutter, it is very important to place the patient in the upright position at least 60 degrees to ensure a smooth and properly

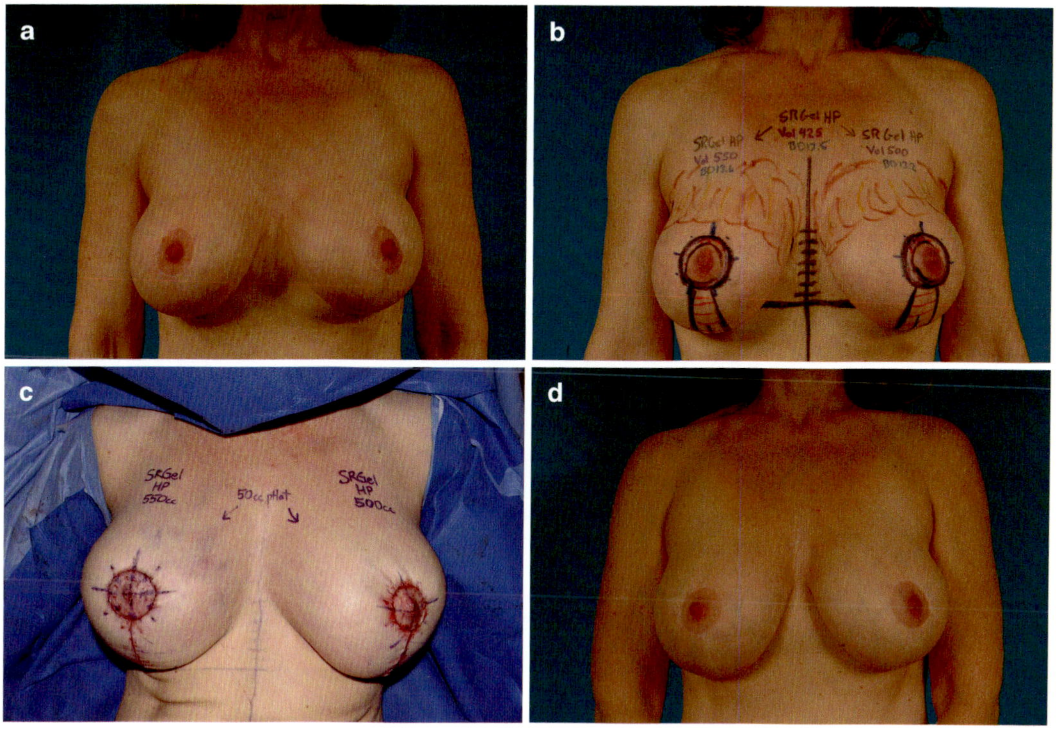

Fig. 20.14 Implant Up-sizing (**a**) Preoperative appearance of a 45 year old woman who presents after bilateral circumvertical augmentation mastopexy with concerns about mild ptosis of the skin envelope and a request for bigger implants. (**b**) Preoperative marks in preparation for bilateral circumvertical skin envelope revision, fat grafting, and bilateral implant exchange for larger devices. (**c**) Immediate postoperative appearance after the placement of high profile smooth round gel implants in a partial subpectoral pocket using a 550 cc device on the right and a 500 cc device on the left, along with bilateral breast fat grafting and circumvertical skin envelope revision. (**d**) Postoperative appearance at 18 months demonstrates an aesthetic result with improvement in the contour of the breast and a properly positioned and symmetric NAC

positioned lateral contour. Making these adjustments with the patient supine can lead to malposition of the lateral border with notching. Once the new implant is in place, the degree of ptosis is reassessed and any re-tightening of the skin envelope or re-lifting of the NAC that might be required can be done using a simple tailor tack technique with de-epithelialization. In this fashion, there is no risk to the blood supply to the skin flaps or the NAC. When managing the NAC, the interlocking technique leaving the dermis intact is very effective at providing a secure NAC position and shape. Here again, the opportunity to address these various size and shape issues a second time can be done with great control providing excellent aesthetic results (Fig. 20.15).

Summary

Augmentation mastopexy remains as one of the more challenging aesthetic procedures performed on the breast. Despite the possibilities for complications to develop postoperatively, accurate identification of the etiology of the deformity allows operative correction to be performed in a manner that can provide aesthetic and long lasting results.

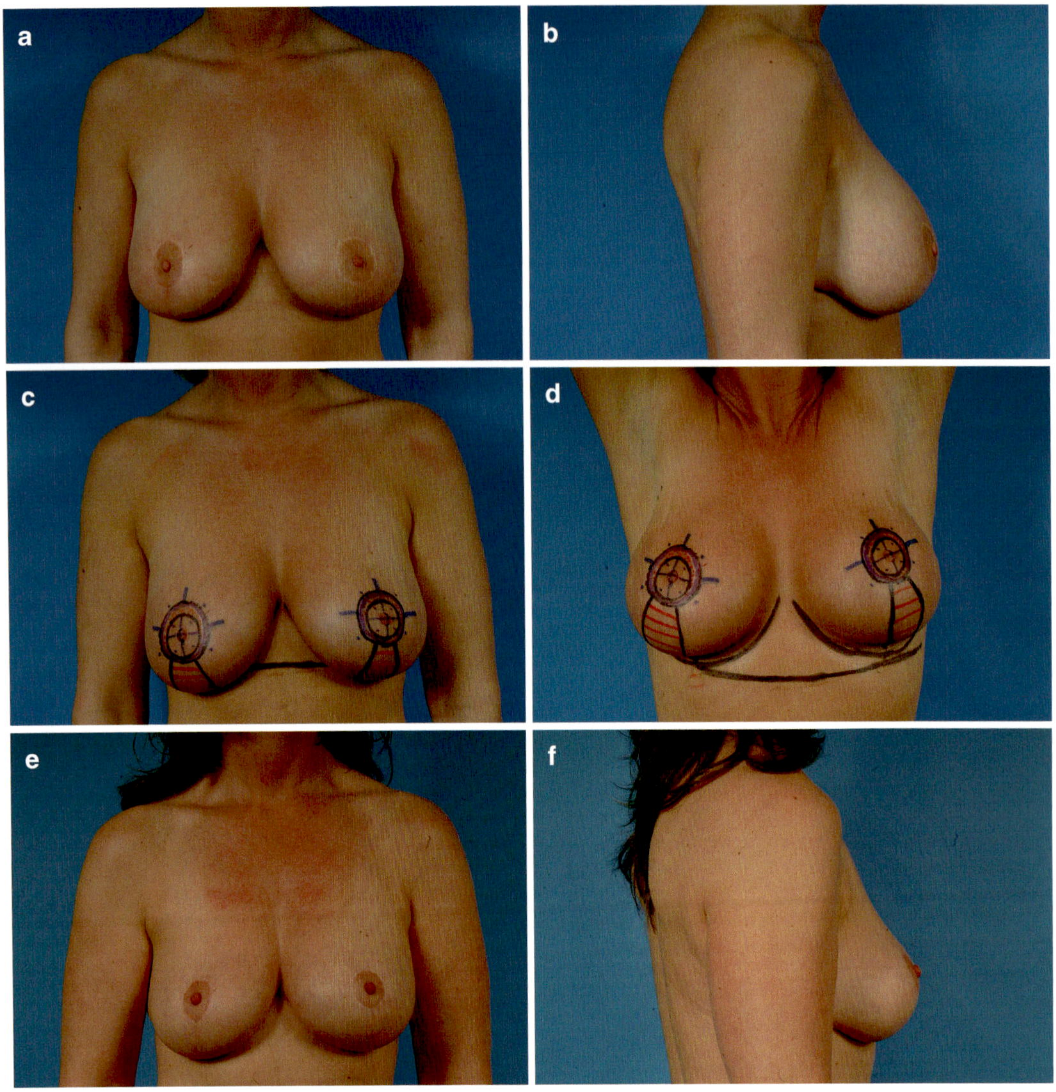

Fig. 20.15 Implant Downsizing (**a**, **b**) Preoperative appearance of a 34 year old woman who presents after previous circumvertical augmentation mastopexy requesting a decrease in implant volume and revision of the mildly ptotic skin envelope. (**c**, **d**) Preoperative marks in preparation for bilateral circumvertical skin envelope revision along with bilateral implant exchange for smaller devices. (**e**, **f**) Postoperative appearance at 8 years after exchange of 350 cc saline implants for 250 cc smooth round gel moderate profile plus implants along with circumvertical skin envelope revision. The patient demonstrates a smaller, more proportional and aesthetic breast shape

References

1. Spear SL, Low M, Ducic I. Revision augmentation mastopexy: indications, operations, and outcomes. Ann Plast Surg. 2003;51:540–6.
2. Friedman RM. Augmentation/mastopexy: 'surgeon beware'. Plast Reconstr Surg. 2004;113:2230–1.
3. Handel N. The double-bubble deformity: cause, prevention, and treatment. Plast Reconstr Surg. 2013;132(6):1434–43.
4. Hammond DC, Khuthaila DK, Kim J. The interlocking Gore-Tex suture for control of the areolar diameter and shape. Plast Reconstr Surg. 2007;119:804–9.
5. Hammond DC, Schmitt WP, O'Connor EA. Treatment of breast animation deformity in implant-based reconstruction with pocket change to the subcutaneous position. Plast Reconst Surg. 2015;135(6):1540–4.
6. Pelle-Ceravolo M, Del Vescovo A, Bertozzi E, et al. A technique to decrease breast shape deformity during musclecontraction in submuscular augmentation mammoplasty. Aesthet Plast Surg. 2004;28:288–94.

Index

M. B. Calobrace et al. (eds.), *Augmentation Mastopexy*,
https://doi.org/10.1007/978-3-030-48226-8

GPSR Compliance

The European Union's (EU) General Product Safety Regulation (GPSR) is a set of rules that requires consumer products to be safe and our obligations to ensure this.

If you have any concerns about our products, you can contact us on ProductSafety@springernature.com

In case Publisher is established outside the EU, the EU authorized representative is:

Springer Nature Customer Service Center GmbH
Europaplatz 3
69115 Heidelberg, Germany

Batch number: 10756384

Printed by Printforce, the Netherlands